# Epidemiology of
# Childhood Cancer

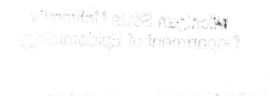

## International Agency for Research on Cancer

The International Agency for Research on Cancer (IARC) was established in 1965 by the World Health Assembly, as an independently financed organization within the framework of the World Health Organization. The headquarters of the Agency are at Lyon, France.

The Agency conducts a programme of research concentrating particularly on the epidemiology of cancer and the study of potential carcinogens in the human environment. Its field studies are supplemented by biological and chemical research carried out in the Agency's laboratories in Lyon, and, through collaborative research agreements, in national research institutions in many countries. The Agency also conducts a programme for the education and training of personnel for cancer research.

The publications of the Agency are intended to contribute to the dissemination of authoritative information on different aspects of cancer research. Information about IARC publications and how to order them, is available via the Internet at: http://www.iarc.fr/

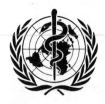

INTERNATIONAL AGENCY FOR RESEARCH ON CANCER
WORLD HEALTH ORGANIZATION

# Epidemiology of Childhood Cancer

By
Julian Little

Epidemiology Group, Department of Medicine and Therapeutics
University of Aberdeen, UK

IARC Scientific Publications No. 149

International Agency for Research on Cancer
Lyon, France
1999

Published by the International Agency for Research on Cancer,
150 cours Albert Thomas, 69372 Lyon cédex 08, France

Distributed by Oxford University Press, Walton Street, Oxford OX2 6DP, UK
(fax: +44 1865 267782) and in the USA by Oxford University Press, 2001 Evans Road, Carey,
NC 27513 (fax: +1 919 677 1303). All IARC publications can also be ordered directly from IARC*Press*
(fax: +33 04 72 73 83 02; E-mail: press@iarc.fr).

**IARC Library Cataloguing in Publication Data**

Little, Julian
Epidemiology of childhood cancer / Julian Little

(IARC scientific publications ; 149)

1. Neoplasms – epidemiology
2. Neoplasms – in infancy and childhood
I. Title    II. Series

ISBN 92 832 2149 4  (NLM Classification W1)
ISSN 0300-5085

Printed in France

# Contents

Contents

# Foreword

Childhood cancers account for less than 2% of the total cancer burden in developed countries. Despite significant progress in therapy, they are of public health importance as they have long-term health implications for survivors.

The pattern of tumours occurring in childhood is distinct from that seen in adults, indicating different etiological factors. The International Agency for Research on Cancer has brought together data on childhood neoplasms from cancer registries, using protocols comparable to those employed in the collection of data previously published in the *International Incidence of Childhood Cancer*. This database has revealed intriguing patterns of geographical variation in incidence, which point to causation by different etiological factors.

Some of the hypotheses regarding the origin of specific types of childhood cancer have been tested in analytical epidemiological studies. Examples of such hypotheses are the possibility that a fraction of leukaemia and brain tumours may be caused by residential exposure to electric and magnetic fields, and that leukaemia may be a rare consequence of infections common in children.

This new publication summarizes the descriptive epidemiology and critically appraises analytical epidemiology data on childhood cancer. There are still many gaps in our understanding of the factors operative in the evolution of tumours in children, and we hope that this book will foster future multicentre and interdisciplinary collaborative research which will lead in the long term to primary prevention.

**P. Kleihues**
Director

# Acknowledgements

In Aberdeen, I would like to thank Seonaidh Cotton for her careful proof-reading, and checking of the references, Kate Dunn for her ever-patient secretarial help, and Paul Lawrence and Wendy Pirie of the Medical School Library. In Lyon, I am indebted to Sheila Stallard for secretarial help, to Helis Miido and Monique Coudert of the IARC library, and to John Cheney. In addition, I would like to thank Max Parkin (IARC) and Peter Boyle (formerly at IARC, now in Milan) for encouragement at different stages of the development of the book, and the two anonymous referees for their constructive criticisms.

# Chapter 1

# Introduction

Cancer is the second commonest cause of death, after accidents, in childhood in developed countries (Higginson et al., 1992; Green et al., 1997). Thus, in these countries, childhood cancer is an important public health problem because not only can the disease prove fatal, but the associated impact on the child, its parents and their immediate circle of relatives and friends can be severe. In developing countries, improvements in the control of communicable diseases and the occurrence of premature delivery may lead to the emergence of cancer in children as a greater public health problem than in the past. In Bombay in the period 1982–84, cancer was the ninth cause of death in boys under the age of 15, and the tenth in girls (Krishnamurthy & Dhar, 1991). The available data from Africa, although limited, suggest that cancer ranks higher among the causes of death in children than in India (Parkin et al., 1988b). This may be attributable to Burkitt's lymphoma and the emergence of HIV-related cancers.

The rationale for considering childhood cancers separately from cancers in adults is that there are differences in the sites of occurrence, in the histological appearance and in their clinical behaviour (Marsden, 1988; Malkin, 1997). Many of the tumours have histological features which resemble fetal tissues at various stages of development and are therefore designated 'embryonal'. Childhood cancers tend to have short latent periods, often grow rapidly and are aggressively invasive, but are generally more responsive to chemotherapy than the tumours typically occurring in adults (Malkin, 1997). The definition of childhood in most studies of childhood cancer is up to and including the age of 14 years, but this is an arbitrary cut-off.

Thus, although specific types of childhood cancer are uncommon, collectively they represent an important public health problem. Much research has been undertaken to document their patterns of occurrence and to investigate possible risk factors. This book reviews the epidemiology of specific types of childhood cancer to the time of writing, mid-1997. The literature has been identified by searches of MEDLINE from 1980 to early 1997, supplemented by searches of the Science Citation Index and EMBASE, and a less systematic review of available journals and books. In appraising individual comparative studies, consideration was given to the extent to which associations might be due to bias, confounding or chance. In considering the totality of the epidemiological evidence regarding a particular association, issues such as the consistency of association between studies, the strength of the association, whether the risk of the disease under consideration increased with the amount of exposure, and the specificity of association were considered (Hill, 1965).

## Design issues

Investigations on the epidemiology of childhood cancer may be classified as descriptive or analytical. Descriptive studies describe the frequency (usually incidence) of childhood cancer in a particular community, and how this varies by geographical area, year of birth or diagnosis, or with personal characteristics such as ethnic group or socioeconomic status. Many such studies have been based on data from paediatric cancer registries. Such data are valuable because (1) referral and treatment of childhood cancers tend to differ from adult cancers, so different sources of ascertainment have to be considered; (2) many registries relating to cancer at all ages have a population base too small to allow the recruitment of sufficient cases for the calculation of reliable incidence rates (Parkin et al., 1988a) and (3) paediatric cancers need to be recorded by morphology rather than topography as is usually done for adult cancers.

The detailed methods of operating childhood cancer registries vary (Parkin et al., 1988a), but in general the sources of ascertainment include hospital records, information from pathology laboratories and lists of deaths certified with a cause of cancer. Another potential source is

1

notification from clinical trials groups. The data from the various sources are collated in order to avoid duplicate registration. In some areas, including parts of Canada, Costa Rica, Cuba, Finland, Israel, Kuwait, New South Wales (Australia), New Zealand, Norway, Poland, Puerto Rica and Sweden, notification of newly diagnosed cancer cases is compulsory (Parkin *et al.*, 1988a). Some registries are based on passive notification of cases, whereas in others cancer registry staff engage in active case-finding by direct contact with medical personnel who see cases of childhood cancer, such as paediatric oncologists, surgeons, radiotherapists and haematologists. The information recorded typically includes site, histopathological diagnosis and morphology of the cancer, the basis of the diagnosis, and basic sociodemographic information. In comparing data between registries, consideration of the basis of diagnosis, usually the proportion of cases that are histologically verified, is an important indication of the data quality and comparability (Parkin *et al.*, 1988a).

Many registries are population-based, that is, they seek to document newly incident cases in a population defined by residence in a specified geographical area during a specified period of time. In some of the older literature and in some less developed countries, only data from hospital series were available. Unless the study includes the hospitals to which most cases were referred and referral rates to these for diagnosis is high, such data may be biased. In some developing countries, many children with cancer never receive hospital treatment, for reasons such as the difficulties of travel to a specialized centre and the use of traditional medicine (Alaoui, 1988; Junaid & Babalola, 1988; Parkin & Sanghvi, 1991). These factors lead to the incidence of cancer being underestimated in some countries. Further difficulties can include poor quality of diagnostic information and lack of stability of the population, leading to difficulty in defining the denominator for calculation of incidence rates (Parkin & Sanghvi, 1991).

There has been considerable interest in small-area variations in incidence of childhood cancers, as a result of concern about excess incidence of haematopoietic malignancies in children and young persons in the vicinity of nuclear installations. This has stimulated a great deal of methodological development in the investigation of clusters and clustering (see Chapter 2). The observations of variation in incidence between small areas, variation by socioeconomic status and variation by age led to the suggestion that childhood leukaemia may be an uncommon response to an unusual pattern of exposure to infection (Kinlen, 1988; see below). Other etiological hypotheses have been developed based on observations in experimental animals, for example regarding the role of *N*-nitroso compounds in the etiology of tumours of the central nervous system, or following a wide-ranging case–control study, for example regarding the role of diethylstilbestrol in the etiology of clear-cell adenocarcinoma of the vagina and endometrium in teenage girls and young women.

Analytical epidemiological study designs applied to childhood cancer include case–control and cohort studies. Many of these have been exploratory in nature, with a wide range of exposures investigated for which there was no *a priori* hypothesis. For example, many of the investigations of the associations with parental occupations have been of this type.

A framework for considering the etiology of childhood cancer is presented in Figure 1. Like any disease, childhood cancer may be caused by genetic and environmental factors. Allelic variation at a number of different genetic loci may affect susceptibility to develop childhood cancer. At some genetic loci, there are rare alleles with autosomal recessive or autosomal dominant modes of inheritance and with high penetrance. For example, about 90% of individuals who have one copy of the Rb gene, which has an autosomal dominant mode of inheritance, manifest the disease. Allelic variation at other loci may give rise to much smaller, or even no detectable, variation in phenotype. For example, genetic variation underlying differences in the metabolism of xenobiotics has been reported to be associated with variation in the risk of various types of cancer (Nebert, 1997). Environmental exposures can cause germ cell mutations. The mechanisms differ for mutations arising in maternal and paternal gametes. New oocytes are not formed after birth, so a germ-cell mutation arising in the index child may be attributable to exposures of the maternal grandmother of the index child before the birth of the mother of the index child. The oocytes are almost mature in the ovaries of a newborn female, but become fully mature much later, one by one, when during each menstrual cycle one egg, or occasionally more than one, is made available for fertilization. In early studies on radiation-induced mutations in female mice and *Drosophila*, virtually no mutations were found in immature resting

# Figure 1.1. Schematic framework for considering etiology of childhood cancer

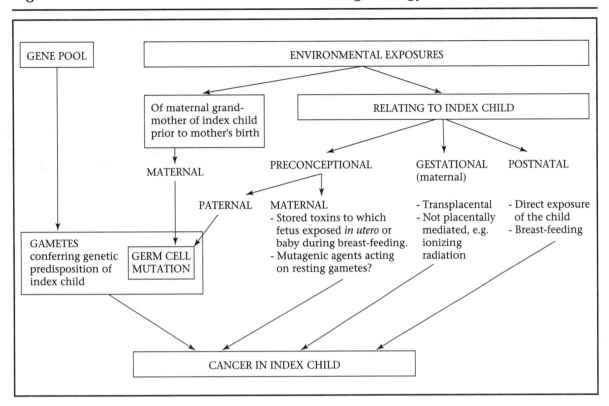

oocytes, but more recent studies indicate that significant levels of genetic damage can result from the irradiation of immature oocytes in the mouse (Chandley, 1991). Point mutations and structural rearrangements appear to occur *de novo* much more commonly in males than females, and arise in the paternal gametes during the preconceptional period. Apart from mutagenic effects, an environmental agent can cause childhood cancer in at least four ways. First, the index child may be exposed to an agent in his or her own lifetime, either directly, or indirectly as a result of breast-feeding. Second, the mother of the index child may be exposed to an agent during pregnancy, thus affecting the embryo or fetus directly. This may be placentally mediated, such as when a metabolite of a drug administered to the mother crosses the placenta, or non-placentally mediated, such as exposure to diagnostic radiation. Third, a soon-to-be-pregnant woman may be exposed to an agent that has slow metabolic clearance, with the result that the woman retains an embryotoxic dose into the early periods of pregnancy (Janerich & Polednak, 1983). Finally, another potential mechanism is that exposures may cause permanent damage to the woman's reproductive system before the index pregnancy, compromising the development of the fetus during pregnancy without necessarily producing clinical disease in the mother (Janerich & Polednak, 1983)

From the epidemiological perspective, the study of childhood cancer provides a unique opportunity to investigate the impact of environmental factors. The periods of exposure to environmental factors are shorter than would be the case in studies of adult chronic disease. As parents are usually aged between 25 and 40 years at the time of the diagnosis of the disease in their child, even the assessment of exposure of parents to potential risk factors in the pre-conceptional period involves consideration of a shorter period of potential exposure than those considered in, for example, lung cancer or prostate cancer studies. In addition, specific exposures are likely to have occurred during a period when their intensity was fairly constant. By definition, intrauterine and postnatal exposures are short, the latter generally less than seven years in view of the age distribution of cases.

## Case–control studies

In view of the rarity of childhood cancer, the majority of studies of etiology have been of a case–control design. Some have been based on deaths due to childhood cancer. A theoretical limitation of this approach is that factors affecting survival could erroneously be interpreted as being of etiological importance. However, many of these studies were initiated before recent improvements in therapy for many types of childhood cancer. For example, the large Oxford Survey of Childhood Cancers, which is an ongoing case–control study of all childhood cancer deaths in Great Britain, was initiated in 1953 (Stewart *et al.*, 1958). A recent report of this study included more than 15 000 cases (Sorahan & Roberts, 1993).

A major issue in the design and interpretation of studies of this type is potential selection bias, depending on the nature of the control group selected and factors determining the participation of both cases and controls. In many studies, controls were selected from birth records. Sometimes, controls were matched with cases on date of birth, sex and area of residence at the time of birth. In certain settings, close matching on the area of residence effectively introduces matching by socioeconomic status, and thereby may introduce overmatching for exposures which relate to socioeconomic status. In a few studies, controls were selected from registers of the general population. This was done in Denmark (Olsen *et al.*, 1991, 1993b), the Netherlands (van Steensel-Moll *et al.*, 1985a,b, 1986, 1992), Spain (Infante-Rivard *et al.*, 1991) and Utah (USA) (Stevens *et al.*, 1990). In the studies in the Netherlands and Spain, the registries of the population were census-based. When censuses are infrequent, there is potential for divergence between the source populations of cases and controls. For example, Infante-Rivard *et al.* (1991) identified cases between January 1983 and June 1985, and controls from the 1981 census. They observed that annual updates of addresses were available, if they had been reported by the family to the census bureau. The comparability of cases and controls in this study, therefore, depended on the mobility of cases and controls, and the level of reporting of change of address. Of 139 unsuccessful attempts to contact controls, 59 (42%) were due to the potential control having moved. This may have compromised the validity of the study.

Multistage sampling of controls has been used in one study in a developing country, in China (Shu *et al.*, 1988, 1995b), and in studies in North America (Graham *et al.*, 1966; Howe *et al.*, 1989) and Australia (McCredie *et al.*, 1994a,b). Although in principle this is a useful method of identifying population-based controls, poor participation rates may compromise the results of the study. For example, McCredie *et al.* (1994b) found that control women who agreed to be interviewed were of higher social class than those who refused to be interviewed. Therefore, the inverse association between brain tumours and high social class found in this study may have been an artefact of the participation bias of control mothers.

In a number of studies of childhood cancer, mainly in North America, controls have been selected by methods which do not depend on a listing of the population. The most commonly used of these methods is random-digit dialling, which generates sets of telephone numbers without relying on a directory that would not have new or unpublished numbers (Wacholder *et al.*, 1992a). Ward *et al.* (1984) described the application of this method to selection of control children in a study of neuroblastoma in the Greater Delaware Valley, the results of which were reported by Kramer *et al.* (1987). Telephone numbers to identify potentially eligible controls were selected by substituting the last two digits of the case family's telephone number with randomly selected digits. Successive random telephone numbers were called until a family was identified, and agreed to participate, in which there was a child matching the case by year of birth plus or minus three years and by ethnic group. To select controls for 101 cases, 3245 telephone numbers were dialled. Among 1908 residential households contacted, 25.5% refused to give information about household characteristics. Of households with known characteristics, 14.9% had a child eligible for study. Among 181 households invited to participate, 101 agreed. A general problem of studies that depend upon random-digit dialling is that it is difficult to define the source populations of controls and to determine the full extent of non-response. The reasons for which a telephone number is unobtainable or not answered are unknown. Robison and Daigle (1984), in a feasibility study of selecting controls matched with cases of Ewing's sarcoma by random-digit dialling, reported that 25% of the numbers generated were not working, and no contact was made in approximately 3.5% of the working telephone numbers. In most applications of this method, if several eligible controls live in a household, only one is selected. Greenberg (1990) noted that this selection process is biased against children from families with multiple eligible controls, that is against families with more children whose births were closely spaced, which in the United States is related to lower social class. Thus, controls may be of higher socioeconomic status relative to the source population than cases. Stratification in numbers of eligible residents in a household could alleviate this problem (Wacholder *et al.*, 1992a).

Other methods used that do not depend on a roster of the population include selection of neighbourhood controls and friends of the cases. With neighbourhood controls, it is difficult to determine the extent of non-response, as the number of eligible subjects in houses for which there is no response is unknown, and there may be over-matching on the exposures under study because of similarities between cases and controls from the same neighbourhood in exposures related to residence (Wacholder *et al.*, 1992a). While selection of friend controls would be expected to match cases on socioeconomic status and/or area of residence, it has been observed that the families of more sociable children tend to be nominated as friends, and that controls have more 'mainstream' social characteristics than their matched cases (Siemiatycki, 1989).

Studies with hospital controls may be classified into two groups. The first group comprises those in which the controls have been selected by hospital at birth. In this type of study, it is relatively easy to ensure the comparability of the source population of cases and controls. The second group comprises studies in which children of the same age range as cases who are admitted to hospital are selected as controls. However, children admitted to hospital may not be a representative sample of the population at risk of developing childhood cancer.

It is possible that illness in a child may act as a stimulus for parents to report exposures which would not be reported by the parents of healthy children. Therefore, recall bias is a potential problem in case–control studies in which data on exposures are collected retrospectively by interview or questionnaire. Few studies have attempted to demonstrate or to quantify such bias directly. Much of the discussion about its possible impact has been in relation to reproductive outcome (Raphael, 1987; Drews *et al.*, 1993), which may be due in part to the frequent use of maternal recall to obtain exposure information in case–control studies of reproductive outcome and concern that a mother's recall or reporting of events may be stimulated by her child's disorder. In a review of four studies in which estimates of odds ratios based on retrospective and on non-retrospective methods could be compared, a total of 56 exposures was considered (Little, 1992). If recall bias acted to produce over-reporting of all exposures by mothers of cases compared with mothers of controls, the retrospectively derived odds ratios would be higher than the others in relative terms; 21 were higher, 33 were lower and one was identical, and the difference for the

remaining one depended on the inclusion of missing information. Thus, the data suggest that relative under-reporting by mothers of cases is more likely.

There appear to be no studies in which possible recall bias in relation to childhood cancer has been investigated directly. In a case–control study of sudden infant death syndrome (SIDS) in which information obtained by interview was compared with information in medical records, case–control differences in recall accuracy did not appear to create spurious associations with SIDS or to bias most associations away from the null value (Drews *et al.*, 1990). As noted by Swan *et al.* (1992), comparison of prospectively and retrospectively collected information assesses reporting consistency, but not reporting accuracy, unless the mother initially reports exposure without error. There has been substantial publicity about some exposures which may be related to childhood cancer, such as residential proximity to nuclear installations or to power lines. The possible impact of recall bias in relation to such exposures has not been investigated. Investigation of the theoretical impact of recall bias shows that even severe recall bias would cause only weak to moderate spurious associations, and that case–control differences in accuracy of exposure assessment may not always bias associations away from the null (Drews & Greenland, 1990; Swan *et al.*, 1992; Drews *et al.*, 1993; Khoury *et al.*, 1994).

The possibility of recall bias has led some investigators to select controls comprising subjects with childhood cancer other than the specific one under investigation. A potential difficulty of this approach is that some of the types of cancer in the control series may also be related to the exposure of interest. For example, Buckley *et al.* (1994) observed that this might account for the association between acute lymphocytic leukaemia (ALL) and exposure of the index child to solvents and insecticides being substantially weaker in comparison with cancer controls than in comparison with healthy controls selected by random-digit dialling.

Swan *et al.* (1992) demonstrated that an association between the exposure of interest and a specific disease which affects only a small proportion of the controls can produce a substantial bias towards a null association. In addition, using the example of congenital anomalies, Drews *et al.* (1993) showed that even when recall bias exists, the observed association can be closer to the true association when a population-based control series is used than when the control group comprises births with anomalies other than those under investigation. Some investigators have sought to strengthen their study design by including two control groups. If consistent associations are found in the comparison of the case group with each of the control groups, the evidence that the association is not explained by non-causal factors is strong. However, if the associations are inconsistent, interpretation becomes very difficult.

A further consideration is matching. In many studies, matching is made on gender, geographical area of residence and age. One reason for matching is to control for unmeasured confounders (Wacholder *et al.*, 1992b). For example, there are small differences in the incidence of a number of types of childhood cancer between boys and girls. Matching by area of residence can aid in the control of potential environmental or socioeconomic differences that are difficult to measure; this was done in many studies of childhood cancer. Matching on year of birth would achieve time comparability between cases and controls for exposures that vary over time. For example, this might be expected to lead to comparability in policies of obstetric and perinatal care. The incidence of specific types of childhood cancer varies by age. The cumulative probability of exposure to any specific agent during the lifetime of the index child increases with age. In studies of adult-onset disease, there may be matching on age in categories such as five-year age groups, or adjustment for age in the analysis using similar categories. Use of such broad categories in studies of childhood cancer might not exclude the possibility of residual confounding by age. In many studies of childhood cancer, matching on age within intervals such as one, two or three years was used. Exposures of the case between birth and diagnosis, or a specified interval before diagnosis, are compared with exposures of the matched control between birth and a reference date. This is chosen so that the length of the period between birth and the reference date is the same as the period of exposure under consideration for the cases. A potential problem is that interviews with control patients may only be sought once an interview has been completed with parents of the matched case. At interview, the control may be somewhat older than the matched case. It is possible that ambiguities may arise in determining the time of exposure of controls, and that exposures

between the reference date and the date of interview may not be excluded. This would act to reduce the relative risks observed, and would bias a true relative risk of unity to being less than unity.

## Cohort studies

In the available cohort studies of childhood cancer, seven main types of exposure have been considered: (1) birth characteristics, as recorded in birth records or in specialized registers of persons with the characteristic; (2) exposures related to area of residence, such as fall-out from explosions of nuclear weapons; (3) diagnostic and therapeutic exposure to ionizing radiation; (4) bacillus Calmette-Guérin (BCG) vaccination; (5) intrauterine infection; (6) parental occupational exposure; and (7) maternal smoking during pregnancy. The main advantages of the cohort design include the avoidance of recall bias and ease of interpretation of the temporal sequence of events. Some of the studies of birth characteristics based on routine records were large. For example, the largest such study included more than 10 000 cases (Hirayama, 1979). In many other studies, the numbers of cases, even for all sites combined, were small, and therefore their statistical power was low. Many of the studies were based on deaths due to childhood cancer, rather than on newly incident cases, so the possible effect of exposure on survival has to be given consideration. Another problem inherent in the cohort approach includes the possibility of incomplete follow-up, which may be related to exposure. An additional possible difficulty is that the information on potential confounding variables may be limited or absent, although this limitation may not be very important in practice, in view of the lack of established risk factors for most specific types of childhood cancer.

## Structure of the review

The next chapter deals with the descriptive epidemiology of childhood cancer. Subsequent chapters are organized by exposure. First, genetic factors and familial aggregation are discussed. Ionizing radiation, electromagnetic fields, chemicals and dusts, and infections which may be of etiological importance during the preconceptional period, during the pregnancy leading to the birth of the index child or during his or her lifetime are then considered. Tobacco smoking, use of marijuana and other 'recreational' drugs, and alcohol consumption by the mother or father before conception, during the index pregnancy or during the lifetime of the index child are discussed. Maternal age and previous reproductive history, other aspects of the previous medical history of the mother, the medical history of the father and of other members of the family are then considered. Finally, perinatal and constitutional characteristics of the index child and exposures experienced during his or her lifetime are considered. In each of these sections, the evidence for specific types of childhood cancer is reviewed in the order of the classification of childhood cancer proposed by Birch and Marsden (1987).

## Hypotheses involving consideration of different possible routes of exposure

Some hypotheses about the causes of specific types of childhood cancer are complex in that their testing involves consideration of different possible routes of exposure. These hypotheses are now outlined. Evidence relating to the various routes of exposure will be collated in the conclusion.

### *Childhood acute lymphocytic leukaemia of the B-cell precursor type: Greaves' hypothesis*

Greaves (1988) suggested that ALL of the common B-cell precursor type, which accounts for the peak in the incidence of childhood leukaemia at the age of two to five years, arises from two spontaneous mutations. The first was postulated to arise *in utero* at a stage of rapid multiplication of the B-cell precursors in the liver and bone marrow when mutation is especially likely to occur—clones of cells capable of responding to a vast range of different antigens are produced. Greaves suggested that lymphoid precursor cells are at a much higher risk of spontaneous mutation than other somatic cells, particularly at early stages of development and infancy, because of developmentally regulated intrinsic mutagenic activity together with a high proliferation rate. The second mutation was postulated to occur after birth during the proliferation of antibody-producing cells following the infant's first contact with a diverse range of antigens. This was postulated to account for the predominance of B-cell precursor ALL over T-cell precursor ALL, the differences in the age distribution of these types, and some evidence that childhood ALL

was not independent of environmental or genetic background, for example, the association with high socioeconomic status observed in some studies. In studies in animals, B-cell precursor turnover in bone marrow was found to be highest in the young. Immune stimulation of mature lymphoid tissue in young mice resulted in a positive feedback proliferation signal to B-cell precursors in the marrow; no equivalent feedback response was detectable in the thymus. This distribution might account for the predominance of the B-cell precursor type, and the distinctive age distribution. Greaves (1988) observed that the steep rise in the incidence rate of ALL occurs shortly after the phase of increasing immunological challenge, as indicated by the increase in serum immunoglobulin levels during the first few years of life, and the fall in incidence after the age of three years occurs concomitantly with the apparent achievement of steady-state conditions in the antibody response. Greaves postulated a promotional effect of the immune response by means of an indirect upregulation of the number of target precursor B-cells at risk. The pattern of exposure to infectious organisms varies according to socioeconomic circumstances, genetic background, vaccination exposure and length of breast-feeding, and these factors would be expected to influence the timing and magnitude of positive feedback stimulation to the lymphoid precursor population in the bone marrow. Greaves suggested that the low incidence of common ALL in the indigenous population of Africa and the Arab population of the Gaza Strip might in part reflect early exposure to infectious organisms and a protective effect of prolonged breast-feeding. The association with higher socioeconomic status and first-born children in developed countries might reflect the effects of delayed exposure to infectious organisms. Greaves suggested that the hypothesis could be tested by case–control studies in which detailed information was collected about the timing of infectious episodes in infancy, vaccination experience and duration of breast-feeding.

### *Childhood leukaemia: the Kinlen hypothesis*

Kinlen (1988) suggested that the excess of leukaemia in young people in the vicinity of two nuclear reprocessing plants in the United Kingdom might be due to the introduction of a new viral exposure into areas that were predominantly rural and sparsely populated until large numbers of people came to work at the installations. These situations would have brought together susceptible and infected individuals, the basis for the transmission of all micro-organisms (Kinlen, 1995). If childhood leukaemia were a rare end result of one or more of the infections, it could have increased in incidence as a result of this population mixing. Elevated proportions of susceptible individuals would have been expected in the areas into which there was population inflow, because of low population density and isolation. A lower level of natural immunization to the infection may occur either because of fewer opportunities for person-to-person transmission than in more densely populated areas, or because the population is not large enough to maintain the infection at endemic levels. Age at exposure may be greater in rural than in urban areas, and this can influence the form of certain viral infections such as maternal rubella and paralytic poliomyelitis (Kinlen, 1988). In addition, Kinlen (1995) postulated that elevated proportions of susceptible individuals might be expected in the incoming professional workers and their children, whose high standards of hygiene and relative social isolation would have tended to limit their exposure to infections. Infected individuals could have been present in any of the groups, and the mixing of infected and susceptible individuals, given a sufficient population density, would have caused outbreaks of the relevant infection or infections. The dose of an infectious agent may also be important, as is the case in several animal models of viral oncogenesis, and large-scale mixing of susceptible with infected people or carriers will increase the likelihood of a susceptible individual being heavily exposed (Kinlen, 1988). Kinlen and colleagues have tested this hypothesis by ecological studies of the associations between leukaemia mortality and incidence rates and measures of population mixing (see Chapter 7).

## Childhood acute lymphocytic leukaemia: maternal fertility problems

In a study in the Netherlands, Van Steensel-Moll *et al.* (1985a) observed positive associations between childhood ALL and a history of two or more miscarriages, hospitalization or consultation for subfertility, prolonged interval between discontinuation of oral contraceptives and the index conception, threatened abortion during the index pregnancy and related use of 'drugs to maintain the pregnancy'. The authors considered that these associations indicated a similar causal pathway, and suggested that

maternal subfertility might be of etiological importance.

## Childhood brain tumours: N-nitroso compounds

Experimental studies have shown that transplacental exposure to a variety of N-nitroso compounds in the rat produces neurogenic tumours in the offspring (Magee *et al.*, 1976). Neurogenic tumours have been produced in the mouse and Syrian golden hamster by administration of N-ethyl-N-nitrosourea to the dam. The effects appear to be independent of route of exposure (subcutaneous, intraperitoneal, intravenous, oral or inhalation) but studies in the rat indicate that the time of administration is a critical factor, with carcinogenic effects being produced only after administration from day 10 to delivery. Tomatis *et al.* (1981) observed neurogenic tumours in the offspring of male BDVI rats treated with N-ethyl-N-nitrosurea before mating. A dose of N-ethyl-N-nitrosourea as low as 2 mg/kg bw (0.8% of the $LD_{50}$ in the rat) can induce a carcinogenic response in the nervous system. A dose corresponding to 2% of the $LD_{50}$ produced a 63% incidence of malignant neurogenic tumours (Ivankovic & Druckrey, 1968). In contrast, a dose of 160 mg/kg bw was necessary to induce a 50% incidence of neurogenic tumours in adult rats, showing that the sensitivity of the nervous system during prenatal development is about 50 times higher than in adults (Druckrey *et al.*, 1969).

Humans are exposed not only to preformed N-nitroso compounds but also to a wide range of nitrogen-containing compounds and nitrosating agents which can react *in vivo* to form N-nitroso compounds (Bartsch, 1991). Exposure to preformed N-nitroso compounds is most intense and widespread in tobacco users (Hecht & Hoffmann, 1991). Beer has been shown to be the main source of the nitrosamine burden in food (Preussmann, 1984). In Germany in 1979, this source was estimated to account for 64% of the total N-nitrosodimethylamine intake, with meat and meat products accounting for 10% and cheese for 1%. Volatile nitrosamines and N-nitrosodiethanolamine have been found in a wide range of concentrations in many commercially available cosmetics. Drugs and pesticides may contain nitrosatable amino groups and can therefore be contaminated with nitrosamines. Rubber materials and manufactured rubber products have been shown to contain volatile nitrosamines; particularly relevant is the observation of these in rubber nipples for babies' bottles, which can migrate into milk or saliva (Havery & Fazio, 1983). Several occupational settings have been found to involve high exposure to exogenous *N*-nitrosamines, notably the rubber, leather, metal and chemical industries, mining, pesticides and detergent production, and fish factories (Preussman, 1984). *N*-Nitroso compounds can be formed *in vivo* by reaction of nitrosatable amines or amides and nitrosating agents, especially nitrite, particularly in the stomach. Nitrite is a normal constituent of human saliva, where its concentration depends largely on the nitrate intake in food and water. Dietary nitrate is absorbed from the gut, and rapidly distributed in the body via the bloodstream before being re-excreted into the oral cavity by the salivary glands. The oral microflora then reduce nitrate to nitrite. The most important source of human nitrate intake is vegetables, followed by drinking water. *N*-Nitrosamines are also found in the infected urinary bladder, and parasitic infection by liver fluke leads to a marked increase in endogenous *N*-nitrosamine synthesis (Bartsch, 1991). In theory, endogenous *N*-nitrosamine synthesis can occur when bacterial enzymes catalyse nitrosation from nitrate or nitrite, but as yet direct experimental support is lacking in relation to other sites. Vitamins C and E, phenolic compounds, and complex mixtures such as fruit and vegetable juices or other plant extracts can inhibit nitrosation (Bartsch *et al.*, 1988).

## Wilms' tumour: overgrowth and fetal growth factors

Olshan (1986) suggested that the association between high birthweight, overgrowth associated with Beckwith–Wiedemann syndrome and hemihypertrophy, and Wilms' tumour may be due to the action of loci additional to the (then) putative Wilms' tumour locus on the short arm of chromosome 11. These genes include insulin, insulin-like growth factor II (IGF-II) and the Harvey *ras* proto-oncogene. Both insulin and IGF-II are postulated to have a promoting influence on fetal growth, and fetal hyperinsulinaemia has been associated with the Beckwith–Wiedemann syndrome. Olshan postulated that the occurrence of high birthweight and certain congenital malformations in a subgroup of patients with Wilms' tumour might be due to abnormal interaction of the IGF-II and possibly the insulin gene with the Wilms' tumour gene.

## Germ-cell tumours: intrauterine exposure to maternal hormones

On the basis of studies of testicular and germ-cell ovarian cancer conducted among adult populations, and animal studies, Shu *et al.* (1995a) suggested that maternal exogenous hormone use and higher endogenous hormone levels may be associated with an elevated risk of malignant germ-cell tumours in childhood. Use of diethylstilbestrol and of oral contraceptives has been associated with malignant testicular and ovarian tumours in the offspring, although the available data are not entirely consistent. Prenatal exogenous hormone exposure has also been associated with cryptorchidism, a well established risk factor for testicular cancer. Estrogen administration induces testicular cancer in certain strains of mice. Testicular and ovarian germ-cell cancer have been associated with conditions related to a high endogenous estrogen level, such as high pregnancy weight, rapid achievement of regular menstruation after menarche, bleeding and spotting during pregnancy and hyperemesis.

# Chapter 2

# Descriptive epidemiology

Linda Sharp, Seonaidh Cotton and Julian Little

In children, as for adults, description and inspection of the epidemiological features of particular neoplasms may provide insights into their etiology. However, the classical descriptive analyses, namely comparisons of the disease burden between countries, between sub-groups of the population and over time, have proved more difficult to undertake for childhood than for adult cancers. Only in the past two decades have high-quality data been available from many parts of the world for such analyses. Most earlier descriptive epidemiological studies of childhood cancer were unsatisfactory, for three reasons that have been detailed by Parkin *et al.* (1988a,b). First, in many studies, the data were derived from registers of all types of cancer, the population bases of which were too small to permit calculation of reliable incidence rates. Second, both incidence and mortality data were often classified by anatomical site, as is appropriate for adult cancers. Childhood tumours are histologically diverse and some occur at several sites. Therefore, classification by histology is more appropriate. Third, many early studies were based on mortality data. These data are subject to the usual problems inherent in studies based on death certificates (Boyle, 1989). In addition, progress in treatment has led to marked improvements in survival for several types of childhood cancer (see, for example, Stiller & Bunch, 1990; Adami *et al.*, 1992; Ajiki *et al.*, 1995; de Nully Brown *et al.*, 1995; Miller *et al.*, 1995). This development further complicates the comparison of mortality rates between geographical areas and over time.

In this chapter, the discussion of geographical variation in incidence is based largely on data from an international study of childhood cancer which included newly incident cases diagnosed around the period 1970–79, registered according to an agreed protocol and coded to a histology-based scheme developed specifically for childhood tumours (Birch & Marsden, 1987; Parkin *et al.*, 1988a). Most of the data in this study were population-based, but in areas where such data were not available, mainly parts of Africa and Asia, hospital or histopathology

laboratory-based data were included. The data from the study are supplemented by reports pertaining to more recent periods. Data on variations in the incidence of childhood tumours by ethnic group are derived mainly from the same sources. For discussion of temporal trends, more diverse sources have been considered, including some older reports in which the data were classified according to versions of the International Classification of Diseases.

Compared with the situation for adult cancer, socioeconomic status has been relatively little studied in relation to cancer in children and most of the investigations have dealt exclusively with leukaemia. In epidemiological studies, gradients in the occurrence of a disease by socioeconomic status can be a starting point for the formulation of more specific hypotheses. The explanations proposed for associations between social class and disease have been grouped under the headings of artefact (i.e., confounding or bias), health selection (i.e., the process whereby health experience affects recruitment for jobs or other aspects of lifestyle) and social causation (i.e., involving direct environmental effects on disease risk) (Macintyre, 1986). In the context of childhood cancer, the possibility of artefact needs to be given particular attention as so many of the studies have been of the case–control design, in which selection bias and/or participation bias can be major concerns (see Chapter 1). Most of the descriptive studies have categorized childhood cases according to a community level indicator of socioeconomic status, usually derived from data recorded in population censuses, rather than according to the socioeconomic status of the individual. In such ecological analyses, the possibility of artefact is also present. In this chapter, the descriptive studies on childhood cancer and socioeconomic status are presented. Findings from case–control studies are considered in some situations where evidence from other sources is limited.

There has been considerable interest in clustering of childhood tumours, particularly leukaemia. Many of the relatively recent investigations have been responses to concern about particular sources of putative hazard (e.g., nuclear installations). These studies are discussed in Chapters 4 and 6. Small-area variations in the incidence or mortality of leukaemia in relation to measures of population mixing have also been undertaken. These are reviewed in Chapter 7. In this chapter, studies which have considered the more general distribution of childhood cancers in space and time, or space only, are reviewed. The studies on clustering of leukaemia and lymphoma are included in the sections on these malignancies. The studies of clustering of other tumours are discussed together at the end of the chapter.

This chapter is organized according to the diagnostic groups in the histology-based classification scheme for childhood tumours (i.e., Birch and Marsden groups I–XI[1]). Within each section, there are sub-sections on geographical patterns, age-specific incidence and sex ratio, ethnic origin, time trends and, where appropriate, socioeconomic status and spatial and temporal clustering. Other distinctive features of the epidemiology of particular tumours are described. The category of all childhood cancer combined has not been considered as this does not have any clear biological significance. Unless otherwise stated, all rates pertain to the 0–14 age range, are standardized to the world standard population (Segi, 1960) and are per million population. Where the term infants has been used, it refers to children under the age of one year.

## Group I: Leukaemias

Leukaemias are the most common cancers affecting children, accounting for, in most populations, between 25% and 35% of malignancies (Parkin *et al.*, 1988a). Acute lymphocytic leukaemia (now usually referred to as acute lymphoblastic leukaemia, or ALL) comprises the overwhelming majority of cases, with acute non-lymphocytic leukaemia (ANLL) the only other sub-type occurring regularly in children. In the mainly white populations of North America, Oceania and Europe, 75–80% of leukaemias are of the acute lymphocytic type and 15–17% acute non-lymphocytic. A higher proportion of cases is accounted for by ANLL in Asia and the black populations of North America. Chronic myeloid leukaemia is universally infrequent, seldom exceeding 4% of cases. The remaining leukaemias fall into the categories of other lymphoid leukaemia and other and unspecified leukaemia.

Variations between cancer registries in the level of ascertainment of leukaemias have been shown (Stiller *et al.*, 1991b), and it has been suggested that the degree of incomplete ascertainment may vary with leukaemia cell type (Bowie, 1987; Alexander *et al.*, 1989a) and over time (Bowie, 1987). There is evidence of miscoding and mis-classification of cell types (Mills, 1979; Bowie, 1987; Glass *et al.*, 1987; Gray *et al.*, 1987; Bessho, 1989; Draper *et al.*, 1993) and a tendency towards more precise classification over time (Stiller *et al.*, 1991b). In addition, in some instances, leukaemia and non-Hodgkin lymphoma represent different stages in the natural history of the same disease. In particular, ALL and lymphoblastic lymphoma share clinical and biological similarities and the distinction between them is arbitrary (Weinstein & Tarbell, 1997). These issues cause difficulties in the interpretation of geographical and temporal variations in the incidence of leukaemia overall and leukaemia sub-types (and non-Hodgkin lymphoma).

## Geographical patterns

During the decade 1970–79, there was an approximately five-fold variation in the incidence, in the 0–14-year age group, of all types of leukaemia combined (Parkin *et al.*, 1988a). For boys and girls together, the highest annual world-standardized rate, 59.4 per million population, was observed in Costa Rica and the lowest, 11.8 per million, in Ibadan, Nigeria. Hispanics in Los Angeles, USA, were the only other population to have a rate in excess of 50 per million. In other central and south American populations, the rates varied substantially. In the white populations of North America and in Australia, Japan, Singapore, the Philippines, north and western Europe and non-Maoris in New Zealand, the incidence was between 35 and 49 per million. In central and eastern Europe it was slightly lower. Among the black populations in the USA, rates were 25–28 per million. An incidence of less than 25 per million was reported in India and Africa and among Kuwaiti natives in Kuwait. However, it is likely that the low rates in India and Africa are underestimates because of diagnostic imprecision which may occur in very young infants in these areas (Parkin *et al.*, 1989). In particular, there may be a lack of resources to perform histopathological examinations on tissue specimens.

### Acute lymphocytic leukaemia (ALL)

As for all leukaemias combined, Costa Ricans and Los Angeles Hispanics had the highest

---

[1.] Diagnostic group XII includes a diverse collection of other and unspecified neoplasms and is not described further in this chapter.

incidences of ALL; the rates were 44.7 and 39.4 per million per annum (Parkin *et al.*, 1988a). The lowest values, of less than 12 per million, were seen among Kuwaiti natives, and in parts of Brazil and India. The most distinctive features of the geographical distribution of this malignancy are (i) a tendency towards higher rates in white North American and European populations than in Asian populations and (ii) substantial variations in incidence across continents and within populations. In Europe there was a two-fold difference in incidence; rates ranged from 17.8 in Slovenia to 36.4 in the former West Germany. The variation was even more extreme among Hispanic populations in the Americas. In Kuwait, the incidence among non-Kuwaitis (mainly immigrants of Arab and Asian origin) was 2.8 times higher than that for Kuwaiti nationals (Table 2.1). A similar pattern was evident among non-Maoris and Maoris in New Zealand. The rates for whites in the USA were approximately twice those for blacks. In Israel, the incidence was almost 50% higher for Jews than non-Jews.

The main immunophenotypic variants of ALL are B-cell precursor ALL of the common (cALL) and null (nALL) types and T-cell precursor ALL. While these are found in diverse geographical locations and ethnic groups (Greaves *et al.*, 1985), their relative proportions are not constant. In white populations in the UK, South Africa and Chile, between 65 and 74% of ALLs are cALL, 11–19% nALL and 2–22% T-cell ALL (Greaves *et al.*, 1993). Common ALL is proportionately less frequent in black African children than in "Caucasian" children and T-cell ALL correspondingly more frequent (Greaves *et al.*, 1993). A deficit in pre-B-cell ALL is also evident among Mapuche Indians in Chile, South Africans of mixed origin (Greaves *et al.*, 1993) and in Kenya, Egypt and the Gaza strip (Ross *et al.*, 1994a). The distribution of sub-types in Taiwan (Greaves *et al.*, 1993) and Hokkaido, Japan (Nishi *et al.*, 1996) differs little from that for white populations.

### Acute non-lymphocytic leukaemia (ANLL)

During the decade 1970–79, rates of ANLL above 10 per million population were observed in New Zealand Maoris (12.7 per million), in Shanghai, China (12.1) and in Kanagawa (11.0) and Miyagi (10.9) in Japan (Parkin *et al.*, 1988a). Elsewhere in Asia, with the exception of Hong Kong and India, the incidence was at least 5 per million. In the Americas, the rates varied from 3.2 per million in the Canadian Atlantic Provinces to 8.8 in Costa Rica and 9.0 among Los Angeles Hispanics. Rates of between 4 and 8 per million were seen in Europe.

In the USA, the incidence rates of ANLL in blacks were only slightly lower than among whites, reflecting the fact that, for black children, a greater proportion of leukaemias are of the acute non-lymphocytic type than for white children. For example, in the black population covered by the Surveillance, Epidemiology and End Results (SEER) Program, ANLL accounted for 22.0% of leukaemia cases and the incidence was 5.2 per million; for whites, the figures were 14.8% and 6.1 per million. This higher frequency of ANLL relative to ALL among blacks compared to whites in the same community has also been observed in South Africa (MacDougall *et al.*, 1986).

### Chronic myeloid leukaemia (CML)

Almost everywhere, too few cases of CML are diagnosed to permit the calculation of reliable incidence rates. Of those series of at least 10 cases, the highest rate, 3.0 per million, occurred in Shanghai, China (Parkin *et al.*, 1988a). In most other populations, the incidence varied between 0.5 and 1.5 per million.

## Age-specific incidence and sex ratio

In most countries the rate of total leukaemia is highest among children under five years and decreases with age (Linet & Devesa, 1991). The decline with age is more rapid under 10 years than after. Almost universally, the age-adjusted incidence for boys exceeds that for girls (Parkin *et al.*, 1988a), with the sex ratio typically between 1.1:1 and 1.4:1.

### Acute lymphocytic leukaemia

In developed countries, the age–incidence curve of ALL is characterized by a peak between the ages of 1 and 4 years. In Britain, during 1971–84, the annual incidence in infants was just below 20 per million, rising to approximately 40 per million in one-year-olds and peaking at over 70 per million in children aged 2 and 3 years. The incidence declined progressively to around 20 per million at age 10 and remained stable thereafter (Draper *et al.*, 1994).

Although this age distribution is well recognized, and attributable to cALL (Greaves *et al.*, 1993), it has not always been present. In England and Wales, the peak was first apparent in mortality data from the 1920s (Hewitt, 1955) and among white Americans featured prominently in mortality data for the 1940s (Gilliam & Walter, 1958). In populations with moderate incidence of ALL in the 1970s, a peak emerged later; in the 1960s in US blacks (Ross *et al.*, 1994a) and Japan (Court-Brown & Doll, 1961; Ajiki *et al.*, 1994); and in the 1970s in Jews and non-Jews in Israel (Katz & Steinitz, 1988). In Kuwait, where leukaemia incidence was low during the 1970s, the age peak has recently been observed (Stiller & Parkin, 1996). In African series, where leukaemia incidence is also low, the peak is not present (Parkin *et al.*, 1988b; Ross *et al.*, 1994a).

The age peak is not equally marked in all communities where it is present. During the 1970s, the peak was less pronounced for US blacks than for US whites (Parkin *et al.*, 1988b; Pratt *et al.*, 1988). Similarly, in Japan during 1971–88 (Ajiki *et al.*, 1994), in Hong Kong in 1984–90 (Alexander *et al.*, 1997), in parts of central and south America in 1970–79 (Parkin *et al.*, 1988b) and among children resident in the former socialist countries of central and eastern Europe during 1980–91 (Parkin *et al.*, 1996), the peak appears to have been less prominent than in western European populations.

In areas of England and Wales which are isolated from urban centres, an exaggerated age peak has been found (Alexander *et al.*, 1990d). This was particularly evident in areas which were also of high socioeconomic status. It appeared to coincide with a relatively low incidence of ALL in older children (Alexander *et al.*, 1991b). A similar pattern has been observed in the rural north of Scotland (Black *et al.*, 1994). These observations led to the hypothesis that elevated risk of ALL is determined by community characteristics, including isolation, high socioeconomic status and population mixing (Kinlen, 1995) which are related to immunological isolation in infancy and which influence patterns of exposure to common infectious agents before the appearance of the leukaemia (Greaves & Alexander, 1993). This is discussed more fully in Chapter 7.

The ratio of the ALL incidence rates for boys and girls is usually between 1.1:1 and 1.3:1 (Parkin *et al.*, 1988b).

*Acute non-lymphocytic leukaemia*

In most series, the sex ratio for ANLL is close to unity (Parkin *et al.*, 1988a). In both sexes, the rates are highest in infants (Linet & Devesa, 1991) and are fairly uniform in older children (Ajiki *et al.*, 1994). In Britain, during 1978–87, the incidence in infants was 9.5 per million, in the 1–4 age group 7.3, in the 5–9 age group 4.1 and 5.6 in children aged 10–14 years (Stiller *et al.*, 1995). Comparable rates have been reported elsewhere in Europe and North America (Mosso *et al.*, 1992; Kaatsch *et al.*, 1995; Gurney *et al.*, 1996a).

*Chronic myeloid leukaemia*

In the largest reported population-based series of CML, consisting of 96 malignancies diagnosed in the period 1978–87 in Britain, the incidence rates were 1.2 per million for infants and 1.6, 0.5 and 0.7 for children aged 1–4, 5–9 and 10–14 years respectively (Stiller *et al.*, 1995). The male to female sex ratio was 1.6:1, which is consistent with other series (Parkin *et al.*, 1988a).

## Ethnic origin

Data on the incidence of ALL and ANLL in series included in Parkin *et al.* (1988a) for which figures by ethnic group were presented are shown in Table 2.1.

*Acute lymphocytic leukaemia*

In the USA, there is substantial variation in the frequency of ALL by ethnic group. The highest rates of ALL are evident among Hispanic populations, Filipinos and Chinese (Linet & Devesa, 1991). Rates among whites are moderate to high by international standards, while those for American Indians are somewhat lower. The lowest rates are among blacks, with the ALL incidence rate ratio approximately 0.5 for blacks compared to whites (Table 2.1).

Two studies in Britain have investigated risk of childhood cancer in relation to ethnicity (Stiller *et al.*, 1991a; Powell *et al.*, 1994). The largest of these included 7638 children with cancer recorded on the register of the United Kingdom Children's Cancer Study and diagnosed from 1981 (Stiller *et al.*, 1991a). Although not population-based, the series was estimated to represent two thirds of all cases of childhood cancer. Because of the lack of a population base and since population data were not available by ethnic group, relative frequencies of specific tumours among white children and those of "West Indian" and "Asian" (mainly Indian subcontinent) origin were calculated. The results of the study are summarized in Table 2.2. There were no significant differences in the risk of ALL, adjusted for treatment centre, age and sex, for West Indian (relative risk (RR) = 0.90) or Asian (RR = 1.08) children, compared with Caucasian (white) children. In addition, the relative frequencies of ALL in the 0–4, 5–9 and 10–14 year age groups were similar for white and Asian children. Moreover, there was no evidence of variation in ALL phenotype with ethnic group, although this information was not available for almost 30% of cases. The second study was conducted in the West Midlands area of England during 1982–91 (Powell *et al.*, 1994).

13

## Table 2.1. Relative risk of specific types of childhood cancer in the United States, Israel, Kuwait, New Zealand and Singapore by ethnic group, based on comparison of age-adjusted incidence rates, using the world standard population for age groups under 15 years

*(a) United States: numbers of cases in smallest ethnic group and risk relative (RR) to largest group*

| Type of tumour | Greater Delaware Valley, 1970–79 | | Los Angeles, 1972–83 | | | New York, 1976–82 | | SEER[a] Program, 1973–82 | |
|---|---|---|---|---|---|---|---|---|---|
| | Number of cases in non-whites | RR, non-whites vs. whites | Number of cases in blacks | RR, Hispanics vs. non-Hispanic whites | RR, blacks vs. non-Hispanic whites | Number of cases in blacks | RR, blacks vs. whites | Number of cases in blacks | RR, blacks vs. whites |
| ALL | 57 | 0.47 | 56 | 0.97 | 0.49 | 75 | 0.53 | 82 | 0.45 |
| ANLL | 17 | 0.73 | 17 | 1.41 | 0.86 | 24 | 0.90 | 31 | 0.85 |
| Hodgkin's disease | 23 | 1.04 | 24 | 1.23 | 0.96 | 30 | 0.89 | 30 | 0.76 |
| Non-Hodgkin lymphoma | 13 | 0.83 | 10 | 0.93 | 0.49 | 17 | 0.76 | 16 | 0.55 |
| CNS tumours | 86 | 0.90 | 59 | 0.83 | 0.67 | 94 | 0.77 | 127 | 0.88 |
| Neuroblastoma | 19 | 0.54 | 27 | 0.59 | 1.04 | 29 | 0.67 | 51 | 0.82 |
| Retinoblastoma | 19 | 1.28 | 13 | 1.27 | 1.00 | 10 | 0.96 | 25 | 1.28 |
| Wilms' tumour | 43 | 1.85 | 32 | 0.81 | 1.20 | 30 | 1.00 | 58 | 1.25 |
| Hepatic tumours | 2 | 0.55 | 5 | 1.57 | 1.14 | 9 | 1.50 | 7 | 0.88 |
| Osteosarcoma | 18 | 1.75 | 17 | 1.48 | 2.00 | 16 | 1.19 | 23 | 1.36 |
| Ewing's sarcoma | 1 | 0.14 | 2 | 0.60 | 0.24 | 1 | 0.08 | 2 | 0.17 |
| Rhabdomyosarcoma | 15 | 0.88 | 12 | 1.08 | 0.82 | 16 | 0.60 | 20 | 0.74 |
| Gonadal and germ cell tumours | 14 | 0.86 | 9 | 1.33 | 0.69 | 14 | 0.73 | 24 | 1.00 |
| Epithelial neoplasms | 13 | 1.24 | 19 | 0.62 | 1.09 | 24 | 1.45 | 25 | 0.87 |

Based on data in Parkin *et al.* (1988a)

[a] Surveillance, Epidemiology and End Results (SEER) Program comprises Connecticut, Detroit (Michigan), Iowa, Atlanta (Georgia), New Mexico, Utah, Seattle (Washington), San Francisco and Oakland (California) and Hawaii

*(b) Israel, Kuwait, New Zealand and Singapore: numbers of cases in smallest ethnic group and risk relative (RR) to largest group*

| Type of tumour | Israel, 1970–79 | | Kuwait, 1974–82 | | New Zealand, 1970–79 | | Singapore, 1968–82 | |
|---|---|---|---|---|---|---|---|---|
| | Number of cases in non-Jews | RR, non-Jews vs. Jews | Number of cases in non-Kuwaitis | RR, non-Kuwaitis vs. Kuwaitis | Number of cases in Maoris | RR, Maoris vs. non-Maoris | Number of cases in Malays | RR, Malays vs. Chinese |
| ALL | 37 | 0.69 | 64 | 2.75 | 14 | 0.39 | 37 | 0.88 |
| ANLL | 13 | 0.76 | 3 | 1.60 | 14 | 1.35 | 16 | 1.35 |
| Hodgkin's disease | 22 | 1.16 | 19 | 0.95 | 8 | 1.79 | 3 | 1.06 |
| Non-Hodgkin lymphoma | 26 | 0.88 | 25 | 1.31 | 11 | 1.47 | 10 | 0.85 |
| CNS tumours | 43 | 0.70 | 23 | 2.41 | 29 | 1.00 | 16 | 0.75 |
| Neuroblastoma | 22 | 0.67 | 20 | 1.89 | 14 | 1.76 | 5 | 0.56 |
| Retinoblastoma | 9 | 1.10 | 8 | 1.67 | 6 | 1.09 | 2 | 0.34 |
| Wilms' tumour | 12 | 0.68 | 12 | 1.58 | 9 | 1.26 | 4 | 0.85 |
| Hepatic tumours | 0 | – | 5 | 5.00 | 2 | 1.07 | 2 | 0.44 |
| Osteosarcoma | 5 | 0.69 | 3 | 0.62 | 2 | 0.50 | 4 | 0.66 |
| Ewing's sarcoma | 2 | 0.40 | 7 | 2.16 | 5 | 1.81 | 1 | 1.40 |
| Rhabdomyosarcoma | 4 | 0.44 | 4 | 0.67 | 4 | 0.79 | 1 | 0.19 |
| Gonadal and germ-cell tumours | 3 | 0.30 | 7 | 7.20 | 10 | 2.00 | 6 | 0.92 |
| Epithelial neoplasms | 5 | 0.35 | 6 | 1.28 | 12 | 1.21 | 4 | 0.44 |

Based on data in Parkin *et al.* (1988a)

## Table 2.2. Number of cases and relative risk of specific childhood tumours in Britain by ethnic group, adjusted for age, sex and centre to which the child was referred for investigation and/or treatment

| Type of tumour | Number of cases (N) and risks relative to whites, by ethnic group | | | |
|---|---|---|---|---|
| | West Indian | | Asian | |
| | N | Relative risk | N | Relative risk |
| ALL | 17 | 0.90 | 121 | 1.08 |
| ANLL | 2 | 0.51 | 21 | 0.94 |
| Hodgkin's disease | 5 | 1.85 | 29 | 2.09** |
| Non-Hodgkin, Burkitt's and unspecified lymphoma | 4 | 0.91 | 26 | 1.04 |
| Brain and spinal tumours | 4 | 0.51 | 36 | 0.75 |
| Neuroblastoma | 8 | 1.78 | 38 | 1.19 |
| Retinoblastoma[a] | 2 | 1.12 | 13 | 1.23 |
| Wilms' tumour | 10 | 2.55* | 16 | 0.51* |
| Osteosarcoma | 1 | 0.85 | 7 | 1.10 |
| Ewing's sarcoma | 0 | 0.00 | 8 | 1.00 |
| Rhabdomyosarcoma | 4 | 0.84 | 10 | 0.44* |

Modified from Stiller *et al.* (1991a)          * *p*<0.05

[a] Not adjusted for centre or age          ** *p*<0.001

The ratio of the standardized incidence rates of ALL among white and Asian children did not differ significantly from unity (RR = 1.14; 95% confidence interval (CI) 0.79–1.65). One-fifth of the Asian cases and 9% of the white children in this study were also included in the analysis by Stiller *et al.* (1991a). In addition, neither of the analyses adjusted for socioeconomic status, which differs markedly among ethnic groups and which is associated with risk of ALL (see below).

The lack of variation in the incidence of ALL between ethnic groups in Britain, in conjunction with the markedly lower frequency of the tumour in the Indian subcontinent and Africa than in Britain (Parkin *et al.*, 1988a; Linet & Devesa, 1991) would suggest that the incidence of ALL depends primarily on environmental factors associated with geographical location. It has been suggested that the more notable ethnic variations apparent in the USA, particularly between black and white children, could reflect a smaller difference in socioeconomic status between ethnic groups in the UK than in the USA (Stiller *et al.*, 1991a). However, it should be noted that the British study included only 17 cases of ALL in West Indian children.

### Acute non-lymphocytic leukaemia

ANLL is consistently less common among black populations of the USA than among whites (Parkin et al., 1988a). The ratio of incidence rates is approximately 0.85 (Table 2.1). In Britain, the malignancy was only half as common among West Indian children as among white children (Table 2.2), but this analysis was based on only two cases in West Indians and 410 in whites (Stiller et al., 1991a). The risk of ANLL among Asian children in the UK does not appear to differ from that for white children (Stiller et al., 1991a; Powell et al., 1994).

## Socioeconomic status

Socioeconomic factors have been proposed as an explanation for the age peak in childhood leukaemia (Ramot & MacGrath, 1982). Specifically, it was postulated that, with economic development, impoverished communities move from a situation where leukaemia is rare, and those ALLs which do occur are of T-cell type, through an intermediate stage where cALL begins to appear, to a state of high socioeconomic status associated with high incidence of ALL and cALL.

The descriptive studies which have investigated the relationship between leukaemia and socioeconomic status are summarized in Table 2.3. In the majority of these, the area of residence of the incident cases (or deaths) was used as a measure of socioeconomic status. A diverse range of measures has been considered, including household income, years of schooling, and composite scores based on variables such as car ownership, social class of the head of household, unemployment and household density. In virtually all of these studies, a weak positive association between leukaemia and high socioeconomic status was observed. Exceptions are the studies of Knox (1964) and Birch *et al.* (1981) in the north of England and those of Muirhead (1995) and Swensen *et al.* (1997) in the USA. In the two English studies, social class was assessed on the basis of paternal occupation rather than on a community-based measure. Alexander *et al.* (1990d) have noted that the observation that associations are more apparent with area than with personal socioeconomic status supports an interpretation involving community behaviour (see Chapter 7). In the two studies in the USA, multiple area-level measures of socioeconomic status were analysed and a modest positive association was found for at least one of these.

The association between leukaemia and lymphoma and measures of the socioeconomic level of the area of residence were considered in the context of an investigation of geographical variation in incidence in Britain (Draper *et al.*, 1991a; Rodrigues *et al.*, 1991). In these analyses, leukaemias of unspecified type were analysed together with lymphocytic leukaemia on the basis that the proportion of unspecified leukaemia had changed over time and the great majority of these were likely to be ALL.

Draper *et al.* (1991a) examined variation in rates between administrative county districts in Britain during the periods 1969–73, 1974–78 and 1979–83 and related these to measures of socioeconomic status derived from 1971 and 1981 census data. The variables used in the analysis were: (i) the proportion of economically active men who were working; (ii) the proportion of households with a car; and (iii) the proportion of households that were owner-occupied. Incidence rates for all leukaemias combined increased with increasing socioeconomic status. The effect was apparent in the 0–4- and 5–9-year age groups, but not in the 10–14-year age group. The effect was due to lymphocytic and unspecified leukaemias, and was not large. When districts were grouped according to quintiles of the socioeconomic score, for the 0–4 age group the rate for the highest quintile was 7–24% greater than the rate for the lowest quintile. For the 5–9 age group, the difference was 12–40%. No effect was found for ANLL. Significant differences

## Table 2.3. Summary of descriptive studies of childhood cancer and socioeconomic status

| Area and period of study | Cases (I) incident, (D) dead, Upper age limit | Total number of cases (% with information on socioeconomic status) | Indicator of socioeconomic status | Contrast | Ratio | References |
|---|---|---|---|---|---|---|
| **Leukaemia** | | | | | | |
| USA, Erie County, (New York), 1943–56 | I, 15 | 137 (99%) | Rent of census tract of residence | Upper half vs. lower half | 1.51 | Pinkel & Nefzger, 1959 |
| England, Northumberland and Durham, 1951–60 | I, 14 | 185 (68%) | Father's occupation at time of diagnosis or death | Social class distribution of cases vs. social class distribution of region | –[a] | Knox, 1964 |
| USA, Denver (Colorado) 1941–59 | D, 14 | 75 (100%) | a) Income of census tract of residence b) Rent of census tract of residence c) Dilapidated houses with inadequate plumbing d) Dilapidated houses with crowding | Upper half vs. lower half Upper half vs. lower half Upper half vs. lower half Upper half vs. lower half | 1.61 1.54 1.81 1.42 | Githens et al., 1965 |
| England, North Western Regional Health Authority area, 1954–77 | I, 14 | 638 | Father's occupation at time of the child's birth | Social class distribution of cases vs. social class distribution of region | –[a] | Birch et al., 1981 |
| England and Wales, 1959–63 and 1970–72 | D, 14 | 1771 (1959–63) 1000 (1970–72) | Occupation of father as recorded on child's death certificate | Administrators, managers, professional, technical workers, artists vs. all occupations, by period of death 1959–63 1970–72 | 141[b] 169[b] | Sanders et al., 1981 |
| England and Wales, 1969–78[c] | D, 24 | 4230 | Distribution of socioeconomic group of county district according to 1971 census | Per 5% increase in proportion of population of social class I compared with increase in proportion of social class V | 1.06 | Cook-Mozaffari et al., 1989a |
| England and Wales, 22 counties 1984–86 | I, 14 | 307 | Socioeconomic index for electoral wards based on social class of head of household, car ownership, household density and unemployment, as recorded in the 1981 census | Quartile 1 (highest) vs. quartile 3 | 1.49 | Alexander et al., 1990b |
| Great Britain, 1969–83[c] | I, 14 | 6691 | Socioeconomic score for districts, based on information from 1971 and 1981 censuses on proportion of economically active men working, proportion of households with a car, and proportion of households that were owner-occupied | Highest vs. lowest quintile, by age group 0–4 5–9 10–14 | 1.11–1.19[d] 1.17–1.38[d] 0.88–1.07[d] | Draper et al., 1991a |
| England and Wales, 1966–83[c] | I, 14 | 7134 | Socioeconomic score derived in similar way to that of Draper et al. (1991a), but analysed by census tract rather than by district | Highest vs. lowest quintile, by age group 0–4 5–14 | 1.34, 0.94[ef] 1.13, 1.61[ef] | Rodrigues et al., 1991 |
| USA, San Francisco-Oakland (California), Detroit (Michigan) and Atlanta (Georgia), 1978–82 | I, 14 | 346[g] | a) Median education among white persons aged 25 years or over in census tracts as recorded in 1980 census b) Median annual white family income in census tracts as recorded in 1980 census | College graduate vs. <12 years of schooling Highest ($30 000) vs. lowest (<$15 000) | 1.27 0.85 | Muirhead, 1995 |
| **ALL** | | | | | | |
| Australia, Queensland, 1973–79[h] | I, 14 | 127 | a) Proportion of population with tertiary qualifications b) Proportion in professional or technical occupations c) Proportion of secondary students attending non-government schools d) Proportion of population in farming, trade, production-processing or labouring occupation | Correlation analysis | r = 0.9, p<0.01 r = 0.8, p<0.01 r = 0.9, p<0.01 r = 0.7, p<0.01 | McWhirter, 1982 |

| Location, period | | No. | Variable | Comparison | Value | Reference |
|---|---|---|---|---|---|---|
| Australia, Brisbane City, 1973–79[h] | I, 14 | 51 | a) Proportion of population in professional or technical occupations<br>b) Proportion of students at non-government schools | 16%+ vs. <8%<br>40%+ vs. <25% | 3.0<br>3.0 | McWhirter, 1982 |
| England and Wales, 22 counties, 1984–88 | I, 14 | 438 | Socioeconomic index for electoral ward of residence at diagnosis, based on social class of head of household, car ownership, household density and unemployment as recorded in the 1981 census | High vs. low | 1.13 | Alexander et al., 1990d |
| Great Britain, 1969–83[c] | I, 14 | 5369 | Socioeconomic score for districts, based on information from 1971 and 1981 censuses on proportion of economically active men working, proportion of households with a car, and proportion of households that were owner-occupied | Highest vs. lowest quintile, by age group<br>0–4<br>5–9<br>10–14 | 1.07–1.24[d,e]<br>1.12–1.40[d,e]<br>0.69–0.97[d,e] | Draper et al., 1991a |
| England and Wales, 1966–83[c] | I, 14 | 5711 | Socioeconomic score derived in similar way to that of Draper et al. (1991a), but analysed by census tract rather than by district | Highest vs. lowest quintile, by age group<br>0–4<br>5–14 | 1.36, 1.10[v,f]<br>1.17, 1.74[e,f] | Rodrigues et al., 1991 |
| England and Wales, 1979–85[c] | I, 14 | 2035 | Socioeconomic score derived in similar way to that of Draper et al. (1991a), for districts | Top 40 districts vs. bottom 40 districts, by age group<br>0–4<br>5–9<br>10–14 | 1.02<br>1.14<br>0.82 | Stiller & Boyle, 1996 |
| USA, 1989–91 | I, 14 | 4411[i] (95%) | Socioeconomic variables for zip code from 1990 census:<br>a) Household income<br><br>b) Educational level of persons aged >25<br><br>c) Occupation of persons aged >16 | a) Proportion of households in zip codes of residence of cases with household income > $50 000 vs. proportion with income < $10 000, by ethnic group<br>Whites<br>African Americans<br>b) Proportion of households in zip codes of residence of cases with persons educated to greater than high school level vs. proportion not completing high school, by ethnic group<br>Whites<br>African Americans<br>c) Proportion of households in zip codes of residence of cases with persons in executive occupations vs. proportion in labour occupations, by ethnic group<br>Whites<br>African Americans | 2.00<br>0.56<br><br><br>2.48<br>1.21<br><br><br>0.85<br>0.61 | Swensen et al., 1997 |

**ANLL**

| Location, period | | No. | Variable | Comparison | Value | Reference |
|---|---|---|---|---|---|---|
| Great Britain, 1969–83[c] | I, 14 | 1107 | Socioeconomic score for districts based on information from 1971 and 1981 censuses on proportion of economically active men working, proportion of households with a car, and proportion of households that were owner-occupied | Highest vs. lowest quintile, by age group<br>0–4<br>5–9<br>10–14 | 0.93–1.32[d]<br>1.16–1.38[d]<br>1.04–1.57[d] | Draper et al., 1991a |
| England and Wales, 1966–83[c] | I, 14 | 1164 | Socioeconomic score derived in similar way to that of Draper et al. (1991a), but analysed by census tract rather than by district | Highest vs. lowest quintile by age group<br>0–4<br>5–14 | 1.21, 1.16[f]<br>1.04, 1.71[f] | Rodrigues et al., 1991 |

**Hodgkin's disease**

| Location, period | | No. | Variable | Comparison | Value | Reference |
|---|---|---|---|---|---|---|
| England and Wales, 22 counties, 1984–88 | I, 24 | 4869[j] | Socioeconomic index for electoral wards as in Alexander et al. (1990d) | High vs. low | 1.22[k] | Alexander et al., 1991c |
| England, West Midlands, 1972–86 | I, 14 | 83 (77%) | Father's occupation at time of child's diagnosis | % of cases in social classes I and II vs. % of West Midlands population in social classes I and II | 0.76 | Parkes et al., 1994 |

## Table 2.3. (contd) Summary of descriptive studies of childhood cancer and socioeconomic status

| Area and period of study | Cases (I) incident, (D) dead, Upper age limit | Total number of cases (% with information on socioeconomic status) | Indicator of socioeconomic status | Contrast | Ratio | References |
|---|---|---|---|---|---|---|
| **Non-Hodgkin and unspecified lymphomas** | | | | | | |
| Britain, 1969–83[c] | I, 14 | 1161 | Socioeconomic score for districts, based on information from 1971 and 1981 censuses on proportion of economically active men working proportion of households with a car, and proportion of households that were owner-occupied | Highest vs. lowest quintile, by age group<br>0–4<br>5–9<br>10–14 | 0.65–2.88[d]<br>0.78–1.39[d]<br>0.85–1.36[d] | Draper et al., 1991a |
| England and Wales, 1966–83[c] | I, 14 | 1273 | Socioeconomic score derived in similar way to that of Draper et al. (1991a), but analysed by census tract rather than by district | Highest vs. lowest quintile, by age group<br>0–4<br>5–14 | 0.98, 1.50[f]<br>1.22, 0.98[f] | Rodrigues et al., 1991 |
| **Central nervous system tumours** | | | | | | |
| England and Wales, 1959–63 and 1970–72 | D, 14 | 1661 (1959–63)<br>760 (1970–72) | Occupation of father as recorded on child's death certificate | Administrators, managers, professional, technical workers and artists vs. all occupations, by period of death<br>1959–63<br>1970–72 | 152[b]<br>136[b] | Sanders et al., 1981 |
| Scotland, 1975–90 | I, 14 | 494 | Socioeconomic score for postcode sectors based on households with no car, male unemployment, households of low social class and household overcrowding, as recorded in 1981 census | Quintile 1 (least deprived) vs. quintile 5 (most deprived) | 1.37 | McKinney et al., 1994 |
| **Neuroblastoma** | | | | | | |
| Denmark, 1946–80[f] | I, 14 | 246 | Socioeconomic group of head of family | Self-employed vs. manual workers | 0.65 | Carlsen, 1986 |
| USA, multicentre (SEER), 1973–78 | I, all ages[m] | 264 | a) Per capita income of county of residence<br>b) Proportion of families below 125% of poverty level in county of residence | $5500 vs. <$3500 per annum<br><br><10% vs. 20%+ | 0.66<br><br>0.90 | Davis et al., 1987 |
| Denmark, 1943–72[f] | I, 14 | 189 | Socioeconomic group of head of family | Self-employed vs. manual workers, by age group<br><1 year<br>1–14 years | 0.59<br>0.74 | Carlsen, 1996 |
| **Renal tumours** | | | | | | |
| England and Wales, 1959–63 and 1970–72 | D, 14 | 270 (1959–63)<br>128 (1970–72) | Occupation of father as recorded on child's death certificate | Administrators, managers, professional, technical workers and artists vs. all occupations, by period of death<br>1959–63<br>1970–72 | 116[b]<br>108[b] | Sanders et al., 1981 |

[a] No figures reported, but paper states that no differences were found.
[b] Proportional mortality ratio.
[c] Studies overlap.
[d] Range for three periods 1969–73, 1974–78, 1979–83.
[e] ALL plus unspecified leukaemia.
[f] Urban, rural.
[g] Leukaemia and non-Hodgkin lymphoma, white children only.
[h] Studies overlap.
[i] Children diagnosed at member institutions of Children's Cancer Group and Pediatric Oncology Group.
[j] 16% of cases aged 14 years (Cartwright et al., 1990).
[k] Adjusted for urban–rural status and distance to built-up area.
[l] Studies overlap.
[m] 88% of cases were aged <15 years at diagnosis.

in rates of lymphocytic and unspecified leukaemia between counties were detected during 1974–78, with the effect mainly evident in the 0–4 age group. While there were substantial differences in the average levels of the socioeconomic variables between counties, it was not possible to determine whether the primary effect was related to county or to socioeconomic differences, although the 'county effect' could not be explained by the socioeconomic variables considered. County districts in England and Wales were also classified into 'predominantly urban' and 'predominantly rural'; these data were not available for Scotland. In general, the rates of lymphocytic and unspecified leukaemias in rural districts were a little higher than those in urban districts, but the difference was statistically significant only for the 5–9-year age group and the effect became less marked after adjustment for socioeconomic status. As the numbers of cases and the populations in the lowest socioeconomic groups in rural districts were very small, it was not possible to determine whether the association with socioeconomic status was confined to urban areas.

Rodrigues *et al.* (1991) undertook a similar analysis at the level of the census tract in England and Wales. A socioeconomic score for the census tract was calculated in a similar way to that derived by Draper *et al.* (1991a) for county districts. The urban or rural classification of the district in which the census tract was located was used, because no urban/rural classification is available for individual census tracts. The age groups 0–4 and 5–14 years were considered. There was a clear trend of increasing incidence of lymphocytic and unspecified leukaemia with higher socioeconomic status of the census tract. This was more marked in the younger age group. There was no clear trend for ANLL. The trend for lymphocytic and unspecified leukaemias was statistically significant for each age group when urban and rural districts were combined, and for urban districts alone. In rural areas, a significant trend was apparent in the older but not in the younger age group, although higher rates were seen in the highest three quintiles compared with· the lowest two. The overall rate of lymphocytic and unspecified leukaemia was higher in rural census tracts than in urban ones, but the differences were not consistent across quintiles of socioeconomic status and were not statistically significant.

Draper and Elliott (1991) observed that since these analyses were ecological, it is possible that the true differences in incidence between different social classes were greater for

individuals than was apparent for areas. On the other hand, it may be that the differences in rates reflect some characteristics of the areas and of the populations living in them, rather than differences between individuals. Alexander *et al.* (1990d) analysed childhood ALL diagnosed in 1984–88 in the 22 counties of England and Wales which contribute data to the Leukaemia Research Fund Data Collection Survey. The effect of socioeconomic status disappeared when combined in an analysis with urban/rural status, settlement classification and distance from a built-up area. However, the classifications were highly intercorrelated, with the majority of wards in the group furthest from a built-up area being both of higher socioeconomic status and classified as villages or towns.

## Time trends

Temporal trends have been more thoroughly investigated for leukaemia than for any other tumour of childhood. Draper *et al.* (1994) summarized the reports which had been published up to 1992. These reports and several recent updates and new analyses are presented in Table 2.4. The findings are difficult to interpret. The studies covered varying time periods and different methods of analysis were used. Some investigators analysed the 0–14 age group as a whole, while others examined trends in specific age groups. In addition, some reported trends for each sex, while others reported both sexes combined. Some of the studies considered only all leukaemias together while others considered the main sub-types separately. In addition, the comments earlier in this section regarding variations in the completeness of registration of leukaemias, problems of miscoding and misclassification and the relationship between leukaemia and non-Hodgkin lymphoma should be borne in mind. In particular, diagnostic improvements have undoubtedly led to more accurate and precise classification of leukaemias over time, which has the potential to produce artefactual changes in the incidence of particular sub-types. For example, it has been shown that the reported increase of ALL between 1973 and 1987 in the populations covered by the SEER registries in the USA (National Cancer Institute, 1990) could be largely accounted for by changes in diagnostic practice and the consequent decrease over time in the proportion of cases of 'acute leukaemia, not otherwise specified' (Miller, 1992).

Of the seven analyses which considered all leukaemias or all acute leukaemia together, six found no evidence of any increase in incidence

## Table 2.4. Temporal trends in the incidence of childhood leukaemia

| Country and area | Data source | Time period | Average number of leukaemia cases per annum, 0–14 years | Main results | Reference |
|---|---|---|---|---|---|
| **Asia** | | | | | |
| Japan, Hokkaido Prefecture | Registry of childhood malignancies | 1969–93 | 43 | Total leukaemia increased by 18% from 1979–83 to 1984–88 then fell slightly during 1989–93; increase due to ALL; rates of ANLL and other leukaemias unchanged; no statistical comparisons made; data prior to 1980 incomplete | Nishi et al., 1996 |
| Japan, Osaka Prefecture | Osaka Cancer Registry | 1971–88 | 73 { 43 ALL, 17 ANLL, 13 other and unspecified leukaemia } | Incidence of leukaemia rose by 18% from 1971–80 to 1981–88; incidence of ALL rose in both sexes, significantly so for boys; ANLL fell in both sexes, significantly for boys; other and unspecified leukaemias unchanged | Ajiki et al., 1994 |
| Europe | 36 cancer registries in 23 countries | 1980–91 | 1980 | +0.6% annual change in leukaemia incidence during 1980–86; +0.4% in 1987–91; rise most evident in 1–4-year age group but annual change by age not reported; ALL not considered separately | Parkin et al., 1996 |
| Denmark | Danish Cancer Registry | 1943–84 | 49 | No change in incidence from 1943–63 to 1964–84; ALL not considered separately | de Nully Brown et al., 1989 |
| Finland | Finnish Cancer Registry | 1966–80 | 48[a] | Incidence of acute leukaemia in boys fell over 1966–70, 1971–75 and 1976–80; no consistent trend for girls; ALL not considered separately | Hakulinen et al., 1986 |
| Germany, former West | Registry of childhood malignancies, population and hospital-based | 1980–92 | 451 | Annual incidence of leukaemia steady over 1980 to 1992; ALL not reported separately; registry completeness estimated to be 80% in 1980–84 and 95% thereafter | Kaatsch et al., 1995 |
| Greece | Search of hospital archives by network of childhood oncologists | 1980–91 | 81 | No change in crude incidence rate over time; ALL not considered separately | Petridou et al., 1994 |
| Italy, Turin Province | Registry of Childhood Cancer | 1967–86 | 22 { 14 ALL, 3 ANLL, 5 other and unspecified leukaemia } | No change in total leukaemia over 1967–69, 70–75, 76–81 and 82–86; incidence of ALL rose from 1970–75 to 1976–81 and more modestly in 1982–86 but trend not significant; ANLL remained stable; other and unspecified leukaemia fell substantially; significant decrease in leukaemia in infants but based on 26 cases over 20 years | Mosso et al., 1992 |
| Netherlands | Dutch Childhood Leukaemia Study Group | 1973–86 | 111 { 90 ALL, 14 ANLL, 3 CML, 3 acute unclassifiable leukaemia } | Temporary increase of ALL during 1979–84, returning to previous level in 1985–86; rates in 1979–84 26% higher than in 1973–78; increase only evident in 1–4-year age group and not significant; possible cohort effect; incidence of ANLL and other leukaemias constant | Coebergh et al., 1989 |
| Netherlands, south-east | Eindhoven Cancer Registry | 1958–92 | 8[b] | Incidence of ALL doubled from 1958–72 to 1973–82 and remained stable in 1983–92; no trends in ANLL or other leukaemias; no statistical comparisons made; registrations before 1973 believed to be less complete than later data | Coebergh et al., 1995 |

| Location | Source | Period | Numbers | Findings | Reference |
|---|---|---|---|---|---|
| Norway | Norwegian Cancer Registry | 1953–80 | 35[b] | No consistent trends in acute leukaemia incidence in boys or girls; ALL not considered separately | Hakulinen *et al.*, 1986 |
| Sweden | Swedish Cancer Registry | 1958–80 | 65[c] | Incidence of acute leukaemia for boys at least 20% higher in 1966–70, 1971–75 and 1976–80 than in 1958–60 and 1961–65; for girls, incidence substantially higher in 1976–80 than either periods; suggestion of rising rates for both sexes in children aged 1–4 years; no formal statistical comparison made; ALL not considered separately | Hakulinen *et al.*, 1986 |
| UK, England, Wales and Scotland | National Registry of Childhood Tumours | 1953–91 | 430 { 343 ALL[d], 80 ANLL | Significant increases in ALL in both sexes over time; most pronounced in 1–4-year age group; rates in boys rose by 1.2% per annum; rates in girls rose by 1.1% per annum; increasing risk of ALL in cohorts born until 1974; significantly falling incidence of ANLL in both sexes for the 5–9 and 10–14-year age groups; registry ascertainment improved over time | Draper *et al.*, 1994 |
| UK, north-west England | Manchester Children's Tumour Registry | 1954–88 | 32 { 25 ALL, 6 ANLL, 0.6 CML | Significant linear trend in ALL consistent with 4% increase per quinquennium; incidence steady over 1954–58, 1959–63 and 1964–68, increased during 1969–73, 1974–78 and 1979–83 and fell during 1984–88; no significant variation in ALL trend by age or sex; significant linear trend in CML | Blair & Birch, 1994a |
| UK, Scotland | Scottish Cancer Registry | 1975–94 | 41 { 33 ALL, 6 ANLL, 2 other and unspecified leukaemia | Significant increase in ALL of 1.9% per annum; evident in both sexes; rates of all other leukaemias combined decreased but could not account for rise in ALL; data rigorously validated for completeness and diagnostic accuracy | McKinney (personal communication) |
| **North America** Canada, Saskatchewan | Cancer Registry of Saskatchewan | 1932–91 | 8 { 6 ALL, 1 ANLL | Increasing incidence of ALL in both sexes since 1930s; rate of increase has attenuated since 1971; compared with children born in 1944–48, relative risk of ALL to age 9 years increased with each successive birth cohort until 1969–73 and has been stable since then; ANLL incidence rose from 1942–51 to 1962–71 for boys and from 1942–51 to 1972–81 for girls aged 0–19 years | Wang & Haines, 1995 |
| USA, Baltimore Metropolitan Area | Review of hospital discharge records, hospital tumour registers, pathology and haematology files and death certificates | 1960–74 | 19 acute leukaemias[e] { 15 ALL, 4 ANLL | Incidence of ALL unchanged over time; significant rise in ANLL in black children based on 3 cases in 1960–64, 3 in 1965–69 and 12 in 1970–74 | Gordis *et al.*, 1981 |
| US, Connecticut | Connecticut Tumour Registry | 1935–79 | 25 { 18 ALL, 7 other leukaemias | Significant increases of ALL in 0–4 and 5–9-year age groups, particularly for boys; decreases in incidence of other leukaemias in all age groups; for girls increase in ALL is counter balanced by decrease in other leukaemias; for boys increase in ALL exceeds decrease in other leukaemias | van Hoff *et al.*, 1988 |
| USA, Greater Delaware Valley | Greater Delaware Valley Paediatric Tumour Registry | 1970–89 | 70 { 54 ALL, 12 acute myelocytic leukaemia (AML) | No significant trends in incidence of ALL or AML over time; no trend in ALL combined with leukaemias classified in non-specific categories; non-specific leukaemias decreased significantly by 10.9% per annum | Bunin *et al.*, 1996 |

## Table 2.4. (contd) Temporal trends in the incidence of childhood leukaemia

| Country and area | Data source | Time period | Average number of leukaemia cases per annum, 0–14 years | Main results | Reference |
|---|---|---|---|---|---|
| USA | Nine cancer registries of the Surveillance, Epidemiology and End Results Program (SEER) | 1974–91 | 207 { 159 ALL, 30 AML, 18 other leukaemias | ALL increased significantly by 1.4% per annum in boys and 1.6% per annum in girls aged 0–14 years; increase evident under 10 years and most pronounced in children under 2; AML rose, non-significantly, by 6.1% per annum; striking decreasing trend in other leukaemias, particularly non-specific acute leukaemias in children aged less than 5 years | Gurney et al., 1996a |
| USA, Upstate New York | New York State Cancer Registry | 1969–80 | 109 | No significant changes in leukaemia incidence over time, by age or sex; ALL not considered separately | Polednak, 1986 |
| **Oceania**<br>Australia | Australian Paediatric Cancer Registry | 1982–91 | 175 { 138 ALL, 29 ANLL, 5 CML, 3 other and unspecified leukaemia | Significant increase in incidence of ANLL | McWhirter et al., 1996 |
| Australia, New South Wales | New South Wales Cancer Registry | 1973–89 | 60 | Significant rise in incidence of ALL in boys from 1973–77 to 1978–82 followed by a decline in 1983–87 and 1988–89; no trend in girls | McCredie et al., 1992 |
| Australia, Queensland | Queensland Childhood Malignancy Register | 1973–88 | 19 ALL[g], 3 ANLL[g] | No significant linear trend in ALL; significant increase in ANLL based on an average of 3 cases per annum | McWhirter & Petroeschevsky, 1991 |
| Australia, Victoria | Victorian Cancer Registry | 1971–89 | 40 { 33 ALL, 6 ANLL, 1 other and unspecified leukaemia | Incidence of ALL rose by 5% for boys and 10% for girls between 1970–79 and 1980–89; ANLL increased in boys and fell in girls; no statistical comparisons made; cancer registration became mandatory in 1981–82 | Giles et al., 1995 |
| New Zealand | New Zealand Cancer Registry | 1948–90 | 37[h] { 27 ALL, 8 ANLL, 2 other and unspecified leukaemia | Significant increase in total leukaemia in 0–4-year age group over 1953–70 to 1988–90; during 1973–77 and 1988–90 this trend due to rise in ALL in under 5s; no trends in ALL incidence in 5–9 or 10–14 age groups; significant decrease in ANLL over 1968–72 and 1988–90, averaging –3.8% per annum; time trends restricted to 1953–90 as earlier data incomplete; data could not be dis-aggregated by sub-type prior to 1968 | Dockerty et al., 1996 |

[a] Average over 1953–70 from data reported in Teppo et al. (1975).
[b] Average over 1978–82 from data reported in Muir et al. (1987).
[c] Average over 1958–74 from data reported in Ericsson et al. (1978).
[d] Includes unspecified leukaemia.

[e] 0–19 years.
[f] Includes acute stem cell/undifferentiated/not otherwise specified leukaemias.
[g] 0–12 years.
[h] Average over 1968–90.

over time. The other study, which collected data from 36 cancer registries in 23 European countries in order to investigate temporal trends in leukaemia following the accident at the Chernobyl nuclear reactor in 1986, found that the age-standardized incidence of leukaemia increased modestly during the 1980s (Parkin *et al.*, 1996). The rate rose by 0.6% per annum in the period 1980–86 and 0.4% in the period 1987–91. The rise appeared to be most evident in children aged 1–4 years, but rates of change by age group were not reported.

The remaining 19 studies analysed the main sub-types separately. Of these, four studies (two in the USA and two in Australia) found no evidence of any change in the incidence of ALL over time (Gordis *et al.*, 1981; McWhirter & Petroeschevsky, 1991; Bunin *et al.*, 1996; McWhirter *et al.*, 1996). However, the most recent US study observed a significant decrease in the incidence of non-specific leukaemias over time (Bunin *et al.*, 1996) and the two Australian studies found that ANLL had decreased significantly (McWhirter & Petroeschevsky, 1991; McWhirter *et al.*, 1996). The 15 remaining analyses found some evidence of at least a temporary increase in the incidence of ALL over time. The rise was observed most commonly among children under five years and appears to have been fairly modest; several reports are consistent with an increase of around 1% per annum. Formal statistical tests were not undertaken in all studies. In those studies where tests were conducted, the increases were not always statistically significant (e.g., Coebergh *et al.*, 1989; Mosso *et al.*, 1992). In most of the reports, the rise in ALL was accompanied by declining rates of ANLL or other leukaemias (van Hoff *et al.*, 1988; Mosso *et al.*, 1992; Ajiki *et al.*, 1994; Blair & Birch, 1994a; Draper *et al.*, 1994; Dockerty *et al.*, 1996; Gurney *et al.*, 1996a; McKinney (personal communication)). Although the rise in ALL must be due in part to diagnostic shifts and more accurate and precise classification, it is not clear how much of the increase can be explained by these factors. In Connecticut, USA, it was reported that the increase in ALL in boys could not be completely accounted for by the decrease in the other leukaemias (van Hoff *et al.*, 1988). In Scotland, the records of the cancer registry were matched with data from other sources to maximize case ascertainment and cases were subject to panel review of diagnosis; in this series also, the increase in ALL could not be explained entirely by the decrease in other types of leukaemia (McKinney, personal communication).

Four reports described an increase in the incidence of ALL in the late 1970s and early 1980s followed by a fall in later years (Coebergh *et al.*, 1989; McCredie *et al.*, 1992; Blair & Birch, 1994a; Nishi *et al.*, 1996). This could be consistent with a cohort effect. In Saskatchewan, Canada, the relative risk of ALL up to age 9, compared with children born in 1944–48, increased with each successive five-year birth cohort until 1969–73 and remained stable thereafter (Wang & Haines, 1995). In a much larger analysis for England, Wales and Scotland, Stiller and Draper (1982) reported an increasing incidence of ALL in children born after about 1964 which was most evident among boys aged 0–4 years. An update of this analysis, which considered ALL plus unspecified leukaemia diagnosed in children born from 1953, confirmed that the most pronounced increase occurred in the under five-year age group, but suggested that this increase did not continue for children born after 1974 (Draper *et al.*, 1994).

## Clustering of leukaemia in space and time

Most of the work on the clustering of childhood cancer has related specifically to leukaemia. Many anecdotal reports are available (Heath, 1988; Alexander, 1993), perhaps the most dramatic of which is the report of eight cases of childhood leukaemia in Niles, Illinois, in a four-year period in a population of about 20 000, nearly five times as many as would have been expected on the basis of the incidence in other parts of the same state (Heath & Hasterlik, 1963). A survey of residents of the parish regarding family church affiliation, school attendance and the recent occurrence of common childhood illness suggested that there were differences in the occurrence of common childhood illnesses such as measles and chicken pox between families of cases with leukaemia and other families. It is noteworthy that the observation of a cluster of cases coincided with a striking growth in the population of the area, and the authors observed that expansion of this community may have been accompanied by abrupt changes in patterns of disease.

Interest in a possible infectious etiology for childhood leukaemia in particular led to developments in statistical methods for the identification of temporo-spatial clustering (Ederer *et al.*, 1964; Knox, 1964; Mantel, 1967). The Knox, Ederer–Myers–Mantel and Mantel methods of detecting spatio-temporal clustering were shown to have low statistical power in the analysis of a simulated data-set relating to Hodgkin's disease in childhood (Chen *et al.*, 1984).

A substantial number of studies were published in the 1960s and early 1970s. Smith (1982) and Linet (1985) reviewed investigations of temporo-spatial clustering of leukaemia and the statistical methods used in these studies. Table 2.5 summarizes the studies on childhood leukaemia included in these reviews, together with more recent studies in Greece (Petridou *et al.*, 1996a), the Netherlands (Van Steensel-Moll *et al.*, 1983), and Britain (Morris, 1990; Gilman & Knox, 1991, 1995).

Of 24 studies, 15 were interpreted by the authors as showing some evidence of clustering. The methods used in most of these studies require arbitrary definitions of closeness in space and time. Therefore, multiple testing was a feature of most of these analyses and the possibility that findings of clustering are no more than would be expected by chance cannot unequivocally be excluded (Alexander, 1993). In a study in Greece, the results of previous investigations were used to define the units of space (5 km) and time (1 year) for which to investigate space–time clustering (Petridou *et al.*, 1996a). For childhood leukaemia in Greece as a whole, the observed number of pairs that were close in space and time exceeded the expected number by 5.2% ($p = 0.004$). This was accounted for by leukaemia diagnosed at under five years of age, for which the observed number of pairs close in space and time exceeded the expected number by 9.4% ($p = 0.004$). There was no evidence of space–time clustering for leukaemia diagnosed at ages of five or more.

It might be expected that clustering would be detected more easily in sparsely populated areas than elsewhere. However, positive reports of clustering include studies in highly urbanized areas such as Liverpool, Greater London, Buffalo City, San Francisco and Metropolitan Atlanta. Petridou *et al.* (1996a) investigated clustering in urban (10 000 or more inhabitants), semi-urban (2000–9999 inhabitants) and rural (less than 2000 inhabitants) areas of Greece. The clustering apparent at all ages and in the 0–4-year age group in the country as a whole was mainly accounted for by the pattern in urban areas. This was especially marked for ALL diagnosed at 2–4 years of age. In rural areas, for leukaemia diagnosed at any age, the observed number of pairs close in space and time exceeded that expected by 27% ($p = 0.13$). In exploratory analysis, this was found to be concentrated in children aged 4–11 years. Thus,

clustering in rural areas appeared to involve cases over a broader and older age range than in urban areas. This would be compatible with a delay in the development of herd immunity against a putative infectious agent involved in the causation of childhood leukaemia (see Chapter 7).

Knox and Gilman (1992a), in a further analysis of the data of Gilman and Knox (1991) relating to leukaemia and lymphoma, observed that the space–time interactions they detected showed geographical heterogeneities. There appeared to be a strong concentration along a corridor stretching from the conurbations of north-west England, through the industrial Midlands, towards the south-east. Standardization for population density made little difference to this pattern. The authors noted that if the critical distance for identifying interaction pairs varied between areas of different population densities, as would be likely if an infectious disease were involved in the etiology of leukaemia, the phenomenon of space–time clustering might be obscured when data from areas of different population density were pooled. There was some evidence of heterogeneity of critical distance; in the densely populated central corridor, the most significant interactions were at 0.1 km and 35 days and at 0.1 km and 10 days, whereas in the north-east region, the most significant interaction was within 0.3 km and 25 days.

In an analysis of deaths due to leukaemia and lymphoma in Great Britain during the period 1953–80, clustering was apparent both by date and place of birth, and date and place of diagnosis (Gilman & Knox, 1995). The clustering by date and place of birth was significant among pairs with different ages at diagnosis, suggesting that the latent period is variable. The clustering by date and place of diagnosis was apparent in pairs comprising children in different age groups (those aged 0–4 years and those aged five or more) as well as in pairs comprising children from the same age groups. Therefore, the clustering by date and place of diagnosis did not appear to be secondary to the birth clustering. The two types of clustering comprised many independent pairs of cases, with little sharing of cases between different pairs. There were no clusters comprising a large number of cases. A limitation of this study is that data on leukaemia mortality may be inappropriate when considered over a time period when survival improved markedly (for further comment, see Chapter 6).

# Table 2.5. Summary of studies of clustering of childhood leukaemia in time and space

| Study population, period of study | Age range/subgroup | Source of ascertainment[a] | Method used | Critical spaces (s) and times (t) | Number of cases | Time frame | Results | Reference |
|---|---|---|---|---|---|---|---|---|
| Czechoslovakia, S. Moravia 1960–68 | 0–15 | | Knox, Pinkel & Nefzger | s: various, t: various | 104 | Diagnosis | Significant excess for distances of 0–12 km and both 0–1 and 0–2 year intervals | Zahalkova et al., 1970 |
| Greece, 1980–89 | 0–14, 0–4, 5–14 | HR | Knox | s: 5 km, t: 1 year | 872, 446, 426 | Diagnosis | Significant clustering / Significant clustering / No clustering | Petridou et al., 1996a |
| The Netherlands 1973–80 | 0–14 | CR | Knox, Mantel | s: 2, 4, 6, 8, 10 km; t: 2, 4, 6, 8, 10, 12 months | 293 | Diagnosis | No significant space–time clustering for total leukaemia, ALL, ALL by sex, or ALL in children aged 0–5 at diagnosis | Van Steensel-Moll et al., 1983 |
| New Zealand 1953–64 | 0–14, 0–5 | DC | Knox | Coordinates to nearest mile; s-t: (a) <1 mile and <2 months; (b) <1 mile and <3 months; (c) <5 miles and <3 months; (d) <10 miles and <6 months. | 288, 159 | Onset | No significant clustering / Significant clusters for combinations (a) and (b) | Gunz & Spears, 1968 |
| | 0–14, 0–5, 2–9 | DC | Knox, Mantel | s: 0.5, 1, 2, 3, 5 miles; t: 0.5, 1, 2, 3, 6 months | 288, 160, 202 | Onset | Significant clustering when s ≤1 mile and t ≤1 month / Strongest evidence of clustering / Weakest clustering | Glass et al., 1971 |
| UK, Northumberland and Durham, 1951–60 | 0–14, 0–5 | H,CR,DC | Knox / Barton et al. | Not specified | 185, 96 | Onset | No clustering for total leukaemia, AML or ALL / Excess for a range of times and distances up to about 2 months and 2 km / No clustering | Knox, 1964 / Barton et al., 1965 |
| UK, Liverpool, 1955–64 | 0–14 | H,DC | Knox | s: 2, 3, 4, 5, 8 km; t: 50–400 days, in steps of 50 days, and 1000 days | 74 | Onset | Significant clustering when s < 4 km and t < 300 days | Mainwaring, 1966 |
| UK, Lewisham 1957–63 | 0–14 | H,CR,DC | Barton & David, Knox | Not specified | NS[b] | Onset | No clustering | Lock & Merrington, 1967 |
| UK, Greater London 1952–61[c] | 0–5, 0–14 | DC | Knox | s: 0.25–2 km in steps of 0.25 km, 2.5, 3.0, 3.5, 4.0 km; t: 15–180 days in steps of 15 days | 292, 444 | Birth, Onset | Weak evidence of clustering of lymphoblastic leukaemia (n = 232) / Weak evidence of clustering of lymphoblastic leukaemia | Till et al., 1967 |
| UK, Greater London,[c] 1952–59 | 0–5 | DC | Pike & Smith | s: 0.25–2 km in steps of 0.25 km, 2.5, 3.0, 3.5, 4.0 km; t: 15–180 days in steps of 15 days | 172 | Birth | There were four significant results among the 144 combinations of space and time examined | Smith et al., 1976 |
| 1961–64 | | | | | 81 | Birth | No clustering | |

## Table 2.5. (contd) Summary of studies of clustering of childhood leukaemia in time and space

| Study population, period of study | Age range/subgroup | Source of ascertainment[a] | Method used | Critical spaces (s) and times (t) | Number of cases | Time frame | Results | Reference |
|---|---|---|---|---|---|---|---|---|
| UK, Worcestershire, Warwickshire, Staffordshire, Shropshire, 1953–60 | 0–9 | CR | Knox | Not specified | 228<br>162 | Onset<br>Birth | Excess when $s = 0.5$ km and $t = 15$ months<br>Excess when $s = 2$ km and $t = 248$ days | Morris, 1990 |
| UK, England, Scotland and Wales 1966–83 | 0–14<br>0–4<br><br>5–14<br>Lymphocytic<br><br>ANLL | CR | Mantel | s: 1 2, 3, 4, 5, 10, 20 km<br>t: 0–6 months in steps of 1 month, 9, 12, 18, 24 and 48 months | 7565 | Anniversary date | Excess when $s = 1$ km and $t \leq 3$ months<br>Excesses when $s \leq 10$ km and $t \leq 2$ months<br>No clustering<br>Large excess in same month and with $s <1$ km<br>Excesses when $s \leq 3$ km and $t \leq 6$ months | Gilman & Knox, 1991 |
| UK, England Scotland and Wales, 1953–80 | 0–15 | OSCC (deaths) | Knox | s: 1, 2, 3, 4, 5, 10, 20 km<br>t: 0, 1, 2, 3, 4, 5, 6, 9,12, 18 24, 48 months | 2478<br>6511<br>7316 | Birth<br>Diagnosis<br>Death | Excess particularly apparent for those born within 1 km and up to five months apart<br>Excess when $s \leq$ km and $t \leq 9$ months<br>No clustering | Gilman & Knox, 1995 |
| USA, Erie County, Buffalo City, 1943–56 | 0–15 | CR | Combinatorial analysis | s 1/3 mile<br>t: 2 years | 95 | Diagnosis or death | No significant clustering, but statistical technique used was inappropriate (Ederer et al., 1964) | Pinkel & Nefzger, 1959 |
| | | | Ridit analysis | s: 1/8 mile–1 mile in steps of 1/8 mile, >1 mile<br>t: time between cases to nearest year | | | Significant clustering when cases <1/8 mile apart | Pinkel et al., 1963 |
| USA, Connecticut 1945–59 | 0–14 | CR | Ederer et al. | s: town (n = 169)<br>t: 1 or 2 years | 333 | Diagnosis | No clustering | Ederer et al., 1964 |
| USA, Oregon, Portland area, 1950–61 | 0–14 | H, DC | Knox | s: 1, 2, 4, 8 km<br>t: 50–350 days in steps of 50 days, 1 year | 69 | Onset | Significant excesses of pairs of cases (a) closer than 1 km and 365 days apart and (b) closer than 5 km and 250 days apart | Meighan & Knox, 1965 |
| USA, New York State, 1943–62 | 0–4<br>0–14 | CR | Ederer et al. | s: city or town (n = 417)<br>t: 1 or 2 years | 616<br>1640 | Birth<br>Year of report | No clustering<br>Clustering for one-year periods in each of four quinquennia | Fraumeni et al., 1966 |
| USA, Michigan 1950–64 | 0–1<br>0–5 | DC | Mantel | s: county<br>t: month, season | 77<br>375 | Birth | No clustering | Stark & Mantel, 1967 |

| Location, period | Age | Source | Test | No. | Space (s) / time (t) | Time basis | Result | Reference |
|---|---|---|---|---|---|---|---|---|
| USA, Los Angeles County, 1960–64 | 0–14 | DC | Ederer et al. | 298 | s: 32 regions each including about 40 census tracts<br>t: 1 year | Death | No clustering | Glass et al., 1968 |
|  | 0–5, 2–5 |  | { Knox, Mantel | 155, 205 | s: 0.5, 1, 1.6, 2.2, 4.4, 6.6, 8.8, 13.2 km<br>t: 0.5, 1, 2, 4, 6, 12 months |  | No clustering | Glass & Mantel, 1969 |
| USA, California 1958–60 | 0–4 | DC,CR | Mantel | 234 | s: hospital of birth<br>t: reciprocal transformation of time difference + 1, 3, 5, 15 or 30 days | Birth | No significant clustering | Klauber, 1968 |
| USA, Ohio, Cuyahoga County, 1955–65 | 0–14 | H | Knox | 168 | s: 2, 4 km<br>t: 60, 90 days | Onset | No clustering | Browning & Gross, 1968 |
| USA, Connecticut, 1935–63 | 0–14 | CR | Permutational test developed by authors | NS[d] | s: town (n=169) | Onset | No clustering | Bailar et al., 1970 |
| USA, San Francisco 1946–65 | 0–14 | H, DC | Mantel | 149 | s: feet (nearest 100) between cases<br>t: 0.5, 1, 2, 4, 12 months | Diagnosis | No significant clustering | Klauber & Mustacchi, 1970 |
|  | 2–14 |  |  |  |  |  | Significant clustering for 12-month interval only |  |
| USA, Georgia (2 counties in metropolitan Atlanta area) 1956–68 | 0–14 (Acute) | CR | $\chi^2$ | 100 | s: census tracts<br>t: 2 years or 3 years | Onset | Significant clustering observed | Evatt et al., 1973 |
| USA, Metropolitan Atlanta 1956–69 | 0–14 (ALL) | CR | Combinatorial test developed by authors | 164 | s: census tracts<br>t: 6 months | Diagnosis | Significant clustering | Larsen et al., 1973 |

NS, Not stated.

[a] CR, cancer registration; DC, death certificates; H, hospital records; OSCC, Oxford Survey of Childhood Cancer.
[b] There was a total of 115 cases with leukaemia aged 2–89 years. Eighteen cases had acute lymphatic leukaemia.
[c] Note: studies of Till et al. (1967) and Smith et al. (1976) overlap.
[d] A total of 4582 cases of leukaemia was reported; the number in children was not specified..
[e] Onset 1952–60.
[f] Restricted to those aged 10 years or less when symptoms first appeared..

## Spatial clustering of leukaemia: no prior hypotheses about sources of putative hazard

Much concern about localized excesses of childhood cancer has arisen in relation to proximity to environmental sources, such as nuclear installations (see Chapter 4). This concern has been a stimulus for the development of statistical methods for investigation of spatial clustering. In addition, the analysis of spatial clustering is more appropriate than the analysis of space–time clustering if infectious agents associated with prolonged and variable latent periods were of etiological importance (Alexander, 1993). Much of the development work has been done in Britain, because of the availability of data for small areas and because of concern about apparent excesses around nuclear sites in Britain.

### — Methods of analysing spatial clustering

Methods of analysing spatial clustering can be grouped into three categories: (i) methods based on cell counts; (ii) methods based on detecting adjacencies of cells with high counts; (iii) distance methods (Cuzick & Edwards, 1990; Little & Elwood, 1992a).

In methods based on cell counts, a grid is placed over a map of the region of interest, and the number of cases in each unit of the grid is counted. The null hypothesis is that the occurrence of cases follows a Poisson distribution. The method does not take into account the distribution of cases in neighbouring cells, which leads to loss of power when cases are rare. An example of such an approach is the ISD method (named after the Information & Statistics Division of the National Health Service in Scotland, where the method was developed; Heasman *et al.*, 1987; COMARE, 1988; Black *et al.*, 1996). Another example is the Potthoff–Whittinghill test, developed for the situation where the units of area are heterogeneous in terms both of population and of geographical size, so that classical methods of testing the goodness of fit of the Poisson distribution are inappropriate (Potthoff & Whittinghill, 1966a,b). These methods aim to provide information on whether the overall distribution of the disease shows clusters and as to the nature of any clustering identified.

The second approach involves the examination of adjacencies of cells with counts at or above a specified level of significance, or observed-to-expected ratio (Barnes *et al.*, 1987). Thus, the method is a test for between-area clustering.

The third approach is based on the consideration of distances between pairs of cases, usually only those between nearest neighbours. It is assumed that, in the absence of clustering, the spatial distribution of cases is uniform. This is not a satisfactory assumption for the denominator population, and methods have been proposed to allow for the non-uniform distribution of the denominator population. With regard to developmental work related to childhood leukaemia and lymphoma, most investigators have taken the non-uniform distribution of the denominator population into account by defining circles of fixed geographical size (the geographical analysis machine of Openshaw *et al.* (1988)), of fixed weighted sums of the numbers of observed and numbers of expected cases (two sample test of Cuzick and Edwards (1990)), of fixed expected numbers of cases (one sample test of Cuzick and Edwards (1990)) or of fixed numbers of observed cases (Besag & Newell, 1991). The probability that each circle is the centre of a cluster is then evaluated. All of these methods aim to provide information on the location of clusters. The geographical analysis machine (GAM) (Openshaw *et al.*, 1988) searches a geographical region for clusters by applying multiple overlapping circles of varying radii on a grid sufficiently fine that a circle can overlap each of its neighbours by 80%. The test described by Besag and Newell (1991) has the same basic aim as the GAM, but may have a more acceptable statistical basis, and is computationally less demanding. Nearest neighbour methods, of which the local nearest neighbour area test is an example, involve measuring the distance from each case $c$ to the nearest (or more generally the $k$th nearest) neighbouring case, and computing the expected number of cases in the circle, centre, radius $r$ (Alexander *et al.*, 1989b). Variations in population density may be taken into account in calculating expected numbers. The local nearest neighbour area test aims to provide information on the proportion of cases occurring in clusters, the number or proportion of cases in the largest cluster, and the location of clusters. In the two-sample test of Cuzick and Edwards (1990), comparison is made of distances between cases and distances between controls, thus obviating the need for information on the distribution of the total denominator population.

In an investigation of the abilities of different methods to detect spatial clustering, these distance methods, together with the cell count approach initially described by COMARE (1988) were applied to 50 simulated data-sets (Alexander & Boyle, 1996). The underlying distributions of the data-sets were known but concealed from the investigators. No simple relationship was found between the parameters used to generate the data-set and the difficulty of detecting clustering. All of the tests had low power to detect clustering when 2.5% of cases occurred in clusters; power increased as the proportion of cases occurring in clusters increased. It proved extremely difficult to detect clustering in urban areas, and it was sometimes difficult to detect clusters which occurred on the edges of urban areas. There were many false positive reports of clustering and clusters. Decisions as to the occurrence of clustering were more difficult when a large number of clusters was involved. A general conclusion is that for the present, it seems appropriate to use more than one method in investigating spatial clustering of disease.

*— Childhood leukaemia and non-Hodgkin lymphoma in Britain, 1966–83*

Several methods of spatial analysis were applied to data on leukaemia and non-Hodgkin lymphoma diagnosed at ages 0–14 years in Great Britain during the period 1966–83. The results of application of the Knox test for space–time clustering to these data (Gilman & Knox, 1991; Knox & Gilman, 1992a) were described above. Seven tests of spatial clustering were applied. Two were cell count methods: (i) the ISD method (Black *et al.*, 1991); (ii) the Potthoff–Whittinghill test (Alexander, 1991). The other five were distance methods: (i) the Cuzick–Edwards method (Alexander, 1991); (ii) the geographical analysis machine (Openshaw & Craft, 1991); (iii) the local nearest neighbour test (Alexander, 1991); (iv) the Besag–Newell test (Besag *et al.*, 1991); and (v) the Knox method as applied to distances (Knox & Gilman, 1992b). All of the analyses except that of Knox and Gilman (1992b) were collected together in a single volume relating to the geographical epidemiology of these diseases, one of the objectives of which was to determine the extent to which results using different methods were consistent and, in particular, whether they agreed as to whether there was evidence for the existence of clustering as a general feature of the specific diseases (Draper *et al.*, 1991b).

Seven diagnostic groups were considered:
(i)   lymphocytic leukaemia;
(ii)  acute non-lymphocytic leukaemia;
(iii) non-Hodgkin lymphoma;
(iv)  lymphocytic and unspecified leukaemia;
(v)   all leukaemia;
(vi)  non-Hodgkin lymphoma and unspecified lymphomas;
(vii) all diagnoses.

The period of study (1966–83) included the years 1971 and 1981, when national censuses were carried out. The enumeration district was the smallest geographical unit for which population data were available (Elliott *et al.*, 1991b). There were approximately 130 000 enumeration districts defined in Britain at each census, giving population counts at ages 0–14 years of about 95–100 persons in each. Cases were analysed according to their address at diagnosis.

The studies are summarized in Table 2.6. The most consistent evidence for clustering was found for lymphocytic leukaemia in children under the age of five years. This was observed when the ISD, Potthoff–Whittinghill and GAM methods were applied (Black *et al.*, 1991; Alexander, 1991; Openshaw and Craft, 1991), and is consistent with the results of the analysis of temporo-spatial clustering by Gilman and Knox (1991).

A concern was the possibility that denominator errors could lead to spurious evidence of clustering. Black *et al.* (1991) found greater than expected heterogeneity of lymphocytic leukaemia and lymphocytic/unspecified leukaemia at almost all aggregation scales. Extra-Poisson variation was observed, suggesting that the effects of denominator errors would have been relatively large in comparison with the phenomenon under study. This problem is likely to apply to all methods using population data derived from censuses.

Alexander (1991) found that, for the overall time period 1966–83, there was evidence of spatial clustering for lymphocytic leukaemia and for the diagnostic groups influenced by this category (i.e., all leukaemias and all cases). This was apparent at ages 0–4 and 0–14. However, when analysis was restricted to one of the two five-year periods surrounding a decennial census, there was a consistent lack of evidence of clustering. Thus, denominator errors may have accounted for the clustering observed over the entire time period.

Besag *et al.* (1991) found that the number of 'database anomalies' was higher than predicted for the period 1974–78; for this intermediate period, the population at risk was estimated by taking averages of the 1971 and 1981 census tract data, whereas in the other analyses of sub-periods, enumeration districts were used. Enumeration districts could not be used for the intermediate period, as in general their boundaries changed between the two censuses. The authors noted that a preliminary analysis of anomalies identified at the 0.01 probability level

## Table 2.6. Summary of studies of clustering and clusters of childhood leukaemia and non-Hodgkin lymphomas in Great Britain, 1966–83

| Reference | Method | Unit of area | Time periods (justification) | Disease categories[a] | Age groups | Null hypothesis rejected for |
|---|---|---|---|---|---|---|
| Black et al., 1991 | ISD[b] | ED[c], aggregated into larger areas until the expected number of cases exceeded a pre-specified threshold. The thresholds considered were 0.5, 0.75, 1.0, 1.5, 2.0, 3.0, 4.0, 6.0, 8.0 and 10.0 | 1966–83 (total) | IV,V,VI,VII | 0–4 / 0–14 | IV,V,VI,VII / IV,VII |
| | | | 1979–83 (completeness of ascertainment greater than in earlier periods; analysis could be based on 1981 EDs without interpolation) | I,III,V,VII | 0–4 / 0–14 | I / I |
| Alexander, 1991[d] | Potthoff-Whittinghill | "Frozen wards", approximating 1981 electoral wards (in order to identify small areas stable over time) | 1966–83 (total) | I,V,VII / I,II,III,V,VI,VII | 0–4 / 0–14[e] | I,V,VII / I,VII |
| | | | 1969–73 (1971 census counts applicable) | I,V,VII / I,II,III,V,VI,VII | 0–4 / 0–14[e] | |
| | | | 1979–83 (1981 census counts applicable) | I,V,VII / I,II,III,V,VI,VII | 0–4 / 0–14[e] | |
| | | | 1969–73 and 1979–83 (1971 and 1981 census counts applicable) | I,V,VII / I,II,III,V,VI,VII | 0–4 / 0–14[e] | I |
| Knox & Gilman, 1992b | Knox | Distance between pairs of cases Identity of postcode co-ordinates | 1966–83 (total) | VII | 0–14 | VII / VII |
| Besag et al., 1991 | Besag–Newell | Circles around index cases defined to include 12 observed cases | 1969–83[f] | V,VI,VII | 0–14 | Number of anomalies in database similar to that predicted for V and VII if (1) cases occur independently and with equal probability for individuals in each risk category; (2) database error-free; number of anomalies fewer for VI |
| | | Circles around index cases defined to include 4 observed cases | 1969–73 (1971 census counts applicable, at ED level); 1974–78 (1971/81 census counts applicable, at census tract level); 1979–83 (1981 census counts applicable, at ED level) | V,VI,VII | 0–14 | Number of anomalies less than predicted for all three groups; Number of anomalies higher than predicted for all three groups; Number of anomalies similar to that predicted for V and VII, fewer for VI |

| Openshaw & Craft, 1991 | | | | | |
|---|---|---|---|---|---|
| GAM/2k, 4 test statistics | Grid of varying origin and size (4, 8, 16, 32 km²) | 1966–83 (total) | VII | 0–14 | 3 out of 4 test statistics indicated significant clustering at the 4 km scale. At the other scales, the results were affected substantially by changing the origin of the grid |

No null hypothesis:
Number of clusters when all cases (VII) considered, at threshold of 0.04

| | 0–14 yrs | 0–4 yrs | 5–9 yrs | 10–14 yrs |
|---|---|---|---|---|
| | 9 | 3 | 1 | 5 |
| | 12 | 5 | 4 | 2 |
| | 12 | 12 | 7 | 6 |
| | 14 | 4 | 4 | 3 |
| | 24 | 16 | 10 | 3 |
| | 23 | 13 | 12 | 7 |
| | 29 | 20 | 9 | 7 |

| GAM-K[h] | (1) Circle of 2 km radius, centred on each intersection of a 500 m grid; if excess, store | 1966–68 (1971 census) 1969–73 (1971 census) 1974–78 (1981 census) 1979–83 (1981 census) | I–VII | 0–4, 5–9, 10–14, 0–14 | |
| | (2) Repeat for slightly larger circle radius based on more widely spaced mesh of points again designed so that circles overlap, to allow for edge effects. | 1966–83 (total, 1971 census) (total, 1981 census) (total, maximum of 1971–81) | | | |

[a] I, lymphocytic leukaemia; II, ANLL; III, non-Hodgkin lymphoma; IV, lymphocytic lymphoma; V, all leukaemias; VI, non-Hodgkin and unspecified lymphomas; VII, all cases (i.e. categories I–VI combined).

[b] In the original ISD method, a chi-square test statistic was used. Subsequently, this was shown to have low power and in this analysis a more sensitive test statistic, the Poisson Index of Dispersion, was used.

[c] ED, Enumeration district.

[d] Only the analysis relating to the full data set is summarized. In exploratory analysis relating to the area of England and Wales which had contributed to an atlas of leukaemia and lymphoma (Cartwright *et al.*, 1990) and to the time period (1979–83) immediately preceding that to which the atlas relates, the Cuzick–Edwards, NNA, and Potthoff–Whittinghill tests, and the test of Barnes *et al.* (1987), were applied to investigate localized clustering. There was a consistent absence of evidence of clustering, but Poisson regression modelling at County District level showed marginally significant heterogeneity for ALL (I), leukaemias (V) and all cases (VII) at ages 0–4 years. After ranking wards by numbers of cases of ALL at ages 0–4 years, the ratio of cumulative values of observed to expected numbers of cases of ALL at ages 0–4 showed an unusual tendency for cases to occur in the least populous wards.

[e] The 5–9- and 10–14-year age-groups were considered for these categories; no clustering was apparent.

[f] 1966–68 not included, as many records were flagged as being uncertain in some respects, there was no obvious way of using census data to estimate populations at risk, and the three-year period was different in length from other periods considered.

[g] Non-overlapping grid-square rather than overlapping circle based version of the original GAM (Openshaw *et al.*, 1989).

[h] GAM with kernel estimation.

for various sizes of circles around the index case, defined in terms of the number of cases included, showed that some occurred in areas where census counts provide poor estimates of the true populations at risk. Such areas included locations where extensive house building had taken place subsequent to the census, and others in the vicinity of military camps, which often receive special status in the census, leading to under-enumeration. Openshaw and Craft (1991) applied (i) tests of clustering (three cell count methods including the ISD method, and a score test of over-dispersion) and (ii) a method aimed at detecting clusters (the GAM with kernel estimation). In the first approach, clustering at the $4 \text{ km}^2$ scale was identified by three out of the four tests. At the larger scales (8, 16 and 32 $\text{km}^2$), the results were affected substantially by changing the origin of the grid. In the second approach, the data analysis was carried out for five different time periods, four of which were intended to localize the effect of population changes since the 1971 or 1981 census, the fifth being the entire study period. All seven disease groupings were considered, but only that for all cases is shown in Table 2.6. There was some weak evidence of clustering in most of the analyses. The number of clusters seemed to be greater in the analyses based on the 1981 census than for those based on the 1971 census, but the results appeared to be reasonably robust to the effects of using different base populations (i.e., the 1971 and 1981 censuses, and the maximum populations for areas included in the 1971 and 1981 censuses defined to be as similar as possible to one another).

The clustering of ALL among young children was confined to sparsely populated areas (Alexander, 1991). The ratio of the incidence at ages 0–4 years to that at 10–14 years was 1.58 for "very sparse" wards (expected number of cases ≤0.004 per year) compared with wards in which the population density was 'normal' (expected number of cases 0.008–0.07 per year). The ratio was 0.65 in wards in which the population density was high (expected number of cases >0.07 per year) compared with wards in which it was normal.

The pattern of clustering of ALL among young children in sparsely populated areas could not be explained by uniformly high rates within them. Adjustment of the expected numbers by the observed relative risk in the different types of area only marginally reduced the values of the test statistic for lymphocytic leukaemia. In every case in which the test gave significantly positive results, the contribution from wards classified as of normal or high population density was around or less than the expected value. The influence of errors in the population denominators could not be assessed as, although similar patterns were not found for diagnostic groups which did not include lymphocytic leukaemia at ages 0–4, these analyses had lower statistical power because of smaller case numbers.

Openshaw and Craft (1991) made a tally of how many of the clusters occurred near to a list of three locations where localized excesses had previously been reported – Gateshead, Seascale (near the Sellafield nuclear plant) and the area around Dounreay nuclear plant. The first two of these were identified in the analysis. Clusters near other nuclear sites and 'new towns' were also considered. Some were identified in the analysis. No clusters were identified near a set of six sites that had been considered for nuclear installations. Most of the clusters appeared to be associated with areas that did not fall into one of these categories. The authors noted that similar levels of association have been found in simulations based on random data.

Knox and Gilman (1992b) tested the same data-set for the presence of short-radius spatial clusters. When the frequency distribution of inter-pair distances was considered, there was a relative excess among case pairs of separation <40 km. The greatest relative excess was at separations >0.5 km. As the registers of co-ordinates for the cases and the controls were not strictly comparable, the authors also undertook a qualitative analysis, based upon counting the numbers of pairs of cases sharing a single postcode map reference. Again, there was a significant excess of pairs sharing common or adjacent postcodes, and this is compatible with the results of the other analysis. The quantitative analysis suggested an excess of 200–300 pairs separated by distances up to 0.5 km. In the analysis of temporo-spatial clustering in the same data-set (Knox & Gilman, 1992a) described above, there were 35 pairs within 0.5 km and 30 days of each other. Therefore, the space–time excess was contained within the geographical excess. While the phenomenon of space–time clustering might have arisen because an epidemic communicable disease had provoked haematological examinations, in turn triggering the near-simultaneous diagnosis of latent leukaemias already existing within the population, such a process could not have accounted for geographical clustering among events aggregated over a long period of time.

*— Other analyses of spatial clustering of leukaemia*

In a study of deaths at ages 0–5 years due to leukaemia in Greater London in the period 1952–65, in which no evidence was found of clustering of the time and place of residence at birth, Smith *et al.* (1976) investigated possible contagion by examining six postulated susceptible periods: the gestational period, each of the three trimesters of pregnancy, the first year of life, and the period from one year before clinical onset to six months before onset. Four periods of infectivity were postulated: onset ±1 month, onset ±3 months, onset ±1 year and onset to death. Areas of susceptibility and infectivity were defined to be circles of one of five diameters (0.25, 0.5, 1.0, 2.0 and 4.0 km) around the places of residence at birth and onset respectively. The observed number of overlapping pairs of cases exceeded expectation at the conventional 5% significance level only for a susceptible period from one year to six months before onset and an infective period of onset ±1 month, with a critical distance of 4 km. Two differences approached this level of statistical significance – the same time periods as above, with critical distances of 0.25 and 0.5 km. When susceptibility *in utero* and infectivity from birth to onset of the disease were considered, the only difference that was statistically significant was associated with a critical distance of 4 km between pairs and cases. The authors acknowledged that these results could well have arisen by chance, given the number of significance tests performed. Also, the tests were not independent.

Using data from a case–control study, in an analysis of residential proximity between cases of leukaemia and non-Hodgkin lymphoma and between controls during the period from one year before birth to diagnosis in three areas in northern England (Cumbria, Gateshead and North Humberside) during the period 1974–88, statistically significant clustering was found using the Cuzick–Edwards test (Alexander *et al.*, 1992a). Alexander *et al.* (1992a) carried out an exploratory analysis to determine which cases gave rise to the excess numbers of case–case pairs, and of the period of linkage for clues as to latency. The analysis was restricted to case children who were both born and diagnosed in the same study area. When the 'target' (i.e., the index child from whose home residential distances to all other homes were computed in order to identify the nearest neighbours) was aged under five years, the nearest neighbour was more likely to be a case than a control. This was not found when the target was aged 5–14 years.

This pattern was not apparent when the analysis was repeated with the ages of nearest neighbours restricted in the same way as for the target children. Inspection of the ages of the nearest neighbours showed that 59% of those involved in case–case pairs were aged 5–14 years, whereas only 39% of cases were in that age range. Thus, there was a tendency for cases with a younger age of onset to have lived close to cases with an older age of onset at some time before the diagnosis of the disease in either child. The relationships between overlap of the time period of residence and dates of birth were similar for case–case and other pairs, but there was a small excess of target cases for whom the period of overlap ended by the date of birth, suggesting that a minority of cases may be susceptible prenatally. When the period of overlap was considered in relation to the date of diagnosis, both targets and nearest neighbours of case–case pairs were somewhat more likely to have an overlap beginning in the second year before diagnosis than other pairs. However, for the vast majority of case–case pairs, the period of overlap extended into periods more than two years before the date of diagnosis of at least one child.

In each of the three geographical areas included in the study, a pattern was apparent whereby an older case was nearest neighbour to a number of younger target cases. However, the periods of overlap between pairs of cases did not coincide and were spread over several years, and the overlap may also have involved different addresses for the older case. Two children were defined to have had school contact if either they or their siblings had attended the same school for at least one term in common. Six pairs of cases and five pairs of controls had had such contact.

On the basis of the results of the exploratory analysis, the authors suggested that some children might have been susceptible around the time of birth. To test this, the spatial analysis in which residential history during the period one year before birth until diagnosis was repeated, with consideration of the residential history restricted to the time between conception and the first birthday. In all three regions in which the study was carried out, there was evidence of excess case to case proximity according to this restricted definition, indicating an excess of case children who, around the time of their birth, had lived close to other children who later developed leukaemia. The authors considered that it was unlikely that the results were due to the localized spatial clustering which had already been identified in these areas, since application of the same methods to test for spatial clustering by location at diagnosis gave significant results only for one of the areas. In addition, the case–case pairs in North Humberside did not include any cases from the postcode sector in which the original reports of clustering had been made.

In a report on the parental occupational exposures of these study subjects (McKinney *et al.*, 1991), it was stated that 11–13% of parents of cases and 17–38% of parents of controls were not interviewed in the main study areas. Control replacement was used. The main reason for non-participation was refusal. If agreement to participate were related to awareness of other cases, non-participation could influence the results of analysis related to case–case interaction. It would be interesting to know if the parental occupational exposures, associations with which were almost exclusively restricted to the time before the child's birth, could account for the observed pattern of interactions between cases.

On the basis of the suggestion that there is a putative childhood leukaemia virus (*Lancet*, 1990) and the hypotheses of Greaves and Kinlen (see Chapter 1), Alexander *et al.* (1992a) postulated that (i) in children exposed to a putative infectious etiological agent *in utero* or very early in life, persistent infection might become established, leading to an increased risk of developing ALL primarily later than the peak years of onset in childhood; (ii) postnatal exposure to the putative agent might contribute to the development of ALL at younger ages; and (iii) ALL in the childhood peak age range may be a rare consequence of recent first exposure to the putative agent. Alexander (1992) tested these hypotheses in an analysis of temporo-spatial interaction of total childhood leukaemia in 131 wards whose contribution to the Potthoff–Whittinghill test of spatial clustering exceeded an arbitrary threshold of 10 in her earlier analysis (Alexander, 1991) of data from Britain during the period 1968–83. In these wards, there were 487 cases with ALL, 6 with acute leukaemia not otherwise stated and 24 with other types of leukaemia. The hypotheses were evaluated by considering the spatial and temporal relationships between the cases, considered to form two series, one the 'infectives' and the other 'susceptibles'. The Knox method was used to evaluate temporo-spatial interactions.

In evaluating the first hypothesis, relating to the persistent infection of children following exposure *in utero* or very early in life, susceptibles were defined to have an age range of 5–14 and their period of susceptibility was their date of birth ±1 year. The relevant analysis showed highly significant temporo-spatial interaction.

Thus, there was evidence that children destined to develop ALL at older ages were exposed *in utero* or perinatally. Examination of the ages at diagnosis of the infectives shows that the excess of observed temporo-spatial interactions compared with that expected was not restricted to older cases.

In evaluating the second hypothesis, relating to the possibility that postnatal exposure to an unspecified agent might increase the risk of ALL in young children, the susceptibles were defined to be in the age range 0–4 and their time of susceptibility to be from their date of birth to the date of their diagnosis. Spatio-temporal interaction of borderline statistical significance was found. The excess appeared to involve infectives who were somewhat older than susceptibles.

In assessing the third hypothesis, relating to ALL in the childhood peak and recent first exposure to the agent, the susceptibles were defined to be in the age range 2–4 years and their period of susceptibility from either 18 months before diagnosis, or the age of 12 months if this was later, to the date of diagnosis. No spatio-temporal interaction was found.

One interpretation of these findings is that horizontal and/or vertical transmission of some infectious agent or agents may contribute to ALL with onset beyond the childhood peak. As indicated by the author, other interpretations are possible, including a common source exposure to a pollutant which is localized in both space and time, but it would then be necessary to postulate an unusual relationship between age at exposure and the length of the latent period. The evidence in support of the hypothesis that infection may contribute to the disease in younger children is weaker. This suggests either that other causes are dominant or that host factors are relevant, as postulated by Greaves (1988).

A number of other analyses of spatial clustering in Britain have been carried out in the context of developing statistical methods for investigation of the phenomenon. No clustering of leukaemia diagnosed at ages up to 24 years was found in Scotland during the period 1968–84, using a variant of the ISD method (COMARE, 1988), but this variant was subsequently shown to lack statistical power (Black *et al.*, 1996). In an analysis of ALL in the north-west of England during the period 1968–88 by the GAM, five clusters were identified, only one of which had been suspected previously (Openshaw *et al.*, 1988). Subsequently, in an analysis of a subset of these cases diagnosed during the period 1975–85 by the Besag–Newell method, no clustering was identified when the whole region was considered (Besag & Newell, 1991). In analyses of residence at diagnosis of leukaemia and lymphoma (Cuzick & Edwards, 1990) and leukaemia (Alexander *et al.*, 1991a) in North Humberside during the period 1974–86, significant clustering was identified using the Cuzick–Edwards method. Using a probability mapping technique in the analysis of data at electoral ward level from the West Midlands Health Authority Region during the period 1980–84, no evidence of spatial aggregation of leukaemia and non-Hodgkin lymphoma was found (Muir *et al.*, 1990b).

Aickin *et al.* (1992) compared data on mortality attributed to leukaemia in children up to the age of 19 years between West Central Phoenix in Arizona, where a childhood leukaemia cluster was suspected, and Maricopa County, excluding West Central Phoenix and three other suspect areas. The choice was based on the perception that the distributions of factors such as ethnic group and socioeconomic status were more comparable to the target area than were the corresponding distributions in national data. The other suspect areas were removed from the comparison region because they contained sites identified by the Environmental Protection Agency as being contaminated by potentially hazardous chemicals. This decision was taken before examining the mortality data. The method of analysis applied, which was developed in response to concern about potential disease clusters, consisted of a formal test of a hypothesis that the standardized rate ratio in the target and comparison regions is unity. This was formulated as a linear hypothesis on Poisson means, and thus some variability of both the numerator and denominator terms was taken into account for both the area of concern and comparison regions. The standardized rate ratio was 1.95, with a *p* value of 0.0002, suggesting that an excess number of childhood leukaemia deaths occurred in West Central Phoenix. The excess appeared to be weakest among the older children. The study period was divided into three (1966–69, 1970–81 and 1982–86) in order to determine if rates were elevated in periods previous and subsequent to the cluster reported in 1982 which stimulated the enquiry. Examination of residuals indicated that the excess was most marked in the middle time period. The method does not seem to resolve the problem of interpreting statistical tests related to areas of concern specified because a cluster was suspected.

Muirhead (1995) investigated spatial clustering of 346 cases of leukaemia and non-Hodgkin lymphoma in white children in three metropolitan regions of the USA (San Francisco–Oakland, California; Detroit, Michigan; and Atlanta, Georgia) during the period 1978–82. Denominator data were obtained from the 1980 census. No evidence of spatial clustering was found, using either the Potthoff–Whittinghill method or that of Breslow (1984) among census tracts with or without adjustment for region, among counties or among regions. Similar results were found when the age range was restricted to zero to four years. The absence of clustering may reflect the greater difficulty of detection in urban than in rural areas (Alexander & Boyle, 1996). Analysis also was made by median education, median family income and population density of the white population of each census tract. There was a statistically significant increasing trend in incidence rates with increasing population density; this trend was observed in all three regions. No trend with education or income was found, although incidence was 27% higher in children resident in the areas of highest education compared with the lowest (Table 2.4).

In an analysis of 1523 cases of childhood leukaemia in Sweden during the period 1973–93, no clustering was found for ALL and ANLL either separately or combined (Hjalmars *et al.*, 1996). The analysis was based on the centroids of 2577 standard parishes, with population data taken as the average of the censuses carried out in 1976, 1982 and 1988. The spatial-scan statistic was used, in which a circular window of variable size, in this instance covering an increasing number of adjacent parishes until 10% of the total population was covered, scans the study area in order to detect clusters without prior knowledge of their location or geographical size. The power of the test has not been fully investigated, but is suggested by the authors to be relatively good.

In an analysis of data on 656 cases of ALL in Sweden during the period 1980–90, no evidence of a tendency for cases to cluster was found when the methods of Turnbull *et al.* (1990) and Besag and Newell (1991) were applied (Waller *et al.*, 1995).

In an analysis of 872 cases of childhood leukaemia in Greece during the period 1980–89, significant clustering was identified using the Potthoff–Whittinghill test (Petridou *et al.*, 1997). As this might have reflected a higher incidence of childhood leukaemia in urban rather than rural areas in Greece (Petridou *et al.*,

1996a), the analysis was stratified among districts classified as 'urban' (districts adjacent to towns of more than 10 000 inhabitants), 'semi-urban' (districts composed of towns with populations between 2000 and 9999 inhabitants) or 'rural' (districts containing villages each with fewer than 2000 inhabitants). Spatial clustering was found in the urban and semi-urban districts, but not in rural districts. When analysis within age groups was performed, the strength of the clustering was stronger for the 0–4-year age group than for the 5–9-year age group, while no clustering was apparent for the 10–14-year age group. The extent to which the proximity of cases from different age groups contributed to the overall clustering was examined; the between-age-group clustering appeared to be stronger than that within age groups. These patterns also were apparent when the analysis was restricted to ALL. In an analysis of space–time clustering of the same data, clustering was apparent only for cases younger than five years (Petridou *et al.*, 1996a; see above).

Data on 261 cases of childhood leukaemia, the majority (79%) of whom had ALL, diagnosed in Hong Kong during the period 1984–90 were analysed by the Potthoff–Whittinghill method (Alexander *et al.*, 1997). There was no evidence of clustering for the entire age range. However, spatial clustering was observed for cases diagnosed at 2–6 years (age group defined *a priori*), and evidence suggestive of clustering was found for the 0–4-year age group. Alternative age bands were considered for the childhood peak in a sensitivity analysis; this showed that the results were not dependent on a precise definition of the childhood peak in terms of age at diagnosis.

— *Summary*

Spatial clustering of childhood leukaemia has been observed in Britain, Greece and Hong Kong, but not in Sweden or in metropolitan areas of the USA. The units of space considered in the study in the USA were larger than in those considered in studies in the other countries, which may have diluted the effects of clustering at a smaller scale. Where spatial clustering was identified, it was strongest for cases diagnosed in young children. However, part of the pattern in Britain may be attributable to errors in the denominator population. In addition, in the British data, the evidence of spatial clustering was confined to sparsely populated areas, whereas in Greece such clustering was found only in urban or semi-urban areas.

## Group II: Lymphomas and other reticuloendothelial neoplasms

A diverse group of neoplasms are included in the category of lymphomas and other reticuloendothelial neoplasms. The most common of these are Hodgkin's disease, Burkitt's lymphoma and non-Hodgkin lymphoma. These exhibit distinctive epidemiological features and are therefore considered separately in this section. Also included among the lymphomas is the rare neoplasm histiocytosis X, which is not recorded by some cancer registries and, in the registries where it is recorded, the data are often incomplete (Stiller & Parkin, 1990a). The remaining tumours in this category are unspecified lymphomas or other reticuloendothelial neoplasms.

### *Relative frequencies of lymphomas and lymphoma types*

There are substantial variations worldwide in the proportion of all neoplasms in children which are lymphomas. The relative frequencies of lymphomas in selected populations, based on the data from Parkin *et al.* (1988a) and covering approximately the decade 1970–79, are shown in Table 2.7. In some of these series, in Africa in particular, leukaemia cases are not enumerated or are likely to be under-ascertained, which has the effect of inflating the apparent relative frequency of lymphomas. Nonetheless, it is evident that in most of Africa, with the exception of the south, lymphomas are the dominant childhood neoplasm, accounting for between 30% and 75% of incident cases. In the south, in Zimbabwe and Namibia, 12–15% of childhood tumours are lymphomas (Parkin *et al.*, 1988a; Wessells & Hesselling, 1996). This geographical pattern is confirmed in other African series (Parkin, 1986; Obafunwa *et al.*, 1992; Tijani *et al.*, 1995; Makata *et al.*, 1996). Lymphomas are also relatively common in countries of the Middle East, Brazil and Papua New Guinea, where they account for between 22% and 33% of malignancies. In north and central America, Australia, New Zealand, eastern Asia and Europe they comprise 8–17% of neoplasms.

To illustrate the distinctive geographical distributions of the main histological types of lymphoma, Table 2.7 also shows the proportions of lymphoma cases which are of these types. Difficulties in the accurate diagnosis and classification of lymphomas are well recognized (Glaser & Swartz, 1990). Therefore, it is possible that some of the disparity in the data, particularly between series from neighbouring

**Table 2.7. Relative frequency of lymphomas and other reticuloendothelial neoplasms and percentages of main sub-types, for selected registries, around 1970–79**

| Country (registry) | Lymphomas and other reticulo-endothelial neoplasms Relative frequency (%)[a] | Hodgkin's disease | Non-Hodgkin lymphoma | Burkitt's lymphoma | Other neoplasms |
|---|---|---|---|---|---|
| | | % of all lymphomas | | | |
| **Africa** | | | | | |
| Malawi | 35.7[b] | 3.5 | 8.2 | 62.4 | 25.9 |
| Morocco | 32.7 | 33.8 | 45.5 | 20.7 | 0.0 |
| Nigeria (Ibadan) | 56.3 | 6.5 | .2 | 82.7 | 5.6 |
| Tanzania | 44.6[b] | 28.7 | 15.7 | 46.1 | 9.6 |
| Tunisia | 35.7[b] | 40.8 | 31.2 | 26.2 | 1.9 |
| Uganda (Kampala) | 29.6 | 18.3 | 45.0 | 28.3 | 8.3 |
| Uganda (West Nile) | 75.6 | 0.6 | 5.8 | 90.3 | 3.2 |
| Zimbabwe (Bulawayo) | 15.3 | 37.3 | 45.8 | 12.0 | 4.8 |
| **Americas** | | | | | |
| Canada (Western Provinces) | 13.0 | 29.6 | 41.5 | 1.9 | 27.0 |
| USA (SEER: whites) | 13.3 | 42.5 | 29.2 | 11.8 | 16.4 |
| USA (SEER: blacks) | 10.2 | 48.4 | 25.8 | 3.2 | 22.6 |
| Brazil (Fortaleza, Recife and São Paulo) | 23.4 | 31.0 | 58.5 | 1.4 | 9.1 |
| Colombia (Cali) | 17.3 | 32.6 | 23.3 | 27.9 | 16.3 |
| Puerto Rico | 15.3 | 42.6 | 29.0 | 8.0 | 20.4 |
| **Asia** | | | | | |
| China (Shanghai and Taipei) | 11.6 | 12.6 | 48.0 | 0.0 | 39.4 |
| India (Bangalore and Bombay) | 17.4 | 37.5 | 40.2 | 3.3 | 18.9 |
| Iraq – Baghdad | 27.6 | 31.4 | 26.6 | 30.9 | 11.1 |
| Israel (Jews and non-Jews) | 21.9 | 27.9 | 40.4 | 17.0 | 14.7 |
| Japan (Kanagawa, Miyagi and Osaka) | 7.6 | 8.0 | 40.6 | 3.4 | 47.9 |
| Kuwait (Kuwaiti and non-Kuwaiti) | 29.5 | 35.7 | 41.1 | 9.8 | 13.4 |
| **Europe** | | | | | |
| Denmark | 11.3 | 35.1 | 21.6 | 20.3 | 23.0 |
| England & Wales | 11.4 | 38.6 | 50.0 | 2.0 | 9.4 |
| Scandinavia (Finland, Norway and Sweden) | 9.2 | 26.9 | 48.5 | 1.2 | 23.4 |
| Slovakia | 14.0 | 39.3 | 33.2 | 1.4 | 26.1 |
| Spain | 15.3[b] | 20.8 | 41.9 | 25.5 | 11.8 |
| **Oceania** | | | | | |
| Australia[c] | 12.3 | 30.4 | 43.6 | 1.3 | 24.8 |
| New Zealand (Maoris and non-Maoris) | 10.4 | 33.6 | 51.6 | 2.5 | 12.3 |
| Papua New Guinea | 32.9 | 3.9 | 31.2 | 54.5 | 10.4 |

Based on data in Parkin *et al.* (1988a).

[a] Percentage of all neoplasms in children.
[b] Series in which leukaemia cases are either not recorded or probably underascertained.
[c] New South Wales cancer registry and Queensland Childhood Malignancy registry.

areas (e.g., within Europe), is due to differences in histopathological classification practice. However, the variations between regions are pronounced and likely to be, in large part, real.

## Hodgkin's disease
### Geographical patterns

In Australia, New Zealand, northern and central Europe, the Middle East and the Americas, Hodgkin's disease represents 27–48% of lymphomas in children (Table 2.7). It is similarly frequent in areas of Africa where Burkitt's lymphoma is not endemic.

The highest recorded annual age-standardized incidence of Hodgkin's disease during the 1970s was 10.8 per million in Costa Rica (Parkin *et al.*, 1988a). Rates of more than 8 per million were observed in Kuwait, Los Angeles Hispanics, Brazil (São Paulo) and the non-Jewish population of Israel. The pattern of high incidence in Israel and Kuwait appears to extend into North Africa, Turkey, Iran, Pakistan and north-west India (Stiller & Parkin, 1990a). It also stretches to the north and west, with registries covering parts of southern Europe reporting rates in the range 5–7 per million. In addition, incidence appears to be generally higher in the Baltic countries and states of central and eastern Europe than those in the European Union (Macfarlane *et al.*, 1995). Moving westward and north in Europe, the incidence falls to 4 per million in Britain and Denmark and to 3 or less in the Scandinavian countries. The pattern of lower incidence in northern than southern parts of Europe is reflected in North America. While rates in US populations were in the range 5–7 per million, those in Canada were 3–4 per million. In eastern Asia, Hodgkin's disease is uncommon, with incidence in most populations less than 2 per million.

Reports of reciprocal geographical patterns in Hodgkin's disease mortality in young adults (Cole *et al.*, 1968) and children (Fraumeni & Li, 1969) in the USA prompted international comparisons of incidence in these age groups. Using data for the early 1960s, Correa and O'Conor (1971) demonstrated an inverse relationship for males. Populations, mainly in developing countries, with high rates of Hodgkin's disease in children (5–14 years) had low rates in young adults (20–34 years). In urban developed communities, the situation was reversed. However, a recent analysis, based on data for the 1980s, found no association between Hodgkin's disease rates in children and young adults (Macfarlane *et al.*, 1995).

### Age-specific incidence and sex ratio

Correa and O'Conor (1971) described different patterns of age-specific incidence of Hodgkin's disease in children in developed and developing countries. Developed communities were distinguished by very low incidence in the youngest children followed by a pronounced increase with age. In contrast, in developing countries, the rates were higher in the younger age groups and rose less steeply with age. These distributions persist in more recent data. In mainly white populations, in Europe, Australia and the USA, very few cases occur in infants, rates in those aged 1–4 years being between 1 and 2 per million. In the 5–9-year age group incidence is in the range 3–6 per million and rises to 8–14 per million in the 10–14-year age group (de Nully Brown *et al.*, 1989, Coebergh *et al.*, 1991; Mosso *et al.*, 1992; Blair & Birch, 1994a; Stiller *et al.*, 1995; Gurney *et al.*, 1996a; McWhirter *et al.*, 1996). In central and south America and in Asia, the age–incidence curves differ from this pattern in two ways: (i) the large increase in older children is not evident, regardless of the overall level of incidence; and (ii) in the areas with high overall incidence, rates in children aged 1–9 years are much higher. For example, in São Paulo, Brazil, a registry with high overall incidence, the rates in the 0, 1–4, 5–9 and 10–14 age groups are 0, 5.1, 10.8 and 12.3 per million respectively (Parkin *et al.*, 1988a). The comparable figures for Osaka, Japan, a registry with low overall incidence, are 0, 0.3, 0.9 and 1.1 per million (Ajiki *et al.*, 1994). In some series, there is a peak in the 5–9 age group (Stiller & Parkin, 1990a).

Almost everywhere, males account for the overwhelming majority of cases, with the male excess around 2:1 in Europe and the Americas and 3.5:1 in Africa and Asia (Stiller & Parkin, 1990a). The sex ratio varies with age, at least in developed countries. In Manchester, UK, the risk for girls relative to boys was 0.27 (0.12–0.63) for those aged 5–9 years and 0.47 (95% CI 0.20–0.73) for those 10–14 years (Blair & Birch, 1994a). This pattern is apparent elsewhere in Europe and the USA (de Nully Brown *et al.*, 1989; Coebergh *et al.*, 1991; Mosso *et al.*, 1992; Gurney *et al.*, 1996a).

### Ethnic origin

In the West Midlands area of England, during 1981–92, the incidence of Hodgkin's disease among Asian children was twice as high as that among white children (RR = 2.16; 95% CI 0.87–5.38) (Powell *et al.*, 1994). During the last four years of the study period (1989–92), the relative risk was 5.04 (95% CI 1.2–20.8). Also in Britain, Stiller *et al.* (1991a) demonstrated significant heterogeneity among ethnic groups in the relative frequency of Hodgkin's disease diagnosed from 1981. This was accounted for by a two-fold raised risk among children of Asian origin, mainly from the Indian sub-continent, compared with white children (Table 2.2). The excess of Hodgkin's disease among Asian children was most pronounced for those aged under five years (RR = 6.7), was substantial for the 5–9-year age group (2.2) and more modest for older children (1.3). The histological sub-types of Hodgkin's disease differed between the ethnic groups. Of the Asian cases, almost 50% were mixed cellularity and one third nodular sclerosis, whereas half of the cases in white children were nodular sclerosis and 25% mixed cellularity.

Many of the migrants to Britain from the Indian sub-continent came from either the Indian state of Gujarat, directly or via East Africa, or the Punjab (Little & Nicoll, 1988). Based on relative frequency data from Ahmedabad in India and Karachi in Pakistan, Stiller and Parkin (1990a) concluded that the incidence of childhood Hodgkin's disease is likely to be high in these regions. In addition, in western Asia, as in most developing countries, the steep rise in incidence during early adolescence does not occur, and mixed cellularity is the dominant sub-type. Hence, the results of the two studies with regard to the overall excess of Hodgkin's disease among Asian children, the age distribution and histological sub-types of the cases provide convincing evidence for an ethnic difference in risk of Hodgkin's disease, which is unaffected by migration and therefore suggestive of a genetic component in the etiology.

There is little other evidence of substantial ethnic variations in Hodgkin's disease (Breslow & Langholz, 1983; Duncan *et al.*, 1986; Spitz *et al.*, 1986; Goodman *et al.*, 1989). In the international study of childhood cancer (Parkin *et al.*, 1988a), there were only relatively minor differences in incidence between ethnic groups in the populations for which these data were available (Table 2.1). For example, in an area of high incidence (Kuwait), among Kuwaiti natives and non-Kuwaitis the rates were 10.3 and 9.8 per million respectively; in an area of low incidence (Singapore), the rates were 1.6 and 1.7 per million for the Chinese and Malay populations respectively.

Incidence was generally slightly lower in the black populations in the USA than other ethnic groups (Table 2.1) and the mainly black population of Jamaica experienced the lowest incidence in central and south America (Parkin *et al.*, 1988a). However, in Britain, no significant difference in the frequency of Hodgkin's disease between West Indian and white children was found (Stiller *et al.*, 1991a) (Table 2.2).

It has been suggested that the particularly low incidence in east Asian populations is related to a genetically determined resistance to Hodgkin's disease (Stiller & Parkin, 1990a). In support of this, the authors quote unpublished data from the SEER program in the USA which shows that in Chinese and Japanese persons of all ages, the rate of Hodgkin's disease is less than one fifth of that for whites.

### Socioeconomic status

It has long been suggested that socioeconomic factors are involved in the causation of Hodgkin's disease (Correa & O'Conor, 1971) and for adults, positive associations between risk and markers of high socioeconomic status have been reported (Grufferman & Delzell, 1984). However, for children it has been suggested that the converse could apply (Grufferman & Delzell, 1984). On the basis of the distinctive geographical and age–incidence patterns in developed and developing countries, an early hypothesis postulated that risk of Hodgkin's disease is closely related to both environmental and economic circumstances (Correa & O'Conor, 1971), with poorer socioeconomic conditions leading to an accelerated onset of the disease via an infectious etiology (Gutensohn & Cole, 1977).

Despite these observations, there have been relatively few studies which have considered directly the relationship between Hodgkin's disease in children and socioeconomic status. In the West Midlands area of England, the occupations of the fathers of 16% of Hodgkin's cases diagnosed during 1972–86 fell into social classes I and II compared with 21% of the population as a whole (Parkes *et al.*, 1994) (Table 2.3). The deficit of cases in social classes I and II was most pronounced for children under 10 years. However, the entire analysis included only 63 cases. The results of a population-based case–control study in the Boston area of the USA are consistent with this finding (Gutensohn & Shapiro, 1982). In this study, cases aged less than 10 years tended to be of lower social class than their controls, as assessed by median household income and occupation of the head of the household, whereas cases aged 10–14 years did not differ in these characteristics from their controls. The study included 14 cases aged under 10 and 52 aged 10–14 years. In contrast, in an investigation of 486 cases of Hodgkin's disease diagnosed in persons under 25 in England and Wales in 1984–88, Alexander *et al.* (1991c) found a positive association between a community-level indicator of socioeconomic status for place of residence of the case at the time of diagnosis and disease risk. After adjustment for urban–rural status and distance from a built-up area, the risk for those resident in areas of higher social class compared with lower social class was 1.22 (95% CI 1.01–1.47). Children accounted for 16% of the cases (Cartwright *et al.*, 1990) and were not analysed separately. A case–control study in three regions of England found no evidence of an association between Hodgkin's disease in children and paternal social class (McKinney *et al.*, 1987).

### Time trends

Advances in immunohistological techniques over the past two decades (Sklar & Costa, 1997) are likely to have improved the diagnostic accuracy for lymphomas. This, in conjunction with changes in pathological criteria for distinguishing Hodgkin's disease and non-Hodgkin lymphoma (Banks, 1992) and the development, and subsequent revision, of lymphoma classifications (Jaffe *et al.*, 1992), renders the interpretation of time trends in the various histological types of lymphomas complex.

The results of investigations of temporal variations in the incidence of Hodgkin's disease are inconsistent. In a study of geographical variations in childhood cancer, based on data from the late 1950s to mid-1960s, upward trends in Hodgkin's disease incidence were evident in the former East Germany and the USA (Breslow & Langholz, 1983). However, the latter finding was attributed to improved case ascertainment. In Connecticut, USA, a three-fold increase in Hodgkin's disease from 1935 to 1979 in females aged 10–14 years and males and females aged 15–19 years was demonstrated, which did not appear to be an artefact of decreasing rates of non-Hodgkin lymphoma (van Hoff *et al.*, 1988). There were no notable trends in younger children. In contrast, recent analyses of SEER data from 1974–91 and Greater Delaware Valley Paediatric Tumour Registry data for 1970–89 found no evidence of any appreciable trend in Hodgkin's disease in children overall, in either sex, or in any age group (Bunin *et al.*, 1996; Gurney *et al.*, 1996a). This is consistent with findings from the Netherlands (Coebergh *et al.*, 1991), Italy (Mosso *et al.*, 1992) and Japan (Ajiki *et al.*, 1994).

In Queensland, Australia, McWhirter and Petroeschevsky (1991) reported a significant fall in Hodgkin's disease between 1973 and 1988; rates of non-Hodgkin lymphoma rose moderately over this time. Meanwhile, in Victoria, Australia, increments in Hodgkin's disease rates of 19% for boys and 39% for girls were evident between 1970–79 and 1980–89 (Giles *et al.*, 1995). However, cancer registration became mandatory in this area in 1981, and this may have increased completeness of ascertainment.

Two studies in England have described a gradual increase in incidence from the mid-1950s to mid-1980s (Parkes *et al.*, 1994; Blair & Birch, 1994a). Age-standardized incidence rates in the West Midlands rose by 40% over a thirty-year period and the linear trend was of borderline statistical significance ($p = 0.06$) (Parkes *et al.*, 1994). In the north-west area, a significant trend was found which was compatible with a 10% increase every five years (Blair & Birch, 1994a). This did not vary substantially by sex or age and there was no evidence of a secular pattern in non-Hodgkin lymphoma.

## Burkitt's lymphoma
### Geographical patterns

In parts of sub-Saharan Africa, Burkitt's lymphoma is endemic. During the 1970s, in some African series it accounted for up to 90% of all lymphomas (Table 2.7) and was the most frequently diagnosed childhood tumour. In the north of the continent, it was also common but less dominant, comprising 20–23% of lymphomas in Morocco and Tunisia. In the south, in Zimbabwe, only 12% of lymphomas were of Burkitt's type. In the international study, age-standardized incidence rates were available for Nigeria (Ibadan) for 1960–69, Uganda (Kampala) for 1968–82 and Zimbabwe (Bulawayo) for 1963–77; these were 79.4, 7.3 and 1.2 per million respectively (Stiller & Parkin, 1990a).

The overwhelming importance of Burkitt's lymphoma in tropical Africa has been well documented (Parkin *et al.*, 1985). The area of highest risk appears to be between 10° north and 10° south of the equator. However, within that region, the frequency of the tumour can vary substantially. For example, in Uganda, 90% of lymphomas in the West Nile area were Burkitt's type compared with 28% in Kampala (Table 2.7). Similarly, in a large histopathology series of 600 solid tumours in western Kenya in 1979–94, Burkitt's accounted for 52% of neoplasms in

Nyanza province, 31% in the Western province and 23% in the Rift Valley (Makata *et al.*, 1996). Nyanza borders Lake Victoria and is hot and moist tropical savannah, whereas the Rift Valley is a semi-arid highland area. This exemplifies the general pattern of Burkitt's lymphoma. It is less common at high altitudes such as Rwanda, Burundi, the Kenya highlands and the plateaux of Zambia and Zimbabwe, and frequency appears to be related to climatic conditions (Parkin *et al.*, 1985).

Burkitt's lymphoma is also extremely common in Papua New Guinea, where more than half of all lymphomas are of this type (Table 2.7). In this population, Epstein–Barr virus (EBV) infection is endemic (Miller, 1990). Likewise, in equatorial Africa, Burkitt's lymphoma is associated with the presence of EBV infection and it has been suggested that holo-endemic malaria acts synergistically with EBV susceptibility to increase risk of the tumour (see Chapter 7).

Stiller and Parkin (1990a) described a zone of intermediate risk for Burkitt's lymphoma which extends across north Africa and Asia as far west as Iraq and the Kuwaiti population of Kuwait. There is some suggestion that it may also extend into European countries bordering on the Mediterranean. In Spain, during 1980–84, in the national childhood cancer registry one quarter of lymphomas were Burkitt's and in Zaragoza in 1973–82 and Valencia in 1983–90 the age-standardized incidence rates were 2.6 and 5.4 per million, respectively (Parkin *et al.*, 1988a; Peris-Bonet *et al.*, 1996). In the area covered by the French Paediatric Registries (south-east France and Corsica), the incidence was 3.7 per million during 1983–85 and 6.1 during 1984–91 (Parkin *et al.*, 1988a; Bernard *et al.*, 1993a). These rates fall within the range observed in the Middle East. Whether risk is indeed higher in southern Europe than elsewhere in the continent will be able to be assessed when larger series accumulate from other European cancer registries.

In most of northern and eastern Europe, the incidence of Burkitt's lymphoma was between 0.1 and 1 per million (Parkin *et al.*, 1988a). The exception was Denmark, where the rate was 2.8 per million in 1978–82 (Parkin *et al.*, 1988a) and still appeared to be high in 1983–90 (European Network of Cancer Registries, 1995). It is possible that this may be due to international variations in histopathological practice (Storm, personal communication). In North America, Australia, New Zealand and eastern Asia, Burkitt's lymphoma is rare.

Geographical variations are apparent in the primary sites at which Burkitt's lymphomas arise (Stiller & Parkin, 1990a). In the high-risk areas, the majority of cases occur in the head and neck. Abdominal tumours predominate in the areas of intermediate and low risk.

*Age-specific incidence and sex ratio*

In equatorial Africa, most cases of Burkitt's lymphoma occur in the 5–9-year age group (Stiller & Parkin, 1990a). In Ibadan, Nigeria, the age-specific incidence was 22.5 per million in children aged under 5, 136.0 per million at age 5–9 and 22.5 per million at age 10–14 years. In series in north Africa and western Asia, more cases were aged 1–4 years than 5–9 years.

Everywhere, Burkitt's lymphoma occurs more often in boys than girls (Stiller & Parkin, 1990a). In the areas of moderate and high risk, the sex ratio is between 1.5:1 and 2.5:1. The male excess is more pronounced in areas of low risk.

*Time trends*

Due to the difficulty in obtaining high-quality cancer registration data and accurate population counts in many parts of Africa and in developing countries elsewhere, there is relatively little information available with which to assess temporal patterns in Burkitt's lymphoma in the areas where the tumour is most common. In addition, many of the longest data series which have been reported derive from searches of hospital records or case-finding activities in the community, and the methods of ascertainment have changed over time.

Miller (1990) suggested that the incidence of the disease was decreasing in Uganda, Natal and New Guinea as a result of malaria eradication programs; however, no data were presented. In the North Mara district of Tanzania, cases of Burkitt's lymphoma during 1964–70 were identified from hospital and cancer registry records and from 1971 were sought by peripatetic field scouts (Brubaker *et al.*, 1973; Geser *et al.*, 1989). The all-ages[2] crude annual incidence rate fluctuated between 2.6 and 6.9 per 100 000 during 1964–76, with an average of 4.2 per 100 000. During 1977–83 incidence varied from 0.5 to 3.0 per 100 000 (average 1.3) and during 1984–87 from 2.5 to 7.1 per 100 000 (average 5.0). A malaria suppression intervention trial operated in the area from 1977–82 and it seems likely that at least part of the reduced incidence in the middle period can be attributed to distribution of chloroquine (Geser *et al.*, 1989).

[2] Rates for children were not reported separately but Burkitt's lymphoma is rare in persons older than 15 years.

In the Mengo Districts of Uganda, the all-ages crude annual incidence of Burkitt's lymphoma fell from an average of 1.03 per 100 000 during 1959–63 to 0.55 per 100 000 for 1964–68 (Morrow *et al.*, 1976). This did not seem to be an artefact of less rigorous case ascertainment, as it was believed that the overall level of completeness of the Kampala Cancer Registry, from which case details had been abstracted, had improved. The authors observed that the amount of chloroquine distributed through government health facilities and private dispensaries had increased greatly during the 1960s.

Among residents of Kyadondo, part of the Mengo Districts, the age-standardized annual incidence of Burkitt's lymphoma in children was estimated to be 7.3 per million during 1968–82 (Stiller & Parkin, 1990a). Figures from the re-established cancer registry indicate that the incidence was 27.0 for boys and 21.1 for girls for 1989–91 (Wabinga *et al.*, 1993). It was speculated that this high incidence could be due to increased prevalence and severity of malaria infection or a consequence of the evolution of AIDS in Uganda (Wabinga *et al.*, 1993).

In the West Nile area of Uganda, there was no evidence of a consistent trend, for either sex, in the incidence of Burkitt's lymphoma for the three periods 1961–65, 1966–70 and 1971–76 (Williams *et al.*, 1978; Siemiatycki *et al.*, 1980). Data are not available for more recent years.

Burkitt's lymphomas comprised three quarters of lymphomas in children in Papua New Guinea in 1967–71 (Wilkey, 1973). The comparable figure for 1979–83 was 55%, but Jamrozik *et al.* (1988) noted that cancer registration for 1979–83 was incomplete.

## Non-Hodgkin lymphoma

The comparison of incidence rates of childhood non-Hodgkin lymphoma either between populations or within populations over time is complicated by the close relationship between non-Hodgkin lymphoma and leukaemia (Weinstein & Tarbell, 1997). In addition, the earlier comments with regard to the classification of lymphoma types are relevant.

### Geographical patterns

Although there was seven-fold variation in the incidence of childhood non-Hodgkin lymphoma reported world-wide during 1970–79 (Parkin *et al.*, 1988a), few clear geographical patterns could be discerned. The three most extreme rates were observed in registries in central and south America (Fortaleza, Brazil 17.8 per million; São Paulo, Brazil 17.6; Cuba 14.5). However, elsewhere in the region the rates ranged from 4.4 to 8.4 per million per annum. In North America the incidence was typically around 3–7 per million, with the only consistent feature being higher incidence among white populations than black. In eastern Asia and most of Europe, rates were between 2 and 9 per million. However, in the western part of Asia, non-Hodgkin lymphoma appeared to be more common. In Israel and Kuwait, the incidence was at least 10 per million (Parkin *et al.*, 1988a) and non-Hodgkin lymphoma occurred relatively frequently in Iran and Turkey (Stiller & Parkin, 1990a). This area of moderately raised incidence in western Asia appears to stretch westwards into the Mediterranean countries of Europe and north Africa (Stiller & Parkin, 1990a) and broadly coincides with the zone of intermediate risk for Burkitt's lymphoma. Incidence of non-Hodgkin lymphoma in Zaragoza, Spain was 13.3 per million and the south-east of France and Corsica 8.7. In Tunisia, where leukaemias are not recorded, and Morocco, where they are, non-Hodgkin lymphoma accounted for 11% and 15% of all childhood neoplasms, respectively.

### Age-specific incidence and sex ratio

Stiller and Parkin (1990a) observed considerable international variation in the age–incidence curves for non-Hodgkin lymphoma. Few cases occur in infants anywhere. In the zone around the Mediterranean and into western Asia, the tumour appeared to be more common in children below age 10 years than in older children. In contrast, elsewhere the incidence rates were higher in children aged 5–14 than those aged 1–4 years.

The most consistent feature of the descriptive epidemiology of non-Hodgkin lymphoma is the marked male excess in incidence, with the sex ratio typically 2:1 or 3:1 (Stiller & Parkin, 1990a; Ajiki *et al.*, 1994; Stiller *et al.*, 1995; Gurney *et al.*, 1996a).

### Ethnic origin

There is relatively little information on ethnic patterns in non-Hodgkin lymphoma, and that which is available suggests that there is no substantial variation in risk among ethnic groups. In the areas of elevated risk in the Middle East, the relative risk for non-Jews compared to Jews was 0.88 and for non-Kuwaitis compared to Kuwaiti natives 1.31 (Table 2.1) (Parkin *et al.*, 1988a).

Powell *et al.* (1994) found a 90% higher age-standardized rate of non-Hodgkin lymphoma among children of Asian origin resident in the West Midlands of England than white children, but this result was not statistically significant. In a larger study in Britain, there was no evidence of different frequencies of non-Hodgkin lymphomas (including Burkitt's and unspecified lymphomas) among Asian, West Indian or white children (Table 2.2) (Stiller *et al.*, 1991a).

In Japanese male children in Hawaii, significantly fewer lymphomas of any type other than Hodgkin's disease were observed than would have been expected based on rates in white children in SEER registries (Goodman *et al.*, 1989). However, there was no reduced risk in Japanese girls.

There is a tendency towards lower rates in black US populations than white (Table 2.1). This holds for boys and girls, but without further evidence it is difficult to assess whether this could be due to ethnic differences in susceptibility, diagnostic bias, environmental factors or chance.

*Socioeconomic status*

Two overlapping ecological analyses of the incidence of non-Hodgkin and unspecified lymphomas in Britain during 1969–83 have been carried out and are summarized in Table 2.3 (Draper *et al.*, 1991a; Rodrigues *et al.*, 1991). Socioeconomic scores for County Districts for Britain as a whole (Draper *et al.*, 1991a), and census tracts for England and Wales (Rodrigues *et al.*, 1991), were derived from census variables and cases assigned to these according to their place of residence at the time of diagnosis. Neither analysis found any notable patterns in incidence with socioeconomic level by age group, period of diagnosis or in urban or rural areas.

*Time trends*

In most parts of the world where long series of high quality cancer registration data are available, the incidence of non-Hodgkin lymphoma in adults has been increasing steadily for many years (Coleman *et al.*, 1993). The situation for children is less clear.

Investigations in the USA (van Hoff *et al.*, 1988; Gurney *et al.*, 1996a), Italy (Mosso *et al.*, 1992), the Netherlands (Coebergh *et al.*, 1991) and Britain (Blair & Birch, 1994a) found no appreciable trend in incidence overall or by sex or age group. However, there have been three reports of increasing incidence. McWhirter and Petroeschevsky (1991) demonstrated a significant linear trend for boys, but not girls, aged 0–12 years

in Queensland, Australia between 1973 and 1988. Over that time, incidence of Hodgkin's disease fell while rates of ALL remained stable. In Osaka where, in the 1970s the incidence of non-Hodgkin lymphoma was substantially higher than elsewhere in Japan (Parkin *et al.*, 1988a), the age-standardized incidence rose from 4.0 per million in 1971–80 to 6.9 in 1981–88 (Ajiki *et al.*, 1994). The rise was statistically significant for both sexes. The rates of Hodgkin's disease were unchanged while incidence of ALL rose, although not significantly. In the Greater Delaware Valley area in the USA, incidence of non-Hodgkin lymphoma rose by an average of 2.9% per annum (95% CI 0.7–5.1) from 1970 to 1989 (Bunin *et al.*, 1996). The rates of other lymphomas and ALL did not change. Bunin *et al.* (1996) considered that AIDS, the effects of which account for part of the rising incidence in adults (Devesa & Fears, 1992), was unlikely to explain the temporal trend in children.

## Histiocytosis X

Based on the few series with reliable data, histiocytosis X is estimated to comprise 3% of all childhood cancers among white European populations (Stiller & Parkin, 1990a). The annual incidence is approximately 3 per million. Infants experience the highest rates and 3 boys are affected for every 2 girls.

## Clustering of lymphomas in space and time

Alexander *et al.* (1991a) analysed data on all childhood lymphomas in the Yorkshire Health Region, England, during the period 1974–86, using the test of Barnes *et al.* (1987) for between-area clustering, the local nearest neighbour area test (Cliff & Ord, 1981), and the Cuzick–Edwards method (Cuzick & Edwards, 1990). Evidence of clustering was found by the former two techniques, but not the third.

Several investigations of clustering in Hodgkin's disease and Burkitt's lymphoma have been carried out. These are summarized in Table 2.8.

*Hodgkin's disease*

In several analyses of Hodgkin's disease in which statistical evaluations of space–time clustering were made in populations unselected with regard to prior observations of clustering, no separate evaluation was made for the disease in children, because such cases are rare (Alderson & Nayak, 1971, 1972; Kryscio *et al.*, 1973). Data specific to children were considered in three analyses. The largest of these related to deaths in the USA in the period 1960–64 (Fraumeni & Li, 1969). This

## Table 2.8. Summary of analytical studies of clustering of childhood cancer other than leukaemia

| Study population, period of study | Incidence per 100000 | Sources of ascertainment | Method | Critical spaces (s) and time (t) | No. of cases | Time frame | Results | Reference | Comment |
|---|---|---|---|---|---|---|---|---|---|
| **Solid tumours** | | | | | | | | | |
| USA, Erie County, Buffalo city, 1943–56 | 105 | CR | Ridit | s: 1/8 mile–1 mile in steps of 1/8 mile, >1 mile; t: time between cases to nearest year | 144 aged 0–15 | Diagnosis or death | Significant clustering when cases <1/8 mile apart. | Pinkel et al., 1963 | Similar clustering was observed for pairs formed by leukaemia cases and solid tumour cases, but not for pairs formed by traffic fatalities, or when a traffic fatality was one member of a pair |
| **Cerebral tumour, neuroblastoma, nephroblastoma** | | | | | | | | | |
| UK, Worcestershire, Warwickshire, Staffordshire, Shropshire, 1953–60 | NS | CR | Knox | Not specified | 142 aged 0–9 | Birth | Excess when s = 3 km and t = 155 days | Morris, 1990 | Clustering was also identified for leukaemia when s=2 km and t=248 days |
| **Hodgkin's disease** | | | | | | | | | |
| USA, 1960–64 | – | DC | EMM | s: State (51); t: 1 year (5) | 359 aged 0–14 | Death | No clustering | Fraumeni & Li 1969 | |
| USA, Greater Boston, 1959–73 | – | H | Knox / Barton & David EMM | s: 0.5 km; t: 6 months; – ; s: 4.12 × 5.45 km (n = 36); t: 5 years (n = 3) | NS aged 0–14 | Diagnosis | No clustering | Greenberg et al., 1983 | The study included cases of ages up to 70 years; a total of 1398 cases was included in the analysis of clustering |
| UK, Greater Manchester, 1962–76 | 0.4 | CR | Knox | s: 0.5, 1.0, 2.0 km; t: 30, 60, 120, 240, 360, 720 days | 39 aged 0–14 | Onset | Significant clustering when s < 1.0 km and t < 721 days | Mangoud et al., 1985 | |
| **Burkitt's lymphoma** | | | | | | | | | |
| Uganda, West Nile District 1961–65 | 1.78 (1961–71) | H | Knox / David and Barton / Knox | Not specified | 36 | Onset | Clustering most marked within 180 days and 40 km; Significant clustering | Pike et al., 1967 | A total of 51 cases was ascertained; 36 had known address and date of onset |
| 1966–67 | | | | s: 1–10 km, in steps of 1 km | 29 | Onset | Significant clustering when s ≥ 5 km; less marked than in previous period | Williams et al., 1969 | |
| 1961–65 | 2.45 | H,CR | Knox | s: 2.5, 5, 10, 20, 40 km; t: 30, 60, 90, 120, 180, 360 days | 35 | Onset | Strong evidence of clustering | Williams et al., 1978 | |
| 1966–70 | | | | | 72 | | No clustering | | |
| 1971–75 | | | | | 81 | | No clustering | | |
| 1961–65 | 1.7/1.4[a] | H | Mantel | 24 combinations of time and space functions | 35 | Onset | Significant clustering with all functions | Siemiatycki et al., 1980 | Re-analysis of data of Williams et al. (1978) with addition of cases accrued in 1976 |
| 1966–70 | 3.2/1.9[a] | | | | 72 | | Clustering for 1/24 functions. Some "marginally significant" clustering | | |
| 1971–76 | 2.9/1.6[a] | | | | 91 | | | | |

| Location, period | Rate | Source | Method | Space/time parameters | No. of cases | Basis | Result | Reference | Comments |
|---|---|---|---|---|---|---|---|---|---|
| Uganda, East and West Mengo Districts 1959–68 | 0.82 | CR | Knox; Barton *et al.* | s: 2.5, 5, 10, 20, 40 km t: 30, 60, 90, 120, 180, 360 days; t: 5, 10, 15, 20, 25, 45, 60, 75, 120 and 180 days | 123 | Onset Diagnosis; Onset Diagnosis | No clustering | Morrow *et al.*, 1976 | Marked decline in incidence over a decade |
| Uganda, Lango and Acholi Districts 1963–68 | 1.87 | CR,H | Knox | s: 2.5,5,10,20, 40 km t: 30,60,90,120, 180,360 days | 82 | Onset | Nominally significant clustering when s=2.5 and t=180, but not considered significant in view of multiple testing | Morrow *et al.*, 1977 | A total of 98 cases was ascertained |
| Tanzania, North Mara District 1964–70 | 2.84 | H | Knox | s: 1,2,4,8,16, 32 km t: 7,14,30,60,90, 120,180 days | 39 | Onset Diagnosis | No clustering | Brubaker *et al.*, 1973 | |
| 1964–70 | 2.80 | H,CR | Mantel | 24 combinations of time and space functions | 40 | Onset | No clustering | Siemiatycki *et al.*, 1980 | Re-analysis of data of Brubaker *et al.* (1973) for 1964–70 period |
| 1971–77 | | | | | 40 | | | | |
| Ghana, Accra 1970–75 | 0.05–1.0 | CR | Knox (modified to take controls into account) | Not specified | 236 | Diagnosis | Suggestion of spatial clustering at 40 km for all time intervals considered | Biggar & Nkrumah, 1979 | |
| Malawi, northern, and central regions 1987–89 | up to 10.0 (Nkhotakota, 1988) | H | Knox | s: 2.5, 5, 10, 15, 20 km t: 10, 30, 60, 90, 180 days | 146; 72[d] | Onset; Onset | Significant clustering at less than 2.5 km and 60 days; Significant clustering for various units of space and time | Van den Bosch *et al.*, 1993a | There appeared to be a chain of cases along the lakeshore. Homes of cases were observed frequently to be in the vicinity of marshy ground and rivers |
| **Central nervous system tumours** | | | | | | | | | |
| UK, Yorkshire Health Region, 1974–86 | – | CR | NNA Cuzick–Edwards | s: enumeration district | 217 | Dg | No localized clustering | Alexander *et al.*, 1991a | Mapping points towards high risk along a particular band of the county |
| **Neuroblastoma** | | | | | | | | | |
| USA, 1960–64 | – | DC | EMM | s: State (51) t: 1 year (5) | 1362 | Death | No clustering | Miller *et al.*, 1968 | |
| USA, North Carolina, 1972–81 | 77.8 | H | EMM | s: Perinatal care region (6) t: 5 years (2) t: 5 years (3) | 85 | Diagnosis Birth | None Modest | Greenberg, 1983 | The space–time clustering for residence and date of birth was due to cases aged >2 years at diagnosis |

## Table 2.8. (contd) Summary of analytical studies of clustering of childhood cancer other than leukaemia

| Study population, period of study | Incidence per 100000 | Sources of ascertainment | Method | Critical spaces (s) and time (t) | No. of cases | Time frame | Results | Reference | Comment |
|---|---|---|---|---|---|---|---|---|---|
| **Retinoblastoma** USA, 1960–67 | – | DC | EMM | s: Division (9) t: 1 year (8) | 269 | Death | No clustering | Jensen & Miller, 1971 | |
| New Zealand, 1948–77 | 5.71 | OR,CR | $\chi^2$ KS | s: District (19) t: 1 year (30) t: 1 year (26) | 95[b] | Diagnosis Diagnosis Birth | No spatial clustering No temporal clustering | Suckling et al. 1982 | |
| **Rhabdomyosarcoma** USA, 1960–64 | – | DC | EMM | s: Division (9) t: 1 year (5) | 418 | Death | No clustering | Li & Fraumeni, 1969 | |
| USA, Gaston County, North Carolina, 1970–89 | 0.11 | CR,H | Combinational test for patchy time series | t: month, year 4-year period | 8 | Diagnosis | The investigators stated that the *p*-values calculated were invalid in the formal sense because the hypothesis was *post hoc*, but would serve to indicate to a concerned community that data had been examined critically | Grimson et al., 1992 | Study motivated by enquiry by father of a case after learning of two other local cases |
| **Bone cancer** USA, 1960–66 | – | DC | EMM | s: Division (9) t: 1 year (7) | 1532[c] | Death | Some clustering of osteogenic sarcoma (*n* = 620) in West North Central division, and of Ewing's sarcoma (*n* = 381) in the Pacific division | Glass & Fraumeni, 1970 | The deaths in the two divisions in which clustering was identified were rather widely scattered in space and seemed unrelated to one another |
| **Liver cancer** USA, 1960–64 | – | DC | EMM | s: Division (9) t: 1 year (5) | 282 | Death | No clustering | Fraumeni et al., 1968 | |

Sources of ascertainment: CR, cancer register; DC, death certificate; H, hospital records; OR, ophthalmology register. Method: EMM, Ederer–Myers–Mantel; KS, Kolmogorov–Smirnov test; NNA, nearest neighbour analysis.

[a] Incidence rates for boys and girls respectively.
[b] Sporadic cases.
[c] Children aged <15 years during 1960–66, and 15–19 years during 1965–66. No data for two states in 1965–66.
[d] Children aged eight years (median age) or more.

analysis could only detect large-scale clustering, as the smallest unit of area was the state, and the smallest unit of time was a year. No clustering was detected. In the other analyses, clustering was also assessed in young adults and older adults. Greenberg *et al.* (1983) reported that there was no significant clustering in children or at older ages, but that there was significant clustering in the 16–45-year age group. By contrast, Mangoud *et al.* (1985) found clustering in children at critical distances of <1 km and <721 days and detected significant clustering for older adults but not for the 15–44-year age group. The clustering in children was attributable to three girls who lived within 150 m of each other and attended hospital within 20 days of one another.

## Burkitt's lymphoma

Strong evidence of temporo-spatial clustering of Burkitt's lymphoma was found in the West Nile district of Uganda during the period 1961–65 (Pike *et al.*, 1967). This was also identified in subsequent re-analyses (Williams *et al.*, 1978; Siemiatycki *et al.*, 1980). However, less marked clustering was found in the period 1966–67 than in the earlier period (Williams *et al.*, 1969) and no clustering was found when the periods 1966–70 and 1971–75/6 were considered (Williams *et al.*, 1978; Siemiatycki *et al.*, 1980). It is noteworthy that in the initial period 1961–65, only 36 of a total of 51 cases ascertained were included; the address and/or date of onset were unknown for the remainder. Seasonal variation in the diagnosis, but not onset, of Burkitt's lymphoma in the West Nile district during the period 1961–65 was reported (Pike *et al.*, 1967). This seasonal variation in month of diagnosis continued in the area during the period 1966–69 (Williams *et al.*, 1974) and seasonal variation in onset was reported in the Mengo Districts of Uganda during the period 1959–68 (Morrow *et al.*, 1976), but not in the Lango and Acholi districts during the period 1963–68 (Morrow *et al.*, 1977). Greenberg and Shuster (1985) interpreted these data as suggesting that symptoms typically arise during the springtime, with excesses of diagnoses during the summer. They suggested the possibility that the observed seasonality may be attributable to seasonal variation in the access to care related to constraints upon transportation to medical facilities. Such a phenomenon would be likely to affect the detection of clustering. Biggar and Nkrumah (1979) attributed their finding of a suggestion of spatial clustering at 40 km for all time intervals considered, to the non-random referral from interested physicians to hospitals.

In Malawi, the peak period for admission of cases of Burkitt's lymphoma coincided with the end of the wettest period of the year, late December to March (van den Bosch *et al.*, 1993a). There was no difference in types of presentation at this time that might have been attributable to delayed referral of abdominal cases. There appeared to be a chain of cases along the shore of Lake Malawi, and the homes of cases were observed frequently to be in the vicinity of marshy ground and rivers. If the peak of admission were connected in some way with the rain and humidity, a co-factor associated with water might account for the onset of endemic Burkitt's lymphoma after a very short induction period. During the period of study (1987–89), an epidemic of Chikungunya fever, due to a mosquito-vectored arbovirus, occurred in Malawi. The authors suggested that this might have contributed to the observed clustering of cases.

# Group III: Central nervous system and miscellaneous intracranial and intraspinal neoplasms

Tumours of the central nervous system (CNS) are the second most frequent form of cancer in children in most populations (Parkin *et al.*, 1988b). They comprise between 17% and 25% of all neoplasms diagnosed in children in North America, most of Europe, Australia and among the non-Maori population of New Zealand (Parkin *et al.*, 1988a). Elsewhere in the Americas and in Asia, with the exception of Israel (18%) and Japan (20%), these tumours are less common, accounting for 8–15% of registrations. In most African populations during the 1970s, CNS tumours comprised a maximum of 5% of neoplasms (Parkin *et al.*, 1988a). This finding is repeated in more recent data from African population-based and clinical series (Obafunwa *et al.*, 1992; Wabinga *et al.*, 1993; Mukiibi *et al.*, 1995; Tijani *et al.*, 1995; Makata *et al.*, 1996). The exceptions to this pattern are Zimbabwe (Bulawayo) and Namibia, where the relative frequencies were 18% during 1963–77 and 17% during 1983–88 respectively (Parkin *et al.*, 1988a; Wessels & Hesseling, 1996). In these two areas, Burkitt's lymphomas were less common than elsewhere in the continent.

## Relative frequencies of histological types of central nervous system tumours

This group of neoplasms is composed of several distinct histological entities. Ependymomas, astrocytomas, medulloblastomas and other gliomas comprise the first four sub-categories. A fifth sub-category refers to miscellaneous intracranial and intraspinal neoplasms, and includes craniopharyngioma, meningioma and pineal tumours. In some recent series, in reflection of current pathological opinion (Kleihues *et al.*, 1993), the sub-category of medulloblastoma has been subsumed by primitive neuroectodermal tumours (PNET)[3] (Stiller *et al.*, 1995; Gurney *et al.*, 1996a). This modification is consolidated in the new International Classification of Childhood Cancer (Kramárová *et al.*, 1996).

It is difficult to draw firm conclusions on whether there are variations between populations or ethnic groups in the relative frequencies of the different types of CNS tumour. The large proportions of miscellaneous neoplasms and, specifically, tumours of unspecified type, in many series (Stiller & Nectoux, 1994) mandates cautious interpretation of the data. Of 494 CNS neoplasms diagnosed in Scotland during 1975–90, which had undergone thorough histo-pathological review, 9.9% were ependymomas, 42.3% astrocytomas, 27.1% medulloblastomas, 12.3% other gliomas and 8.3% miscellaneous neoplasms (McKinney *et al.*, 1994). In series in the USA, France and Australia, with at most 13% miscellaneous neoplasms, the frequency of ependymomas was 10–16%, astrocytomas 40–54%, medulloblastomas 19–24% and other gliomas 8–9% (Bernard *et al.*, 1993a; Giles *et al.*, 1995; Miller *et al.*, 1995).

Of the miscellaneous group of neoplasms, Stiller and Nectoux (1994) report that craniopharyngioma is most frequent, particularly in Africa, where it accounts for 12% of CNS tumours. In the 1970s, pineal tumours were more common in Japan than other populations (Stiller & Nectoux, 1994). This confirmed earlier observations (Koide *et al.*, 1980).

### Factors pertinent to the interpretation of geographical variations and time trends

Until recently, few studies had considered the epidemiological features of the different types of CNS tumour. The interpretation of geographical variations and time trends in these tumours is complicated by several factors. Firstly, in some populations, neurosurgical services were still scarce during the 1970s (Stiller & Nectoux, 1994), which is likely to have resulted in under-diagnosis of brain tumours. Secondly, there have been considerable advances in the technology for the diagnosis of CNS tumours with the introduction of computerized tomography in the 1970s and magnetic resonance imaging in the 1980s. These advances have the potential to improve the completeness of ascertainment and the accuracy of cancer registration and, therefore, to affect both the overall incidence rate of this group of tumours and the incidences of the individual tumour types. This technology is unlikely to have become widely available in different populations simultaneously, and therefore the effects on registration would have occurred at different times. Thirdly, it can be difficult to distinguish between malignant and benign tumours in some cases (Marsden, 1988). Therefore, some benign tumours may have been included in series of meningiomas, ependymomas and astrocytomas (Stiller & Nectoux, 1994). The proportions of these benign tumours are likely to vary between registries. Moreover, some registries, for example, the Danish Cancer Registry, collect data on CNS tumours which are explicitly stated to be benign and these may be included in reported data (e.g., Stevens *et al.*, 1991; Martos *et al.*, 1993). Finally, the histological classification of childhood brain tumours has changed substantially over time (Heidemann *et al.*, 1993) and continues to evolve (Kramárová *et al.*, 1996). The use of different classifications makes it difficult to compare the results of studies.

### Geographical patterns

The combined annual age-standardized incidence of CNS tumours in the three African registries in the international study of childhood cancer for which incidence could be computed was 11.2 per million, the lowest rate worldwide (Stiller & Nectoux, 1994). Rates of less than 20 per million were also observed in Chinese populations, India, central and South America, Canada and Germany during 1970–79 (Stiller & Nectoux, 1994). The relatively low incidence in Germany compared with the rest of western Europe is probably due to under-reporting of these tumours in the national registry of childhood tumours (Kaatsch *et al.*, 1995). In Canada, the apparently low rate is likely to be partly due to the fact that three registries in the Atlantic provinces record only malignant CNS neoplasms (Nimmagadda *et al.*, 1988). Incidence rates of between 20 and 30 per million were reported in Japan, most of Europe, Australia, New Zealand and the USA (Stiller & Nectoux, 1994). The highest rates were observed in the Nordic countries, where the combined incidence was 31.4 per million (Stiller & Nectoux, 1994).

---

[3.] Medulloblastomas comprise the majority of PNET.

## Ependymoma

In the countries of central and South America and Asia, the annual incidence of ependymoma was generally less than 2 per million (Parkin *et al.*, 1988a). Rates between 2 and 4 per million were observed in North America, Oceania and most of Europe. In Denmark, Sweden, Finland, the former East Germany and Slovenia, the incidence was at least 4 per million.

## Astrocytoma

The lowest rates of astrocytoma were observed in Hong Kong (2.5 per million) and Shanghai, China (2.7) (Parkin *et al.*, 1988a). In other parts of Asia, the incidence was always below 5 per million, with the exception of the Jewish population in Israel, in which the rate was 8 per million. There was considerable variation in the rates observed in central and South America, ranging from 3.3 per million in Cuba to 9.2 in Puerto Rico. The highest rates, in excess of 10 per million were observed in the white populations of the USA, Australia, France and the Nordic countries.

## Medulloblastoma

This tumour has a similar geographical distribution to those for ependymoma and astrocytoma. Rates of at least 5 per million were seen in Oceania, North America, western and northern Europe (Parkin *et al.*, 1988a). In Asia and central and South America, the incidence was generally between 2 and 4 per million.

## *Age-specific incidence and sex ratio*

In Europe, the USA and Japan, the incidence of all CNS tumours in infants falls in the range 24 to 27 per million (de Nully Brown *et al.*, 1989; Mosso *et al.*, 1992; Ajiki *et al.*, 1994; Stiller *et al.*, 1995; Gurney *et al.*, 1996a). The rate is a little higher for children aged 1–5 years (30–36 per million) and declines slightly in older age groups (26–34 for children aged 5–9 and 23–29 in the 10–14-year age group).

The age distributions of the main types of tumour vary. In Scotland, during 1975–90, 8% of ependymomas were diagnosed in infants, 51% in the 1–4-year age group, 10% in those aged 5–9 and 31% in those aged 10–14 (McKinney *et al.*, 1994). The comparable figures for astrocytoma were 5%, 30%, 34% and 32% and for medulloblastoma were 3%, 29%, 40% and 28%. This propensity of ependymomas to occur in younger children is demonstrated in other series in Britain and the USA (Stevens *et al.*, 1991; Blair & Birch, 1994b; Gurney *et al.*, 1996a).

More boys are affected with CNS tumours than girls in most populations. The sex ratio is approximately 1.2:1 (Parkin *et al.*, 1988a). The ratio for astrocytoma is similar (Stiller & Nectoux, 1994). A moderate male excess of ependymoma is also evident: the sex ratio is between 1.1:1 and 1.7:1 (Parkin *et al.*, 1988a). The data on medulloblastoma are consistent with a sex ratio of 2:1 (Stiller & Nectoux, 1994).

## *Ethnic origin*

In Britain, two studies of childhood cancer among ethnic groups in Britain have reported a moderately lower risk of CNS tumours among Asian children, most of whom originate from the Indian sub-continent, than white children (Table 2.2) (Stiller *et al.*, 1991a; Powell *et al.*, 1994). One further British study has suggested that these tumours are relatively less common among Asians than non-Asians (Muir *et al.*, 1992). However, the results were not statistically significant in any of the three studies. Two of the analyses were based on relative frequencies (Stiller *et al.*, 1991a; Muir *et al.*, 1992) and, in the other, it is likely that the Asian population was underestimated (Powell *et al.*, 1994). In addition, one study was based on a large clinical register in which children with CNS tumours are known to be under-represented (Stiller *et al.*, 1991a) and the three study data-sets were not independent (Powell *et al.*, 1994). However, the observed deficits of CNS among Asians in Britain are consistent with the lower rates in the countries of southern Asia than in the mainly white populations of western Europe (Parkin *et al.*, 1988a).

In New Mexico, during 1970–82, the relative risk of a tumour of the CNS was 0.5 (95% CI 0.3–0.9) for Hispanic boys and 0.7 (0.4–1.2) for Hispanic girls compared with white SEER populations (Duncan *et al.*, 1986). This is probably due, in part, to the lower incidence of glial neoplasms in the New Mexico population than in US whites (Breslow & Langholz, 1983). In 1973–77, the numbers of glial tumours and medulloblastomas in Puerto Rico were 51% and 75% lower than expected on the basis of incidence in US whites (Breslow & Langholz, 1983). Comparison of the age-standardized incidence rates among Hispanic and other white children in Los Angeles yields rate ratios of 0.8 for both sexes (Parkin *et al.*, 1988a). Again this is consistent with the moderately lower rates in central and South America than among whites in the USA (Parkin *et al.*, 1988a).

Also in the USA, the incidence of CNS tumours in white populations is 22% higher than in black populations (26.4 per million for whites compared with 21.7 for blacks) (Stiller & Nectoux, 1994). For West Indian children in Britain, the risk of CNS neoplasms was half of that for white children (Table 2.2), although this analysis included only four cases in West Indian children (Stiller *et al.*, 1991a). In African populations for which incidence is available, the rates are generally low (Parkin *et al.*, 1988b; Wabinga *et al.*, 1993; Mukiibi *et al.*, 1995).

In summary, there is limited evidence of ethnic variations in the risk of CNS tumours in children, consistent with higher risk in white than in non-white populations. This conclusion, taken in conjunction with observations of familial aggregations of CNS tumours and their occurrence in several genetically determined disorders (Kuijten & Bunin, 1993; for further comment, see Chapter 3), has led to speculation that genetic predisposition may play a dominant role in the etiology of these neoplasms (Stiller & Nectoux, 1994).

## Socioeconomic status

Socioeconomic status has been relatively little studied with regard to childhood CNS tumours. In Scotland, McKinney *et al.* (1994) demonstrated a statistically significant inverse trend in risk associated with residence in areas with increasing levels of deprivation. The incidence among those resident in the least deprived areas was 37% higher than that for those in the most deprived areas (Table 2.3). This finding arose from an ecological analysis which ascribed the characteristics of an area to individuals resident within that area. The cases analysed had been ascertained by cross-checking cancer registry records with several other data sources and had undergone rigorous validation. It seems unlikely, therefore, that the association was an artefact of differential levels of ascertainment in deprived and more affluent areas. In addition, the comprehensive nature of the National Health Service in the UK would imply that the finding is unlikely to be a result of diagnostic bias.

Results from two studies are in accord with the finding in Scotland. Basing socioeconomic status on paternal occupation, as stated on the death certificates of children dying from brain neoplasms during 1959–63 and 1970–72 in England and Wales, Sanders *et al.* (1981) reported proportional mortality ratios of 137 and 130 associated with professional or managerial jobs (Table 2.3). Both mothers and fathers of children with astrocytoma participating in a case–control study in New Jersey and Delaware, USA, were

more likely than parents of control children to have completed college or graduate school (Kuijten *et al.*, 1992). In contrast, in a case–control study of brain tumours in Ontario, Canada, parental high school education was associated with a significant reduction in risk (Howe *et al.*, 1989). In addition, in two studies in the USA, parents of cases tended to be less highly educated than parents of controls (Wilkins & Sinks, 1990; Norman *et al.*, 1996) and in another, more cases than controls were from lower-income households (Bunin *et al.*, 1994b). However, in these three studies, controls were selected by random-digit dialling, which can result in controls of higher socioeconomic status relative to the source population than cases (see Chapter 1). In a recent population-based case–control study in Australia, increased risk was also associated with longer parental education, but the control mothers who were interviewed were of a higher social class than control mothers who were approached and refused to participate (McCredie *et al.*, 1994a). Two further case–control studies, both with controls selected from population registers, found no significant association between years of parental education and risk of CNS tumours in children (Nasca *et al.*, 1988; Cordier *et al.*, 1994).

The potential contribution of socioeconomic factors in the causation of these malignancies remains to be clarified.

## Time trends

On the basis of data abstracted from the first four volumes of *Cancer Incidence in Five Continents*, Breslow and Langholz (1983) observed that the incidence of brain and CNS tumours had increased substantially over the period from the late 1950s to mid-1970s in a number of regions, but remarked that this could reflect changes in pathological diagnosis or reporting practices. An upward trend is evident in more recent data in most series in Europe, the USA, Japan and Australia (de Nully Brown, 1989; Mosso *et al.*, 1992; Ajiki *et al.*, 1994; Blair & Birch, 1994b; Draper *et al.*, 1994; McKinney *et al.*, 1994; Giles *et al.*, 1995; Bunin *et al.*, 1996; Gurney *et al.*, 1996a). In Britain, for example, over the period 1962–91, significant increases in CNS tumours were observed in all childhood age groups. The estimated annual percentage increase in incidence in infants was 2.1% and in older age groups 0.6% (Draper *et al.*, 1994). However, the authors noted that the level of ascertainment of childhood cancer had increased over time. The situation reflects that for adult brain tumours, the recorded incidence of which is increasing worldwide (Desmeules *et al.*, 1992; Coleman *et al.*, 1993), in that it is not clear to what extent the observed rises are an artefact of diagnostic advances leading to improved ascertainment.

In some areas of Britain, secular trends have been investigated for specified tumours. The average annual increase in all CNS neoplasms in Scotland during 1975–90 was 2.6% (95% CI 0.3–4.9) (McKinney *et al.*, 1994). Although this trend was evident for the four main histological types, it was statistically significant only for medulloblastoma, which increased by 3.4% per annum (0.3–6.6). This finding conflicts with a report of declining rates of medulloblastoma in the south-west and north of England: in these regions incidence fell from 5.5 in 1976–84 to 2.8 in 1985–91 (*p* = 0.006) (Thorne *et al.*, 1994). In a detailed analysis of data from the Manchester Children's Tumour Registry for the period 1954–88, significant increases were observed in the incidence rates of medulloblastoma, particularly for girls, astrocytoma of the juvenile type for boys and a miscellaneous group of intracranial and intraspinal neoplasms (Blair & Birch, 1994b). There was no evidence of changes in the incidence of ependymoma, astrocytoma of the adult type, craniopharyngioma or meningioma, although some of these analyses included relatively few cases (Blair & Birch, 1994b). The authors argued that divergent temporal patterns between the sexes imply that the observed increases in incidence cannot be explained entirely by improved surgical or radiological techniques.

In the Greater Delaware Valley area in the USA, the incidence of all CNS tumours rose by 2.7% per annum (95% CI 1.6–3.8) over the years 1970 to 1989 (Bunin *et al.*, 1996). Increases were apparent in all three tumour sub-groups considered, namely glioma, PNET/medulloblastoma and other tumours. However, when the data were examined by ethnic group, sex and age, divergent trends became apparent. The increases in glioma were limited to white males (annual percentage change +3.6% (95% CI 1.7–5.5) and white females aged 0–4 years (+6.2% (95% CI 2.8–9.9)). No change in incidence among blacks was evident. For whites, the rate of PNET/medulloblastoma increased by 4.3% per annum (95% CI 1.8–6.8), while for blacks, incidence fell by 4.6% per annum (95% CI –10.1, 1.1). In an analysis of SEER data for 1974–91, the rates of PNET in blacks decreased by an average of 2.8% per annum, while those for whites showed little change (+0.8% per annum) (Gurney *et al.*, 1996a). Neither of these results

reached statistical significance. In contrast to the finding of Bunin *et al.* (1996), in this data-set, significant increases in astroglial tumours were evident for both blacks and whites. Age- and sex-specific analyses revealed annual increases in astroglial tumours which were most pronounced among children aged 3 and younger. Increases in ependymoma were observed only for the 0–4-year age group. It was suggested that the disparate trends in PNET and astroglial tumours, which are usually diagnosed with the same type of imaging equipment, support the hypothesis that factors other than changing diagnostic practice are contributing to these trends (Gurney *et al.*, 1996a). No explanations are obvious for the different patterns among black and white children.

## Group IV : Sympathetic and allied nervous system tumours

The category of sympathetic and nervous system tumours encompasses neuroblastoma and ganglioneuroblastoma and other sympathetic nervous system tumours. Neuroblastoma and ganglioneuroblastoma account for at least 96% of these tumours (de Nully Brown *et al.*, 1989; Ajiki *et al.*, 1994; Miller *et al.*, 1995; Stiller *et al.*, 1995). In the only large series which has reported neuroblastoma and ganglioneuroblastoma separately (the USA SEER data-set for 1973 to 1987), neuroblastoma was five times as frequent as ganglioneuroblastoma (Miller *et al.*, 1995). The majority of the other sympathetic nervous system tumours are peripheral neuroectodermal tumours (Stiller *et al.*, 1995).

### *Neuroblastoma*

Neuroblastoma and ganglioneuroblastoma tend to be considered together under the heading 'neuroblastoma'. Together they constitute the most frequent individual type of solid tumour and can occur at many sites in the body. The most common primary site is the adrenal gland (Green *et al.*, 1997).

#### *Geographical patterns*

Between 6% and 10% of all tumours diagnosed in children in Europe, North America and Australia are neuroblastomas (Parkin *et al.*, 1988a). Among most of the populations of eastern Asia, with the exception of Japan, they occur somewhat less frequently (Parkin *et al.*, 1988a; Ajiki *et al.*, 1994; Nandakumar *et al.*, 1996; Sriamporn *et al.*, 1996). Several reports have suggested that neuroblastoma is rare in most of tropical Africa (Massabi *et al.*, 1989; Lucas & Fischer, 1990; Miller,

1989; Mukiibi *et al.*, 1995; Obafunwa *et al.*, 1992; Tijani *et al.*, 1995; Makata *et al.*, 1996). However, this finding should be interpreted with caution as (i) reliable population-based incidence rates are not available for most of these populations; (ii) studies reporting relative frequencies of a particular tumour are influenced by the occurrence of other tumour types (in these series the substantial contribution of Burkitt's lymphoma); and (iii) difficulties can be experienced with clinical diagnosis of neuroblastoma (Aikhionbare *et al.*, 1988), a problem exacerbated by the late stage diagnosis and poor prognosis of most cases (Green *et al.*, 1997) and leading, potentially, to under-ascertainment. In the three African series for which incidence rates are available, the annual age-standardized rate of neuroblastoma was 1.1 per million in Uganda (Kampala), 6.0 in Nigeria (Ibadan) and 8.0 in Zimbabwe (Bulawayo) (Stiller & Parkin, 1992). These figures pertained to the time periods 1968–82, 1960–69 and 1963–77, respectively, and were each based on fewer than 12 cases. Parkin *et al.* (1988b) concluded that while there did appear to be low incidence of neuroblastoma in African populations, it was impossible to determine whether this was of etiological significance or a consequence of diagnostic difficulties.

Elsewhere in the world, during the 1970s, rates below 6 per million were reported by registries in central America, among the Hispanic population of Los Angeles and in parts of eastern Asia (Parkin *et al.*, 1988a). In most of western and northern Europe and Australia the incidence varied between 7 and 10 per million (Parkin *et al.*, 1988a). The rates in the black populations of the USA and in Japan also fell in this range (Stiller & Parkin, 1992). Rates in excess of 11 per million were experienced by white populations in the USA, Israeli Jews, New Zealand Maoris and in France and Italy.

### Age-specific incidence and sex ratio

Neuroblastoma is predominantly a tumour of very young children. 80% of cases present in children aged under five years, 15% in the 5–9 age group and 5% in those 10 and older (Stiller, 1993b). During the 1970s, in most populations, the rate of neuroblastoma in infants under one year was between 25 and 50 per million, in the 1–4-year age group was in the range 15–20 per million, in the 5–9-year age group between 2–4 per million and in the 10–14-year age group 1–1.5 per million (Stiller & Parkin, 1992). In the 0–5-year age group, the incidence is highest in infants and declines steadily year on year (Stiller, 1993b).

Data from the Manchester Children's Tumour Registry suggest that during the 1950s significantly fewer boys than girls were diagnosed with neuroblastoma (RR = 0.6, 95% CI 0.33–0.93) whereas, by the 1980s, the situation had reversed (RR = 1.3, 0.80–2.13) (Blair & Birch, 1994b). Internationally, in the 1970s, the sex ratio of boys to girls was around 1.3:1 (Parkin *et al.*, 1988a).

### Ethnic origin

During the 1970s, the age-standardized incidence of neuroblastoma among black children in the USA was on average 26% lower than that for white children (Table 2.1) (Stiller & Parkin, 1992). This confirmed earlier reports of a reduced risk in Afro-Americans (Breslow & Langholz, 1983; Davis *et al.*, 1987). However, other evidence on ethnic variations in risk of neuroblastoma is inconsistent. In the West Midlands area of England, the tumour was reported to be rare in children of Afro-Caribbean extraction (Muir *et al.*, 1990a). However, this finding was not confirmed in a more comprehensive study of childhood cancer and ethnic group in Britain (Stiller *et al.*, 1991a). In this analysis, summarized in Table 2.2, neuroblastoma was 1.8 times as frequent in children of West Indian origin than white children, although this result was based on only 8 cases among West Indian children and was not statistically significant. In the same study there was no difference in the relative frequencies of neuroblastoma in Asian and white children.

In a combined group of non-white children in the USA, including native American, Chinese, Japanese, Filipino and Hawaiian children, the incidence of neuroblastoma in children under five years was 15.7 per million (9 cases), compared with 24.2 (170 cases) in white children (Davis *et al.*, 1987). The observed numbers of neuroblastomas diagnosed in New Mexico during 1970–82 among non-Hispanic white, Hispanic and American Indian children were each lower than would have been expected based on the incidence in white children elsewhere in the USA, but again these analyses included small numbers of cases (Duncan *et al.*, 1986). In Hawaii, from 1960 to 1984, there were no systematic differences in observed numbers of sympathetic nervous system tumours in the white, Japanese, Filipino, Hawaiian and Chinese ethnic groups compared with numbers expected based on the white SEER population (Goodman *et al.*, 1989). In conclusion, with the exception of the suggestion of modestly lowered risk among blacks in the USA compared with whites, there is only very limited evidence of within-population ethnic variations in risk of neuroblastoma.

## Socioeconomic status

Studies in two locations have suggested that neuroblastoma may be associated with lower socioeconomic status (Table 2.3). In Denmark, a lower crude incidence was observed among children of self-employed parents (annual rate 4.2 per million) than children of manual workers (6.5). This relationship held for both infants and older children (Carlsen, 1996). However, there was no clear trend in incidence by socioeconomic group; the incidence among children of salaried employees was 8.8 per million (Carlsen, 1986). An ecological analysis in the USA found a significant inverse trend in incidence according to county-level per capita income (Davis *et al.*, 1987). These associations, and the generally lower socioeconomic position of the black population in the USA, led Stiller and Parkin (1992) to postulate that, while blacks could have a weaker genetic predisposition to neuroblastoma, their low average social class acts to increase risk and thus results in rates among black US populations which are only moderately lower than those for white populations.

## Time trends

Information on the incidence of neuroblastoma is available from the 1930s (van Hoff *et al.*, 1988). However, some of the older data for this tumour should be interpreted with caution. Since neuroblastomas occur at a number of primary sites, accurate incidence figures can only be obtained from series which are classified by histology rather than anatomical site. It is likely that the frequency with which tumours were investigated histologically has changed over time. Methods of diagnosis have improved (Marsden & Steward, 1968) and classification of tumour types has become more accurate (Stiller, 1993b). These changes could have influenced the recorded incidence of neuroblastoma. In addition, in Japan experimental screening for neuroblastoma, based on measuring urinary levels of catecholamine metabolites in children at around six months of age, started in the 1970s and a national programme was introduced in 1985 (Chamberlain, 1996). Population-based screening trials are planned or under way in North America and Europe (Stiller, 1993b). Such screening, if effective, would be expected to lead to an increase in the disease incidence in infants, as a result of earlier diagnosis. It has been suggested that some of the tumours detected by screening are biologically

benign and may never have presented clinically (Bessho *et al.*, 1991).

While bearing these comments in mind, there is considerable evidence of a persistent increase in the incidence of neuroblastoma, apparent both in the longest data series and in data-sets from the 1970s and 1980s. In an analysis of data from the Connecticut Cancer Registry for the period 1935–79, statistically significant increases in the incidence of neuroblastoma in both boys and girls aged under five years were found (van Hoff *et al.*, 1988). Incidence rose by an estimated 14% in boys ($p<0.01$) and 19% in girls ($p<0.001$) per quinquennium. During 1935–39, 69% of all cancers in persons aged 0–19 years included in the study were histologically confirmed; for 1940–44 this was 75% and for the remainder of the study period, 90%. In Denmark, a review of death certificates and hospital records was conducted to ascertain definite or probable cases of neuroblastomas occurring during 1943 to 1980 (Carlsen, 1986). Incidence rose steadily throughout this period, accounted for solely by an increase in children under five years and which was most pronounced in infants. The rate in infants grew from 7.0 per million during 1946–50 to 18.2 in 1956–60, 33.0 in 1966–70 and 51.3 during 1976–80. Modelling of data from the Manchester Children's Tumour Registry revealed a continual increase in the incidence of neuroblastoma during the period 1954–88 (Blair & Birch, 1994b). This was apparent, and statistically significant, only for girls and represented a 17% increase in incidence per quinquennium. In this registry, the overwhelming majority of solid tumours undergo panel review of pathological material to optimize diagnostic accuracy (Birch, 1988).

Elsewhere in the USA and western Europe, similar rises in incidence have been documented. Bunin *et al.* (1996) demonstrated an annual percentage increase in neuroblastoma of 1.9% (95% CI 0.0–3.7) for the Greater Delaware Valley area. In the SEER data-set, a significant average annual percentage change in incidence of +3.1% (95% CI 0.9–5.2) for infants during 1974 to 1991 was apparent (Gurney *et al.*, 1996a). However, in the 1–2- and 2–3-year age groups, incidence fell year upon year. In Sweden, significant increases in both sexes for the 0–14-year age group were found over the period 1958 to 1974 (Ericsson *et al.*, 1978). In Turin, Italy, a 49% increase in the age-standardized incidence of neuroblastoma between 1970–75 and 1976–81 and a 14% increase from 1976–81 to 1982–86 were described (Mosso *et al.*, 1992). Bernard *et al.* (1993b) reported that the incidence of neuroblastoma in south-east France during 1984–91 was 15.5 per million. This compared with the incidence of 12.9 for the same registries during 1983–85 (Parkin *et al.*, 1988a). Comparing neuroblastoma incidence for all England, Wales and Scotland for the periods 1971–75 and 1986–90, Stiller (1993b) found a 26% increase for children of all ages; among infants and children aged 1–9 years the incidence rose by 36% and among older children it fell by 70%. Longer-term analysis of the British data suggests a pattern of decreasing incidence for children born from 1962 to 1973, followed by a steady increase (Draper *et al.*, 1994). No upward trend has been observed in Australia (McWhirter & Petroeschevsky, 1991; Giles *et al.*, 1995).

It is possible that the early increase in neuroblastoma incidence could be, in part, an artefact of improvements in diagnosis resulting from the measurement of catecholamine levels. However, the use of this technique was widespread by the early 1970s (Marsden & Steward, 1968) and cannot explain the increase which has continued more recently. The patterns observed in the SEER data, of a rising incidence in infants in parallel with falling rates in children aged 2–4 years, is consistent with a trend towards earlier detection. But screening is not systematically practised in the populations contributing to this program (Woods *et al.*, 1996). Moreover, the observed association between neuroblastoma and lower socio-economic status (Carlsen, 1986, 1996; Davis *et al.*, 1987) suggests that incidence should be falling rather than rising in a time of improving living standards (Stiller, 1993b). To date, no plausible explanation of the growing burden of neuroblastoma has been proposed.

## Group V: Retinoblastoma

In Europe, North America and Australia, retinoblastoma accounts for 2–4% of neoplasms in children (Parkin *et al.*,1988a). The relative frequency is similar in Asia (Parkin *et al.*, 1988a; Ajiki *et al.*, 1994; Nandakumar *et al.*, 1996; Sriamporn *et al.*, 1996). In contrast, in African population-based and clinical series, retino-blastoma represents 10–15% of tumours (Parkin *et al.*, 1988a; Mukiibi *et al.*, 1995; Wessels & Hesseling, 1996).

A substantial proportion of cases of retinoblastoma is hereditary, arising through germ-line mutations in tumour-suppressor genes (see Chapter 3). From of a series of almost 1600 cases of retinoblastoma diagnosed in Britain between 1962 and 1985, it was estimated that

44% were hereditary (Draper *et al.*, 1992). This proportion agrees with those reported in other studies (Higginson *et al.*, 1992) and does not appear to have changed over time.

### Geographical patterns

The highest annual age-standardized incidence rates of retinoblastoma, in excess of 7 per million population, have been observed in the Fortaleza area of Brazil, Nigeria (Ibadan) and Uganda (Kampala) (Parkin *et al.*, 1988a). Data from the 1970s and more recent publications suggest that the incidence in most of Europe, North and South America, Oceania and Asia falls in the range 3–6 per million (de Nully Brown *et al.*, 1989; Drut *et al.*, 1990; Mosso *et al.*, 1992; Bernard *et al.*, 1993a; Ajiki *et al.*, 1994; Kaatsch *et al.*, 1995; Miller *et al.*, 1995; Stiller *et al.*, 1995; McWhirter *et al.*, 1996; Nandakumar *et al.*, 1996; Sriamporn *et al.*, 1996). Rates below 3 per million have been reported in China, Hungary, New York (both black and white populations) and the Atlantic Provinces of Canada (Parkin *et al.*, 1988a).

### Age-specific incidence and sex ratio

Retinoblastoma has the lowest median age of all childhood malignancies (approximately 15 months) (Kaatsch *et al.*, 1995) and bilateral cases tend to be diagnosed at a younger age than unilateral cases (Draper *et al.*, 1992). Incidence peaks in the first year of life, at between 18 and 26 per million, and declines gradually with age thereafter (de Nully Brown *et al.*, 1989; Kaatsch *et al.*, 1995; Stiller *et al.*, 1995; Gurney *et al.*, 1996a; McWhirter *et al.*, 1996). The tumour is extremely uncommon in children aged 10 and over. On the basis of data from the Manchester Children's Tumour Registry, UK, for 1954–88, the relative risk of retinoblastoma in those aged 1–4 years compared with those under one year was 0.39 (95% CI 0.26–0.58), in those aged 5–9 years compared with those under 1 was 0.03 (95% CI 0.01–0.07) and in those aged 10–14 years is 0 (Blair & Birch, 1994b). The male to female ratio fluctuates around unity (Parkin *et al.*, 1988a).

### Ethnic origin

The relative frequency of retinoblastoma is at least as high among the black populations of the United States as the white (Table 2.1), although the tumour occurs less frequently in these black populations than in Africa (Parkin *et al.*, 1988a; Miller *et al.*, 1995). Analysis of data from the SEER program in the United States for 1974 to 1991 indicated a slightly higher incidence of retinoblastoma among black children than white: the incidence rates (standardized to the

US 1980 standard population) were 4.3 and 3.7 per million for black and white children, respectively (Gurney *et al.*, 1996a). However, in the New York registry area there was little difference in incidence among the black and white populations (Parkin *et al.*, 1988a). In a nationwide study of 269 death certificates for American children with retinoblastoma from 1960–67, the mortality rate for black children was 2.2 times that for white children (Jensen & Miller, 1971). However, it was impossible to distinguish whether the excess of deaths among black children reflected a greater risk of the disease, or the same risk as experienced by white children but increased mortality due to factors related to diagnosis and/or therapy.

In a study conducted in the West Midlands area of England, cases of retinoblastoma diagnosed during 1982–92 were categorized by ethnic group. The standardized rate ratio for the group designated as Asian (of Indian, Pakistani or Bangladeshi origin) compared with those categorized as white was 2.14 (95% CI 0.77–5.90) (Powell *et al.*, 1994). This analysis was based on 8 and 33 cases in the Asian and white groups respectively. An investigation of childhood cancer and ethnic group based on the data of the UK Children's Cancer Study Group, which includes two thirds of all childhood cancers diagnosed in Britain since 1981, considered 196 children with retinoblastoma (Stiller *et al.*, 1991a). In the relative frequency analysis, the relative risk of retinoblastoma of any type among Asian (Indian sub-continent) children compared with "Caucasians" was estimated to be 1.23 (Table 2.2), and the relative risk of unilateral retinoblastoma was 1.86. Again the number of Asian cases was small.

In combination, the results of these analyses suggest a small increased risk of retinoblastoma in the black population in the United States and the Asian population in Britain.

*Laterality*

Ethnic differences in the frequencies of unilateral and bilateral retinoblastoma are apparent. In the series of cases in Britain, the overwhelming majority of which would have been in white children, 40% of retinoblastomas occurred bilaterally and 90% of the hereditary cases were bilateral (Draper *et al.*, 1992). In two, relatively small, African series in which laterality was reported, no bilateral cases were observed (Obafunwa *et al.*, 1992; Tijani *et al.*, 1995). In addition, in the Asian population of Britain, less than one quarter of cases were bilateral (Stiller *et al.*, 1991a). This is consistent with the low frequencies of bilateral retinoblastoma described in those registries in Asia which were included in the international study of childhood cancer and for which laterality was recorded for the majority of cases (Parkin *et al.*, 1988a).

## Time trends

There is little evidence of any significant change in the incidence of retinoblastoma over time. Analyses of trends from 1954 to 1988 in Britain showed no consistent temporal pattern by year of diagnosis (Blair & Birch, 1994b). In accord with this, Sanders *et al.* (1988) found no trend by year of birth in incidence in children aged 0–4 years during 1962 to 1975 in Britain. Similarly, data from Queensland and Victoria, Australia (McWhirter & Petroeschevsky, 1991; Giles *et al.*, 1995) and the Turin Province, Italy (Mosso *et al.*, 1992) do not indicate any regular time trends. In the USA, a rise in retinoblastoma incidence from 1974 to 1991 has been described (Gurney *et al.*, 1996a). This was most pronounced in infants aged under one year at diagnosis (average annual percentage change +5.4%). However, there was a concomitant fall in incidence in children aged 1–2 years (average annual percentage change –2.1%) The same age-specific time trends have been observed in data from 1970 to 1989 for the Greater Delaware Valley Paedatric Tumour registry in the USA (Bunin *et al.*, 1996) and suggest that the increasing incidence in infants is explained, at least in part, by a shift towards earlier diagnosis.

## Group VI: Renal tumours

In most populations in Europe and Australia and among white Americans, renal tumours represent approximately 5–6% of all cancers diagnosed in children (Parkin *et al.*, 1988a). In central and South America and Asia, the frequency is slightly lower (Parkin *et al.*, 1988a; Ajiki *et al.*, 1994; Sriamporn *et al.*, 1996). In contrast, among US black populations and in African case series, around 10% of tumours arise in the kidney (Parkin *et al.*, 1988a; Miller *et al.*, 1995; Obafunwa *et al.*, 1995; Wessels & Hesseling, 1996). In almost all populations, the relative frequency in girls exceeds that in boys.

Wilms' tumour, or nephroblastoma, is an embryonal malignancy which arises from remnants of immature kidney. It comprises approximately 95% of all renal neoplasms (Kaatsch *et al.*, 1995; Miller *et al.*, 1995; Stiller *et al.*, 1995). The remainder are renal carcinomas and other and unspecified renal tumours.

## Wilms' tumour
### Geographical patterns

Wilms' tumour was originally proposed as an 'index tumour' of childhood which could serve to gauge quality of case ascertainment on the grounds that it was thought to have almost constant incidence throughout the world (Innis, 1972). However, it is now clear that there is considerable international variation in the incidence of this neoplasm. During the 1970s, the lowest annual rates, below 2 per million population, occurred in Taipei, Taiwan and Kanagawa, Japan (Parkin *et al.*, 1988a). Incidences in the range 2–4 per million have been reported for other east Asian and Indian registries in the 1970s and more recently (Parkin *et al.*, 1988a; Ajiki *et al.*, 1994; Nandakumar *et al.*, 1996; Sriamporn *et al.*, 1996). The incidence among Asian-Americans is also in this range (Breslow *et al.*, 1994). Intermediate incidence rates, varying between 6 and 9 per million, have been observed in the mainly white populations of Europe, North and South America and Oceania (Parkin *et al.*, 1988a). The highest documented rates are among the non-white population of Greater Delaware Valley, USA (13.7 per million), the black population of Los Angeles (11.8) and the SEER black population (11.1).

Few population-based data are available for Africa on which to base incidence calculations. For the three registries for which incidence was available in the international study of childhood cancer, tumours classified as Wilms' were considered together with renal tumours of unspecified type on the basis that the majority of this latter group were without histological investigation and were likely to be Wilms' tumour (Stiller & Parkin, 1990b). The combined incidence in Nigeria (Ibadan) was 10.9 per million, in Zimbabwe (Bulawayo) 8.3 and in Uganda (Kampala) 7.9. It has been suggested that incomplete case ascertainment may have led to these latter two rates being underestimates (Stiller & Parkin, 1990b). However, they were still within the upper third of the range of rates reported worldwide.

### Age-specific incidence and sex ratio

In series in Europe and the USA, the highest rates of Wilms' tumour (between 12 and 20 per million) are experienced by children under five years old (Kaatsch *et al.*, 1995; Stiller *et al.*, 1995; Gurney *et al.*, 1996a). The incidence declines to around 5–6 per million in children aged 5–9 years and approximately 1 per million for those aged 10–14 years. There is some evidence of a difference in age distribution between ethnic groups, in that a greater proportion of cases in east Asian populations present in infants than in European or American series (Stiller & Parkin, 1990b). This is consistent with the observation from the US National Wilms' Tumour Study (NWTS) that the median age at onset of cases in Asian American children is 24 months compared with 37 months in white non-Hispanic children (Breslow *et al.*, 1993). In black children in the NWTS, the median age at onset was 41 months (Breslow *et al.*, 1993). While Stiller and Parkin (1990b) did not find any difference in age distribution between the sexes, data from both the NWTS (Breslow *et al.*, 1993) and the Brazilian Wilms' Tumour Study Group (Franco *et al.*, 1991) suggest that the age at diagnosis is slightly higher for girls than boys (between 6–9 months later).

In most series in eastern Asia, there appeared to be a modest male excess of cases, in a ratio of 1.4:1 (Stiller & Parkin, 1990b). Elsewhere, there is little evidence of a consistent pattern in the ratio of the incidence in boys to that in girls.

### Ethnic origin

Data from cancer registries suggest substantial ethnic variations in the risk of Wilms' tumour. Asians have a reduced risk and blacks an elevated risk compared with whites (Table 2.1). In the large study of childhood cancer among ethnic groups in Britain, described in earlier sections and summarized in Table 2.2, the relative risk of Wilms' tumour for children of Asian origin compared with "Caucasians", adjusted for centre, age and sex, was 0.51 and the adjusted relative risk for West Indian children compared with whites was 2.55 (Stiller *et al.*, 1991a). Both of these relative risks were statistically significant. Although based on relatively few cases, the deficit for Asian children was apparent in both the 0–4 and 5–9-year age groups. The excess among West Indian children was most apparent in children aged 5–9 years. These results, in conjunction with the international disease rates, suggest that the incidence of Wilms' tumour is unaffected by migration and, therefore, genetic rather than environmental factors are most significant in determining risk. Some cases of Wilms' tumour are known to be of genetic origin, arising either as part of familial aggregations or in association with congenital anomalies thought to have an underlying genetic etiology (see Chapter 3). However, these account for only a minority of such tumours. Therefore, it would appear that the variation by ethnic group may reflect variation in genetic disposition rather than variation in the incidence of Wilms' tumour associated with specific genetic syndromes.

## *Laterality*

Wilms' tumours may occur unilaterally or bilaterally, but few population-based series have reported proportions of these. In the SEER, Finnish, British and Hungarian data, between 3% and 6% of tumours for which laterality was known were bilateral (Stiller & Parkin, 1990b). These tumours tended to occur earlier than unilateral Wilms' tumours, a finding confirmed in analyses of the USA and Brazilian clinical series (Franco *et al.*, 1991; Breslow *et al.*, 1993). In addition, bilateral tumours tend to occur in association with congenital anomalies, including aniridia, hemihypertrophy, cryptorchidism and Beckwith–Wiedemann syndrome (Breslow *et al.*, 1993).

## *Socioeconomic status*

The one available investigation of renal tumours and socioeconomic status categorized deaths in England and Wales according to paternal occupation as recorded on the child's death certificate (Sanders *et al.*, 1981). The proportionate mortality ratios for children whose fathers were administrators, managers, professionals, technical workers and artists compared with all occupations were 116 in 1959–63 and 108 and 1970–72 (Table 2.3).

## *Time trends*

The only report of a marked change in the incidence of Wilms' tumour originates from Sweden (Ericsson *et al.*, 1978). Over the period 1958–74, the incidence rose significantly for the 0–14-year age group for both sexes. Results of analyses in Britain (Blair & Birch, 1994b; Draper *et al.*, 1994), Australia (Giles *et al.*, 1995), the USA (Bunin *et al.*, 1996; Gurney *et al.*, 1996a) and Japan (Ajiki *et al.*, 1994), which covered periods during 1954 to 1991, found no evidence of any change in the incidence over time.

## Renal carcinoma

Renal carcinomas occur very rarely in children, typically with an annual age-standardized incidence of less than 0.2 per million population (Parkin *et al.*, 1988a). The largest combined group of these tumours to have been analysed are the 153 recorded by the registries contributing to the international study of childhood cancer (Stiller & Parkin, 1990b). The pattern of renal carcinomas is very different to that of Wilms' tumour. In the 0–9-year age group, renal carcinomas were twice as common in males as in females, but equal numbers of each sex were affected in the 10–14 age group. At each year of age until age 12, the numbers of cases were fairly constant. A modest rise was evident at ages 13 and 14 years.

## Group VII: Hepatic tumours

Although uncommon, hepatic tumours constitute a clearly defined group of childhood neoplasms. The relative frequency of these tumours ranges from 0.8% to 1.3% in Europe, Australia and the USA (Parkin *et al.*, 1988a). In Japan and Thailand, relative frequencies of approximately 2.5% have been reported (Ajiki *et al.*, 1994; Sriamporn *et al.*, 1996).

This group includes hepatoblastoma, hepatic carcinoma and other and unspecified hepatic tumours. In the full childhood age range (0–14 years), hepatoblastoma accounts for between 60% and 85% of liver neoplasms (de Nully Brown *et al.*, 1989; Australian Paediatric Cancer Registry, 1994). In infants and those aged 1–4 years, hepatoblastoma is by far the most common hepatic tumour; above that age hepatic carcinoma occurs more frequently than hepatoblastoma (Stiller *et al.*, 1995).

### *Geographical patterns*

During the period 1970–79, the highest annual age-adjusted incidence rates of hepatic tumours, around 4 per million, were observed in China (Shanghai), Hong Kong, Taiwan (Taipei) and for the Fijian population in Fiji (Parkin *et al.*, 1988a). In the Osaka and Miyagi registry areas of Japan and among Singapore Chinese, the incidence was approximately 3 per million. Childhood hepatic tumour incidence rates in Europe, North America, Australia and New Zealand were in the range 1–2 per million (Parkin *et al.*, 1988a).

The incidence of hepatoblastoma appeared to be relatively constant worldwide, with rates between 0.5 and 1.5 per million (Parkin *et al.*, 1988b).

The populations with high or intermediate rates of childhood hepatic tumours correspond to those in which raised rates of adult hepatocellular neoplasms have been recorded (Muir *et al.*, 1987; Parkin *et al.*, 1992). The highest rates of liver cancer in adults occur in sub-Saharan Africa (Muñoz & Bosch, 1987). This suggests that the incidence of childhood hepatic tumours in these areas is also likely to be relatively high. There are few data available on this, although it has been observed that hepatocellular carcinoma is more frequent among children in sub-Saharan Africa than hepatoblastoma (Parkin *et al.*, 1988b).

### *Age-specific incidence and sex ratio*

The incidence of hepatic tumours is highest in children aged under 1 year. In Europe, Australia and Japan, rates of between 5 and 7 per million population have been described (de Nully Brown *et al.*, 1989; Ajiki *et al.*, 1994; Blair & Birch,

1994b; Stiller *et al.*, 1995; McWhirter *et al.*, 1996). In those aged 1–4 years, the incidence is somewhat lower (1 to 6 per million) and, for older children, falls to less than 1 case per million population.

Few registries report sufficient numbers of hepatic tumours to estimate the male to female incidence ratio with confidence. However, the largest population series suggest a modest male excess, with the ratio in the range 1.1 to 1.9 (Parkin *et al.*, 1988a; de Nully Brown *et al.*, 1989; Kaatsch *et al.*, 1995; Stiller *et al.*, 1995).

### Ethnic origin

The series which disaggregate incidence by ethnic group are summarized in Table 2.1 and do not show any consistent pattern (Parkin *et al.*, 1988a).

### Time trends

Relatively little information is available on temporal trends in the incidence of tumours of the liver in children. Data from the Danish Cancer Registry suggest an increase in incidence for both sexes between 1943–63 and 1964–84 (de Nully Brown *et al.*, 1989). The incidence rate for boys rose from 1.0 to 1.9 per million over this period and that for girls from 0.6 to 1.3 per million. Increases in incidence are also apparent in data from Manchester, UK, and the SEER program (Parkin *et al.*, 1988a; Miller *et al.*, 1995). In contrast, in Osaka, Japan, there was no change in incidence between 1971–80 and 1981–88 (Ajiki *et al.*, 1994).

### Group VIII: Malignant bone tumours

The category of malignant tumours of the bone includes osteosarcoma, chondrosarcoma, Ewing's sarcoma and other and unspecified malignant bone tumours. Of these, osteosarcoma and Ewing's sarcoma are the most common but display rather different incidence patterns. For this reason, they are described separately in this section.

Bone tumours in their entirety comprise around 5% of all cancers in childhood in European and North American populations (Parkin *et al.*, 1988a). In Japan, Thailand, India and China and central and South America, these tumours appear to be somewhat less common, accounting for between 2.5% and 4% of malignancies (Parkin *et al.*, 1988a; Drut *et al.*, 1990; Ajiki *et al.*, 1994; Nandakumar *et al.*, 1996; Sriamporn *et al.*, 1996). The highest relative frequency which has been described is 16.3%, by the Paediatric Cancer Registry of Australia for the

period 1982–91 (McWhirter *et al.*, 1996). This was the result of an unusually high occurrence of Ewing's tumour.

### Relative frequencies of bone tumour sub-types

There are considerable international variations in the percentages of the main types of bone tumours. Of 639 bone tumours diagnosed in England, Wales and Scotland from 1978 to 1987, 50% were osteosarcomas, 44% Ewing's sarcomas, 3% chondrosarcoma and 3% other types (Stiller *et al.*, 1995). Similar frequencies have been observed in Denmark (de Nully Brown *et al.*, 1989), in the western part of Germany (Kaatsch *et al.*, 1995) and in the white populations in the USA (Miller *et al.*, 1995). In contrast, among the black US population, osteosarcoma predominates and Ewing's tumour is rare, accounting for only 7% of malignancies (Miller *et al.*, 1995). This observation was first made by Fraumeni and Glass (1970) following a review of death certificates in the USA during the 1960s. The low relative frequencies of Ewing's sarcoma in African registries and hospital series are consistent with this pattern (Parkin *et al.*, 1988a, 1993b). Previous analyses have also suggested that Ewing's tumours are uncommon among Chinese and Japanese (Li *et al.*, 1980; Bone Tumour Committee of Japanese Orthopedic Association, 1982). More recent and extensive data confirm this and, further, indicate that the tumour is also rare in other parts of eastern and south-east Asia (Parkin *et al.*, 1993b). In addition, the frequencies of Ewing's sarcoma also appear to be relatively low in most Hispanic populations (Parkin *et al.*, 1988a). However, in two series, in Valencia, Spain (Peris-Bonet *et al.*, 1996) and Australia (McWhirter *et al.*, 1996), Ewing's sarcomas comprise the majority of bone tumours. In both analyses, thorough histological review of the cases was conducted and the authors concluded that the findings were unlikely to be due to mis-classification of bone or other tumours.

### Osteosarcoma
#### Geographical patterns

There is relatively modest geographical variation in the incidence of osteosarcoma. In the 1970s, and more recently, the annual age-standardized incidence rates of osteosarcoma were between 1 and 2 per million in India, Thailand, China, Hong Kong, Cuba, and Hungary (Parkin *et al.*, 1988a, 1993b; Nandakumar *et al.*, 1996; Sriamporn *et al.*, 1996). In most of Europe and white North American populations, rates ranged from 2 to 3.5 per million (Parkin *et al.*, 1988a). Rates of more than 3.5 per million were seen in US black populations, Italy, Brazil, Germany, and Spain.

## Age-specific incidence and sex ratio

Based on data from Britain and the USA, the incidence of osteosarcoma is very low below the age of five years, but increases steeply thereafter reaching, typically, 2 per million in those aged 5–9 years and around 6–7 per million in the 10–14-year age group (Blair & Birch, 1994b; Stiller *et al.*, 1995; Gurney *et al.*, 1996a). The incidence is similar between the sexes.

## Ethnic origin

In Britain, osteosarcomas occurred at similar frequencies among white, Asian and West Indian children (Table 2.2) (Stiller *et al.*, 1991a). These analyses were based on small numbers of cases. In the four US series which provide data by ethnic group (Table 2.1), osteosarcomas were more frequent among non-white than white populations (Parkin *et al.*, 1988a).

## Time trends

Analysis of osteosarcomas and chondrosarcomas diagnosed from 1954 to 1988 in Manchester, UK, provided no evidence of any secular trend in incidence (Blair & Birch, 1994b). Similarly, no consistent pattern was observed in Victoria, Australia (Giles *et al.*, 1995), However, Bunin *et al.* (1996) tentatively suggested that osteosarcoma rates in white males were rising in Greater Delaware, USA, while those in white females and blacks were falling. However, small numbers of cases were included in the analysis and the annual percentage changes in rates did not reach statistical significance. In a larger study, which included 305 osteosarcomas registered with the SEER program from 1974 to 1991, an annual percentage increase of 2.4% (95% CI 0.3–4.7) in incidence in the 0–14-year age group was found (Gurney *et al.*, 1996a). The rise was most pronounced in the 5–9-year age group and among white children. In addition, the age-standardized incidence of osteosarcoma in Osaka registry area, Japan, rose significantly from 1.5 per million during 1971–80 to 2.6 for 1981–88 ($p<0.05$).

## Skeletal sub-site distribution

81% of osteosarcomas arise in the long bones of the leg (Parkin *et al.*, 1993b). This percentage increases with age at diagnosis, consistent with the postulated association between risk of osteosarcoma and bone growth (Miller, 1981). A further 12% of cases occur in the long bones of the arms, with 3% in the skull and jaw and 3% in the pelvis. There is little evidence of important differences in sub-site distributions between the sexes or across populations.

# Ewing's sarcoma
## Geographical patterns

The incidence of Ewing's sarcoma was less than 1 per million in eastern and south-east Asian populations, including Chinese populations, India, Thailand and Japan in the 1970s and more recently (Parkin *et al.*, 1993b; Ajiki *et al.*, 1994; Nandakumar *et al.* 1996; Sriamporn *et al.*, 1996). Similarly low rates have been observed in Africa and US blacks (Parkin *et al.*, 1993b). Intermediate rates, in the range 1–2 per million have been reported in Cuba, Puerto Rico and the Hispanic population of Los Angeles (Parkin *et al.*, 1993b). In predominantly white populations, including those in Canada, the USA, New Zealand non-Maoris and much of Europe, the rates were in the range 2–3 per million (Parkin *et al.*, 1988a).

## Age-specific incidence and sex ratio

The tumour is rare in those under five years and incidence increases with age, but less markedly than for osteosarcoma. In populations with the highest 0–14-year age-standardized incidence, the age-specific rate in those aged 5–9 years was around 2 per million, rising to 4 per million for those aged 10–14 years (Stiller *et al.*, 1995; Gurney *et al.*, 1996a; McWhirter *et al.*, 1996). The reported data are consistent with a slight male excess of cases.

## Ethnic origin

The relative risks in black US populations compared with whites range from 0.08 to 0.24 (Table 2.1). For Hispanics in Los Angeles, the risk is 60% of that for whites. In Britain, there was no difference in the risk of Ewing's sarcoma among white and Asian children, but this analysis included only 8 cases in Asian children (Table 2.2) (Stiller *et al.*, 1991a). Thus, the available evidence on variation in the incidence of Ewing's tumour by ethnic group suggests a pattern consistent with the distinctive geographical distribution in risk. This would be compatible with a genetic component in the etiology.

## Time trends

There is little evidence of any notable temporal pattern in the incidence of Ewing's sarcoma. Two studies suggest higher incidence during the 1980s than 1970s, but the observed increases were not statistically significant (Ajiki *et al.*, 1994; Giles *et al.*, 1995). In a further three studies, no significant trend was found (Blair & Birch, 1994b; Bunin *et al.*, 1996; Gurney *et al.*, 1996a).

## Skeletal sub-site distribution

Of Ewing's sarcoma, 39% and 17% arise in the long bones of the leg and arm respectively, 18% in the pelvis, 13% in the ribs, 5% in the spine, 4% in the skull and jaw and 4% in the hand and foot (Parkin *et al.*, 1993b). With increasing age, there is a relative decline in frequency of tumours of the arm and skull with age and an increasing proportion of pelvic cancers. As for osteosarcoma, the sub-site distribution varies little between the sexes or geographically.

## Chondrosarcoma

Chondrosarcoma is extremely rare and few series contain sufficient cases to permit conclusions to be drawn regarding its descriptive epidemiology. Analysis of the aggregated set of cases arising in the international study suggests that the age-standardized incidence is between 0.1 and 0.4 per million and that 6% of cases occur in children aged under five years at diagnosis, 18% in children aged 5–9 and 76% in those aged 10–14 (Parkin *et al.*, 1993b).

## Group IX: Soft-tissue sarcomas

The soft-tissue sarcoma group contains three sub-categories: (*a*) rhabdomyosarcoma, embryonal sarcoma and soft-tissue Ewing's tumour (together commonly referred to under the heading rhabdomyosarcoma), (*b*) fibrosarcoma, neurofibrosarcoma and other malignant fibromatous neoplasms (referred to as fibrosarcoma) and (*c*) other and unspecified soft-tissue sarcoma. This third category includes Kaposi's sarcoma and such rare neoplasms as synovial sarcomas, mesenchymoma and leiomyosarcoma. In two of the largest population-based series of soft-tissue sarcomas which have been reported, in the USA (number of cases = 660; Miller *et al.*, 1995) and Britain (*n* = 794; Stiller *et al.*, 1995), the percentages of rhabdomyosarcoma (category (*a*)) were 51% and 67% respectively, of fibrosarcoma (category (*b*)) were 24% and 14% and of other and unspecified soft-tissue sarcomas were 25% and 19%. Most of the data relevant to the descriptive epidemiology of soft-tissue sarcomas pertain to the entire group. However, some series provide data on rhabdomyosarcomas separately. This section therefore considers, firstly, all soft tissue sarcomas and, secondly, the rhabdomyosarcoma sub-group.

## All soft-tissue sarcomas
### Geographical variations

Soft-tissue sarcomas account for between 4% and 8% of all childhood neoplasms in most populations outside Africa (Parkin *et al.*, 1988a). The relative frequency of these tumours in countries in eastern Asia and central and South America tends be in the lower half of this range (Parkin *et al.*, 1988a; Ajiki *et al.*, 1994; Nandakumar *et al.*, 1996; Sriamporn *et al.*, 1996). In most African populations for which recent data are available, soft tissue sarcomas are rather more common, comprising between 8% and 16% of tumours in children. This is, in part, a consequence of the high frequencies of paediatric Kaposi's sarcoma which have been observed in regions of eastern and central Africa in particular (Parkin *et al.*, 1988a; Obafunwa *et al.*, 1992; Wabinga *et al.*, 1993; Stiller & Parkin, 1994; Chintu *et al.*, 1995; Mukiibi *et al.*, 1995; Tijani *et al.*, 1995; Makata *et al.*, 1996; Wessels & Hesseling, 1996).

Incidence rates were available for three African registries in the international study of childhood cancer. All three had rates which were in the upper part of the range reported worldwide; these were (*a*) Kampala, Uganda, 1968–82, 8.0 per million, (*b*) Bulawayo, Zimbabwe, 1963–77, 8.6 and (*c*) Ibadan, Nigeria, 1960–69, 8.7 (Parkin *et al.*, 1988a). In the Uganda series, 47% of the cases were rhabdomyosarcoma, 18% fibrosarcoma and the majority of the others Kaposi's sarcoma. In Zimbabwe, 20% of cases registered were rhabdomyosarcoma, 24% fibrosarcoma and 25% Kaposi's sarcoma. In contrast, in Nigeria, 59% were rhabdomyosarcoma, 20% fibrosarcoma and 22% other types, of which only one was a Kaposi's sarcoma, perhaps a reflection of the fact that this is an older data series (see Time trends).

Outside Africa, during the decade 1970–79, the highest annual incidences of soft-tissue sarcomas were observed in France, among the Hispanic and other white populations of the USA and in Israeli Jews. The rates in these populations were greater than 8 per million (Parkin *et al.*, 1988a). Rates in the range 5–8 per million occurred elsewhere in the Americas and Europe and in Oceania (Stiller & Parkin, 1994). In areas of China, India and Japan, the incidence of soft-tissue sarcomas was below 5 per million.

### Age-specific incidence and sex ratio

In Europe, Australia and Japan, the incidence of soft-tissue sarcomas is highest in infants and is typically in the range 11–17 per million (de Nully Brown *et al.*, 1989; Ajiki *et al.*, 1994; Kaatsch *et al.*, 1995; Stiller *et al.*, 1995; McWhirter *et al.*, 1996).

In the 1–4-year age group, incidence falls to 7–12 per million and is between 4–7 per million in the 5–9 and 10–14-year age groups. In most series, more boys are affected than girls. The sex ratio of the incidence rates varies between 1.1:1 and 1.8:1 (Parkin *et al.*, 1988a).

## Ethnic variations

There are relatively few data available on ethnic variations in the incidence of soft-tissue sarcomas, probably because of the comparative rarity of these neoplasms. In all of the populations which reported rates by ethnicity in the international childhood cancer study, other than those in the USA, the rates for at least one ethnic group are based on fewer than 10 cases (Table 2.1) (Parkin *et al.*, 1988a). In the USA, rates were higher among white children than black children for girls, but similar among white and black children for boys (Stiller & Parkin, 1994). In addition, there is some evidence that the distribution of sub-types differs among black and white children: fibrosarcoma was more common among black children than white (Stiller & Parkin, 1994).

Hispanic children have the highest incidence in the USA; 10.2 per million in Los Angeles Hispanics compared with 7.3 in Los Angeles blacks (Parkin *et al.*, 1988a). However, no excess among Hispanics was found in a study in New Mexico, but this included small numbers of cases (Duncan *et al.*, 1986). Similarly, in a comparison of incidence in several ethnic groups in Hawaii with incidence among the white SEER population, no significant differences were detected (Goodman *et al.*, 1989).

## Time trends

The most striking temporal trends in soft-tissue sarcomas relate to Kaposi's sarcoma in tropical Africa. Uganda is one of the areas of Africa most severely affected by AIDS and recent data from the Kampala cancer registry suggest that Kaposi's sarcoma accounted for 27% of all childhood neoplasms during 1989–91 (Wabinga *et al.*, 1993). The age-standardized incidence in children, for this period, was approximately 85 per million, more than ten times higher than the rate in 1968–82. An increase in the burden of Kaposi's sarcoma of a similar magnitude is apparent in Zambia, where HIV has been prevalent since 1983–84 (Chintu *et al.*, 1995). Following review of all histopathological records for children at the University Teaching Hospital in Lusaka, an eight-fold increase in the relative frequency of Kaposi's sarcoma between 1980–82 (relative frequency 2.6%) and 1990–92 (19.5%) was described.

Statistically significant increases in the incidence of all soft-tissue sarcomas have been reported in Britain (Draper *et al.*, 1994), Italy (Mosso *et al.*, 1992) and Japan (Ajiki *et al.*, 1994). Draper *et al.* (1994) found rising rates in all age groups other than infants over the period 1962–91. Annual increases of 1.9%, 1.6% and 1.6% were evident in the 1–4, 5–9 and 10–14-year age groups respectively. In Turin, Italy, the 0–14-year incidence rate of soft-tissue sarcomas rose steadily from 6.7 per million in 1962–69 to 11.0 in 1982–86 (Mosso *et al.*, 1992). In Osaka, Japan, the age-standardized incidence rose from 4.1 in 1971–80 to 7.9 in 1981–88 (Ajiki *et al.*, 1994). The rate was similar in the first period to rates reported from other east Asian registries and in the second period similar to rates in western Europe and North America. The increases were apparent for all three sub-categories of soft-tissue sarcoma.

## *Rhabdomyosarcoma*

The most common anatomical sites at which rhabdomyosarcomas arise are in the head and neck, in particular the orbit. They also occur at intra-abdominal or genitourinary sites, in the thorax or in soft tissue in the extremities (Green *et al.*, 1997).

## Geographical patterns

The international pattern in rhabdomyosarcoma incidence is likely to be influenced to some extent by the proportions of soft-tissue sarcomas which are of unspecified type. This proportion exceeds 10% in data from several population-based registries (Stiller & Parkin, 1994) and it is possible that if thorough histological investigation of these unspecified tumours were undertaken, a substantial proportion would prove to be rhabdomyosarcomas. Therefore, the incidence of this tumour may be under-reported in some series. Of the series with under 10% of unspecified tumours during 1970–79, incidence rates of more than 5 per million were seen in France and Australia. Elsewhere, the incidence was generally between 2 and 5 per million. Rates in the lower part of this range were observed in most Asian registries, but several of these had relatively high proportions of soft-tissue sarcomas of unspecified type (Parkin *et al.*, 1988a).

## Age-specific incidence and sex ratio

In western Europe and Australia, the highest incidence of rhabdomyosarcoma occurs in the 1–4-year age group (Blair & Birch, 1994b; Kaatsch *et al.*, 1995; Stiller *et al.*, 1995; McWhirter *et al.*,

1996). In infants, the incidence is around 5–6 per million, increasing to 7–9 per million in children aged 1–4 years, and falling to 3–5 per million and 2–3 per million in the 5–9 and 10–14-year age groups, respectively (Blair & Birch, 1994b; Kaatsch *et al.*, 1995; Stiller *et al.*, 1995; McWhirter *et al.*, 1996). This age-specific peak is not apparent in data from most registries in eastern Asia (Parkin *et al.*, 1988a; Ajiki *et al.*, 1994). In these series, the incidence is highest in infants and declines with age.

Data from Manchester, UK, show a relative risk of rhabdomyosarcoma of 0.68 (95% CI 0.47–0.96) for girls compared with boys (Blair & Birch, 1994b). This is consistent with the moderate male excess of cases observed in most other data-sets (Parkin *et al.*, 1988a).

### Ethnic variations

In a relative frequency analysis, summarized in Table 2.2 and involving data from the UK Children's Cancer Study Group, the risk of rhabdomyosarcoma among Asian children resident in the UK was significantly lower than for white children (RR = 0.44, *p*<0.05) (Stiller *et al.*, 1991a). The tumour was particularly infrequent in Asian children aged under 10 years, although this was based on 7 cases in Asian children under 10 years and 316 in white children. In another study in England, the ratio of the age-standardized incidence rates of rhabdomyosarcoma in Asian and white children was 0.37 (95% CI 0.15–0.95) (Powell *et al.*, 1994). This analysis included 44 cases in white children and 2 in Asian children. These findings of a lower risk in Asian than white children accord with the international variations in tumour incidence. In addition the suggestion of a deficit of cases in children below 10 years of age is consistent with the lack of a peak in incidence in the 1–4-year age group in data from Asian cancer registries. This evidence is supportive of ethnic variations in the risk of rhabdomyosarcoma which are unaffected by migration.

In data from the US registries, a similar incidence of rhabdomyosarcoma among black and white children was observed for boys (Stiller & Parkin, 1994). Among girls, however, the incidence for black children was half that among white children. In the UK study of childhood cancer and ethnic group, described above, there was no difference in the relative frequencies of rhabdomyosarcoma between white and West Indian children (Table 2.2) (Stiller *et al.*, 1991a). The results were not presented separately by sex. No other studies of ethnicity and rhabdomyosarcoma are available.

### Time trends

The evidence for temporal trends in incidence of this tumour is inconsistent. Analyses in England (Manchester) and the USA (Greater Delaware Valley) found no evidence of changing incidence (Blair & Birch, 1994b; Bunin *et al.*, 1996). In contrast, Ajiki *et al.* (1994) described a significant increase in the rate of rhabdomyosarcoma in Osaka, Japan from 1.9 per million in 1971–80 to 4.3 per million in 1981–88. There was no decrease in the rate of soft-tissue sarcomas of unspecified type. Modelling of the USA SEER data for 1974 to 1991 revealed an average annual percentage change in incidence of +2.2% (95% CI 0.3–4.1) (Gurney *et al.*, 1996a). This was most pronounced in children under five years for whom the average increase was 3.1% per annum (0.2–6.1). The data also suggested an increase of a similar magnitude among children 10–14 years of age, but this was not statistically significant.

## Group X: Germ-cell, trophoblastic and other gonadal neoplasms

Germ-cell, trophoblastic and other gonadal neoplasms comprise a relatively rare but distinct group of tumours occurring in children. They account for 2–4% of all childhood tumours (Parkin *et al.*, 1988a). As germ cells are the precursors of the sperm and egg cells of the gonads, these tumours most commonly arise in the testes and ovaries. However, they can also arise at extragonadal sites. Of 159 non-gonadal germ-cell tumours diagnosed in Britain during 1978–87, 55% presented at intracranial sites, 27% in the pelvis, 9% in abdominal sites and 5% in intrathoracic sites (Stiller *et al.*, 1995).

This group includes four sub-categories of tumours (*a*) non-gonadal germ-cell and trophoblastic neoplasms, (*b*) gonadal germ-cell and trophoblastic neoplasms, (*c*) gonadal carcinoma and (*d*) other and unspecified malignant gonadal tumours. There are considerable international variations in the ratio of gonadal to non-gonadal germ-cell tumours, although, in most series, gonadal tumours are more frequent than non-gonadal (Parkin *et al.*, 1988a). In two large series in Britain (*n* = 385) and the USA (*n* = 299) combined, 54% were gonadal germ-cell tumours, 41% non-gonadal germ-cell tumours, 2.5% gonadal carcinomas and 2.8% other and unspecified types (Miller *et al.*, 1995; Stiller *et al.*, 1995).

### Geographical patterns

During the decade 1970–79, in most population-based series, the annual age-adjusted incidence of germ-cell and gonadal tumours varied between 2 and 5 per million (Parkin *et al.*, 1988a). In a few populations, rates exceeding 5 per million were reported. The Maori population of New Zealand had the highest incidence at 8.8 per million, followed by rates of 6.4 and 6.3 in two Japanese registries (Osaka and Miyagi respectively) and 5.6 among Los Angeles Hispanics. Rates of less than 2 per million were observed in Cuba, Bombay and the former West Germany. Both the raised and lowered rates were accounted for by the incidence of tumours of gonadal origin. World-wide the incidence of non-gonadal germ-cell tumours was fairly uniform, with rates lying in the range 1–2 per million.

## Age-specific incidence and sex ratio

In a series of 368 germ-cell tumours from the SEER program, Gurney *et al.* (1996a) reported rates of 5.5 per million in the 0–4-year age group, 2.0 per million in children aged 5–9 and 4.7 per million in those aged 10–14 years. Similar incidence rates have been described elsewhere (Parkin *et al.*, 1988a; Stiller *et al.*, 1995).

In Britain, 47% of non-gonadal tumours were diagnosed in children under five years, 16% in those 5–9 years and 37% in those 10–14 years (Stiller *et al.*, 1995). For gonadal tumours, there is some evidence that the age distributions vary by sex. 85% of gonadal tumours in boys occurred in the 0–4-year age group, whereas 74% in girls occurred in the 10–14-year group (Stiller *et al.*, 1995). In other series a similar pattern emerges (Parkin *et al.*, 1988a; de Nully Brown *et al.*, 1989; Blair & Birch, 1994b). However, it should be noted that these findings are based on small numbers of cases in the age–sex categories.

In most data-sets, the sex ratio of the incidence of germ-cell and gonadal tumours is around unity. In the populations with the highest rates, however, a male excess of cases is apparent (Parkin *et al.*, 1988a; Ajiki *et al.*, 1994). When gonadal germ-cell neoplasms are considered separately, more males are affected than females, the sex ratio being between 1.1:1 and 1.8:1 (Parkin *et al.*, 1988a; de Nully Brown *et al.*, 1989; Blair & Birch, 1994b; Stiller *et al.*, 1995).

## Ethnic origin

There has been little investigation of ethnic variations in the incidence of germ-cell tumours, no doubt due to their rarity. In a study in the West Midlands of England, the ratio of the incidence of germ-cell tumours in Asian children compared with white children was 3.29 (95% CI 1.06–10.2) (Powell *et al.*, 1994). Although based on only 9 cases in Asian children and 27 in whites, this result was statistically significant at the 5% level. It is consistent with an earlier finding by Stiller *et al.* (1991b) of a two-fold higher frequency of germ-cell tumours in Asian children across Britain compared with white children (Table 2.2).

## Time trends

In the north-west of England, between 1954 and 1978 a significant increase in the annual incidence of malignant germ-cell tumours (from 1 to 4 per million) was observed (Birch *et al.*, 1982). More recent data for that area show that this trend has continued into the 1980s and appears to be due to rising rates of gonadal tumours (Blair & Birch, 1994b). A study in the West Midlands region of England demonstrated a doubling in the incidence of malignant germ-cell tumours between 1957–74 and 1975–92 (Muir *et al.*, 1995). It was thought unlikely that this was due to increased ascertainment. Analysis of data from the National Registry of Childhood Tumours, which covers all of Britain, confirmed these trends at the national level (Mann & Stiller, 1994). In the periods 1962–76 and 1977–91, the age-standardized rate of malignant germ-cell tumours at all extra-cranial sites rose from 1.9 to 2.8 per million per annum for boys and from 2.2 to 2.8 for girls. For gonadal germ-cell tumours, the incidence increased from 1.5 to 2.2 for boys and from 1.3 to 1.5 for girls. Further analysis of this data-set by age revealed that the annual increase in incidence was statistically significant for the 1–4-year age group (annual percentage increase: boys 2.1%; girls 3.9%) (Draper *et al.*, 1994).

In Australia, in both sexes, the incidence of germ-cell and other gonadal tumours rose by more than 50% between 1970–79 and 1980–89 (Giles *et al.*, 1995). A rise of similar magnitude was detected in Osaka, Japan between 1971–80 and 1981–88 and was due to increasing rates of non-gonadal tumours (Ajiki *et al.*, 1994). Gurney *et al.* (1996a) described an average annual percentage change in the incidence of germ-cell tumours of +2.2% (95% CI 0.2–4.2) in the SEER data-set over the period 1974–91. This increase was most evident in females aged 0–4 years (+10.2%; 4.5–16.1) and males aged 10–14 years (+7.2%; 1.2–13.6). In contrast, however, no evidence of rising rates of gonadal tumours was found in Greater Delaware Valley, USA between 1970 and 1989 (Bunin *et al.*, 1996).

These results can be viewed against the background of the temporal trends in adult testicular and ovarian cancers. Almost universal increases in the incidence of testicular tumours in adults have been observed (Coleman *et al.*, 1993). Although the pattern for adult ovarian cancer is more complex, rates are rising in parts of North America and Asia (Coleman *et al.*, 1993) and increasing incidence of ovarian teratomas in women aged 0–44 years born between 1935 and 1969 in England and Wales has been reported (dos Santos Silva & Swerdlow, 1991). It has been suggested that some of the risk factors implicated in the trends in these adult tumours may also be involved in the childhood neoplasms (Mann & Stiller, 1994).

### Gonadal carcinomas

The largest series of these very rare tumours for which the descriptive epidemiology has been considered are those recorded by registries participating in the international childhood cancer study (Parkin *et al.*, 1988a). On the basis of these data, Stiller (1994) noted that these tumours are at least twice as common among girls as among boys; the age-standardized rate is well below 1 per million for each sex.

## Group XI: Carcinomas and other malignant epithelial neoplasms

Epithelial tumours account for the great majority of malignant disease in adults. In children, however, they are rare, particularly so at the sites which dominate in adults (i.e., lung, breast, stomach and bowel). Childhood carcinomas tend to occur in the adrenal cortex, thyroid, nasopharynx and skin (including melanoma). A few are gonadal or arise in the kidney or liver; these are discussed in earlier sections (Groups VI, VII, X).

### Adrenocortical carcinoma

Carcinomas of the adrenal cortex have an annual incidence of less than 0.5 per million in all populations with the exception of São Paulo, Brazil, where the rate is 1.5 per million (Parkin *et al.*, 1988a). The tumour appears to be particularly uncommon in Asia. The majority of cases present in children aged less than five years (Stiller, 1994). Overall, three girls are affected for every two boys.

### Thyroid carcinoma

In the USA during the 1970s, the age-standardized incidence rates of thyroid carcinoma were relatively high; among whites the annual rate was 1.3 per million, among blacks 0.9 and among Hispanics 1.4 (Stiller, 1994). The incidence was of similar magnitude in the Scandinavian countries and in Turin, Italy, for Jews in Israel and non-Kuwaitis in Kuwait. Elsewhere, the rates were below 1 per million.

The incidence of cancers of the thyroid increases with age in both sexes. In a population-based series of 154 thyroid carcinomas in England and Wales, which have been investigated in detail, 72% were diagnosed in children aged 10–14 years (Harach & Williams, 1995). The tumour is much more common among girls than boys and the sex ratio varies with age (Stiller, 1994). For example, in the series in England and Wales, in children under 10 years the ratio of male to female cases was 0.8:1, while in the 10–14-year age group it was 0.3:1 (Harach & Williams, 1995).

In England and Wales, the number of registrations of thyroid carcinoma rose in each decade during 1963 to 1992 (Harach & Williams, 1995). This was attributed to the introduction, from 1976, of screening for familial medullary thyroid carcinoma.

In Belarus, which experienced high levels of radioactive fallout from the accident at the Chernobyl nuclear reactor in 1986, dramatic increases in the frequency of childhood thyroid cancers have been reported from 1990; incidence reached 80 per million in 1991–2 (Baverstock *et al.*, 1992; Kazakov *et al.*, 1992). However, intensive surveillance for thyroid cancer began in the area only in 1990 and it is not clear how many of the tumours might never have been detected otherwise, particularly as occult papillary carcinomas may be present without symptoms for many years (Beral & Reeves, 1992; see Chapter 4 for further comment).

### Nasopharyngeal carcinoma

Although rare, nasopharyngeal carcinoma has a distinctive geographical and ethnic distribution. It is generally infrequent in the predominantly white populations of Europe, North America and Oceania, where the incidence rarely exceeded 0.4 per million per annum in the 1970s (Parkin *et al.*, 1988a). In the area covered by the Paediatric Registries of France (the south-east and Corsica), the incidence was relatively high (0.7 per million), which has been attributed to the fact that 10% of the population are of north African extraction (Bernard *et al.*, 1993a). In the USA, the rate experienced by blacks was 1.1 per million, 11 times that for whites (Stiller, 1994), confirming an earlier observation based on mortality data (Greene *et al.*, 1977).

Based on data for the 1970s and more recent publications, in Chinese populations, and in the Philippines, Thailand and India, the incidence was 0.6–0.8 per million (Stiller, 1994; Nandakumar *et al.*, 1996; Sriamporn *et al.*, 1996). The tumour appeared to be at least as common elsewhere in eastern Asia, with the exception of Japan. Reliable incidence rates are not available for most of Africa, but cancers of the nasopharynx seem to be seldom diagnosed south of the Sahara. They were particularly frequent in Tunisia and Sudan, accounting for 7–15% of all childhood neoplasms. This area of high risk appears to extend across north Africa and into western Asia (Stiller, 1994).

Among adults, rates of nasopharyngeal cancer are moderately raised in north Africa, with higher incidence in south-east Asia and the most extreme risk in populations of southern Chinese origin (Higginson *et al.*, 1992). Reasons for the differences in the geographical distributions of this tumour between children and adults are not clear.

Few nasopharyngeal carcinomas occur in children under 10 years of age. In the areas of north Africa and Asia where the tumour is most common (Stiller, 1994), approximately 85% of cases are in children aged 10–14 years. In virtually all populations, the incidence among boys exceeds that among girls (Parkin *et al.*, 1988a).

## Melanoma

During the 1970s, exceptionally high rates of melanoma in children were reported in New South Wales, Australia (4.6 per million) and among the non-Maori population of New Zealand (3.7 per million) (Parkin *et al.*, 1988a). During the nine years from 1973 to 1981, only three cases of melanoma were diagnosed in children resident in Queensland, Australia (Parkin *et al.*, 1988a). In the following ten years, 63 melanomas occurred (McWhirter *et al.*, 1996), giving a crude annual incidence of 10 per million in 1982–91 compared with 0.6 per million in 1973–81. The incidence in Queensland children in 1982–91 was twice that of Australia as a whole, reflecting the pattern of adult melanomas (McWhirter *et al.*, 1996). No rise was seen in New South Wales.

During 1970–79, in other series comprising at least 10 cases (mainly white populations in North America and Europe and Israeli Jews), the incidence varied from 0.9 to 1.8 per million.

The incidence of melanoma increases with age (Stiller *et al.*, 1995). In Australia, 6% of cases diagnosed from 1977 to 1986 were aged under five years at diagnosis, 14% aged 5–9 and 79% aged 10–14 (Australian Paediatric Cancer Registry, 1994). The sex ratio is around unity (Parkin *et al.*, 1988a).

## All carcinomas

In two regions of England, the incidence of childhood carcinomas more than doubled over a thirty-year period (Birch & Blair, 1988; Al-Sheyyab *et al.*, 1993). In an update of the earlier of these reports, Blair and Birch (1994b) described significant increases in the incidence of skin neoplasms (carcinomas and melanomas combined) and epithelial tumours except skin over the period 1954–88. However, these analyses were based on small numbers of cases, with only 9 skin and 11 other epithelial neoplasms diagnosed in the most recent quinquennium. In the Netherlands also, a doubling of carcinomas was observed between 1958–72 and 1983–92 (Coebergh *et al.*, 1995), but it was not reported whether this was due to any particular tumour. It is noteworthy that registration in the earlier period was believed to be incomplete. In contrast, in both Denmark (de Nully Brown *et al.*, 1989) and Italy (Mosso *et al.*, 1992) rates of carcinomas appear to have decreased over time.

## Clustering of malignancies other than leukaemia or lymphoma in space and time

Studies of clustering of childhood cancer other than leukaemia are summarized in Table 2.8. In all but two of the studies (that of Suckling *et al.* (1982) relating to retinoblastoma, in which spatial and temporal clustering were assessed separately, and that of Grimson *et al.* (1992) relating to rhabdomyosarcoma, in which temporal clustering was assessed), the analysis related to temporo-spatial clustering. None of the more recently developed techniques of investigating spatial clustering, whose application to studies of childhood leukaemia and non-Hodgkin lymphoma was described in earlier sections, has been used.

In the two studies in which temporo-spatial clustering of different types of childhood cancer combined was assessed, some clustering was identified which was similar to that also identified for leukaemia in the same areas and time periods (Pinkel *et al.*, 1963; Morris, 1990). A possible interpretation is that the results are attributable to uneven distribution of the general population of children with respect to time and space. It is interesting that in the analysis of Pinkel *et al.* (1963), no clustering was identified when pairs formed by traffic fatalities, or by one traffic fatality and one case of cancer, were considered.

With the exception of three investigations (Suckling *et al.*, 1982; Greenberg, 1983; Grimson *et al.*, 1992), all of the studies have been based on death certificates in the USA during the early to mid-1960s. The unit of time considered in each has been one year, and the unit of area either the state (*n* = 51) or division (*n* = 9). No clustering was identified in any of the studies except in that related to bone cancer, in which some clustering of osteogenic sarcoma was identified in the West North Central Division, and of Ewing's sarcoma in the Pacific Division (Glass & Fraumeni, 1970). However, these authors consider that the deaths were rather widely scattered in space and seemed unrelated to one another.

## Conclusions

In early studies, it was difficult to exclude the possibility that geographical variation in incidence of childhood cancer was attributable to differences in completeness of ascertainment. Moreover, for some tumours, such as neuroblastoma, it was not possible to determine incidence accurately since data were available only by anatomical site. From the data accumulated in the international study of childhood cancer in the 1970s (Parkin *et al.*, 1988a) and more recently, it is now clear that there is approximately two- to five-fold variation in the incidence of virtually all types of childhood cancer. Exceptions to this are osteosarcoma, hepatoblastoma and non-gonadal germ-cell tumours, the incidence of which vary relatively little, and the lymphomas, for which more pronounced variation is apparent.

Although variation in incidence by ethnic group has been relatively little studied, some tumours show substantial differences in risk between ethnic groups. In particular, this is apparent for some tumours which have been associated with genetic syndromes (e.g., Wilms' tumour, retinoblastoma), although these syndromes account for only a small proportion of cases. Ethnic variation in risk is also apparent for cell-types of ALL, Ewing's sarcoma, rhabdomyosarcoma and Hodgkin's disease and there is weak evidence that this is also the case for CNS tumours.

Most of the tumours in children occur more frequently in boys than girls, although for ANLL, osteosarcoma, retinoblastoma and melanoma the sex ratio is around unity. The only two tumours which are more frequent in girls are carcinomas of the adrenal cortex and thyroid. Rates are highest for infants for neuroblastoma, retinoblastoma, soft-tissue sarcoma and hepatic tumours and a distinctive peak in the range 1–5 years is well documented for ALL. Wilms' tumours and germ-cell tumours are more common in children under five years than in older age groups.

Socioeconomic status has been relatively little investigated in relation to childhood cancer, with the exception of leukaemia. There is a consistent positive association between ALL and high socioeconomic status. In studies in two locations, neuroblastoma was associated with low socioeconomic status. In the available descriptive and analytical studies of CNS tumours, no consistent association with socioeconomic status is apparent.

The interpretation of temporal trends in childhood cancer is particularly complex. For several tumours, there have been diagnostic advances that are likely to have led to more complete ascertainment and more precise diagnosis. In addition, diagnostic criteria and classifications have evolved over time. While many studies suggest increasing rates of ALL over time, this tends to be accompanied by decreasing rates of leukaemia of other types. Overall, it appears that rates of ALL have risen modestly in children aged 0–4 years. Several studies have shown an increasing incidence of CNS tumours in children, but it is not clear what sub-groups are involved and, as is the case for adults, the possibility that this is an artefact of changes in ascertainment cannot be excluded. There are consistent reports of an increase in the incidence of neuroblastoma. In most areas in which this has been observed, no systematic screening for neuroblastoma has been in operation. In several areas, the incidence of soft-tissue sarcoma is increasing. In particular, in the two available series from parts of Africa, there has been an eight- to ten-fold rise in the frequency of Kaposi's sarcoma as a result of the AIDS epidemic. In several locations, the incidence of germ-cell tumours appears to be rising.

There has been considerable interest in small-area variations in the incidence of childhood cancers, particularly leukaemia. Spatial clustering of leukaemia has been observed in the UK, Greece and Hong Kong and appears strongest in young children. However, in Sweden and the USA, no clustering of leukaemia is apparent. In Malawi and parts of Uganda, where Burkitt's lymphoma is endemic, strong evidence of clustering has been found for this tumour. There is no convincing evidence of clustering of other tumours of childhood.

# Chapter 3

# Genetic factors and familial aggregation

In this chapter, for each type of childhood cancer, the proportion of cases that are accounted for by specific genetic syndromes and familial aggregation are discussed. In addition, second primary neoplasms occurring after a first primary haematopoietic malignancy, tumour of the nervous system or retinoblastoma are considered. Although most second primary neoplasms occurring in individuals who had a first tumour diagnosed in childhood are thought to represent a late effect of treatment, about a quarter to a third of second primary neoplasms in such individuals have been associated with genetic factors (Kingston *et al.*, 1987, Meadows *et al.*, 1985). Associations with genetic markers are discussed. Also, the occurrence of congenital anomalies and other conditions in close relatives of cases with specific types of childhood cancer is considered. Such associations may be attributed to a shared genetic susceptibility. Finally, the available evidence on the role of environmental factors in the occurrence of germ-cell mutations associated with childhood cancer is evaluated.

Most studies in which reported family history has been compared with medical records indicate a high level of agreement for the occurrence of cancer in first-degree relatives (Love *et al.*, 1985; Bondy *et al.*, 1991, 1994).

## Leukaemia

A number of specific genetic syndromes are associated with susceptibility to leukaemia. These include Down's syndrome (see Chapter 10), neurofibromatosis type 1 (Bader & Miller, 1978; Stiller *et al.*, 1994), chromosome breakage syndromes such as ataxia telangiectasia and Fanconi's anaemia, and certain types of hereditary immunodeficiency (Harnden, 1985; Pendergrass, 1985).

Few data are available on the proportion of cases of leukaemia or other specific types of childhood cancer that are of known genetic etiology or associated with genetic syndromes. Narod *et al.* (1991) reviewed the records of 5564 cases of childhood leukaemia in Great Britain during the period 1971–83 for the presence of genetic disease. A total of 142 (2.6%) of the children were recorded as having a recognized genetic condition. This was almost entirely accounted for by Down's syndrome (131 cases; 2.3% of the total). This proportion is similar to that found in studies in the USA (Robison *et al.*, 1984; Watson *et al.*, 1993). In the British study, only two of the cases of leukaemia were associated with hereditary immunodeficiency states. In an extension of the British study covering the period 1976–92, five (9%) of 58 children with chronic myelomonocytic leukaemia (RR = 221, 95% CI 71–514), and 12 (0.2%) of 5725 children with lymphoblastic leukaemia (ALL) (RR = 5.4, 95% CI 2.8–9.4), had neurofibromatosis type 1 (Stiller *et al.*, 1994). There was no evidence for an increased risk of the adult, Philadelphia chromosome-positive type of chronic myeloid leukaemia or of ANLL. In three out of five cases with chronic myelomonocytic leukaemia, a parent was recorded also as having neurofibromatosis type 1, whereas only four of the 12 cases of ALL had an affected parent.

### Concordance for childhood leukaemia in twins

Assessment of concordance for childhood leukaemia in twins may provide clues about etiology. If childhood leukaemia were of a predominantly genetic etiology, monozygotic twins would be expected to be concordant for leukaemia more frequently than dizygotic twins, because of their genetic similarity. If childhood leukaemia were caused by an abnormal intra-uterine environment, it would be expected that if one member of a dizygotic twin pair were affected, the other would be affected more often than a non-twin sib, because of the common environment. Virtually no details are available of the zygosity of twin pairs in which one twin is affected or both twins are. Therefore, the association between zygosity and concordance has to be considered by the indirect method of comparing concordance rates between pairs of like and unlike sex. All pairs of unlike sex are dizygotic, whereas pairs of like sex may be dizygotic or monozygotic. If childhood leukaemia were of a predominantly genetic etiology, twins from pairs of like sex would be expected to be concordant more frequently than twins from pairs of unlike sex.

Keith *et al.* (1973) compiled case reports of leukaemia in 71 pairs of twins, in 60 of which the zygosity had been determined. Some 54% (25 of 46) of monozygotic pairs were concordant, compared with 29% (4 of 14) of dizygotic pairs. However, data from consecutive series of leukaemia cases, and from series of twins occurring in a defined geographical area, show much lower concordance rates for pairs of like sex, 6.3% (95% CI 3.1–11.0) in pooled data (Table 3.1). More recently, in a study of leukaemia in pooled series from Canada, the USA and the UK, only three concordant pairs (1.5%) were found among 197 pairs in which one or both twins had leukaemia (Buckley *et al.*, 1996). The discrepancy between the two types of data may be attributed to preferential publication of case reports of concordant pairs. Concordance rates reported from other studies in North America are also higher than those reported from Europe; this may be a chance finding, and/or an artefact of differences between case series and population-based studies, and difference in length of follow up may also be relevant (MacMahon & Levy, 1964). Although the concordance rate in twins of like sex clearly is higher than the zero concordance reported for twins of unlike sex, the concordance rate in twins of like sex is quite variable. This may be attributable to chance or may be taken as suggesting that genetic factors play a relatively small part in etiology. In the study of Buckley *et al.* (1996), the concordance rate for monozygotic pairs was 3.9% (95% CI 0.8–11.1, 3 of 76 pairs).

Clarkson and Boyse (1971) suggested that the occurrence of concordant leukaemic pairs may be due to parallel expansions of clones descended from a single, ancestral cell transformed *in utero*. Thus, a clone of leukaemia precursor cells arising in one monozygotic twin may enter the circulation of the co-twin through placental vascular anastomoses. This would explain similarities in age at onset between pairs concordant for leukaemia and is supported by cytogenetic evidence (Chaganti *et al.*, 1979; Hartley & Sainsbury, 1981) and DNA analysis of the immunoglobulin gene configuration in Siamese twins (Pombo de Oliveira *et al.*, 1986). Inskip *et al.* (1991) commented that the hypothesis also would explain why like-sex pairs concordant for leukaemia tend to have an early age of onset, and why cytogenetic observations on like-sex pairs concordant for leukaemia with a later age of onset do not support monoclonality. Unequivocal support for the hypothesis of Clarkson and Boyse (1971) is provided by the recent observation of shared clonal, but non-constitutional, HRX rearrangements in the leukaemic cells of three pairs of monozygotic twins concordant for infant acute leukaemia (Ford *et al.*, 1993). The evidence that the rearrangements were not inherited as structural anomalies or restriction site polymorphisms is that the rearrangements were not observed in non-leukaemic cells of the twins or in the maternal and paternal blood for two of the three pairs. Other explanations proposed to account for increased concordance in monozygotic compared with dizygotic twins include increased intrauterine exposure of twins to ionizing radiation because of diagnostic radiological procedures, shared chromosomal anomalies and direct metastasis of leukaemia from the mother, but there is little evidence in support of any of these (Danis & Keith, 1982).

## Leukaemia and cancer in the families of children with leukaemia

Studies of the occurrence of childhood cancer in first-degree relatives of children with leukaemia, in which the number of index cases was at least 50, are summarized in Table 3.2. In the studies of leukaemia of all types combined, no excess of cancers in sibs, parents or offspring was observed. In studies of acute leukaemia, an excess of acute leukaemia was observed in sibs, but the expected number of cases was very low. The very high ratio reported from Egypt (Hafez *et al.*, 1985) is difficult to interpret in the absence of information about the way in which the expected frequency in sibs was calculated, about the participation rate, and about the method of obtaining data on cancer in sibs.

Linet (1985) reviewed studies of the familial aggregation of leukaemia occurring at all ages. She noted that in the earlier studies, cases tended to be a select group from a single hospital or may have been somewhat more representative but incompletely followed up. Relatives more distant than those of the first degree tended to be included, which, in the absence of verification from medical records and other sources, introduced the possibility of recall bias. The studies tended to be small. In a few studies from Australia and New Zealand which are not subject to these limitations, familial excesses of leukaemia at all ages were observed (Gunz, 1964; Gunz *et al.*, 1975). These studies suggest that familial aggregation is most marked for chronic

# Table 3.1. Selected reports of concordance and discordance for leukaemia in twins

## (a) By sex type of pair

| Area and period of study | Deaths (D) or newly incident (I) cases, upper age boundary | Type of series[a] | Total number of cases | Total number of twin pairs | Discordant pairs | | | | | Like-sex concordant pairs[b] | Concordance rate (%) in like-sex pairs (95% CI) | Reference |
|---|---|---|---|---|---|---|---|---|---|---|---|---|
| | | | | | Like-sex | | Unlike-sex | | Total | | | |
| | | | | | Mm | Ff | Mf | Fm | | | | |
| Denmark, 1946–57 (ALL) | I, 14 | C | 516 | 11 | 7 | 1 | 1 | 2 | 11 | 0 | 0.0 (0–28) | Iversen, 1966 |
| Great Britain, 1953–79 | D, 15 | P | – | 126 | 36 | 36 | 27 | 24 | 123 | 3 | 4.0 (0.8–11.2) | Knox et al., 1984 |
| Norway, 1967–79 (births) | I, 14 | P | 329 | 4 | 4 | | | 0 | 4 | 0 | 0.0 (0–60) | Windham et al., 1985 |
| Sweden, 1952–83 | I, 16 | P | – | 31 | | | | | 31[c] | 0 | 0.0 | Rodvall et al., 1990 |
| USA Boston, circa 1940–50 | I, 16 | C | 449 | 9 | 3[d] | 3[e] | 0 | 3 | 9 | 0 | 0.0 (0–46) | Steinberg, 1960 |
| North-east, multicentre and California 1947–61 | D, 15 | C | 4679 | 72 | 18 | 24 | 12 | 13 | 67 | 5 | 10.6 (3.5–23.1) | MacMahon & Levy, 1964 |
| California, 1940–67 | D, 15 | P | – | 48[f] | 15 | 11 | 10 | 10 | 46 | 2[f] | 7.1 (0.9–23.5) | Jackson et al., 1969 |
| Boston, 1947–65 | I, 15 | C | 1263 | 27 | | | | | 26[g] | 1 | – | Fraumeni et al., 1971 |
| Connecticut, 1935–80 | I, 15 | P | – | 11[f] | 5 | 4 | 4 | | 9 | 2[f] | 28.6 (3.7–71) | Inskip et al., 1991 |
| **Total** | | | | 337 | 79 | 75 | 50 | 52 | 326 | 11 | 6.3 (3.1–11.0) | |

Like-sex discordant total 163; unlike-sex discordant total 106.

F affected female; M affected male; f unaffected female; m unaffected male.
[a] C, consecutive series of cases of childhood leukaemia; P, series of twins in a defined geographical area.
[b] No concordant pairs of unlike sex have been reported.
[c] In one pair, one twin had leukaemia, the other a tumour of the CNS.
[d] One of these pairs was monozygotic.
[e] Two of these pairs were monozygotic.
[f] One of these pairs was included in the study of MacMahon and Levy (1964), and therefore is not counted in the total.
[g] Eight pairs were monozygotic, and 18 were dizygotic.

## (b) By zygosity (Buckley et al., 1996)

| Area and period of study | Prevalent (P) or newly incident (I) cases, upper age boundary | Type of series[a] | Type of leukaemia | Number of twin pairs | | | | Concordant pairs | | Concordance rate % in MZ pairs (95% CI) |
|---|---|---|---|---|---|---|---|---|---|---|
| | | | | Total | DZ | MZ | ZU | MZ | ZU | |
| USA, International Twin Study | P, 20 | Adv | ALL | 167 | 90 | 63 | 14 | 2 | 1[b] | 3.2 (0.04–11.0) |
| USA and Canada, CCG, 1972–89 | I, 20 | C | AML | 30 | 14 | 13 | 3 | 1 | 0 | 7.7 (0.02–36.0) |
| UK, CCSG, 1977–86 | I, 14 | P | Any | 197 | 104 | 76 | 17 | 3 | 1[b] | 3.9 (0.8–11.1) |
| USA, SJCRH | I, 20 | C | | | | | | | | |

CCG, Children's Cancer Group; CCSG, Children's Cancer Study Group; SJCRH, St Jude Children's Research Hospital.
[a] Adv, twins recruited by advertising; C, consecutive series of cases of childhood cancer; P, series of twins in defined geographical area.
[b] ALL in one member of pair, "lymphoma and leukaemia" in the other.

## Table 3.2. Selected reports of cancer in first-degree relatives of cases with childhood leukaemia

| Area and period of study | Deaths (D) or newly incident (I) cases, upper age boundary | Population (P) or hospital (H) series | Index cases Total | Index cases Percentage for whom data on relatives obtained | Method of obtaining data on cancer in relatives[a] | Type of relatives | Number of relatives with cancer Expected[b] | Observed | O/E | Percentage of affected relatives with same type of tumour as index cases | Reference |
|---|---|---|---|---|---|---|---|---|---|---|---|
| **Leukaemia** | | | | | | | | | | | |
| USA, 1960–67 | D, 14 | P | 16130 | NS | DC | Sibs | 9 | 10 | 1.1 | 100 | Miller, 1971 |
| Great Britain, 1953–74 | D, I[c],14 | P | NS | NS | I, VR, HR | Sibs | 21.1 | 27 | 1.3 | 56 | Draper et al., 1977 |
| UK, South Glamorgan, NS | I, NS | H | 303 | 66 | HR, I, VR | Mothers / Fathers | 4.4 / 4.4 | 5 / 5 | 1.1 / 1.1 | | Thompson et al., 1988 |
| Denmark, 1943–85 | I, 14 | P | 2067 | 99 | R | Mothers / Fathers | 258.9 / 269.6 | 243 / 242 | 0.9 (0.8–1.1) / 0.9 (0.8–1.0) | 2.5 / 2.1 | Olsen et al., 1995 |
| Great Britain, 1940–NS[d] | I, 14 | P | 885 | 87 | Q | Offspring | 0.36 | 0 | 0.0 | – | Hawkins et al., 1995a |
| **Acute leukaemia** | | | | | | | | | | | |
| USA, Boston, circa 1940–50 | I, 15 | H | 249 | 99 | I, VR[e] | Sibs / Mothers / Fathers | 0.3–0.4 / 0.9 / 0.8–1.0 | 2 / 0 / 0 | 5.0–6.7 / 0.0 / 0.0 | 50 / – / – | Steinberg, 1960 |
| Egypt, Mansoura and Cairo, 1980–85 | I, 15 | H | 166 | NS | NS | Sibs | 0.01[f] | 5[f] | 471[f] | 45 | Hafez et al., 1985 |
| Nordic countries, 1966–85 | I, 14 | P | 3789 | NS | HR | Sibs | 0.68[f] | 4[f] | 5.9[f] | NS | Perkkiö et al., 1990 |
| **ALL** | | | | | | | | | | | |
| Denmark, 1968–92 | I, 14 | P | 704 | –[g] | R | Sibs | NS | 0[h] | 0.0 | – | Westergaard et al., 1997 |
| **AML** | | | | | | | | | | | |
| Denmark, 1968–92 | I, 14 | P | 114 | –[g] | R | Sibs | NS | 0[i] | 0.0 | – | Westergaard et al., 1997 |

NS, Not stated.

[a] DC, death certificates; HR, hospital and other medical records; I, interview; R, cancer registry record linkage; VR, positive reports verified from medical records; Q, questionnaire to hospital consultant responsible for clinical follow-up of proband, or to general practitioner

[b] Calculation of expected numbers of affected relatives:

Miller, 1971  Sib-years at risk calculated assuming two sibs for index case, followed for 8-year study period, and mortality rates of specific types of cancer under age 15 applied.

Draper et al., 1977  Not specified.

Thompson et al., 1988  Age-specific cumulative incidence rates from the West Midlands Region applied for each parent using age at last follow-up or death.

Olsen et al., 1995 and Hawkins et al., 1995  National rates, adjusted for sex, age and calendar period.

Steinberg, 1960  Expected numbers of affected sibs and parents dying of cancer calculated using (a) US data for 1940 and 1950 (b) Massachusetts data for the periods 1939–41 and 1949–51.

[b (contd.)]
Hafez et al., 1985a  Not specified.
Perkkiö et al., 1990  National rates.

[c] Since 1962; twins and cases with a known genetic component excluded.

[d] Leukaemia and non-Hodgkin lymphoma.

[e] As expected numbers relate to deaths from cancer, only deaths from cancer in siblings or parents are included in the table. No living sib had developed cancer. The mean age of sibs at follow-up was 8.1 years. Two mothers alive at follow-up had developed cancer. The mean maternal age at follow-up was 34.6, and the mean paternal age 37.2 years.

[f] These figures relate to acute leukaemia only.

[g] All children who were alive on 1 April 1968, or later and born before 1 January 1993 were included in a population-based sibship database.

[h] ALL only.

[i] AML only.

lymphocytic leukaemia (the type primarily affecting the elderly), less so for the acute leukaemias affecting children and adults, and there is probably no substantial aggregation for chronic myelocytic leukaemia that affects predominantly middle-aged adults (Gunz & Veale, 1969; Gunz *et al.*, 1975).

Kurita *et al.* (1974) ascertained 20 families where familial leukaemia occurred in siblings from case reports in the Japanese literature and questionnaires sent to hospitals throughout the country; the cases were diagnosed during the period 1930–68. Parental consanguinity was found in 10 of the families; in six, the parents were first cousins, and in two they were first cousins once removed. In seven of the 20 families, the onset of the disease was in childhood in one or more sibs; in four (57%) of these families, the parents were first cousins, and in one, second cousins. It is possible that these families were reported preferentially because of parental consanguinity. By contrast, only 4.5% of parents of 200 cases with non-familial leukaemia seen in two major hospitals during the period 1955–67 were first cousins. Estimates of the proportion of births whose parents were first cousins in Japan of 2.1% (Imaizumi *et al.*, 1975) and 6.2% (Schull & Neel, 1965) have been reported. In a small Syrian Jewish community in Brooklyn, New York, five girls were diagnosed with ALL at ages between 17 and 41 months during the period 1960–74; a sixth girl was diagnosed with lymphosarcoma at the age of 15 years and 4 months (Feldman *et al.*, 1976). The parents of three of the cases were related to each other. In addition, the parents of one case were first cousins and each set of grandparents of another case were first cousins. Thus, some degree of consanguinity was identified for all but one of the cases. Among 24 female control children, matched with cases on year of birth and order of birth within the community, one child's parents were first cousins.

## Cancer in the offspring of patients treated for leukaemia in childhood

There have been few studies of the frequency of cancer in the offspring of patients treated for leukaemia, or other types of cancer, in childhood, because until recently too few patients survived for the numbers of offspring to be adequate to estimate their risk of developing malignant neoplasms. The evidence provided by such observations as to the possible genetic component to etiology is limited because (*a*) survival may in part be genetically determined and (*b*) the treatment may have an effect on the health of the

offspring. As of 1995, data were published on 709 known offspring of survivors of childhood and adolescent leukaemia or non-Hodgkin lymphoma, 382 from Great Britain and 327 from studies in France, Sweden and the USA, who have been followed up to a median of six years of age (Hawkins *et al.*, 1995a). Only one of these offspring developed childhood cancer – a female survivor of ALL who was treated with multiple chemotherapy had a daughter who was reported to have died of acute leukaemia (not otherwise specified) at six months of age (Mulvihill *et al.*, 1987). On the basis of the data from Great Britain, it is unlikely that the risk of malignant neoplasm in the offspring of patients treated for leukaemia or non-Hodgkin lymphoma in childhood is more than eight times that of the general population (Hawkins *et al.*, 1995a). Using these data, these authors also calculated a one-sided upper confidence limit of the proportion of cases with an autosomal dominant mode of inheritance. Assuming that the age of onset of all heritable cases is 15 years or less, then, if the diseases had a penetrance of 70% or more, the proportion of heritable cases among the survivors is unlikely to exceed 5%.

## Other conditions in relatives of cases with childhood leukaemia

Based on parental report, Miller (1963) found that among a thousand sibs of children with leukaemia, five had Down's syndrome as compared with 1.4 expected. However, this observation was not confirmed in a study in Great Britain (Barber & Spiers, 1964). Karhausen and Hutchison found no excess of leukaemia among the sibs of children with Down's syndrome in a study designed to detect an increase of greater that five-fold (unpublished data cited by Miller, 1966). Again in the study of Miller (1963), there was no difference in the frequency of congenital anomalies other than Down's syndrome between the sibs of leukaemic children and the sibs of matched neighbourhood controls. Savitz and Ananth (1994) reported an excess of major birth defects among the sibs of cases with ALL (RR = 3.2, 95% CI 1.3–7.7, adjusted for age at diagnosis, sex and year of diagnosis).

Mann *et al.* (1993) observed that there was a significant excess of congenital anomalies reported at interview with the parents, in uncles, aunts, cousins, half-aunts and half-uncles of cases with ALL compared with community controls. Neural tube defects accounted for about half of the excess. Among the parents of 1620 children with Down's syndrome, three fathers died from leukaemia compared with an expected 1.2 (Holland *et al.*, 1962).

In studies of reproductive outcome in survivors of childhood cancer, it is difficult to separate the effects of the disease, and/or susceptibility to it, from the effects of therapy. In a multicentre study in the USA and Canada, the offspring of adult survivors of childhood ALL were not found to be at increased risk of congenital anomalies compared with the offspring of sibling controls (Kenney *et al.*, 1996). Other studies do not suggest any difference in the prevalence at birth of congenital anomalies between the offspring of survivors of childhood cancer of all types and controls (Little *et al.*, 1995).

In the study of Buckley *et al.* (1994), excesses of a number of conditions were observed in sibs, parents or grandparents of index cases with various sub types of ALL. For common ALL, there was a familial excess of bone and joint diseases; for the pre-B-cell type, an excess of gastrointestinal, haematological, bone and joint diseases, or allergy was observed; for the T-cell type, an excess of gastrointestinal disorders; and for null-cell ALL, an excess of congenital heart and lung disorders.

## Second primary tumours in patients whose first primary tumour was leukaemia

The occurrence of second primary tumours may be the result of an interaction of age, genetic predisposition, radiation exposure and chemotherapeutic exposure (Neglia *et al.*, 1991; Robison, 1993). In the largest available study, Neglia *et al.* (1991) found that tumours of the central nervous system (CNS) were the most common second cancers in patients whose first cancer was ALL diagnosed in childhood, accounting for 24 of the 43 second cancers in their series. All of the CNS neoplasms developed in children who had previously undergone irradiation. There was a clustering of CNS tumours among children five years of age or less when diagnosed with ALL, despite the less frequent use of the more intensive regimens of chemotherapy, radiation, or both in this younger group. In other studies, an excess of tumours of the CNS developing as a second primary tumour after leukaemia has been observed (Meadows *et al.*, 1985; Kingston *et al.*, 1987; Olsen *et al.*, 1993a).

## Leukaemia and the major histocompatibility complex

In experimental animals, virally induced leukaemia in mice was the first disease shown to be associated with the major histocompatibility complex (MHC) genes (Lilly *et al.*, 1964). This stimulated investigations of associations between HLA antigens and leukaemia in humans. In early studies, no consistent association between ALL and HLA was observed (Dausset *et al.*, 1982). In more recent studies, leukaemia patients appeared to have a higher frequency of HLA-Cw3 and Cw4 antigens than controls (Dorak & Chalmers, 1992). Most other antigens reported to occur at increased frequency in leukaemia patients are in strong linkage disequilibrium with these two antigens. In addition, the HLA-Cw3 and Cw4 associations, and the association with HLA-DP, is most apparent in patients with ALL. In a preliminary study, there was a positive association between ALL of the common subtype and the HLA-DPB1 locus allele *0201 (Taylor *et al.*, 1995). Children with ALL of the common subtype were more likely than controls to be heterozygous for the *0201, *0301, *0401 and *0402 alleles.

Interest in homozygosity at the various HLA loci of patients with cancer has been stimulated by the hypotheses that: (1) there is genetic susceptibility to certain types of cancer which have a recessive mode of inheritance with linkage to the HLA system; and (2) there is a more direct link between the HLA system and susceptibility to cancer because the immunological defences of homozygotes are weaker than those of heterozygotes (Dausset *et al.*, 1982). However, no excess homozygosity at HLA loci has been observed in cases with ALL (Dausset *et al.*, 1977; von Fliedner *et al.*, 1983) or myeloblastic leukaemia (Dausset *et al.*, 1977).

Reduced genetic heterogeneity in parents of cases with leukaemia, as evidenced by increased compatibility for one or more of the HLA loci, might be indicative of the existence of a gene or genes linked to the HLA system with a recessive mode of inheritance conferring susceptibility to the disease. However, studies of a possible excess of pairs of parents of cases of ALL sharing HLA antigens or haplotypes are inconsistent (Werner-Favre & Jeannet, 1979; MacSween *et al.*, 1980; Betuel *et al.*, 1981; von Fliedner *et al.*, 1983). In these studies, the methods of selection of study subjects were not fully described, so the possibility that selection bias accounts for this inconsistency cannot be excluded.

In several studies, unaffected sibs of patients with ALL have been found to share more HLA haplotypes with the patients than the 25% expected on the basis of Mendelian inheritance or the frequency in control families (Betuel *et al.*, 1981; Chan *et al.*, 1982; von Fliedner *et al.*, 1983; de Moor & Louwagie, 1985; O'Riordan *et al.*, 1992). In order to exclude restricted heterogeneity as the cause of the excess of healthy sibs who are HLA-identical with the index case, de Moor and Louwagie (1985) studied separately the 22 (out of a total of 33) sibships of leukaemia patients who each expressed four different haplotypes. The distribution of haplotypes was still abnormal, a case with acute leukaemia having an HLA-identical sib 3.6 times more often than a healthy child. It has been suggested that this observation of HLA haplotype sharing indicates that the HLA system itself is not involved in the development of leukaemia, and is compatible with segregation distortion (Dorak & Burnett, 1992).

Dorak and Burnett (1992) postulated that a human analogue of the t-complex in the mouse includes genes with a recessive mode of inheritance which confer susceptibility to leukaemia. Dorak and Burnett considered that the most compelling evidence establishing a link between cancer and the mouse t-complex is the demonstration that if embryos homozygous for the lethal factor tw18 were rescued and transplanted to an amenable environment, they could produce histologically malignant neuro-ectodermal growths resembling medulloblas-toma–neuroblastoma (Artzt & Bennett, 1972). The mutant factor tw18 is a partial t-haplotype which contains the major histocompatibility complex. Dorak and Burnett argued that evidence in humans in support of their hypothesis included (*a*) the increase in the risk of haemopoietic-lymphatic cancer in the sibs of children with tumours of the CNS, and (*b*) that tumours of the CNS were the most common second cancers in patients whose first cancer was ALL diagnosed in childhood. The other associations that these authors suggested supported the hypothesis do not appear to be well substantiated.

## Associations between leukaemia and other genetic markers

Associations between ALL and the two allele properdin B (Budowle *et al.*, 1982, 1985) and leukocyte group 5A systems (Warren *et al.*, 1977) have been reported. The complement component C4A6 phenotype was significantly associated with ALL in American blacks (Budowle *et al.*, 1985).

## Mutation in the paternal gametes and childhood leukaemia in the offspring

There has been considerable debate about the possibility that mutation in the paternal gametes may cause childhood leukaemia in the offspring, following the observation that paternal precon-ceptional occupational exposure to ionizing radiation was associated with childhood leukaemia and non-Hodgkin lymphoma in Seascale (Gardner *et al.*, 1990a). In other studies carried out specifically to attempt to replicate this observation, the association was not confirmed (McLaughlin *et al.*, 1992, 1993b; Kinlen *et al.*, 1993b; Michaelis *et al.*, 1994; Pobel & Viel, 1997; see Chapter 4 for further discussion). There was no excess of childhood leukaemia among the offspring of Japanese men who survived the atomic bomb explosions; these men received a mean radiation dose of 492 mSv (Ishimura *et al.*, 1981).

In two studies (Graham *et al.*, 1966; Shu *et al.*, 1988) but not in a third (Magnani *et al.*, 1990) of pre-conceptional X-ray exposure of the father, there was a positive association with leukaemia in the offspring. It is possible that the X-ray doses received in the study of Magnani *et al.* (1990) were lower than in the other two studies. However, all of the studies are limited by the fact that the part of the body X-rayed was not considered, and by possible selection bias or inadequate control of confounding (see Chapter 4 for detailed comment). Leukaemia has not been described among offspring of fathers treated with radiotherapy in the available cohort studies (Narod, 1990). In the world literature, four cases of leukaemia have been reported in the offspring of treated parents, three of which are thought to be due to a genetic condition (Li–Fraumeni syndrome) (Draper, 1989).

If paternal germ-cell mutation were an important cause of childhood leukaemia, a paternal age effect would be expected. In the majority of the available studies, no association with paternal age has been found (Kwa & Fine, 1980; Shaw *et al.*, 1984; McKinney *et al.*, 1987; Shu *et al.*, 1988; Magnani *et al.*, 1990; Urquhart *et al.*, 1991; Roman *et al.*, 1993; Westergaard *et al.*, 1997).

## Lymphoma

Susceptibility to lymphoma is associated with a number of specific genetic syndromes, including certain types of hereditary immunodeficiency (Harnden, 1985), neurofibromatosis type 1 (Stiller *et al.*, 1994), and ataxia telangiectasia (Taylor, 1992). In a study of childhood cancer associated with genetic syndromes in Great Britain (described above), among 1781 cases of childhood lymphoma 17 (1%) had genetic syndromes (Narod *et al.*, 1991). Seven of the 17 cases of lymphoma associated with genetic syndrome had ataxia telangiectasia. The risk of lymphoma among children with ataxia telangiectasia was 400 times greater than in the general population. In an extension of this study, five (0.4%) of 1275 children with non-Hodgkin lymphoma had neurofibromatosis type 1 (RR = 10.0, 95% CI 3.3–23.4; Stiller *et al.*, 1994)

## Concordance in twins

In combined data from five series, none of the co-twins of 31 twins with Hodgkin's lymphoma, 18 with non-Hodgkin lymphoma and 11 with lymphoma not otherwise stated, was affected (Buckley *et al.*, 1996).

## Cancer in the families of children with lymphoma

Data on the risks of cancer to first-degree relatives of children and young persons with lymphoma are summarized in Table 3.3. No overall excess of cancer was observed. In the study of cancer risks for parents of children who developed cancer in Denmark, while the overall risk of cancer in the parents of individuals who had non-Hodgkin lymphoma in childhood was not increased, excess risks of brain tumours (standardized incidence ratio (SIR) = 2.9, 95% CI 1.1–6.3 ) and cancer of the cervix uteri (SIR = 2.0, 95% CI 1.1–3.3) in the mother were found (Olsen *et al.*, 1995). There have been reports of lymphoma and brain tumours occurring in the same family (Grundy *et al.*, 1973). In a population-based study of 1577 cases of Hodgkin's disease diagnosed before the age of 45 years in the Greater Boston area (USA) in the period 1959–73, five sibs developed Hodgkin's disease (SIR = 7.1, 99% CI 1.6–3.0; Grufferman *et al.*, 1977).

## Second primary tumours

In a population based study in Piedmont, Italy, three of 105 cases of Hodgkin's lymphoma registered at ages up to 14 years during the period 1967–89 and followed up to December 1995, developed a second primary tumour (SIR = 10.5, 95% CI 2.2–30.9; Magnani *et al.*, 1996). In one of the 151 cases of non-Hodgkin lymphoma, a second primary tumour occurred (SIR = 5.6, 95% CI 0.1–30.9).

## Tumours of the central nervous system

Genetic syndromes established as associated with tumours of the CNS include the autosomal dominant disorders neurofibromatosis (mainly NF-1) (Bader & Miller, 1978; Seizinger, 1993; Ragge, 1993), tuberous sclerosis (Monaghan *et al.*, 1981), Gorlin syndrome (Evans *et al.*, 1991), and the autosomal recessive disorder Turcot's syndrome

(CNS tumours associated with familial polyposis of the colon) (Turcot *et al.*, 1959; Bishop & Hall, 1994). In a study of childhood cancer associated with genetic syndromes in Great Britain (described above), of 3872 cases with tumours of the brain and spinal cord, 79 (2%) had genetic syndromes (Narod *et al.*, 1991). Sixty of the cases had neurofibromatosis and 18 had tuberous sclerosis. In an extension of this study to cases diagnosed during the period 1953–93, seven of 225 families, in each of which two children had been diagnosed with cancer before the age of 15 years, had neurofibromatosis type 1 (Draper *et al.*, 1996). Eight of the children in these seven families, including one pair of monozygotic twins, developed an optic nerve glioma. In three of the 225 families, patients were recorded as having Turcot's syndrome. In a study in New York state, five sibs of 328 cases with CNS tumours were reported to have neurofibromatosis, compared with no sibs of controls (Baptiste *et al.*, 1989). In Great Britain during the period 1971–86, four cases of CNS tumours were associated with cystic fibrosis, compared with 1.35 expected (ratio 3.0, 95% CI 0.8–7.6; Robertson & Hawkins, 1995). There was no overall excess of childhood cancer connected with this genetic condition. In a population-based series of 173 cases of medulloblastoma in the Manchester area (UK), five (2.9%) had autosomal dominant conditions known to predispose to neoplasia (Evans *et al.*, 1993).

## Concordance in twins

In combined data from five series, none of the co-twins of 16 cases with medulloblastoma had childhood cancer (Buckley *et al.*, 1996). In 51 pairs in which one or both members had other types of CNS tumours, one like-sex pair was concordant for glioblastoma and in a further like-sexed pair, one twin had a mixed glioma and the other an optic nerve tumour.

## Cancer in the families of children with central nervous system tumours

In most studies, an excess of cancer in sibs of index cases with tumours of the brain and CNS has been found (Table 3.4). The highest concordance between sibs for brain tumours was reported in the early mortality-based study of Miller (1971). In other studies, an increased risk of leukaemia in sibs of cases with brain tumours has been found (Draper *et al.*, 1977; Farwell & Flannery, 1984a).

Farwell and Flannery (1984a) observed a five-fold excess risk of tumours of the nervous system in parents of children with CNS tumours, of a similar order to the risk of such tumours in sibs observed in the same study. Children with a history of cancer in first-degree relatives were older at

## Table 3.3. Summary of studies of cancer in first-degree relatives of cases with lymphoma diagnosed in childhood

| Area and period of study | Deaths (D) or newly incident (I) cases, upper age boundary | Population (P) or hospital (H) series | Index cases | | Method of obtaining data on cancer in relatives[a] | Type of relatives | Number of relatives with cancer | | | Percentage of affected relatives with same type of tumour as index cases | Reference |
|---|---|---|---|---|---|---|---|---|---|---|---|
| | | | Total | Percentage for whom data on relatives obtained | | | Expected[b] | Observed | O/E | | |
| USA, 1960–67 | D, 14 | P | 2629 | NS | DC | Sibs | 2.2 | 1 | 0.5 | 100 | Miller, 1971 |
| Great Britain, 1953–74 | D, F, 14 | P | NS | NS | I, VR, HR | Sibs | 6.0 | 4 | 0.7 | 75 | Draper et al., 1977 |
| Denmark, 1943–85 | I, 14 | P | 541 | 99 | R | Mothers | 70.2 | 87 | 1.2 (1.0–1.5) | 0.0 | Olsen et al., 1995 |
| | | | | | | Fathers | 73.6 | 73 | 1.0 (0.8–1.2) | 1.4 | |

NS, Not stated.

[a] DC, death certificates; HR, hospital and other medical records; I, interview; R, cancer registry record linkage; VR, positive reports verified from medical records.

[b] Calculation of expected numbers of affected relatives:
Miller, 1971 — Sib-years at risk calculated assuming two sibs for index case, followed for 8-year study period, and mortality rates of specific types of cancer under age 15 applied.
Draper et al., 1977 — Not stated.
Olsen et al., 1995 — National rates, adjusted for sex, age and calendar period.

[c] Since 1962; twins and cases with a known genetic component excluded.

## Table 3.4. Summary of studies of cancer in first-degree relatives of children with tumours of the central nervous system

| Area and period of study | Deaths (D) or newly incident (I) cases, upper age boundary | Population (P) or hospital (H) series | Index cases | | Method of obtaining data on cancer in relatives[a] | Type of relatives | Number of relatives with cancer | | | Percentage of affected relatives with same type of tumour as index cases | Reference |
|---|---|---|---|---|---|---|---|---|---|---|---|
| | | | Total | Percentage for whom data on relatives obtained | | | Expected[b] | Observed | O/E | | |
| USA, 1960–67 | D, 14 | P | 5221 | NS | DC | Sibs | 3.8 | 11[c] | 2.9 | 73 | Miller, 1971 |
| Great Britain, 1953–74 | D, F[d], 14 | P | NS | NS | I, VR, HR | Sibs | 10.8 | 30 | 2.8 | 27 | Draper et al., 1977 |
| USA, Connecticut, NS | I, 19 | P | 667 | 96 | R | Sibs | 3.0 | 11[e] | 3.7 | 36 | Farwell & Flannery, 1984a |
| | | | | | | Parents | 1.6 | 8 | 5.0[f] | | |
| UK, North West, West Midlands and Yorkshire 1980–83 | I, 14 | P | 78 | NS | I, VR | Mothers | 5 | 6 | 1.2 | | Birch et al., 1990a |
| | | | | | | Fathers | 1 | 2 | 2.0 | | |
| USA, Texas, 1944–83 | I, 14 | H | 243 | 95 | I, VR | Sibs | 3.8 | 6 | 1.6 | NS | Bondy et al., 1991 |
| | | | | | | Mothers | 10.8 | 7 | 0.7 | | |
| | | | | | | Fathers | 10.2 | 11 | 1.1 | | |
| Denmark, 1943–85 | I, 14 | P | 1368 | 99 | R | Mothers | 166.4 | 153 | 0.9 (0.8–1.1) | 3.9 | Olsen et al., 1995 |
| | | | | | | Fathers | 173.8 | 184 | 1.1 (0.9–1.2) | 3.8 | |
| USA, Philadelphia[g] | I | H | 165 | 99 | HR | Sibs | NS | 0 | 0.0 | 0 | Jones et al., 1995 |

NS, Not stated.

[a] DC, death certificates; HR, hospital and other medical records; I, interview; R, cancer registry record linkage; VR, positive reports verified from medical records;

[b] Calculation of expected numbers of affected relatives.
Miller, 1971 — Sib-years at risk calculated assuming two sibs for index case, followed for 8-year study period, and mortality rates of specific types of cancer under age 15 applied.
Draper et al., 1977 — Not stated.
Farwell & Flannery 1984 — Expected numbers of siblings affected in childhood, defined as up to the age of 20 years. Each index case was assumed to have two sibs, one two years older and one two years younger. Age- and year-specific incidence rates for Connecticut were applied.
Birch et al., 1990a
Bondy et al., 1991 — Case-control study. Person-years at risk were determined from the date of birth to the date of death, first cancer diagnosis, date of interview or age 75, whichever came first. Age-, sex- and calendar year-specific rates from Connecticut were applied.
Olsen et al., 1995 — National rates, adjusted for sex, age and calendar period.

[c] An additional pair had astrocytoma; the surnames were different but the mother's maiden name and address were the same.

[d] Since 1962; twins and cases with a known genetic component excluded.

[e] Includes two affected sibs of one index case.

[f] Tumours of the nervous system only.

[g] Children with neurofibromatosis type 1 were excluded.

diagnosis than children without such a history. By contrast, in a population-based study in Denmark, only a weak excess of CNS tumours (SIR in mothers 1.2, in fathers 1.3) was observed in the parents of 1368 patients who developed brain and nervous system tumours in childhood (Olsen *et al.*, 1995). No overall excess of cancer in the parents was observed in this study. In a registry-based study, Sussman *et al.* (1990) found that children with a brain tumour whose grandparents and great-grandparents had a history of any kind of tumour were younger at the time of presentation than affected children without this family history. No association between brain tumours in children and a family history of cancer has been observed in other studies (Gold *et al.*, 1979, 1994; Preston-Martin *et al.*, 1982; McCredie *et al.*, 1994a).

In a case–control study of astrocytoma in Pennsylvania, New Jersey and Delaware, the relative risk associated with having a first- or second-degree relative with cancer was 1.7 (95% CI 1.0–2.7, based on 86 discordant pairs; Kuijten *et al.*, 1990). The association was strongest for the age group 0–4 years. However, the overall excess was accounted for by second-degree relatives (RR = 1.6, 84 discordant pairs). No association between astrocytoma and a history of cancer in parents, grandparents or great-grandparents was found in a larger (169 cases) multicentre population-based study in the USA (Gold *et al.*, 1994). In a multicentre hospital-based study in the USA and Canada, there were non-significant excesses of brain tumours, leukaemia and lymphoma and childhood cancer among relatives of cases with astrocytoma (*n* = 155) compared with controls selected by random-digit dialling, but not compared with the general population (Kuijten *et al.*, 1993). In this study, first- and second-degree relatives of children with primitive neuroectodermal tumours (166 cases) were more likely to be reported as having childhood cancer than relatives of controls or the general population. There was no excess of total brain tumours or of leukaemia and lymphoma. 81% of the tumours reported in the families of the subjects were validated from medical records or death certificates. Fewer tumours reported in the families of controls could be validated, as more parents of controls than of patients refused to release medical information.

## Congenital anomalies in relatives of children with tumours of the central nervous system

Van der Wiel (1960) reported on the occurrence of malformations of the CNS among 3557 close relatives of 100 patients with glioma, compared with 1687 controls from 50 families; the method of selection was not described. There were 29 cases of neural tube defects or hydrocephalus in the relatives of cases with glioma, as compared with one among the relatives of the controls. In case–control studies in the USA and in northern England, no association between CNS tumours and the reported occurrence of congenital anomalies of any type in sibs was observed (Baptiste *et al.*, 1989; Mann *et al.*, 1993; Gold *et al.*, 1994; Savitz & Ananth, 1994). In one of these studies, the occurrence of congenital anomalies in other family members was investigated (Gold *et al.*, 1994). There were statistically significant associations with congenital anomalies reported in the mother and her grandmother and great-grandmothers. No particular type of anomaly accounted for the excess. No association was reported with congenital anomalies in the father and his relatives. The reported prevalence of anomalies at birth was similar as between mothers and fathers of controls, and as between matrilineal and patrilineal relatives of controls, arguing against better reporting of family history in maternal relatives as an explanation for the finding. Furthermore, as noted by the authors, the lack of association with congenital anomalies in the father and his relatives argues against recall bias. In a study in northern England, no excess of congenital anomalies was observed among parents, grandparents, uncles, aunts, cousins, half-aunts or half-uncles of 78 children with CNS tumours compared with the relatives of community or hospitalized controls (Mann *et al.*, 1993).

## Second primary tumours

In view of some reports of an excess of cancer in the families of children with tumours of the CNS, it might be expected that children with CNS tumours would have an increased risk of developing a second primary neoplasm. Farwell and Flannery (1984b) found that nine of a total of 670 children diagnosed with CNS tumours before age 20 developed a second neoplasm; the ratio of observed to expected numbers of second neoplasms was 9.1 (95% CI 4.0–17.3). Five cancers occurred in the parents or sibs of these nine patients, compared with an expected number of 0.91 (RR = 5.5, 95% CI 1.2–10.0). Three of these relatives had developed leukaemia, whereas only 0.04 cases were expected. Kingston *et al.* (1987) found that among 45 children with CNS tumours who subsequently developed a second cancer, fifteen had a known genetic disease and a further four children had a first-degree relative with cancer. Two of these families had features of the

Li–Fraumeni syndrome. However, in this same study base, among survivors of CNS tumours receiving neither radiotherapy nor chemotherapy, the incidence of subsequent malignant tumours was very similar to that expected (Hawkins *et al.*, 1987). In a population-based study in Piedmont, Italy, none of 532 cases of malignant CNS tumour registered at ages up to 14 years during the period 1967–89, and followed up to December 1995, developed a second primary malignant tumour (Magnani *et al.*, 1996). In the 3319 person years of follow-up, 0.61 cases would have been expected.

Meadows *et al.* (1977) observed that the combination of glioma with leukaemia or lymphoma was the most frequent combination in their series and occurred in five patients for whom no etiology for a second primary neoplasm was known. In addition, three patients developed leukaemia or lymphoma following radiotherapy for a glioma. Sibs of three of these eight patients were affected with tumours of the same type. The authors suggested that the association might be part of a new genetic cancer syndrome. Kingston *et al.* (1987) also observed a high frequency of leukaemia occurring as a second tumour in patients whose first tumour was of the CNS. Further support for a genetic relationship between these neoplasms is provided by the observation of an excess of haemato-poietic–lymphatic cancer in the sibs of children with tumours of the CNS (Farwell & Flannery, 1984a).

## Paternal age and CNS tumours in the offspring

No paternal age effect has been reported for tumours of the CNS (Gold *et al.*, 1979; Johnson *et al.*, 1987; Nasca *et al.*, 1988; Wilkins and Koutras, 1988; Birch *et al.*, 1990b; Kuijten *et al.*, 1990; Wilkins and Sinks, 1990).

## Neuroblastoma

Neuroblastoma does not appear to be associated with specific genetic syndromes (Miller *et al.*, 1968; Carlsen, 1996). In a study of childhood cancer associated with genetic syndromes in Great Britain (described above), out of 985 tumours of the sympathetic nervous system, two (0.2%) had genetic syndromes (Narod *et al.*, 1991). One was a case of neuroblastoma and the other of malignant phaeochromocytoma; both cases had neurofi-bromatosis (type unspecified).

## Concordance in twins

In combined data from five series, one of 11 pairs of monozygotic twins, one or both members of which had neuroblastoma, was concordant for the disease; none of 20 dizygotic pairs or two pairs of unknown zygosity was concordant (Buckley *et al.*, 1996). Kushner and Helson (1985) reviewed earlier published case reports on concordance for neuroblastoma in twins. In five concordant pairs reported to be monozygotic, the diagnosis was made during the first few months. By contrast, in two discordant monozygotic pairs, the age of diagnosis was greater than 30 months, similar to the median age at diagnosis in unselected series. These observations may be compatible with hereditary factors predominating in neuroblastoma diagnosed in infants, whereas other factors may predominate in neuroblastoma diagnosed after infancy.

## Cancer in families of cases with neuroblastoma

There is no clear evidence of familial aggregation of neuroblastoma (Table 3.5). Kushner *et al.* (1986) reviewed reports of familial neuroblastoma. The data on the 23 families in their compilation conform to an autosomal dominant mode of inheritance. The median age of diagnosis was nine months, with 60% of cases being diagnosed before one year. This pattern contrasts with a median age of diagnosis of 2.5 years in the series of Hayes and Green (1983), and 30% or less of cases being diagnosed before one year in population-based studies (Miller *et al.*, 1968; Kinnier-Wilson & Draper, 1974; Stiller & Parkin, 1992). In the compilation of Kushner *et al.* (1986), eleven cases of multiple primaries (23% of the total) occurred in eight families; in selected series a proportion of around 5% with multiple primaries has been observed (Knudson & Strong, 1972). In records of childhood cancer in Great Britain during the period 1953–93, the risk for a sib of a neuroblastoma patient of developing this tumour was about 1 per 1000 (Draper *et al.*, 1996).

## Other conditions in relatives of children with neuroblastoma

In a case–control study of 35 cases of neuroblastoma in northern England, a higher proportion (18 of 416; 4.3%) of uncles, aunts, cousins, half-aunts and half-uncles of cases than community controls (13 of 648; 2.0%) was reported to have congenital anomalies (Mann *et al.*, 1993). In a case–control study of neuroblastoma in parts of Germany with high

## Table 3.5. Summary of studies of cancer in first-degree relatives of children with neuroblastoma

| Area and period of study | Deaths (D) or newly incident (I) cases, upper age boundary | Population (P) or hospital (H) series | Index cases — Total | Index cases — Percentage for whom data on relatives obtained | Method of obtaining data on cancer in relatives[a] | Type of relatives | Number of relatives with cancer — Expected[b] | Number of relatives with cancer — Observed | Number of relatives with cancer — O/E | Percentage of affected relatives with same type of tumour as index cases | Reference |
|---|---|---|---|---|---|---|---|---|---|---|---|
| USA, 1960–67 | D, 14 | P | 2383 | NS | DC | Sibs | 2.1 | 3 | 1.4 | 0 | Miller, 1971 |
| Great Britain, 1953–74 | D, F, 14 | P | NS | NS | I, VR, HR | Sibs | 2.6 | 10 | 3.8 | 30 | Draper et al., 1977 |
| Italy, 1979–81 | I, NS | H | 145 | 70 | I | Sibs / Mothers / Fathers | 0.1[d] / 0.4 / 0.5 | 1[d] / 0 / 0 | 10 / 0.0 / 0.0 | NS | Pastore et al., 1985 |
| USA, Greater Delaware Valley, 1970–79 | I (median 1 year) | RDD | 104 | 75 | I | Mothers / Mother's sibs | 1 / 2.7 | 4 / 4 | 4.0 (0.7–21.9)[e] / 1.3 | | Kramer et al., 1987 |
| UK, South Glamorgan, NS | NS | H | 30 | 57 | HR, I, VR | Mothers / Fathers | 0.06 / 0.04 | 2 / 0 | 33.3 / 0.0 | | Thompson et al., 1988 |
| Denmark, 1943–85[f] | I, 14 | P | 319 | 99 | R | Mothers / Fathers | 25.1 / 25.7 | 29 / 22 | 1.2 (0.8–2.7) / 0.9 (0.5–1.3) | – | Olsen et al., 1995 |

NS, Not stated.

[a] DC, death certificates; HR, hospital and other medical records; I, interview; R, cancer registry record linkage; VR, positive reports verified from medical records.

[b] Calculation of expected numbers of affected relatives:

Miller, 1971: Sib-years at risk calculated assuming two sibs for index case, followed for 8-year study period, and mortality rates of specific types of cancer under age 15 applied.

Draper et al., 1977: Not stated.

Pastore et al., 1985: Age-sex-period-specific mortality rates for Italy applied to sibs up to time of diagnosis of index child.

Kramer et al., 1987: Case-control study.

Thompson et al., 1988: Age-specific cumulative incidence rates from the West Midlands Region applied for each parent using age at last follow-up or death.

Olsen et al., 1995: National rates, adjusted for sex, age and calendar period.

[c] Since 1962; twins and cases with a known genetic component excluded.

[d] Only deaths in sibs were considered.

[e] 90% CI.

[f] Tumours of the sympathetic nervous system.

levels of caesium-137 fall-out resulting from the Chernobyl accident, congenital anomalies were more frequently reported among the sibs of cases than of controls (RR = 3.4, 95% CI 0.8–16.6; Michaelis *et al.*, 1996). In a population-based study in Denmark in which neuroblastomas presenting in the first year of life were compared with those presenting later (Carlsen, 1996), no hereditary disease was observed in the families of the 75 cases presenting in the first year of life, whereas such disease was observed in the families of 11 of the 175 cases presenting later. Asthma was reported in four families, and rheumatic history in two; no other conditions occurred in more than one family.

## Second primary cancer

De Vathaire *et al.* (1992) studied the incidence of thyroid tumours occurring after cancer in childhood in a cohort of 592 children treated before 1970. Six of the children later developed a thyroid carcinoma, and 18 developed a thyroid adenoma. The frequency of thyroid neoplasm was five times more frequent after irradiation for neuroblastoma than after irradiation for any other first primary neoplasm. This ratio did not vary by sex, time since irradiation, or dose of radiation received by the thyroid gland. These findings were interpreted as suggesting a common mechanism for the occurrence of neuroblastoma and of differentiated thyroid tumour. An excess of thyroid carcinoma after neuroblastoma was also found in the hospital-based studies of Tucker *et al.* (1984, 1991), but was not observed in population based studies in Great Britain (Hawkins *et al.*, 1987) or Italy (Magnani *et al.*, 1996). As acknowledged by de Vathaire *et al.* (1992), as a rule more second cancers, and particularly more thyroid cancers, are found in hospital-based studies than in population-based studies because of differences in treatment intensity and in the extent of diagnostic investigations during follow-up.

## Paternal age and neuroblastoma in the offspring

No paternal age effect has been observed for neuroblastoma (Johnson & Spitz, 1985; Neglia *et al.*, 1988).

## Retinoblastoma

Knudson (1971) proposed a two-mutation hypothesis to explain the occurrence of retinoblastoma in both hereditary and sporadic forms with differing frequencies of bilaterality, and this model has become a paradigm for considering the role of genetic factors in the etiology of cancer in general. Knudson postulated that all retinoblastomas occur as the result of two mutations. In hereditary cases, the first mutation is in a germinal cell, while in non-hereditary cases, the first mutation is in a somatic cell. The second mutation always occurs in somatic cells. In carriers of the germinal mutation, the mutation is present in all the cells of the individual, and in consequence a bilateral tumour, or indeed multiple primary neoplasms, are more likely to occur. In the non-hereditary form, both mutations take place post-zygotically in the same somatic cell, and as a result the tumours are more likely to be unilateral and unifocal, with a later age of onset.

Between 40 and 50% of retinoblastoma patients have the heritable form of the disease; one quarter of these are familial cases and the remaining three quarters are thought to be sporadic, arising from new mutations in the parental germ cells (Bunin *et al.*, 1989a; Narod *et al.*, 1991). The majority of heritable cases are bilateral and all bilateral cases are heritable. All of the predictions of Knudson's model have been confirmed following molecular cloning and characterization of a candidate retinoblastoma susceptibility gene (Goodrich & Lee, 1990).

In a study of childhood cancer diagnosed during the period 1971–83 in Great Britain, some 37% (162 of 436) cases were bilateral and therefore presumed to be hereditary (Narod *et al.*, 1991). Genetic forms of retinoblastoma other than bilateral include unilateral familial tumours, unilateral tumours in individuals carrying 13q deletions, and unilateral sporadic tumours associated with new germ-cell mutations which are not detectable by cytogenetic techniques. Using published reports, Narod *et al.* (1991) estimated that the total hereditary proportion for retinoblastoma was 48.8%.

## Concordance in twins

In combined data from five series, four of seven monozygotic twin pairs, and two of ten dizygotic pairs, were concordant for retinoblastoma (Buckley *et al.*, 1996).

## Cancer in families of cases of retinoblastoma

Data on the risk of cancer in non-twin relatives of cases with retinoblastoma are presented in Table 3.6.

## Table 3.6. Summary of studies of cancer in non-twin sibs and parents of children with retinoblastoma

| Area and period of study | Population (P) or hospital (H) series | Proportion for whom data on relatives obtained (%) | Subgroup | N | Method of obtaining data on cancer in relatives[a] | Type of relatives | Expected[b] | Observed | O/E (95% CI) | Reference |
|---|---|---|---|---|---|---|---|---|---|---|
| France, multicentre, NS | H | 91 | All | 308 | I, Q | Grandparents | 110.6[c] | 148 | 1.3 | Bonaiti-Pellié & Briard-Guillemot, 1980 |
| | | | Unilateral sporadic | | | | 61.6[c] | 81 | 1.3 | |
| | | | Bilateral sporadic | | | | 34.5[c] | 51 | 1.5 | |
| | | | Familial | | | | 10.5[c] | 16 | 1.5 | |
| USA, Texas, 1944–80 | H | 86 | All Unilateral sporadic | 93 | I/Q, VD | Sibs | 0.2[c] | 0 | 0.0 | Strong et al., 1984 |
| | | | | | | Mothers | 0.4[c] | 1 | 2.3 | |
| | | | | | | Fathers | 0.9[c] | 1 | 1.1 | |
| | | | Bilateral familial | | | Sibs | 1.7[c] | 1 | 0.6 | |
| | | | | | | Mothers | 1.2[c] | 1 | 0.9 | |
| | | | | | | Fathers | 1.4[c] | 7 | 4.9 | |
| The Netherlands, 1945–70 | P | 100 | Hereditary | 145 | I, VR | Brothers | 1.5 | 1 | 0.7 (0.0–2.7) | der Kinderen et al., 1988 |
| | | | No family history | 103 | | Sisters | 3.4 | 2 | 0.6 (0.1–1.7) | |
| | | | | | | Mothers | 11.1 | 10 | 0.9 (0.4–1.6) | |
| | | | | | | Fathers | 11.4 | 13 | 1.1 (0.6–1.9) | |
| Denmark, 1943–84 | P | 98 | All | 176 | R | Sibs | 0.02[d] | 5[d] | 268 (96–583)[d] | Olsen et al., 1990a |
| | | | | | | | 2.19[e] | 1[e] | 0.5 (0.02–2.3)[e] | |
| | | 95 | Genetic[g] | 61 | | Mothers[f] | 11.3 | 8 | 0.7 | |
| | | 94 | Non-genetic | 115 | | Fathers[f] | 12.4 | 14 | 1.1 | |
| | | | | | | Parents[f] | 6.4 | 3 | 0.5 (0.1–1.3) | |
| | | | | | | | 17.3 | 19 | 1.1 (0.7–1.7) | |
| Great Britain, 1963–85 | P | 83 | All | 918 | I, VR, HR | Sibs | 2.7[h] | 2[d] | 0.7 | Draper et al., 1992 |
| | | | Unilateral sporadic | 512 | | Sibs | 54[i] | 51[d] | 0.9 | |
| | | | Bilateral familial | 109 | | | | | | |

[a] DC, death certificates; HR, hospital and other medical records; I, interview; Q, questionnaire; R, cancer registry record linkage; VD, positive reports and status of dead siblings verified from death certificates; VR, positive reports verified from medical records;

[b] Calculation of expected numbers of affected relatives:
Bonaiti-Pellié and Briard-Guillemot, 1980  National rates.
Der Kinderen et al., 1988  National rates.
Strong et al., 1984  Sib-years at risk were determined from date of birth to 31 December 1980, date of death, or date of last observation. Age–sex–ethnic group–year-specific US mortality rates were applied.
Olsen et al., 1995  National rates, adjusted for sex, age and calendar period.

[c] Only deaths due to cancer in relatives considered.
[d] Retinoblastoma.
[e] Tumours other than of the eye.
[f] Parents who had retinoblastoma in childhood excluded from analysis.
[g] Bilateral, multifocality in unilateral tumour, or familial.
[h] One per cent recurrence risk estimated by Vogel (1979).
[i] Risk to offspring of cancer patient (50%), times penetrance (90%).

In a hospital-based study in Texas, no excess mortality due to cancer was observed among first-degree relatives, aunts, uncles or grandparents of cases with the unilateral-sporadic form of retinoblastoma. A significant excess of cancer deaths occurred in fathers of cases with the bilateral form of the disease and in relatives aged under 55 years. This excess was not associated with the occurrence of second tumours in patients who had had bilateral retinoblastoma, but was to some extent accounted for by families in which more than one child had retinoblastoma (Strong *et al.*, 1984).

In a study in the Netherlands of cancer incidence in first-degree relatives of patients with retinoblastoma, no excess of non-ocular tumours was found (der Kinderen *et al.*, 1988). Among the fathers of 103 cases with hereditary retinoblastoma, three developed pancreatic cancer, compared with 0.4 expected (RR = 8.3, 95% CI 1.5–20.8). No excess of pancreatic cancer has been reported in other studies.

In a population-based study in Denmark, there was no overall excess of non-ocular cancer in the parents (Olsen *et al.*, 1990a, 1995) or sibs (Olsen *et al.*, 1990a) of cases with retinoblastoma. An excess of melanoma was observed in the fathers of unilateral sporadic cases. Melanoma has been reported as a second primary tumour in patients with the hereditary form of retinoblastoma (Draper *et al.*, 1986; Eng *et al.*, 1993; Moll *et al.*, 1996) and was found in excess (*p*<0.02) in relatives of patients with the bilateral familial form of the disease in the study of Strong *et al.* (1984).

In a study in Great Britain, the proportion of sibs of retinoblastoma cases who developed the disease was close to that expected according to the modes of inheritance for the two forms of the disease (Draper *et al.*, 1992; Table 3.6). Among 75 offspring born to patients with retinoblastoma that was either bilateral or accompanied by family history of the disease, 32 developed retinoblastoma and one a malignant testicular teratoma (Draper *et al.*, 1992). The proportion of offspring affected with retinoblastoma is very close to what would be expected with an autosomal dominant mode of inheritance with a penetrance of approximately 90%. The authors estimated a risk of retinoblastoma in the offspring of cases of sporadic unilateral retinoblastoma of 0.7–0.8%, with a standard error of the same magnitude. For each unaffected child born to a possible carrier, the estimated probability that subsequent children will be affected decreased.

In the study of Mulvihill *et al.* (1987), 47 offspring were born to patients with retinoblastoma, two of whom also developed retinoblastoma; one parent of each child had bilateral retinoblastoma. When these cases are excluded, the number of observed cases of cancer in the offspring is close to that expected on the basis of the frequency in the offspring of sib controls.

## Second primary tumours

Parents with the hereditary form of retinoblastoma have a much higher excess risk of second primary tumours than those with the non-hereditary form (Draper *et al.*, 1986; der Kinderen *et al.*, 1988; Eng *et al.*, 1993). In studies with a short follow-up period, most of the second primary tumours are osteosarcomas and soft-tissue sarcomas (Moll *et al.*, 1996). Other types of second primary tumour, including melanoma, are found in studies with longer follow-up.

## Environmental exposures and the occurrence of retinoblastoma mutations

There are two main mechanisms whereby environmental exposures are believed to lead to germ-cell mutations (Figure 1.1). First, mutations may arise in the paternal gametes during the pre-conceptional period. In males, spermatogenesis continues from puberty to old age. Thus, mutations may arise and accumulate with time. Second, the mechanism by which mutation may occur in maternal germ cells is different from that in the father. New oocytes are not formed after birth, so exposures of the maternal grandmother of the index child before the birth of the mother of the index child may be relevant. The oocytes are almost mature in the ovaries of a newborn female, and become fully mature much later, one by one, when during each menstrual cycle one, or occasionally more than one, egg is made available for fertilization. Thus, there is less opportunity for the accumulation of mutant genes in female than in male gametogenesis (Cavalli-Sforza & Bodmer, 1971). If a mutagenic agent were to act on resting gametes and its intensity were constant over time, even in the absence of division of gamete-forming cells, a linear accumulation of mutant genes with age might also be expected in females. There are about 380 mitosis states involved in the formation of sperm, compared with 23 in egg production (Bradley, 1992). Mutations are most likely to arise in mitosis, because the repair activity of cells appears to stop during this stage.

## Preconceptional exposures of the father

If paternal germ-cell mutation were an important cause of retinoblastoma, a paternal age effect would be expected. While the mutation rate may also increase with maternal age, this is likely to be at a lower rate than for paternal age, because in females there is no possibility of accumulation of mutant genes associated with the division of gamete-forming cells (see above).

In studies of the parental origin of *de novo* germ-line mutation in retinoblastoma, 31 such mutations were found on the paternal allele and only two on the maternal allele (Kato *et al.*, 1994). No strong paternal age effect has been observed in retinoblastoma (Jadayel *et al.*, 1990; Kato *et al.*, 1994). Therefore, apart from the much greater number of cell divisions involved in spermatogenesis as compared with oogenesis, environmental factors or a deficiency in DNA repair in sperm may account for the paternal predominance of *de novo* mutation (Kato *et al.*, 1994). In a combined total of 33 non-hereditary retinoblastoma tumours, 17 had lost the maternal allele and 16 had lost the paternal allele of the *RB* gene (Kato *et al.*, 1994).

It would be expected that the risk of the sporadic heritable form of retinoblastoma would be associated with preconceptional exposures of the father, whereas the non-heritable form would be associated with exposures after conception. Bunin *et al.* (1989a) found that in a comparison of 67 sporadic heritable cases and age–sex–area matched controls selected by random-digit dialling, there were nonsignificant positive associations with preconceptional gonadal X-rays of the father, and older paternal age. The weak association with paternal age is in accord with previous studies. In contrast to the prediction of the hypothesis, a statistically significant protective effect of multivitamins consumed by the mother during the pregnancy leading to the birth of the index child was found. In multivariate analysis, only one variable, 'father with a graduate or professional education' was 'selected' by conditional stepwise logistic regression. A higher proportion of control fathers had received such education, suggesting that the results reflect participation bias in controls resulting from recruitment by random-digit dialling. Further analysis of these data showed statistically significant positive associations with paternal employment in the armed forces and in the metal industry, and a nonsignificant association with the mother's father having held jobs in a 'cluster' including welding, machining and paper-processing occupations (Bunin *et al.*,

1990a). For 115 non-heritable cases, Bunin *et al.* (1989a) found a positive association with low maternal educational level, which again may be an artefact of recruitment of controls by random-digit dialling. In the later analysis relating to occupation, there were positive associations with paternal employment before or after conception in a job cluster consisting mostly of welders and machinists, and with the mother's father having worked in farming at the time of her birth (Bunin *et al.* 1990a).

In addition to a possible paternal origin of mutation, preferential transmission of paternal mutant RB-1 alleles from one generation to the next has been reported (Munier *et al.*, 1992). In a study of 51 individuals from eight kindreds with hereditary retinoblastoma, the odds of transmitting a mutant allele to children of male carriers was 18:4 ($p < 0.005$) whereas no difference from a 1:1 segregation ratio was detected among the children of female carriers.

## Exposures of maternal grandmother of index child before mother's birth

In the one available study of 67 cases of sporadic heritable (i.e., bilateral or unilateral with 13q deletion, without family history) retinoblastoma and controls matched on age, sex and area and selected by random-digit dialling, no association was found with grandmaternal employment, medication or X-rays during the pregnancy leading to the birth of the mother of the index child (Bunin *et al.*, 1989a, 1990a). However, many mothers were not able to answer these questions.

## Preconceptional exposures of the mother

Using the same classification of cases as discussed in relation to preconceptional exposures of the father, Bunin *et al.* (1989a) found that the sporadic heritable form of the disease was associated with maternal preconceptional X-ray of the lower abdomen or pelvis. No such association was apparent for the non-heritable form of the disease.

## Wilms' tumour

Initially, a two-mutation model, developed from observations on retinoblastoma, was proposed to explain the etiology of Wilm's tumour (Knudson & Strong, 1972). Subsequently, it has been shown that several genes are involved (Pritchard-Jones & Hawkins, 1997). First, missense mutations of *WT1* at 11p13, are associated with Denys–Drash syndrome (a triad of nephrotic syndrome, ambiguous genitalia and Wilms' tumour). *WT1* appears to be mutated in less than 10% of cases (Rainier & Feinberg, 1994). Second, 11p15 contains the gene or genes responsible for Beckwith–Wiedemann syndrome. About 8% of cases with the syndrome develop malignant tumours, about half of which are Wilms' tumours. Third, in linkage studies carried out in families in which familial Wilm's tumour occurred, linkage with chromosome 11 was not found (Grundy *et al.*, 1988; Huff *et al.*, 1988).

In a pedigree with seven cases of Wilm's tumour, a gene for a familial form of the tumour was localized to chromosome 17p (Rahman *et al.*, 1996). In addition, there is thought to be a gene predisposing to Wilms' tumour at chromosome 7p (Pritchard-Jones & Hawkins, 1997).

Comparison of constitutional and tumour genotypes has shown loss of alleles from chromosome 11p in a substantial proportion, but less than half, of cases with Wilms' tumour (Smith, 1992). Most of the cases involving loss of alleles from 11p13 lose the maternal alleles (Schroeder *et al.*, 1987). In seven of eight children who had a *de novo* mutation at 11p13, the *de novo* deletion occurred on the paternally derived chromosone (Huff *et al.*, 1990). Some Wilms' tumours not associated with Beckwith–Wiedemann syndrome have been shown to have undergone loss of heterozygosity at 11p15.5 (Koufos *et al.*, 1989).

It has been suggested that preferential loss of maternal alleles from chromosome 11p may be due to inactivation of a tumour-suppressor gene by genomic imprinting (Wilkins, 1988). A cluster of genes on chromosome 11p15.5 shows monoallelic expression despite the presence of two genetically identical copies of these genes (Issa & Baylin, 1996). This cluster includes the *IGF2* gene, which is normally expressed from the paternally derived allele and encodes a fetal growth promoter, and the *H19* gene, which is expressed from the maternal allele, and whose expression is thought to play a critical role in the imprinting (monoallelic expression depending on the parental origin of the allele) of *IGF2* and other genes on 11p15.5 (Barlow, 1995). Whereas in normal human kidney, the paternal allele of *IGF2* is expressed and the maternal allele is transcriptionally inactive, 70% of Wilms' tumours show loss of imprinting and thus express both maternal and paternal alleles (Ogawa *et al.*, 1993; Rainier *et al.*, 1993). In addition, some of these patients had biallelic *IGF2* expression in their normal kidney tissue, suggesting that a somatic failure of imprinting may have occurred (Issa & Baylin, 1996). Loss

of imprinting of *H19* occurred in some of the Wilms' tumours (Rainier *et al.*, 1993). Therefore, loss of imprinting of *H19* may also be involved in the etiology of Wilms' tumour (Rainier & Feinberg, 1994).

In addition to the Denys–Drash and Beckwith–Wiedemann syndromes, specific syndromes associated with Wilms' tumour include WAGR syndrome (Wilms' tumour with congenital aniridia, genitourinary abnormalities and mental retardation), Perlman syndrome and Wilms' tumour with hemihypertrophy (Sharpe & Franco, 1995).

In a study of childhood cancer diagnosed during the period 1971–83 in Great Britain, of 984 cases of kidney tumour, 71 (7.2%) had genetic conditions (Narod *et al.*, 1991). 51 cases (5.2%) were bilateral; four of the cases had aniridia. The assumption that all bilateral cases are hereditary has been questioned (Narod & Lenoir, 1991; Sharpe & Franco, 1995; Breslow *et al.*, 1996). Eight of the unilateral cases had aniridia (two also with hemi-hypertrophy), and twelve additional cases had hemihypertrophy.

As of 1981, 24 families with two or more cases of Wilms' tumour had been reported in case reports (Matsunaga, 1981). The highest proportion of familial cases reported is 2.4% (Sharpe & Franco, 1995), observed in a French multicentre study (Bonaïti-Pellié *et al.*, 1992). None of the 12 cases, all of which were unilateral, had an affected first-degree relative.

### Concordance in twins

In a population-based study in Norway, Windham *et al.* (1985) observed that two out of five twins, all from like-sex pairs, with renal cancer were members of a concordant twin pair; no concordance for any other type of childhood cancer was seen in this study. In 71 patients in the National Wilms' Tumour Study in the USA, with a twin sibling, the only instance of concordance was for a dizygotic pair (Olson *et al.*, 1993a). One other case had a co-twin with medulloblastoma. In combined data from five series, none of the 60 twins with Wilms' tumour had an affected co-twin (Buckley *et al.*, 1996). In one like-sex dizygotic pair, the co-twin was diagnosed with ALL at about the same time as the index twin (three years of age). Thus, concordance for Wilms' tumour in twins is rare.

### Cancer in relatives of cases with Wilms' tumour

The risks to relatives are summarized in Table 3.7. There was no consistent excess risk of cancer of all types combined.

## Table 3.7. Summary of studies of cancer in relatives other than co-twins and offspring of children with Wilms' tumour

| Area and period of study | Deaths (D) or newly incident (I) cases, upper age boundary | Population (P) or hospital (H) series | Index cases | | Method of obtaining data on cancer in relatives[a] | Type of relatives | Number of relatives with cancer | | | Percentage of affected relatives with same type of tumour as index cases | Reference |
|---|---|---|---|---|---|---|---|---|---|---|---|
| | | | Total | Percentage for whom data on relatives obtained | | | Expected[b] | Observed | O/E | | |
| USA, 1960–67 | D, 14 | P | 1774 | NS | DC | Sibs | 1.6 | 3 | 1.9 | 67 | Miller, 1971 |
| Great Britain, 1953–74 | D, F, 14 | P | NS | NS | I, VR, HR | Sibs | 16 | 0 | 0.0 | – | Draper et al., 1977 |
| France, multicentre, 1982–89 | I, P, NS | H | 501 | NS | I, Q | Sibs | 0.9[d] | 1[d] | 1.2[e] | – | Moutou et al., 1994 |
| | | | | | | Mothers | 0.8 | 2 | 2.5[e] | – | |
| | | | | | | Fathers | 2.3 | 6 | 2.6 (p=0.012)[e] | – | |
| | | | | | | Cousins | 2.6 | 5 | 1.9[e] | – | |
| | | | | | | Grandparents | 133.1 | 172 | 1.3 (p<0.001)[e] | – | |
| | | | | | | Aunts & uncles | 19.6 | 28 | 1.4 (p=0.04)[e] | – | |
| | | | | | | Sibs | 0.9 | 1 | 1.2[f] | – | |
| | | | | | | Mothers | 2.2 | 2 | 0.9[f] | – | |
| | | | | | | Fathers | 5.3 | 6 | 1.7[f] | – | |
| | | | | | | Cousins | 3.7 | 5 | 1.4[f] | – | |
| | | | | | | Grandparents | 150.1 | 172 | 1.2[f] | – | |
| | | | | | | Aunts & uncles | 24.8 | 28 | 1.1[f] | – | |
| Denmark, 1943–85 | I, 14 | P | 381 | 99 | R | Mothers | 43.0 | 44 | 1.0 (0.7–14) | 0 | Olsen et al., 1995 |
| | | | | | | Fathers | 49.5 | 33 | 0.7 (0.5–0.9) | 9 | |

NS, Not stated.

[a] DC, death certificates; HR, hospital and other medical records; I, interview; R, cancer registry record linkage; VR, positive reports verified from medical records; Q, questionnaire to hospital consultant responsible for clinical follow-up of proband, or to general practitioner

[b] Calculation of expected numbers of affected relatives:

Miller, 1971    Sib-years at risk calculated assuming 2 sibs for index case, followed for 8-year study period, and mortality rates of specific types of cancer under age 15 applied.

Draper et al., 1977    Not stated.

Moutou et al., 1994    National rates.

Olsen et al., 1995    National rates, adjusted for sex, age and calendar period.

[c] Since 1962; twins and cases with a known genetic component excluded.

[d] Deaths due to cancer for all classes of relatives.

[e] Standardized proportional mortality ratio method.

[f] Standardized mortality ratio method.

No case of childhood cancer was reported in 179 offspring of patients surviving Wilms' tumour after treatment in seven centres in the USA and France (Li *et al.*, 1988), and followed to a median age of six years. In a study of 146 offspring of 78 survivors of unilateral Wilms' tumour in Great Britain and followed to a median age of 6.8 years, three offspring developed Wilms' tumour (RR = 287, 95% CI 59–837; Hawkins *et al.*, 1995b). Two of these were offspring of one female survivor. In a study of 37 offspring of survivors of unilateral Wilms' tumour followed to a median age of under five years, one child developed Wilms' tumour (Byrne *et al.*, 1988).

## Paternal age and Wilms' tumour

In a multicentre study in the USA, an association between sporadic Wilms' tumour (that is without a family history of the disease) and paternal age was found, with a relative risk of 2.1 of the tumour in children of fathers aged over 55 years compared with children of fathers aged under 20 (Olson *et al.*, 1993b). Of a total of 3054 eligible cases, data on paternal age were not recorded for 20%. Little difference in the paternal age distribution was found between patients with bilateral and unilateral disease. Patients with congenital anomalies, evidence of nephrogenetic rests or with early or late age of onset had fathers and mothers substantially older than other cases. In other studies of Wilms' tumour, no paternal age effect has been found, but these were too small to be informative (Wilkins & Sinks 1984b; Bunin *et al.*, 1987; Olshan *et al.*, 1993).

## Congenital anomalies in relatives of patients with Wilms' tumour

The frequency of congenital anomalies in relative of cases with Wilms' tumour has been investigated in two small studies. First, the frequency of congenital anomalies was not increased in a total of 59 liveborn offspring of 27 women and the wives of nine men who survived unilateral Wilms's tumour in childhood (Green *et al.*, 1982). Second, in a study of survivors of unilateral disease, wives of male survivors had no apparent excess risk of problem pregnancies (Byrne *et al.*, 1988). Fifteen of 26 female survivors had a total of 33 pregnancies. Six of 18 liveborn babies born to 12 women had congenital anomalies. Three were compatible with anomalies seen as part of the Wilms' tumour complex – cryptorchidism, umbilical hernia and hypospadias. A fourth was a ventricular septal defect in a child who developed Wilms' tumour. The remaining two cases were of hip dislocation and are compatible with intrauterine constraint

following radiation-induced fibrosis. Among 36 infants of sisters of cases, three had congenital anomalies.

## Liver tumours

In a study of childhood cancer diagnosed during the period 1971–83 in Great Britain, three (2.2%) of 135 cases with liver tumours (102 hepatoblastoma, 33 liver carcinoma) had genetic conditions (Narod *et al.*, 1991). Hepatoblastoma has been associated with familial adenomatous polyposis (Bishop & Hall, 1994).

## Bone tumours

In a study of childhood cancer diagnosed during the period 1971–83 in Great Britain, none of 850 cases of bone tumours was recorded as having a genetic condition (Narod *et al.*, 1991). In combined data from five series, one of 16 twins with osteosarcoma (who also was diagnosed with retinoblastoma) had a co-twin who developed retinoblastoma (Buckley *et al.*, 1996). None of 21 twins with Ewing's sarcoma, or 10 twins with a bone tumour not otherwise specified had an affected co-twin.

No consistent excess of cancer of all types counted was observed in first-degree relatives of cases with bone tumours (Table 3.8). In the study of parents of cases of childhood sarcoma in Denmark described above, there was an excess of breast cancer in mothers aged 45 years when the sarcoma in the child was diagnosed at ages under three years (Olsen *et al.*, 1995).

Following a change in the classification of Ewing's sarcoma to include Ewing's sarcoma of bone and soft tissue and peripheral primitive neuroectodermal tumours of bone and soft tissue, an increased risk of melanoma (O/E 1.9, 95% CI 1.2–2.8), brain tumours (O/E 1.9, 95% CI 1.1–3.0) and stomach cancer (O/E 2.0, 95% CI 1.4–2.8) was observed in first-degree relatives of patients with this group of tumours in a study in the USA (Novakovic *et al.*, 1994). In earlier studies of Ewing's sarcoma, there was no association with a family history of congenital anomalies (Holly *et al.*, 1992; Winn *et al.*, 1992), or bone diseases (Winn *et al.*, 1992).

## Osteosarcoma and genetic markers

In a multicentre study in the USA and Canada, seven of 235 (3.0%) children with osteosarcoma had germ-line *p53* mutations (McIntyre *et al.*, 1994). Such germ-line mutations were first identified in children with

## Table 3.8. Summary of studies of cancer in non-twin sibs and parents of children with bone tumours

| Area and period of study | Deaths (D) or newly incident (I) cases, upper age boundary | Population (P) or hospital (H) series | Index cases Total | Percentage for whom data on relatives obtained | Method of obtaining data on cancer in relatives[a] | Type of relatives | Number of relatives with cancer Expected[b] | Observed | O/E (95% CI) | Percentage of affected relatives with same type of tumour as index cases | Reference |
|---|---|---|---|---|---|---|---|---|---|---|---|
| **Bone tumours** | | | | | | | | | | | |
| USA, 1960–67 | D, 14 | P | 1218 | NS | DC | Sibs | 1.0 | 4 | 4.0 | 25 | Miller, 1971 |
| Great Britain, 1953–74 | D, F, 14 | P | NS | NS | I, VR, HR | Sibs | 0.6 | 0 | 0.0 | – | Draper et al., 1977 |
| UK, North West, West Midlands and Yorkshire, 1980–83 | I, 14 | P | 30 | 100 | I, VR | Mothers<br>Fathers | 1.0<br>1.0 | 5<br>1 | 5.0<br>1.0 | 0<br>0 | Hartley et al., 1988b |
| **Osteosarcoma** | | | | | | | | | | | |
| USA, Texas, 1944–83 | I, 19 | H | 383 | NS | I, VR | Sibs | 7.6 | 17 | 2.3 | 24[d] | Strom & Strong, 1991 |
| USA, New York State, 1978–88 | I, 24 | P | 130 | NS | I | First-degree relatives | NS | NS | 1.0[h] | – | Gelberg et al., 1997 |
| **Ewing's tumour** | | | | | | | | | | | |
| UK, Manchester, 1965–88 | I, 14 | P | 66 | 95 | I, HR | Sibs<br>Mothers<br>Fathers | 0.78<br>4.0<br>5.0 | 1<br>3<br>6 | 1.3 (0.03–7.2)<br>0.7 (0.2–2.2)<br>1.2 (0.4–2.6) | 0<br>0<br>0 | Hartley et al., 1991a |
| USA, multicentre, NS | I, 22 | H | 204 | 76 | I | Mothers<br>Fathers<br>Other[e] maternal<br>Other[e] paternal | 9<br>4<br>85<br>64 | 8<br>9<br>85<br>72 | 0.9 (0.3–2.4)<br>2.3 (0.7–7.3)<br>1.0 (0.7–1.1)<br>1.2 (0.0–1.8) | NS<br>NS<br>NS<br>NS | Winn et al., 1992 |
| **Sarcomas (not otherwise specified)** | | | | | | | | | | | |
| USA, Boston, 1948–76[f,g] | I, 17 | H | 104 | 85 | Q, VR | Sibs<br>Mothers<br>Fathers | 3.2<br>9.6<br>11.0 | 2<br>14<br>10 | 0.6<br>1.5<br>0.9 | NS<br>0<br>0 | Burke et al., 1991 |
| UK, Manchester, 1968–86 | I, 15–24 | P | 165 | 97 | HR | Mothers | 12.3 | 11 | 0.9 (0.4–1.6) | 0 | Hartley et al., 1991b |

NS, Not stated.

[a] DC, death certificates; HR, hospital and other medical records; I, interview; Q, questionnaire; VR, positive reports verified from medical records.

[b] Calculation of expected numbers of affected relatives:

Miller, 1971  Sib-years at risk calculated assuming two sibs for index case, followed for 8-year study period, and mortality rates of specific types of cancer under age 15 applied.

Draper et al., 1977  Not stated.

Hartley et al., 1988b  Matched case-control study.

Strom & Strong, 1991  Person-years at risk were determined from the date of birth to the date of death, first cancer diagnosis, date of interview or age 35, whichever came first.

Gelberg et al., 1997  Age-, sex- and calendar year-specific rates from Connecticut were applied. Case-control study

Hartley et al., 1991a  Age-sex-time period-specific rates for the defined geographical area were applied. The median age of sibs at exit from analysis was 27 years.

Winn et al., 1992  Case-control study.

Burke et al., 1991  Expected numbers of affected siblings calculated using SEER data 1973–77.

Hartley et al., 1991c  Age-sex-time period-specific rates for the defined geographical area were applied. Follow-up was truncated at the age of 75 years.

[c] Since 1962; twins and cases with a known genetic component excluded.

[d] Sarcomas of bone or soft tissue.

[e] Grandparents, aunts, uncles and cousins.

[f] Excludes Ewing's sarcoma: 61 patients had a soft-tissue sarcoma, and 27 an osteosarcoma.

[g] Long-term survivors – median survival 22 years.

[h] The authors stated that there was no significant association with a history of cancer in first-degree relatives.

Li–Fraumeni syndrome (Malkin *et al.*, 1990). In a study of 24 unrelated patients with osteosarcoma (age range 7.5–18.3 years) from various regions in Spain, who were typed for HLA-AB7 and HLA-A antigens, there was a significant increase in HLA-A11 and HLA-B7 in osteosarcoma patients compared with a control group consisting of 1000 blood donors from different regions of Spain (Barona *et al.*, 1993). An increased frequency of the HLA-ALL antigen was observed in a series of 20 patients in Japan (Shimizu *et al.*, 1990c) but increases in the frequency of the HLA-B7 antigen have not been reported in other studies (Tabacchi *et al.*, 1982; Shimizu *et al.*, 1990c).

## Soft-tissue sarcoma

Soft-tissue sarcomas are associated with the Li–Fraumeni syndrome (Li *et al.*, 1988). This syndrome was first defined when review of the medical records and death certificates of 648 childhood rhabdomyosarcoma patients resulted in identification of four families in which siblings or cousins had a childhood sarcoma (Li & Fraumeni, 1969). In these four families, there was a striking aggregation of breast cancer and other neoplasms. Since the original description of the syndrome, its existence has been demonstrated in various geographical and ethnic groups (Li *et al.*, 1988). Since the original association between rhabdomyosarcoma and breast cancer was defined, the range of cancer types included in the syndrome has been extended to include brain tumours, osteosarcoma, leukaemia and adrenocortical carcinoma (Malkin *et al.*, 1990). Additional possible component tumours include carcinomas of the lung, prostate and pancreas, melanoma and gonadal germ-cell tumours. These diverse types of tumours in family members typically develop at unusually early ages, and multiple primary tumours are frequent (Malkin *et al.*, 1990). Germ-line mutations of the *p53* gene have been identified in some families with Li–Fraumeni syndrome, but the extent to which this accounts for the familial aggregation of the component tumours is uncertain (Strong *et al.*, 1992; Birch, 1994; Malkin, 1994). There may be a subset of Li–Fraumeni syndrome families with a distinct pattern of cancers (high frequency of multiple primary cancers, osteosarcoma and brain tumours) associated with specific germ-line *p53* mutations (Santibañez-Koref *et al.*, 1991).

Soft-tissue sarcoma also is associated with neurofibromatosis type 1 (Yang *et al.*, 1995). In a study of childhood cancers diagnosed during the period 1971–83 in Great Britain, of 1003 cases of soft-tissue sarcoma, 20 (2.0%) had genetic conditions (Narod *et al.*, 1991). Eighteen of the cases had neurofibromatosis; the other two had tuberous sclerosis. In a multicentre case–control study of rhabdomyosarcoma in the USA, five of 249 cases (2%) had neurofibromatosis type 1, compared with none of 302 controls ($p = 0.02$; Yang *et al.*, 1995). In a study of 440 cases with rhabdomyosarcoma in Japan, six (1.4%) had neurofibromatosis type 1 (Matsui *et al.*, 1993).

### Concordance in twins

In combined data from five series, none of 46 twins with soft-tissue sarcoma had an affected co-twin (Buckley *et al.*, 1996).

### Cancer in relatives of cases with soft-tissue sarcoma

The available data appear to be compatible with a modest excess of cancer of all types in first-degree relatives of cases with soft-tissue sarcoma (Table 3.9). In the one available study relating to second-degree relatives of affected children, there was no excess risk (Hartley *et al.*, 1991b). A stronger excess has been observed for mothers of small subgroups of cases with second malignant neoplasms (Strong *et al.*, 1987; Burke *et al.*, 1991).

In a population-based study in Denmark of 1135 parents of 580 children with soft-tissue ($n = 306$) or osteogenic ($n=274$) sarcomas diagnosed during the period 1943–85, the SIR for cancer of all types in the mother was 1.1 (95% CI 0.9–1.3), and that for the father 0.8 (95% CI 0.7–1.0; Olsen *et al.*, 1995). Apart from a reduced rate of lung cancer in the father and a slight elevation of risk of multiple myeloma in the mother (SIR = 4.3, 95% CI 1.1–12, based on three cases), there was no deviation of observed numbers compared with expected numbers for any category of cancer. There was an increase in the risk of breast cancer before the age of 45 years in mothers who had a child with cancer of any type before the age of three. The SIR when the child was diagnosed with a sarcoma was 2.9 (95% CI 1.4–5.3), while that when the child had other types of cancer was 1.7 (95% CI 1.0–2.6). This finding is compatible with the familial syndrome of soft-tissue sarcoma, breast cancer and other neoplasms in young adults and children initially described by Li and Fraumeni (1969). Excesses of breast cancer in mothers of children with soft-tissue sarcoma (Birch *et al.*, 1990a) and in mothers of children with osteosarcoma and chondrosarcoma (Hartley *et al.*, 1986; Garber *et al.*, 1991) have been observed in other studies.

## Table 3.9. Summary of studies of cancer in non-twin sibs and parents of children with soft-tissue sarcoma

| Area and period of study | Reference | Deaths (D) or newly incident (I) cases, upper age boundary | Population (P) or hospital (H) series | Index cases | | Method of obtaining data on cancer in relatives[a] | Type of relatives | Number of relatives with cancer | | | Percentage of affected relatives with same type of tumour as index cases |
|---|---|---|---|---|---|---|---|---|---|---|---|
| | | | | Total | Percentage for whom data on relatives obtained | | | Expected[b] | Observed | O/E | |
| Italy 1979–85 | Pastore *et al.*, 1985 | I, NS | H | 203 | 84 | I | Sibs | 0.2[c] | 3[c] | 15 | NS |
| | | | | | | | Mothers | 0.6 | 0 | 0.0 | |
| | | | | | | | Fathers | 1.1 | 1 | 0.9 | |
| USA, Texas, 1944–76 | Strong *et al.*, 1987 | I[d], 15 | H | 163 | 98 | I, VR, VD | Sibs | NS[e] | 8 | NS | NS |
| | | | | | | | Parents | NS[e] | 25 | NS | |
| UK, North West, West Midlands and Yorkshire, 1980–83 | Hartley *et al.*, 1988b | I, 14 | P | 43 | 100 | I, VR | Mothers | 1.5 | 3 | 2.0 | 0 |
| | | | | | | | Fathers | 1.0 | 0 | 0.0 | – |
| UK, Manchester, 1954–87 | Birch *et al.*, 1990a | I, 14 | P | 177 | NS | I, VR | Sibs[f] | 0.78 | 7 | 9.0 | NS |
| | | | | | | | Sibs[g] | 2.20 | 10 | 4.5 | 10[h] |
| | | | | | | | Mothers | 10.8 | 18 | 1.7 | 0 |
| | | | | | | | Fathers | 11.8 | 12 | 1.0 | 8 |
| **Rhabdomyosarcoma** | | | | | | | | | | | |
| UK, South Glamorgan, NS | Thompson *et al.*, 1988 | NS | H | 37[i] | 46 | HR, I, VR | Mothers | 0.08 | 2 | 26.7 | 0 |
| | | | | | | | Fathers | 0.05 | 0 | 0.0 | – |

NS, Not stated.

[a] HR, hospital and other medical records; I, interview; VD, positive reports and status of dead siblings verified from death certificates; VR, positive reports verified from medical records.

[b] Calculation of expected numbers of affected relatives.
  Pastore *et al.*, 1985  Age-sex-period-specific mortality rates for Italy applied to sibs up to time of diagnosis of index child.
  Strong *et al.*, 1987  Person-years at risk were determined from the date of birth to the date of death, first cancer diagnosis, date of interview or age 75, whichever came first. Age-, sex- and calendar year-specific rates from Connecticut were applied
  Hartley *et al.*, 1988b  Case-control study.
  Birch *et al.*, 1990a  Age-sex-specific rates for the defined geographical area were applied to 30 June 1988 or the date of death.
  Thompson *et al.*, 1988  Age-specific cumulative incidence rates from the West Midlands Region applied for each parent using age at last follow-up or death.

[c] Only deaths in relatives were considered.
[d] Index patients alive at least three years after diagnosis; mean years since diagnosis 13.6.
[e] Expected numbers of affected sibs not presented. O/E for first-degree relatives aged <35, 2.9; for those aged 35–74, 1.3.
[f] At ages <20 years.
[g] At all ages.
[h] Sarcomas of soft tissue or bone.
[i] Overall total includes cases of soft-tissue sarcoma other than rhabdomyosarcoma.

## Second primary tumours

In an international combined anaylsis of 1770 children diagnosed at ages up to 21 years with rhabdomyosarcoma and recruited into clinical trials, 22 second primary tumours were reported (Heyn *et al.*, 1993). A complete family history was obtained for 16 of these patients. Three of the patients had neurofibromatosis, and two of these had a family history of this disorder. Among the other 13 families no family history of cancer was reported in one family only. Three parents died of malignancies between the ages of 30 and 40 years. The family history may be compatible with the Li–Fraumeni syndrome.

In studies of families of children with soft-tissue sarcoma alive at least three years after diagnosis in Texas, segregation analysis was applied under the mixed model, that is comprising independent effects of a major gene, a multifactorial familial aggregation component and a random environmental component acting additively (Lustbader *et al.*, 1992; Strong *et al.*, 1992). The cancer distribution in 159 families (125 with an affected first-degree relative) was found to be more compatible with a rare autosomal dominant gene than with random occurrence or a multifactorial mechanism. It was estimated that the postulated major gene was transmitted in nine of the families, whereas in most families the cancer distribution could be explained by chance. If confirmed, this would suggest that relatives of most patients with childhood soft-tissue sarcoma are not at an increased risk of cancer.

## Other conditions in families of cases with soft-tissue sarcoma

In a population-based study of soft-tissue sarcoma (181 cases) in the North Western region of England during the period 1954–91, 14 (4.0%) of 357 sibs had serious congenital malformations, a somewhat higher prevalence than that at birth in surveys based on multiple sources of ascertainment on extended follow-up in Great Britain and the USA (Hartley *et al.*, 1994a). In this study group, miscarriages occurred in 60% (3 out of 5) of the families in which the index case and/or a close relative had been diagnosed with or showed diagnostic features of neurofibromatosis, 33% (15 of 45) of the families with Li–Fraumeni syndrome or features of the syndrome, and in 18% (23 of 107) of the other families (Hartley *et al.*, 1994b). In a study in Denver, Colorado, USA, four of 31 liveborn sibs of cases with soft-tissue sarcoma were reported to have major birth defects,

compared with 20 of 361 sibs of controls (RR = 2.7, 95% CI 0.9–8.6; Savitz & Ananth, 1994).

## Paternal age and sarcomas

No paternal age effect has been reported for bone tumours or soft-tissue sarcoma (Hartley *et al.*, 1988b) or rhabdomyosarcoma (Grufferman *et al.*, 1982; Magnani *et al.*, 1989; Ghali *et al.*, 1992).

## Gonadal and germ-cell tumours

In a study of childhood cancer diagnosed during the period 1971–83 in Great Britain, three (0.7%) of 430 cases with gonadal and germ-cell tumours had genetic conditions (Narod *et al.*, 1991). Two had 46XY gonadal dysgenesis and one had Down's syndrome. In a population-based study in Denmark of 125 cases of germ-cell, trophoblastic or other gonadal neoplasm in childhood, no excess risk of cancer in either parent was observed (Olsen *et al.*, 1995).

## Epithelial tumours

In a study of childhood cancer diagnosed during the period 1971–83 in Great Britain, ten (1.9%) of 524 cases with epithelial tumours had genetic conditions (Narod *et al.*, 1991). Six of these cases were from families with multiple endocrine neoplasia type 2. In a population-based study in Denmark of 176 cases of carcinoma or other malignant epithelial neoplasm, no excess risk of cancer in either parent was observed (Olsen *et al.*, 1995).

## Conclusions

Cancers with a Mendelian mode of inheritance, or associated with disorders with a Mendelian mode of inheritance, constitute only a small fraction of childhood cancer. No strong evidence of familial aggregation is apparent for the commoner types of childhood cancer. Retinoblastoma is known to be of genetic etiology. Strong familial aggregation has been observed for a range of tumour types in the Li–Fraumeni syndrome. There is a genetic basis to the etiology of Wilms' tumour; at least three genes are known to be involved in the development of the tumour. Studies of second primary neoplasms indicate that there is a genetic relationship between retinoblastoma and osteosarcoma, and that there may be such a relationship between leukaemia and CNS tumours, and also between thyroid tumours and neuroblastoma.

# Chapter 4
# Ionizing radiation

## Residential exposure

Residential exposures to ionizing radiation may be classified as those arising from point sources in both space and time, such as the atomic bomb explosions in Japan and accidents at nuclear plants, from point sources in space, i.e. nuclear installations, and those of a more diffuse origin such as fallout from nuclear weapons tests and domestic radon exposure.

### *Effects of doses received after isolated episodes of exposure: the atomic bomb explosions at Hiroshima and Nagasaki, August 1945*

*Offspring of women exposed during pregnancy*

A total of 1630 children exposed *in utero* to the atomic bomb explosions, i.e. whose mothers were resident in Hiroshima on 6 August 1945 or in Nagasaki on 9 August, and who were born between this date and 31 May 1946, were enumerated as alive on 1 October 1950; the great majority (1401) were exposed in Hiroshima. Only two individuals developed cancer before the age of 15 years, one of whom died at the age of six with liver cancer and the other developed Wilms' tumour at age 14 and subsequently died of stomach cancer at the age of 35 (Yoshimoto *et al.*, 1988). Both had been heavily exposed. The analysis was limited to subjects alive on 1 October 1950 because of the confusion in vital statistics records immediately after the war, with a possible bias whereby deaths may have been identified as exposed *in utero* shortly after notification of the fact of death. In some 1263 children aged under 15 years, the risk of cancer could be followed completely from birth. Dosimetry was based on shielding histories, distances from the sites of the explosions, and transmission factors averaged over all stages of fetal development without regard to orientation or posture at the time of exposure. The mean dose to the uterus was 0.184 gray (1 gray = 100 rad). As already mentioned, two children developed cancer, giving an estimated increase in the risk of childhood cancer of 279 per 10 000 population-gray. Yoshimoto *et al.* (1988) noted

that this is compatible with the excess risk associated with exposure to diagnostic X-rays *in utero*, estimated as 572 per 10 000 population-gray (Bithell & Stewart, 1975). An earlier analysis had suggested a much smaller effect in the Japanese data, based on the occurrence of one case of cancer before the age of 10 years (Jablon & Kato, 1970). Kneale and Stewart (1978) attributed this apparent disparity to damage to the reticuloendothelial system in infants exposed *in utero* to the atomic bomb explosions, leading to a risk of death at an early age from infectious diseases. Mortality in children aged less than 1 year was high in the group that received the highest dose, but there is no evidence as to the risk of infectious disease. Mortality may have been underestimated because of a tendency in Japan to report early neonatal deaths as stillbirths, but there is only limited evidence from Nagasaki of an association between fetal mortality and distance of the mother from the hypocentre of the explosion; the data on childhood cancer are mainly from Hiroshima, there are no data specifically relating stillbirth and dose, and vital statistics records are incomplete for the period immediately following the bombing.

Yoshimoto *et al.* (1988) also presented data on an overall 40-year follow-up of the 1630 survivors exposed to the bombing *in utero*. In addition to the two cases of childhood cancer already discussed, 16 cases of cancer were ascertained in adults. Incidence increased, and age of onset decreased, with increasing dose. The estimated relative risk of cancer at any age associated with a dose of one gray absorbed by the uterus was 3.8 (95% CI 1.1–13.5), the estimated average excess risk per 10 000 person-year-gray among survivors receiving 0.01 Gy or more was 6.6 (95% CI 0.5–14.5), and the estimated attributable risk was 40.9% (95% CI 2.9–90.2). These indices were 30–40% lower when estimation was limited to cancer in subjects aged 15–39 years. The increase was not confined to any specific type of cancer. Only two cases of leukaemia were observed, associated with doses to the uterus of 0.02 and 0.04 Gy.

90

This contrasts with the pattern for survivors of the bombing in general, among whom leukaemia is the main cancer seen. It is noteworthy that the number of deaths from non-cancer causes was three times that expected for doses of 0.6 gray or more, but only three of the 10 deaths were from infection. The migration rate appears to have increased with exposure, and this differential migration may have led to underestimation of the absolute risk of cancer by 15–20%.

## Other offspring of exposed individuals

The occurrence of cancer up to the age of 20 years in the offspring of parents from Hiroshima and Nagasaki born between 1 May 1946 and 1982 has been investigated (Yoshimoto, 1990; Yoshimoto *et al.*, 1990). Among 31 150 children born to parents one or both of whom were less than 2000 m from the hypocentres of the explosions, and thereby received a dose of more than 0.01 Sv, 43 malignant tumours were ascertained, giving an incidence of 7.8 per 100 000 person years. This is slightly greater than the incidence of 6.7 per 100 000, 49 cases among 41 066 offspring matched on age, sex and city, born to parents both of whom were either more than 2500 m from the hypocentre or not in the city at the time of the bombings. There was no statistically significant dose–response association with combined parental gonadal dose. Specific types of childhood cancer were considered in three groups: (1) leukaemia; (2) tumours considered to be heritable, comprising retinoblastoma, Wilms' tumour, osteosarcoma, renal sarcoma, embryonal carcinoma of the testes, and neuroblastoma. On the basis of family studies, all of these tumours could be viewed as the result of germ-line mutation in the preceding generation ($F_0$) and a somatic cell mutation, or as a double somatic mutation in the $F_1$ generation; (3) other tumours. There was no trend in risk with dose for any of these groups. Follow-up of this population is continuing (Yoshimoto, 1990).

## Children who were exposed postnatally

Jablon *et al.* (1971) investigated the incidence of cancer in 15 584 survivors alive on 1 October 1950 who were in Hiroshima and Nagasaki at the time of the explosions and aged under 10 at that time, and 5025 controls who were normally resident in the cities but not there at that time. Leukaemias greatly outnumbered other cancers from 1950 to about 1960. The first cancer death not ascribed to leukaemia was in 1954, of a control subject. Thus, as there was no evidence of radiation carcinogenesis other than leukaemia in the early years of follow-up, the authors considered mortality and morbidity only after 1955. During the period 1955–69, there was a small excess of mortality from leukaemia (O/E = 2.9) but not other cancers (observed = 0, expected = 3.7) for those with dose estimates of 0.1–0.99 Gy. For higher doses, there were significant excesses of both leukaemia (O/E = 19.1, eight cases observed) and other cancers (O/E = 7.3, eight cases observed). There was no specificity as to the site of cancers other than leukaemia.

Subsequently, the method of estimating individual doses has been questioned. Re-analysis has been carried out using a revised method of calculation, and the period of follow-up has been extended to 1985 (Shimizu *et al.*, 1990b). The revised dose estimates were available for 15 895 subjects aged under 10 years at the time of bombing (Shimizu *et al.*, 1990c), 77% of the total investigated by Jablon *et al.* (1971). In the group for which the estimated dose was greater than 1 gray, the cumulative death rate due to cancer was 25.9 per 1000, four times the rate of 6.5 per 1000 in subjects either not in the cities at the time of the bombing, or in the cities but with exposures estimated as less than 0.1 Gy (Shimizu *et al.*, 1990b). The age of onset of cancer was earlier in the former group. The group with exposures of 0.50–0.99 Gy exhibited an intermediate pattern. The relative risk of leukaemia peaked 6–8 years after the bombing, and tended to decrease with years after exposure, irrespective of age at the time of the bombing. For other cancers, the relative risk was higher the younger the age of the subject at the time of bombing, and there was no statistically significant change with years after exposure after adjusting for age at exposure. Although overall it appears that radiation-induced cancers increase significantly only when survivors attain the ages at which the specific cancers occur in unexposed populations, these data suggest that exposure at high doses before age 10 years is followed by early onset. However, although follow-up in this group was largely complete to age 40, the majority of survivors had not yet reached the age of 50.

Jablon *et al.* (1971) also reported data on cancers other than leukaemia or thyroid tumours ascertained from cancer registries and surgical-pathology files from hospitals in the cities, and from medical files on a subsample of 20 000 (18%) of the total cohort of 109 000 subjects (82 000 atomic bomb survivors and

27 000 not in the cities at the time of the bombings) identified from the national census in 1950 in whom mortality is being monitored. The authors acknowledge that follow-up is incomplete, since if the subject did not seek treatment or received medical care outside the two cities, the diagnosis would not have been notified unless it were later identified as a cause of death. A significant trend of increase with increasing dose was identified, based on 24 cases, the relative risk associated with doses estimated to have been greater than 1 Gy being 6.1 as compared to subjects not in the cities at the time of bombing or having received doses less than 0.1 Gy. The rate increased rapidly after 1960 in all categories of dose as the children came into adulthood. There was no specificity as to the type of tumour. The investigators also considered thyroid cancer detected by clinical examination in the subsample whose medical records were reviewed. These subjects were examined every two years. Among 1819 subjects aged under 10 years at the time of the bombing, with the baseline defined as above, the relative risk associated with estimated exposures of 0.1–0.99 Gy was 1.9, and with higher exposure 5.8. For the remainder of the subjects ($n$ = 18 698), no cases were observed in the group estimated to have exposures of 1 Gy or more, but numbers were small; the relative risk associated with exposures of 0.1–0.99 Gy was 6.1.

### Overall comment on data from Hiroshima and Nagasaki

No substantial increase in the overall risk of cancer has been observed in the survivors' offspring who were not exposed *in utero*. Therefore, the emphasis of concern has moved from genetic to somatic effects (Yoshimoto, 1990). Increased risks of cancer in adult life have been observed in individuals exposed *in utero* and in childhood. Based on incidence data, the average excess risk of cancer associated with exposure for those exposed *in utero* is 6.6 per 10 000 person-year-gray, and those exposed at ages 0–9 years, based on mortality data, 5.2 per 10 000 (Yoshimoto *et al.*, 1988). These excess risks are quite similar, although one estimate is based on incidence and the other on mortality, and both are based on small numbers of cases of cancer. With continuing follow-up, an increase in the frequency of radiation-induced cancer may become apparent as the individuals exposed *in utero* age and it will be interesting to subdivide the analysis for the 0–9-year age group (Shimizu *et al.*, 1990b). An important difference between the two groups lies in the risk of

leukaemia, this being substantially lower in the group exposed *in utero*. The apparently low risk associated with intrauterine exposure has been considered inconsistent with studies which show an association between childhood leukaemia and prenatal diagnostic X-ray exposure (Boice, 1990). No significant difference in risk of radiation-related cancer has been found following exposure in different gestational periods (Yoshimoto *et al.*, 1988).

In considering the effects on childhood cancer, the data are limited by the delay between exposure and forming the cohort, and this delay will have included a period of considerable social and economic upheaval at the end of the Second World War. Cancer risk in survivors may have been influenced by thermal and blast effects, malnutrition, sanitary conditions, infectious disease, and other health problems (Boice, 1990). For individuals exposed as children, the rates of cancer were higher in those not in the cities at the time of bombing than in those who received the lowest exposure (0–0.09 Gy); the difference was not accounted for by associations with city, sex or use of medical services (Jablon *et al.*, 1971). The group of subjects not in the city at the time of bombing comprised immigrants from rural areas and individuals returning from Korea, Manchuria, China and south-east Asia. The authors considered that the differences between these subjects and subjects who were in the cities at the time of bombing are likely to be much larger than those within the latter group—geographic stratification of residence by income level is stated not to have been prominent, but it is not clear whether this was assessed at the time of bombing, which seems implausible, or at the time of the 1950 census, when the cohort was identified. The main argument against confounding by socioeconomic factors is that the difference in risk between subjects receiving high and low doses is much greater than that between subjects receiving low doses and those not in the cities. Additional difficulties are that many of the analyses are based on death certification rather than measures of cancer incidence, and that there are doubts about the accuracy of dose estimates.

### Doses received after isolated episodes of exposure: accidents at nuclear plants

Three reactor accidents are known to have caused measurable exposures to the public: Windscale in 1957, Three Mile Island in 1979, and Chernobyl in 1986 (UNSCEAR, 1988).

## The Windscale reactor fire, October 1957

The fire began during a routine release of energy stored in the graphite of one of the piles whose main use was the production of material for the British weapons programme (UNSCEAR, 1982). The fire lasted for three days and major releases of $^{131}$I occurred on two occasions, once when air flow was directed to the core in an attempt to cool it, and again when water was pumped into the reactor which extinguished the fire. The other radionuclides released in significant quantities were $^{210}$Po and $^{137}$Cs (NRPB, 1984). The reactor has not been used since. The National Radiological Protection Board (NRPB, 1984) estimated the contribution of different sources to the total risk of radiation-induced leukaemia for persons up to the age of 20 or until 1980, in seven cohorts assumed to have been born at five-year intervals from 1945 to 1975. Among five sources—the fire, routine discharges, fallout from atmospheric tests of nuclear weapons, diagnostic and therapeutic irradiation, and natural background radiation — the smallest estimated contribution was from the fire (1.6% overall), varying between a maximum of 3.5% for the 1950 cohort and a minimum of 0.1% for the 1975 cohort. Regarding other fatal cancers, the only type for which the fire is estimated to have made a substantial contribution is thyroid cancer because of the release of $^{131}$I, 54% of which is attributed to the fire for all seven cohorts. The authors conclude that in a hypothetical population of 1225 children born in Seascale between 1945 and 1975, and followed to 1980, a total of 0.1 radiation-induced leukaemias would be expected in children under 20 years. The expected number is of a similar order, or less, for specific types of radiation-induced solid cancer. The numbers expected as a result of the fire are even lower. Empirical data for West Cumbria, the area in which Sellafield and Seascale are located, are discussed below.

## The Three Mile Island accident, March 1979

As a result of the Three Mile Island accident, a total of 370 GBq of noble gases, mainly $^{133}$Xe, and 550 GBq of $^{131}$I, were released into the atmosphere (UNSCEAR, 1982). Individual levels of dose averaged $1.5 \times 10^{-5}$ gray within 50 miles (80 km) of the plant, approximately 1% of the background level, and the official estimate of the maximum absorbed dose received by a member of the public is $85 \times 10^{-5}$ gray (Kemeney, 1979). Pregnant women and those with pre-school children resident within 8 km of the plant were advised to leave the area two days after the accident; this advice was rescinded 10 days later (Tyror, 1989).

Following a request by the Three Mile Island Public Health Fund, a court-supervised fund created to address concern about public health issues among residents of the area surrounding the plant, the association between cancer occurrence in the area and radiation releases from the plant was investigated by an ecological analysis of cancer incidence and accidental and routine releases from the plant (Hatch *et al.*, 1990), and of background radiation (Hatch & Susser, 1990). The analysis covered 69 study tracts within a 16 km radius of the plant during the period 1975–85. Cases were ascertained from records of all 19 hospitals within 48 km (30 miles) of the plant, and of six referral hospitals in the nearby cities of Philadelphia, Pittsburgh and Baltimore. The addresses of 4% of all cases (children and adults; details are not given separately for children) could not be assigned with certainty, and such cases were apportioned among likely tracts according to the relative population size of each tract. Relative exposures of the study tracts were assigned, the absolute values being uncertain but thought to be low. Releases due to the accident and routine emissions were estimated by dispersion modelling. In this modelling as applied to exposures from the accident, estimates of radioactive release were derived from the only monitors within the plant that remained on scale during most of the period of the accident. Good agreement (correlation coefficient 0.92) was observed between exposures predicted from 20 dosimeters located around the plant during the accident and the dispersion model. The distribution of background gamma radiation was derived from measurements made in an aerial survey in 1976, and exposure estimates were based on absolute measurements. Annual exposures of this type were in the range 0.5–1.0 mSv, compared with an average of 0.1 mSv from accidental releases over four days (median exposure in highest quartile 0.4 mSv) and 0.001 mSv per year from routine emissions.

The results relating to childhood cancer are summarized in Table 4.1. National rates from the SEER for 1978–81 were used to estimate expected incidences in the calculation of standardized incidence ratios, and are generally comparable with cancer registration rates reported for south-central Pennsylvania. The incidence of total childhood cancer in the Three Mile Island area was similar to national rates, but that of childhood leukaemia was well below national rates, despite the inclusion of regional referral units in case-finding. Analysis was performed for the pre-accident period (1975–March 1979) and

**Table 4.1. Summary of results of ecological study of incidence of childhood cancer (ages 0–14 years) and residential exposure to ionizing radiation from various sources in the area around the Three Mile Island nuclear plant (Hatch *et al.*, 1990; Hatch & Susser 1990)**

| Category | Total number of cases | Standardized incidence ratio by quartile of exposure[a] | | | | RR[b] (95% CI) quartile 4 versus quartile 1 |
|---|---|---|---|---|---|---|
| | | 1 | 2 | 3 | 4 | |
| **Total childhood cancer** | | | | | | |
| Emissions due to the accident | | | | | | |
| 1975–79 | 19 | 1.7 | 0.2 | 1.0 | 0.9 | 0.7 (0.2–2.5) |
| 1981–85 | 18 | 0.5 | 0.9 | 0.9 | 1.2 | 1.1 (0.4–2.8) |
| 1984–85 | 6 | 0.6 | 0.4 | 1.3 | 0.0 | 0.4 (0.0–12.0) |
| Routine emissions | | | | | | |
| 1975–79 | 19 | 0.6 | 1.4 | 0.6 | 3.0 | 2.0 (0.6–6.7) |
| 1979–85 | 30 | 0.7 | 1.1 | 1.4 | 1.2 | 1.2 (0.4–3.9) |
| 1975–85 | 49 | 0.7 | 1.2 | 1.1 | 1.9 | 1.5 (0.7–3.5) |
| Background gamma radiation | | | | | | |
| 1975–85 | 49 | 0.6 | 1.2 | 1.1 | 1.8 | 2.7 (1.3–5.6) |
| **Childhood leukaemia** | | | | | | |
| Emissions due to the accident | | | | | | |
| 1975–79 | 1 | 0.5 | 0.0 | 0.0 | 0.0 | |
| 1981–85 | 4 | 0.4 | 0.0 | 1.1 | 1.3 | 2.3 (0.4–12.8) |
| 1984–85 | 1 | 0.0 | 0.0 | 1.4 | 0.0 | |
| Routine emissions | | | | | | |
| 1975–79 | 1 | 0.1 | 0.3 | 0.0 | 0.0 | |
| 1979–85 | 7 | 0.0 | 0.3 | 2.5 | 2.0 | 2.5 (0.6–10.3) |
| 1975–85 | 8 | 0.1 | 0.3 | 1.6 | 1.3 | 2.3 (0.6–9.7) |
| Background gamma radiation | | | | | | |
| 1975–85 | 8 | 0.5 | 0.4 | 0.5 | 1.2 | 3.2 (0.5–19.3) |

[a] Expected numbers for calculation of standardized incidence ratios were based on data from SEER for the period 1978-81.
[b] For emissions due to the accident and routine emissions, these were adjusted for age, sex, population density, median income and proportion of high-school graduates in study tracts. For background gamma radiation, adjustment was made only for the first four of these variables.

the post-accident period, allowing for two-year (1981–85) and five-year (1984–85) latency intervals after the accident. No association was apparent between emissions due to the accident and total childhood cancer. A relative risk of 2.3 (95% CI 0.6–10.3) of leukaemia for the highest versus the lowest quartile of exposure was seen, based on one case in each category.

Data on routine emissions were considered for the periods 1975–March 1979, when the plant was in operation, and April 1979–85, when the plant was not in operation. For total childhood cancer, a relative risk of 2.0 was found for the highest quartile of exposure versus the lowest during the period the plant was in operation, based on 3 and 4.4 exposed cases respectively. The fractional number of observed cases is a result of the allocation of cases across study tracts where address information did not specify exact location. No dose–response pattern is apparent from consideration of standardized incidence ratios. For childhood leukaemia, a raised relative risk was observed for the period when the plant was not in operation, but the confidence intervals are extremely wide.

For the overall eleven-year period 1975–85, the relative risk for total childhood cancer associated with background gamma radiation was 2.7 (95% CI 1.3–5.6), based on 9.7 cases in the highest

quartile of exposure and 13 in the lowest. For leukaemia, the relative risk was 3.2 (95% CI 0.5–19.3) based on 2 and 3 cases respectively. Hatch and Susser (1990) observed that conventional risk models would not predict a detectable increase in the incidence of childhood cancer from background gamma radiation. The association for childhood leukaemia, which is based on very small numbers of cases, has to be viewed in the context of the rate being well below the national rates, and the possibility of incomplete ascertainment cannot be excluded. Thus, the data on childhood leukaemia are inadequate to assess a possible association with emissions arising from the accident. For total childhood cancer, no association is apparent with emissions due to the accident.

### The Chernobyl accident, April 1986

To date, the most serious accident in a nuclear power station is that which occurred at the Chernobyl plant, about 100 km north-west of Kiev and 310 km south-west of Minsk, in the former USSR, on 26 April 1986 (UNSCEAR, 1988). The official death toll by the first anniversary of the accident was 31, most of whom were emergency workers and plant personnel who died of acute radiation sickness (Gale, 1987; WHO,

1987). Other than the workers in the plant, the groups thought to be most at risk from radiation are the 115 000 people living within a 30-km radius, who were evacuated (WHO, 1987), and about 245 000 decontamination workers (Dickman, 1991).

Data on the geographical distribution of radiation exposures occurring as a result of the fallout have been reviewed by the United Nations Scientific Committee on the Effects of Atomic Radiation (UNSCEAR, 1988). Release of material over a ten-day period, together with wind changes over Europe, led to areas of highest deposition in (1) the western part of the former USSR, Finland and Sweden (2) central Europe, notably Poland, Austria, Bavaria, eastern Switzerland and northern Italy and (3) Romania, Bulgaria and parts of Yugoslavia and Greece. Outside the former USSR, the highest effective dose equivalents in the first year after the accident were 760 μSv in Bulgaria, 670 μSv in Austria, 590 μSv in Greece and 570 μSv in Romania. The average annual effective dose equivalent from natural sources is 2400 μSv. Overall, 75% of exposure resulted from the consumption of contaminated food, while the main source of external exposure was from deposition of radionuclides on the ground. However, deposition of radionuclides on the ground was higher in areas which experienced heavy rainfall at the time of the accident, notably Austria and some of the Nordic countries, while food-chain exposure in southern European countries was the major pathway of exposure, as several crops were ready for harvesting and dairy cattle were grazing on new forage (Bertazzi, 1989). The principal radionuclides involved were iodine-131 (half-life 8 days), caesium-134 (half-life 2.1 years) and caesium-137 (half-life 30 years). The caesium isotopes continue to be a source of exposure because of their longer half-life and accumulation in foodstuffs.

*— The Chernobyl accident and childhood leukaemia*

Ivanov *et al.* (1993) reported that there was no appreciable change in the incidence of acute leukaemia in children either in Belarus as a whole or in the Gomel and Mogilev regions, the most highly contaminated areas, during the period 1986–91 compared with the period 1979–85. Cases were ascertained from haematology departments, oncology centres, autopsies and vital records.

No marked change in the incidence of childhood leukaemia or all other childhood cancers except that of the thyroid was observed during the period 1981–90 in Polesskoye,

Naroditchy and Ovrutch in Ukraine, the areas with the highest levels of radioactive caesium in the soil outside the 30 km zone of evacuation around the plant (Prisyazhiuk *et al.*, 1991).

Gibson *et al.* (1988) compared observed and expected numbers of registrations of childhood leukaemia in Scotland in 1981–86 and 1987, expected numbers being calculated from data for 1971–80, to follow-up clinical observations of an unusually high number of children diagnosed with leukaemia in Scotland from 1987 onwards. Some 48 cases were observed in 1987 in comparison with an expected 35. This excess was entirely accounted for by cases under the age of five years. The observed numbers for the period 1981–86 were similar to those expected for this age group, and for older children were somewhat below those expected. The authors considered that bias of ascertainment was unlikely to explain the findings. Indeed, any bias would have been expected to arise from late registration of recent cases, which would result in the observed number of cases in 1987 being an underestimate. No evidence of small-area clustering of cases in the 0–4–year age group was found—the excess was spread over a large part of central Scotland. In view of concern about the effects of the Chernobyl accident, whole-body scanning for radiocaesium was done in some children and their mothers, but no increased levels were found compared with control subjects.

Cartwright *et al.* (1988) subsequently examined registrations in the under-five-year age group in a system especially designed to ascertain leukaemia in Cumbria, South Wales and Yorkshire (higher fallout areas) and in the Trent and the South Eastern regions of England (lower fallout areas) during the period 1984–88. No evidence for higher rates in birth cohort data related to the accident was found, but the authors noted that follow-up was insufficient.

The International Agency for Research on Cancer is co-ordinating a study of childhood leukaemia and non-Hodgkin lymphoma (the European Childhood Leukaemia/Lymphoma Incidence Study; ECLIS) based on registries in 16 countries in Europe outside the former USSR and in five areas within the former USSR, (Parkin, 1990). The areas within the former USSR comprise Belarus (formerly Byelorussia), where the annual first-year effective dose equivalent is estimated to have been 1950 μSv, five oblasts in the Russian Federation with an estimated dose of 440 μSv, a further five oblasts in the Federation with a dose of 135 μSv, and Estonia and Lithuania, each with doses of 135 μSv. The study does not include the highly exposed areas in Greece or Romania. On the basis of estimates of effect made by the US National Research Council Committee on Biological Effects of Ionizing Radiations (1990), in turn based on data from the follow-up of survivors of the bombings in Japan using the estimates of dose revised in 1986, Parkin estimated that an average increase in the number of cases of 0.8% was expected, with a maximum in Belarus of around 6%. These estimates were based on first-year effective dose equivalents and doses in subsequent years would be less. Several evaluations suggest that increases of this order are unlikely to be detectable (e.g., Pershagen, 1988; Gale & Butturini, 1991), but there remains considerable public concern about the health effects of the accident (Darby & Reeves, 1991) and in the evaluation made for the Commission of the European Communities (1990), it was suggested that it might be possible to detect an effect if the estimates of risk were too low by a factor of five (Mole, 1991). Mole (1991) has commented on the considerable problems of ensuring comparability in this study. Uncontrolled confounding would be a major difficulty if areas were compared, but is less of a problem in the analysis of time trends within areas, which is the main focus of the study. In addition, he observed that inadequate data for the period before the accident, lack of information about the evacuation of individuals, and inadequate detail about deposition of debris from the explosion would make a survey of childhood leukaemia in the 25 000 most highly exposed individuals who lived or worked near Chernobyl worthless. There is some uncertainty about the dose–response relationship between childhood leukaemia and postnatal exposure to ionizing radiation because of the lack of data for the first five years following the atomic bombings in Japan (Parkin *et al.*, 1993a). Unless current knowledge of the effects of low doses of ionizing radiation is grossly incorrect, the main benefits of surveys of the health effects of the accident are to be seen to respond to public concern, to stimulate registration in areas where this has not been extensively developed, and to stimulate contact between registries.

In a preliminary analysis of data from 30 regions, there was a 41% increase in the leukaemia incidence in 1987–88 compared with 1980–85, but this may have been accounted for by improvements in the quality of the incidence data (Parkin *et al.*, 1993a). In addition, there was no association between the change in incidence and effective dose in the first year estimated for the individual regions. Subsequently, in an analysis of data from 35 regions during the period 1980–91, an average annual increase of 0.06% in the overall age-standardized rate of childhood leukaemia was observed in the period 1980–86 (Parkin *et al.*, 1996). There was no indication of an increase in the gradient of this trend in the period 1987–91 (average annual increase 0.4%), following the Chernobyl accident. Moreover, the overall geographical pattern of change was unrelated to environmental exposure to ionizing radiation resulting from the accident. As acknowledged by the authors, the study had low power to detect a trend in risk with dose at this stage of follow-up.

Country-specific results have been published from four of the countries participating in the ECLIS study, namely Finland, Germany, Greece and Sweden (Auvinen *et al.*, 1994; Hjalmars *et al.*, 1994; Petridou *et al.*, 1994; Michaelis *et al.*, 1997a). While in some, detailed exposure assessment was possible, the statistical power of these analyses was low (Ambach & Rehwald, 1994; Parkin *et al.*, 1996).

Auvinen *et al.* (1994) assessed external exposure as the cumulative dose over the two-year period following the Chernobyl accident in 455 Finnish municipalities. Values specific to municipalities were corrected for shielding, based on the population of blocks of flats in each municipality, and for fallout from atomic weapons testing. Internal exposure was estimated from whole-body measurements on a random sample of 81 children in June 1986 and April 1988. The mean effective dose for the two-year period after the accident was calculated from these measurements. The population weighted mean effective dose was 4.0 µSv for the whole country and 9.70 µSv for the fifth of the population with the highest dose. Data on childhood leukaemia were obtained from the Finnish National Cancer Registry and verified through hospitals treating childhood cancers for the period 1976–92. Overall, no clear increase in the incidence of childhood leukaemia in the period after the accident was detected. In the population with the highest quintile of exposure, the standardized incidence ratio (SIR) for the period 1989–92 was 1.2 (95% CI 0.9–1.6). This finding was based on one to two extra cases per year in 1990–92, but not in 1989. The SIRs for the period 1978–85 and 1986–88 were below unity.

In Greece, parts of which were exposed to fallout from the Chernobyl accident at levels as high as those in countries bordering the former Soviet Union, 17 regions were defined according to levels of caesium-137 fallout radiation from the accident and radium-226 background radiation (Petridou *et al.*, 1994). Cases of childhood leukaemia were ascertained from patient discharge data from all hospitals in the country in which childhood leukaemia was treated. The incidence was compared between the pre-accident period (1980–June 1986), the immediate post-accident period (July 1986 to June 1988) and the period July 1988 to June 1991, this being considered to accommodate the presumed latent period of the disease. It was postulated that no biologically relevant increase in the incidence of leukaemia would have occurred in the immediate post-accident period, but that increased awareness and scrutiny for leukaemia might have occurred. There was no evidence of an increased incidence of childhood leukaemia in any of the regions during either of the two post-accident periods. In addition, there was no association between childhood leukaemia by region and either fallout or background radiation. However, the authors acknowledged that the study did not have adequate power to rule out an increase in leukaemia as a result of the accident. Subsequently, Petridou *et al.* (1996b) reported a significant excess of leukaemia in children diagnosed at ages under one year exposed to fallout from Chernobyl *in utero*, defined as born in the period July–December 1987, compared with those born in the periods 1980–85 and 1988–90 = 2.6, 95% CI 1.4–5.1). There was no excess for this birth cohort between the ages of one and four years.

In Sweden, radiation exposure was measured using an airborne spectrometer during the period May–October 1986 (Hjalmars *et al.*, 1994). The incidence of childhood leukaemia in areas with a ground-level caesium-137 activity of 10 kBq/m$^2$ or more after the accident was compared between the period 1980–May 1986 and June 1986–92. The method of ascertainment of cases was not specified. There was no statistically significant difference in rate either overall, for acute lymphocytic leukaemia (ALL), or for subgroups defined by age. In addition, the association between the incidence of leukaemia with the level of contamination in the period after the accident was investigated. No association was found either when residence at diagnosis or residence at birth was considered.

In the USA, where levels of fallout due to the Chernobyl accident were much lower than in Greece, the incidence of leukaemia diagnosed in the first year of life in cancer registration areas covering 19% of births in the country was 30% higher for those born in 1986–87 than for those born in the remainder of the period 1980–90 (Mangano, 1997). There was no such increase for leukaemia diagnosed at age 1–4 years.

In Germany, an increase in the incidence of infant leukaemia in children born in the period 1 July 1986 to 31 December 1987 in the former Federal Republic after the Chernobyl accident compared with those born in the period 1980–85 and 1988–90 was observed (rate ratio 1.5, 95% CI 1.0–82.2; Michaelis *et al.*, 1997a). However, when the analysis was stratified according to level of deposition of caesium-137 on the ground, no relationship between level of exposure and incidence was apparent. In addition, it was noted that the dose rate in the first days after the accident were 23 times higher than in the last month of 1987, because of decline in the activity of short-lived radio-nuclides and because surface contaminations in the environment and on food were quickly washed out. Michaelis *et al.* (1997a) postulated that levels of radiation exposure *in utero* would have been higher for children born in the period July 1986 to March 1987 than in the period April to December 1987. The rate ratio for leukaemia in children born in the former period was 1.29, compared with 1.67 for those born in the later period, which is not consistent with an effect of fallout from Chernobyl.

In addition to these studies, investigations of time trends in the incidence of leukaemia in Bulgaria during the period 1981–93, Bavaria (Germany) during the period 1983–93 and in leukaemia mortality in Romania during the period 1980–92, in relation to the Chernobyl accident were summarized by Sali *et al.* (1996). No changes in leukaemia incidence or mortality which could be clearly related to the accident were observed, but the statistical power of these analyses was low.

— *The Chernobyl accident and thyroid cancer in childhood*

A substantial increase in the incidence of thyroid cancer in childhood has been reported in the areas that received the highest exposures in Belarus (Kazakov *et al.*, 1992; Baverstock *et al.*, 1992). There was a marked increase in frequency from 1990 onwards compared with the average for the period 1986–90. In the Gomel region, Belarus, over which the plume passed in the first few hours after the major release of radioactivity, and in consequence received the highest fallout from Chernobyl, the incidence in 1991 and the first part of 1992 was approximately 80 per million children per year. In most studies, the incidence of thyroid cancer in children has been reported to be of the order of 1 per million per year. The authors considered that improved ascertainment could have had only a limited role in the increase in reported incidence, as the proportion of resected thyroid nodules that were malignant was high and the type of tumour was aggressive. The histopathological findings of cases undergoing surgery between 1986 and 1991 were described by Furmanchuk *et al.* (1992). Histological examination of thyroid glands removed from 93 of 101 cases diagnosed in Belarus between 1986 and 1991 confirmed the diagnosis of malignancy in 92.5% of patients. The pathological characteristics of the tumours were similar to those reported for other series of thyroid cancer in children (Williams *et al.*, 1993). The ratio of thyroid cancer in children to that in adults increased dramatically, although the investigators commented that the incidence in adults was also beginning to increase. However, in a study conducted four and a half years after the accident, there was no difference in the incidence, prevalence and characteristics of thyroid nodules detected by ultrasonagraphy between subjects living in seven highly contaminated villages around Chernobyl and those living in six control villages (Mettler *et al.*, 1992). The findings were similar to those reported for unexposed populations in other countries.

As well as in southern Belarus, a high frequency of thyroid tumours in children has been reported in northern Ukraine and more recently in the Bryansk region in the Russian Federation, close to Chernobyl (Williams, 1994; Stsjazhko *et al.*, 1995). Prisyazhiuk *et al.* (1991) considered trends in the incidence of thyroid cancer in children in Poleskoye, Naroditchy and Ovrutch in Ukraine, the areas with the highest levels of radioactive caesium in the soil outside the 30-km zone of evacuation around the plant. No cases of thyroid cancer in the 0–14–year age group were observed in 1981–89, but three cases were observed in 1990. The data were obtained from record review in regional and district hospitals and specialist institutes, and death registrations. Screening for thyroid cancer began after the accident and was intensified after 1988, especially among children from contaminated areas. It is not known whether the three cases observed in 1990 were detected at screening or presented with symptoms.

In Belarus and Ukraine, a substantial proportion of the thyroid cancers detected in children were detected within five years of the accident (Boice & Linet, 1994). This apparently short latent period is inconsistent with data on the effects of fallout from nuclear weapons on inhabitants of the Marshall Islands, where the first thyroid tumour occurred nine years later than the weapons tests there (Conard, 1984), and with a combined analysis of all major studies of childhood irradiation, where fewer thyroid tumours than expected occurred within five years of exposure (Ron *et al.*, 1995).

With regard to the apparent increase in incidence of thyroid cancer in children in areas heavily contaminated by fallout from Chernobyl, some commentators considered that the potential importance of changes in ascertainment had been underestimated, particularly as no data were presented on the relative proportions of cases detected as a result of screening and as a result of clinical symptoms (Beral & Reeves, 1992; Shigematsu & Thiessen, 1992). Later it was stated that between 40% and 70% of all cases diagnosed in Belarus were found through a programme of annual screening by palpation of the neck, ultrasound imaging and thyroid hormone testing (Stsjazhko *et al.*, 1995). Beral and Reeves (1992) observed that the great majority of the children had papillary carcinomas, whereas work elsewhere has shown that fewer than half the thyroid cancers which cause clinical disease are papillary. At autopsy, the prevalence of occult papillary carcinoma has been found to be 2% at ages 0–15 and 22% at ages 16–30 years (Franssila & Harach, 1986). Most occult lesions found at autopsy with a diameter of greater than 2 mm show invasion into the surrounding tissue. In a study of the morphological and clinical features of tumours from 86 cases of thyroid cancer in children aged 5–14 years at diagnosis treated in Minsk in 1991–92, Nickiforov and Gnepp (1994) found papillary carcinoma in 83 cases and medullary carcinoma in one. The tumours usually were aggressive, often demonstrating diffuse intrathyroidal tumour dissemination, thyroid capsular and adjacent soft-tissue invasion and cervical lymph-node metastases.

Ron *et al.* (1992) compared incidence rates of thyroid cancer in adults before and after the implementation of a screening programme for thyroid cancer in the USA. The screening programme was implemented following publication of newspaper articles drawing attention to the excess of thyroid cancer among people treated with head and neck radiation, and was directed to patients who had received such treatment. In the six-year period after the introduction of screening, compared with a previous period of unspecified length, the age–sex-adjusted incidence rates of malignant thyroid nodules increased seven-fold, and of total thyroid cancer 17-fold, similar to the magnitude of increase observed in Belarus. To minimize the effect of radiation exposure, the analysis was repeated for subjects who had received less than 50 centigray exposure. In this group, the difference was even greater. Therefore, work is needed to clarify the effect of screening on the recorded incidence of thyroid cancer in children in Belarus. Ultrasound equipment, which would aid diagnosis, was installed only after the Chernobyl accident (Bertin & Lallemand, 1992). There is also a need for analyses of changes in incidence by recorded level of exposure (Beral & Reeves, 1992; Shigematsu & Thiessen, 1992). No relationship between individual dose and the rate of thyroid cancer has been found (Boice & Linet, 1994).

The area of southern Belarus, northern Ukraine and the Briansk region of Russia is low in natural iodine salts and is recognized as an area of mild endemic goitre (Williams *et al.*, 1993). In the late 1970s, the diet of the population had been supplemented with iodine, but this practice had fallen into abeyance by the time of the accident. As a consequence of the low level of natural iodine in the diet, any additional iodine, including radioactive, would have been taken up rapidly by the thyroid. While potassium iodine tablets were reported to be widely distributed in the affected regions, a prophylactic measure intended to block the uptake of radioactive iodine in the thyroid, it is thought that this was too late to have had the desired effect among those living in northern Ukraine and southern Belarus, who suffered the first exposure to radioactive iodine (Williams *et al.*, 1993).

Sali *et al.* (1996) summarized studies of time trends in incidence or mortality due to thyroid cancer in infants in Croatia, Greece, Hungary, Poland and Turkey. No clear changes in rates were apparent in relation to the accident.

— *The Chernobyl accident and other types of childhood cancer*

In Bavaria during the period 1983–93, no changes in the incidence of tumours of the central nervous system or of embryonal tumours (defined to include neuroblastoma, nephroblastoma, retinoblastoma and malignant tumours of the germ cells) occurred that could be linked to the Chernobyl accident (Sali *et al.*, 1996). In a case–control study of neuroblastoma diagnosed at up to four years of age in the former West Germany during the period 1988–92, there was no association with parental consumption of locally grown foods likely to have been contaminated by the accident, either for a summary indicator or for specific foods, particularly deer and mushrooms (Michaelis *et al.*, 1996). The analysis was based on data relating to 64 cases and 109 population-based controls obtained by a combination of postal questionnaires and telephone interviews. The participation rate for mothers of cases was 86% and for mothers of controls 72%.

## Fallout from weapons tests

The effects of fallout from weapons testing have been investigated in detailed studies in Utah and Nevada, in the USA in general, in the United Kingdom, in the Nordic countries and in Kazakstan.

### Childhood leukaemia

Between January 1951 and the end of October 1958, at least 97 atomic devices were detonated above ground in the Nevada desert at a site approximately 160 km west of the Utah–Nevada border (Lyon *et al.*, 1979). Fallout from at least 26 of the tests, amounting to over half of the total yield, was carried by winds into Utah. Deaths due to leukaemia in Utah between 1952 and 1981 were cross-matched with the Deceased Membership File of the Church of Jesus Christ of Latter Day Saints for the period 1950–58 (Stevens *et al.*, 1990). For children, at least one parent had to be a member of the Church. All deaths from causes other than leukaemia that met the above selection criteria were eligible for selection as controls. Living controls were not used because the census records of the Church were not complete. An age-stratified random sample sufficient to provide five controls for each case was selected from the Deceased Membership File of the Church, and each case was individually matched with controls by year of death, age and sex, resulting in the inclusion of 5330 of the potential controls. Of a total of 1836 leukaemia cases identified for the state of Utah, 1195 (65%) were linked with the Deceased Membership File of the Church. This proportion was similar to the proportion of the total population who were members of the Church (70%), although the authors acknowledged that this did not take account of differences in distribution by age, year, sex and area. The residence history during the period of fallout from tests at the Nevada test site was determined for each subject using information from the Deceased Membership File, in the census records maintained by the Church, and from telephone and city directories. As absorbed dose to active bone marrow is considered to be involved in the mechanism whereby radiation exposure leads to leukaemia, and the most significant contribution of dose to bone marrow was derived from external exposure from deposition of fallout on ground surfaces, sources of information on exposure at residence location were used in estimating dose. Absorbed dose to active bone marrow was then estimated using age- and dose-conversion factors and taking into account shielding by buildings.

For leukaemias of all types, no notable significant trend with dose was found. The relative risk for subjects with the highest doses (6–30 mGy) compared with those who received low doses (0–2.9 mGy) was 1.7 (95% CI 1.0–2.8). Individuals who were aged less than 20 years in 1953 were considered *a priori* to be at high risk of leukaemia from external radiation. The relative risk of dying from acute leukaemia during the period 1952–63 was 1.3 (95% CI 0.6–2.7) for the group receiving an intermediate dose (3–5.9 mGy) and 7.8 (95% CI 1.9–32.2) in the group receiving the high dose, in which five cases of leukaemia were observed. Subjects whose gestational period occurred during the period of maximum fallout (1952–58) also were considered to be at high risk. In 99 cases and 329 controls who were so exposed, no association was observed with doses received *in utero*, during the first year of life, or between the ages of one and nine years.

As the control group comprised deceased subjects, variations in all-cause mortality by geographical area could have biased the results, but adjustment for differences in all-cause mortality rate between counties had little effect on the results observed. The results are applicable only to leukaemia mortality, but the authors pointed out that before 1968 acute leukaemia was uniformly fatal within three years of diagnosis. A comparison of the prevalence of exposure to therapeutic and diagnostic X-rays reported in a study of thyroid disease and fallout showed no difference between Washington County, the area of highest exposure within Utah, and comparison counties in Nevada and Arizona. The low elevation of the county suggests that confounding by cosmic radiation is unlikely, and limited data suggest that terrestrial background radiation was low in the county. In addition, limited data were available on occupational exposures, prior cancer treatment, migration and genetic syndromes, none of which appeared to be systematic confounders. It is also possible that limitation of the study to members of the Church of Jesus Christ of Latter Day Saints may have produced a group relatively homogeneous with respect to health behaviour, thereby reducing the possible extent of uncontrolled confounding. The observed risks in the study were approximately double those predicted by equations developed by the National Research Council (NRCCBEIR, 1990), based largely on the data from the atomic bombing victims in Japan.

Other studies in Utah relevant to childhood cancer (Lyon *et al.*, 1979; Land *et al.*, 1984; Machado *et al.*, 1987) have been of an ecological design and were based on approximately the same cases as those included in the study by Stevens *et al.* (1990). These studies therefore make little additional contribution. They have been reviewed in detail by Linet (1985) and the National Research Council (NRCCBEIR, 1990).

Archer (1987) carried out an analysis of trends in leukaemia mortality during the period 1950–77 in the USA as related to peaks in fallout in 1951, 1953, 1957 and 1962. Death rates for all leukaemias among whites showed a statistically significant increase in all of the States included in the study during and shortly after the period of above-ground nuclear testing, followed by a fall several years after the limited test ban treaty. Regional age-adjusted death rates for all leukaemias in whites were positively associated with a composite exposure index, based on concentrations of strontium-90 in milk, food and bone, and time trends in leukaemia death rates were similar between the regions. For acute and myeloid leukaemia, which were thought to be more closely related to radiation than other types on the basis of the data on Japanese atomic bombing survivors, there was a positive association between the peak periods of fallout and mortality in 5–9-year-old children, 5.5 years later. However, no leukaemia mortality peak was associated with the second of the fallout peaks (1953), although there was an elevated mortality rate between the peaks associated with the first and third fallout peaks. For the age range 5–19, mortality attributed to leukaemias of these types began rising in 1954, three years after the start of testing at the Nevada site, and exhibited a marked elevation that persisted until 1963. No elevated risk was apparent for other types of leukaemia in this period. There was a wide peak between 1957 and 1962, which the author considered as corresponding to fallout from 1951 to 1958, and a second peak in 1968 to 1969, 6–7 years after the fallout peak of 1962. Overall, an excess of leukaemia deaths at ages 5–19 years associated with fallout of 6.5 ± 0.2 per million person years per cGy was estimated. Although the specific associations with peaks of fallout in children were apparent only for subtypes of leukaemia that had been associated with ionizing radiation, there are some limitations to this analysis. The subtype distribution before 1958 had to be estimated indirectly. Moreover, there were marked changes in the outcome of treatment, especially for acute leukaemia, during the period studied which complicated interpretation of time trends in mortality. Trends for children under the age of five were not reported.

In the context of evaluating a possible association between the excess of leukaemia around Dounreay in northern Scotland and radioactive discharges from the plant, Darby and Doll (1987) considered time trends in leukaemia in the 0–24–year age group in the United Kingdom, Denmark and Norway in relation to fallout from atmospheric testing of nuclear weapons. The doses from both low and high linear energy transfer radiation due to fallout rose to a maximum in the mid-1960s and then declined. In England and Wales and in Scotland, an increase in leukaemia incidence started about 1971 and persisted until 1979, when the recorded incidence fell to the level of mortality in the 1950s. The increase may possibly be attributable to improvements in diagnosis. National cancer registration has been established for a longer period in Denmark and Norway than in the United Kingdom. The estimated doses of high linear energy transfer radiation and fallout in these countries are similar to those in the United Kingdom, and those due to low linear energy transfer radiation are higher, especially in Norway because of its high rainfall. Measured concentrations of caesium-137 in Norwegian milk have been about six times those in the United Kingdom, and concentrations of strontium-90 about three times. In Denmark, the values for caesium-137 are similar to the United Kingdom, and those for strontium-90 are intermediate between those for the other two countries. In both Scandinavian countries, the leukaemia incidence declined slightly after 1960, during the period of highest exposure to fallout. Thus, there was no consistent evidence of an increase in incidence that could be attributed to fallout.

Subsequently, Darby *et al.* (1992) considered data on childhood leukaemia from cancer registries in Denmark and Norway, as before, and also in Finland, Iceland and Sweden. These registries started sufficiently early for stable registration practices to have been established, enabling the effects of the peak period of atmospheric testing to be evaluated. In addition,

the radioactive fallout from weapon testing was relatively high in these countries. In view of possible problems of completeness of registration in the initial years of operation of the registries, data for the first five years of operation from the three registries which started earliest (Denmark, Finland and Norway) were excluded, and data for the first three years from Iceland and Sweden were also excluded. Thus, data were included from 1948 from Denmark, 1961 from Sweden, and from 1958 for Finland, Iceland and Norway.

Trends were considered through to the end of 1987. In addition to doses to the red bone marrow resulting from nuclear weapon fallout, the authors also considered doses to the testes, in view of the finding of Gardner *et al.* (1990a) relating to paternal occupational exposure. Estimates of annual doses to these tissues from fallout had not been published for any of the Nordic countries. Therefore, estimates of the dose equivalent to the red bone marrow of a fetus and to a one-year-old child in Britain were applied. Although doses in Nordic countries were of a different magnitude from those in Britain because of the effects of latitude, rainfall and dietary habits, it was considered that the pattern of variation with time should be similar in all six countries. The authors estimated doses to the testes by combining the annual effective dose equivalent to an adult through external radiation in Britain with the annual internal dose from caesium-137. The average dose equivalent from weapon fallout to the testes of an adult man in the year before conception was estimated as 140 $\mu$Sv. This is much lower than that reported to be associated with an increased risk in the vicinity of Sellafield.

The possible effects of radiation from fallout after birth, *in utero* and to the fathers' testes during the year before the year in which the child was born, for children aged 0–14 and for children aged 0–4 years, were examined. There was little evidence for an increase risk of leukaemia associated with the periods of highest fallout, irrespective of the grouping of birth cohorts into exposure categories, and there was no association between fallout dose and either year of birth or year of diagnosis.

In New Zealand, where there are no nuclear power stations or reprocessing plants, concentrations of strontium-90 and caesium-137 in cow's milk due to fallout from weapon testing peaked in 1965 and had decreased to the limits of detection by 1986 (Dockerty *et al.*, 1996). If fallout were to have had an effect on the incidence of leukaemia in New Zealand, a peak would have been expected soon after 1965, followed by a decline. Instead, there was an increase in incidence from 1953–57 to 1988–90, particularly in the 0–4–year age group. Thus, data on leukaemia time trends in New Zealand are not consistent with an effect of fallout from atmospheric weapons testing.

Nuclear weapon testing was carried out in Kazakstan above ground between 1946 and 1963, and underground between 1963 and 1988 (Zaridze *et al.*, 1994). The risk of cancer in children aged up to 14 years was estimated in relation to distance from (1) a site where airborne testing was performed before 1963; (2) a site where underground testing took place thereafter and (3) a reservoir created by four nuclear explosions in 1965. The populations at risk were estimated by linear interpolation between the censuses of 1979 and 1989. The risk of acute leukaemia increased with increasing proximity to the testing areas. The relative risk for those living within 200 km of the air testing site was 1.8 (95% CI 1.2–2.6) compared with those living 400 km or more from the site. Similar relative risks were observed for the underground site and the reservoir. There was also substantial regional variation in the rate of acute leukaemia that was not accounted for by distance from the test sites. This may in part have been due to under-ascertainment of cases in rural areas, although notification of cancer was compulsory. In addition, high levels of chemical pollution from a large chemical industry are thought to have occurred, and these may also have contributed to the regional variation in incidence. A significant positive association between non-Hodgkin lymphoma and proximity to the reservoir was observed (RR associated with distance of less than 200 km compared with 400 km or more 2.4, 95% CI 1.0–5.6). Non-significant elevations of risk were observed with decreasing distance from the other test sites. In addition, a positive association between proximity to the test sites and brain tumours was found. No association was apparent for Hodgkin's lymphoma, bone tumours or kidney tumours.

### Thyroid cancer in children

Rallison *et al.* (1974, 1975) examined schoolchildren in Lincoln County, Nevada, and Washington County, Utah, annually from 1965–71. During 1965–68, 1378 children in grades 6 to 12 who were born or who had resided during infancy or early childhood in these counties were examined. A further 1313 children in the same schools who moved into the area after the major nuclear testing and were considered to be unexposed were also examined. An additional comparison group comprised 2140 children in a county in the south-east of Arizona, remote from fallout. During the last three years of the survey, only children in the 12th grade were examined. In reporting the results of the investigation, the authors emphasized the findings from the first three years of the survey. Each child was independently examined by three physicians. Children who were suspected of having a thyroid abnormality by two or more of the three examiners, or who were thought definitely to have an abnormality by one examiner, were referred for a more detailed examination.

The authors concluded that no relation existed between fallout exposure and thyroid disease, but Rothman (1984) has shown that their data indicate a positive association when the categories of thyroid disease are combined. The prevalence of all abnormalities of the thyroid among exposed children was 37 per 1000 compared with 29 per 1000 among unexposed children. The prevalences among children in Arizona and in those considered as unexposed in Utah and Nevada were similar to one another. Except for malignant neoplasms of the thyroid, of which only two were found, the prevalence of each type of thyroid abnormality was greater among exposed children than among either unexposed group. The overall prevalence ratio was 1.3 (90% confidence interval 1.0–1.7). In the second paper, the only comparison relevant to the possible effect of fallout relates to nodular goitre without accompanying abnormality of the thyroid. Of 28 such cases, 20 were benign neoplasms and two were malignant. The prevalence of nodular goitre among exposed children was 8.7 per 1000, compared with 4.6 for children considered as unexposed in Utah and Nevada, and 4.7 in Arizona. The corresponding prevalence ratio was 1.9 (90% confidence interval 1.0–3.5). There were no malignant neoplasms in the exposed group.

The effect was small and substantially lower than predictions in the literature. Rothman suggested that iodine-131, a fallout product concentrated in cow's milk, which is subsequently concentrated in the thyroid gland, may not be as effective as external radiation in inducing thyroid tumours. In addition, the follow-up period of 14 years may have been too short to observe a substantial effect, and children with serious thyroid disease may have been under-ascertained either because they did not attend the schools included in the survey or because they were over-represented among the 14% who did not comply (Rothman, 1984).

In a study of cases recorded in the childhood cancer registry for Turin province, Italy, during the period 1967–88, a decrease in the incidence of thyroid cancer was found, which was reported to parallel dilution of radioactive pollution from nuclear tests carried out in the early 1960s (Mosso *et al.*, 1992). However, there were only 13 cases of thyroid cancer in the 0–14-year age group, and the trend was not statistically significant. Sala and Olsen (1993) assessed time trends in the incidence of thyroid cancer in the 0–19-year age group in Denmark during the period 1943–88 in relation to trends in strontium-90 levels in bones in infants and children. In contrast to the findings from Turin, there was a marked increase in incidence, especially in girls, during the period 1983–88. All children and most teenagers who contributed to the period of high incidence were born after 1968, i.e. after the substantial reduction in strontium-90 levels.

## Proximity to nuclear installations

### Nuclear reprocessing plants: Sellafield, West Cumbria

Much of the research on possible associations between childhood cancer and radioactive emissions from nuclear plants was stimulated in the UK by a television documentary "Windscale; the Nuclear Laundry" in November 1983. The original intention of the documentary was to discuss the health effects of workers of occupational exposure to radiation in the nuclear industry, but the focus of the discussion was reoriented to the local children when residents in the area near Sellafield (Windscale) told the producer that they believed there was an unusually high frequency of childhood leukaemia and other cancers (Gardner, 1991). Awareness of the scale of radioactive discharge from the nuclear waste reprocessing operation at Sellafield led to the suggestion in the television documentary of a linkage between childhood cancer and environmental contamination from the site. The following day, the British Government announced that it would set up an independent enquiry into the allegations. Most people considered that the excess was concentrated in the village of Seascale, on the coast about 3 km south of Sellafield. The first reactor at the Sellafield site became operational in October 1950 and the first spent fuel reprocessing plant in January 1952.

— *The initial investigations made by the Independent Advisory Group*

Using data from the children's cancer register for the Northern Region of England and Wales during the period 1968–82, the Independent Advisory Group (1984) established that four cases of childhood cancer in children under the age of 15 years had occurred in Seascale. Among the 765 wards studied, Seascale ranked sixth highest in terms of the incidence of childhood cancer of all types combined. The four cases all had lymphoid malignancies, and Seascale had the third highest incidence rate of this particular type of malignancy, and ranked highest in terms of Poisson probability. In estimating incidence, the denominator was calculated using data from the 1981 census. This is likely to have been a source of error as the population of children undoubtedly changed during the total 15-year period (Craft *et al.*, 1985), as was later established in the cohort studies of school-children (Gardner *et al.*, 1987a,b; see below). Craft *et al.* (1985) reported that Sellafield was not the only ward in the Northern Region in the period 1968–82 with an elevated incidence of childhood malignancy. Other such wards were scattered throughout the region and were not confined to coastal areas of Cumbria.

Millom Rural District, the administrative area which includes Seascale, had the second highest mortality rate for leukaemia among people under the age of 25 years among 152 rural districts of comparable size in England and Wales during the period 1968–78 (Independent Advisory Group, 1984). Six deaths were recorded, compared with an expected number of 1.4. Mortality due to all causes was very similar to that expected from national rates. Data from Ennerdale Rural District, which includes the Sellafield site, were also considered. During the period 1968–78, there was a modest excess of total childhood cancer (14 deaths recorded versus 9.3 expected; standardized mortality ratio 150); this was not apparent for leukaemia (4 observed cases versus 3.3 expected). Mortality data for the period 1959–67 did not show an excess of either total childhood cancer or leukaemia in either area.

The Advisory Group recommended four areas for further epidemiological investigation: (1) a case–control study of risk factors for leukaemia and lymphoma in West Cumbria; (2) a birth cohort study; (3) determination of the incidence of cancer in schools in the area; (4) further work using cancer registries. The study (Gardner *et al.*, 1990a,b) carried out in response to the first recommendation is described in the section on paternal occupational exposure to ionizing radiation. The studies on cancer in children born in Seascale and resident in Seascale but born elsewhere, made in response to the second and third recommendations, are described below. We next describe the work carried out in response to the fourth recommendation, as this is an extension of the initial work (Independent Advisory Group, 1984; Craft *et al.*, 1985).

*— Further work using cancer registries*

Craft *et al.* (1993) considered cancer in the 0–24-year age group during the period 1968–85 in the Northern and North Western Regional Health Authority regions and in two health districts within the Mersey region, thus including the whole western coastline, on which Sellafield is located, from the Solway to the Mersey. Cases were identified from the three regional cancer registries, which have a high level of ascertainment. Population data were derived from the 1971 and 1981 censuses, and rankings of census wards by relative incidence rate and Poisson probability values were made using each of these population bases. Seascale remained the ward the most highly ranked by Poisson probability for the incidence of ALL for the entire study period (1968–85) and the earlier half of the period (1968–76), but was not among the top five wards when only the later half (1977–85), or only the older age group (15–24 years) were considered. Between 1972 and 1985, only one case of ALL occurred. In some analyses, non-Hodgkin lymphoma was included, as in the past it may have been difficult to distinguish this disease from leukaemia and the diseases may have etiological factors in common. The excess of leukaemia and non-Hodgkin lymphoma in Seascale was apparent using either the 1971 or 1981 census data, suggesting that large population changes are unlikely to be an explanation. In Seascale, most cases of ALL occurred in the first part of the study, and most cases of non-Hodgkin lymphoma in the second. In the wider context of other types of childhood cancer, Seascale was not the most highly ranked ward and there was no excess of other cancers. It was among the highest ranking for total childhood cancer, but this was due to the excess of ALL and non-Hodgkin lymphoma. Contrary to the original allegations of the Yorkshire Television programme, there was no suggestion of an increase in the number of highly ranked wards in West Cumbria apart from Seascale.

Although the report of the Independent Advisory Group (1984) did not include any specific statement about the period of investigation covered, none of the analyses on which it was based related to cases diagnosed or dying after 1983 (Draper *et al.*, 1993). Draper *et al.* (1993), in analyses based on more complete data than were available to the Independent Advisory Group, confirmed the excess of cancer, and leukaemia in particular, in the 0–24-year age group in Seascale during the period 1963–83. During the period 1984–90, there was an excess of total cancer in this age group, based on four cases, two of whom had non-Hodgkin lymphoma but none of whom had leukaemia. One of the other cases had Hodgkin's disease and the other had a pinealoma. There was no excess of leukaemia and lymphoma at older ages in Seascale, in the two country districts nearest to Seascale (Allerdale and Copeland) or in the rest of Cumbria during the period 1984–90. In addition, the excess of cancer in young persons was not apparent in the two adjacent districts or in Cumbria as a whole, in either the period 1963–83 or 1984–90. Subsequently, data for 1984–92 have been analysed (COMARE, 1996). A further case of ALL was diagnosed in a boy aged 16 in 1991. Thus, in the period 1984–92, three cases of lymphoid leukaemia/non-Hodgkin lymphoma occurred, compared with 0.16 expected (O/E = 19.1, $p$ = 0.0006). Two cases of cancers of other types occurred, compared with 0.62 expected (O/E = 3.2, $p$ = 0.129).

*— Birth cohort study and incidence in schools in the area*

Gardner *et al.* (1987a,b) reported cohort studies in children born in the period 1950–83 or later who were resident in Seascale village at any age. Some 1068 live births to mothers resident in Seascale were identified and the information was cross-matched with the National Health Service Central Register in order to obtain data on deaths, cancer registrations and emigration. In addition, information on all Family Practitioner Committee areas in which the children had been recorded since birth allowed estimates to be made of durations of residence in the area. By the end of 1984, 56% of the children appeared to have moved out of Cumbria. This information was supplemented by a search for the parents' names in the annual Seascale electoral registers and by information from the local authority's school register. Some 43% of the children who would have attained school age by late 1984 were not found on the school register and were assumed not to have stayed to attend the local school, while a similar percentage of parents came off the electoral register within five years of their child's birth. Thus, the population was highly mobile. The mortality and cancer follow-up was made to 30 June 1986. Forty-three children had left the country by this date, and 27 had died. Five deaths attributable to leukaemia were recorded compared with 0.53 expected from national rates (O/E = 9.4, 95% CI 3.0–21.8). Four of these cases were known to the Independent Advisory Group (see above), while the fifth was a death from leukaemia that occurred after the child had left Seascale. There was one death from non-Hodgkin lymphoma, compared to 0.1 expected. There were three other deaths from cancer compared to 0.9 expected (O/E = 3.4, 95% CI 0.7–10.0). There was a deficit of deaths from other causes: 18 compared with 30.7 expected (O/E = 0.6, 95% CI 0.4–0.9). This deficit was largely for infants (i.e., under one year of age).

In addition to the nine deaths from cancer, a further three cases were notified from the National Health Service Central Register. One was a case of ALL diagnosed in a five-year-old girl, one a case of non-Hodgkin lymphoma in a girl aged one year, and one a case of malignant melanoma diagnosed in a man aged 28 years after he left Seascale. The authors considered that it was unlikely that the excess apparent for leukaemia could be attributed to social class factors, although this is likely to have explained the deficit of infant mortality and also of stillbirths (rate 8.4 per 1000 compared with a national rate of 15 per 1000).

In a closely related study (Gardner *et al.*, 1987b), records on children born since 1950 outside Seascale who were identified as having attended three out of the four schools in the village up to November 1984 were cross-matched as before with the National Health Service Central Register. A total of 1546 children were thus identified. The records of one school which had taken 150 pupils were not included because a full date of birth had not been recorded and children who moved to the village after birth but left before school age or went to boarding school elsewhere would not have been included. 107 children could not be traced, and 65 had left the United Kingdom. The majority of children who could not be traced were born before 1963, when the central register index was compiled from applications for welfare foods, and it is thought that about 15% of parents nationally did not complete the application form issued at birth registration. Out of 1173 children for whom the date of leaving school was recorded, 545 (46%) had left the area before the usual age of 11 years. Thus, as was the case for children born in Seascale, the population was highly mobile.

A total of 10 deaths were observed, compared with 12.7 expected. One of these was certified as due to cancer, compared with 2.0 expected, and was due to malignant melanoma in a man aged 33 years who had moved away from Seascale. Three cases of non-fatal cancer were registered, compared with 2.0 expected; these were a case of non-Hodgkin lymphoma in a boy aged 9 years, a case of Hodgkin's disease in a man aged 26 years and a carcinoma of the lung diagnosed in a woman aged 21 years. Therefore, Gardner *et al.* (1987b) concluded that the excess of leukaemia in Seascale appeared to be attributable to environmental factors acting before birth or early in life on a locality-specific basis. The case–control study (Gardner *et al.*, 1990a,b), described in detail in the section on paternal occupational exposures to ionizing radiation, was interpreted by the authors as suggesting an effect of preconceptional ionizing radiation in the fathers that may be leukaemogenic in their offspring.

In an analysis based on incidence rather than mortality, and over a longer period (1951–91), Kinlen (1993) found that the excess of leukaemia and non-Hodgkin lymphoma in Seascale was apparent for individuals born outside the area. In contrast to the findings of Gardner *et al.* (1987b), the excess was not confined only to persons born in Seascale. The assumptions used in making population estimates were such as to err towards overestimating the numbers born outside Seascale, leading to a conservative estimate of any excess in this group. The observed/expected ratio of leukaemia for persons born outside Seascale was 5.2 (3/0.58, *p* < 0.05), while that for people born in the district was 12.9 (4/0.31, *p* < 0.001). The corresponding ratios for non-Hodgkin lymphoma were 12.5 (2/0.16, *p* < 0.05) and 28.5 (2/0.07, *p* < 0.01). All but one of the five cases born outside Seascale were born outside West Cumbria. Paternal preconceptional exposure to ionizing radiation does not explain the excess in individuals born outside Seascale. The excess appears to be too large to be explained by the association between childhood leukaemia and high socioeconomic status or geographical isolation (Draper *et al.*, 1993).

— *Other studies*

The association between leukaemia in young people and discharges from Sellafield into the Irish Sea has been investigated in several studies. Heasman *et al.* (1984) considered leukaemia in Scotland in the 0–24-year age group during the period 1968–81. A higher registration rate for myeloid leukaemia between 1968 and 1974 was observed in coastal areas, but this was not apparent during 1975–81. There was a lower registration rate for lymphoid leukaemias during the earlier period, so the overall registration rate for leukaemia was not substantially in excess of that for the rest of Scotland. Subsequently, Gillis and Hole (1984) showed that rates of leukaemia in children aged under 15 years in coastal areas of the west of Scotland were not consistently higher than in inland areas.

Cook-Mozaffari *et al.* (1987) compared mortality due to cancer in the 0–24-year age group between a group of coastal Local Authority Areas to the north and south of Sellafield and coastal areas matched on Standard Region, urban–rural status and population size. The coastal areas had some overlap with areas around Sellafield, Springfields, Capenhurst and Wylfa, considered in the analysis of possible effects of residential proximity to nuclear installations (discussed below). No excess mortality due to total cancer, or to any specific type of cancer, was apparent in coastal areas in this age group. An excess of myeloid leukaemia in subjects aged 25–74 years was accounted for specifically by an excess in the Wirral, and the authors considered that it was unlikely that this could be linked to discharges from Sellafield in the absence of excess for coastal areas closer to the plant.

In Northern Ireland, the incidence of leukaemia in children under 15 years of age during the period 1977–85 and mortality in children in this period and in the earlier period 1968–76 was compared between coastal and inland areas by an independent committee (Department of Health and Social Services, 1989). Acute leukaemia and all leukaemias thought to be associated with radiation were studied. Newly incident cases of leukaemia were ascertained from hospital laboratory records, the cancer registry, and the leukaemia mortality file maintained by the General Registrar Office. The latter provided details of all leukaemia deaths for the mortality study. Case-finding was initially attempted for the period 1975–85; bone marrow records were available for only 67.7% of cases. The study period was subsequently restricted to 1977–85 because of concerns about the quality of data in the first two years of the study. A total of 153 cases in childhood was ascertained in the nine-year period, all but two of whom had acute leukaemia. The incidence of acute leukaemia in coastal areas was 4.7 per 100 000 per year, compared to 4.3 in inland areas. Nine deaths from acute leukaemia were recorded in the period 1977–85, and 90 in the period 1968–76. The total of 159 deaths corresponds to a

mortality rate of 2.1 per 100 000 per year. In each period, the mortality rate in coastal areas was less than that in inland areas, although the difference was not substantial. A further 18 deaths from other types of leukaemia in children were recorded; the small differences between coastal and inland areas for total leukaemia were similar to those for acute leukaemia. A difficulty with the study was that data on the denominator population were available only for the censal years 1971 and 1981. Although some monitoring of radiation levels was carried out during the study period, it was not detailed enough to be correlated reliably with epidemiological data collected by the committee.

Alexander *et al.* (1990b) postulated that the incidence of leukaemia at all ages would be higher in areas adjacent to estuaries than elsewhere. Part of the rationale of the hypothesis was that levels of radiation in estuarine silts and other fine sediments, rather than in sand, were increased. These high levels were not localized in Cumbria but dispersed along the entire west coast of Britain. The hypothesis was tested using the Data Collection Study (DCS), a specialist registry of haematopoietic malignancies covering approximately 40% of the population of England and Wales for the period 1984–86. Estuaries were defined as all river-mouths with a substantial amount of mud marked on an Ordnance Survey map. Some 36 estuaries were identified in the areas covered by the DCS, and 477 electoral wards with contact (other than a point contact) were classified as estuarine. The remaining wards were classified as inland (2922) or coastal (234), depending on whether they had a contact with the coast. There were 40 cases of childhood leukaemia in estuarine wards, 11 in coastal wards, and 256 in inland wards. The risk in estuarine wards relative to inland wards was 1.20 (95% CI 0.8–1.7), adjusted for urban–rural and socioeconomic status, and differing incidence at county level. The relative risk in coastal wards was 0.69 (95% CI 0.4–1.3). The elevated risk of childhood leukaemia in estuarine wards was higher than that observed for any of the categories of leukaemias at all ages (acute lymphocytic, acute or chronic myeloid, and total excluding chronic lymphocytic).

Five cases of retinoblastoma have been documented whose mothers were resident in Seascale at some time during the period 1950–90, representing an excess of approximately twenty-fold (Morris *et al.*, 1993a). One of the cases was bilateral and associated with a partial deletion of chromosome 13, including the *RB1* locus, which was not present in either parent and therefore represents a new germ cell mutation (Morris *et al.*, 1993b). The other unilateral cases are likely to have been non-hereditary (Stiller, 1993a). The maternal grandfathers of three of the children had worked at Sellafield (Morris *et al.*, 1993b). Three further cases have occurred among children born in Copeland, the district which includes Seascale and Sellafield, but whose mothers had never lived in Seascale; the father of one and the paternal grandfather of another had worked at Sellafield (Morris *et al.*, 1993b).

## Nuclear reprocessing plants: Dounreay, Caithness

The second reprocessing plant in the United Kingdom, at Dounreay, commenced active operation in 1960. In the study relating predominantly to leukaemia in the west of Scotland during the period 1968–91 of Heasman *et al.* (1984), described above, the incidence of leukaemia near the three nuclear power stations in Scotland, namely Dounreay, Chapel Cross in Dumfriesshire and Hunterstone in Ayrshire, was also considered. The observed number of registrations of leukaemia in the 0–24-year age group within a 16-km radius of Dounreay was similar to that expected.

Subsequently, in preparation for the public enquiry held in 1986 concerning the planning application for a new nuclear reprocessing plant at Dounreay, Heasman *et al.* (1986a,b) extended the period covered by three years to include 1968–84. Census enumeration districts whose centroids fell within 12.5 km or within 25 km of the Dounreay installation, other districts falling within 25 and 75 km of Dounreay, and the islands of Orkney (range 35–120 km) and Shetland (range 160–300 km) were considered. Population data were obtained from the 1971 and 1981 censuses. During the overall period, 15 cases of leukaemia were registered in the 0–24-year age group in the entire area considered, compared to 14 expected on the basis of registration rates for Scotland as a whole. Five of the cases lived within 12.5 km of Dounreay compared to 1.6 expected, a further case (1.4 expected) lived between 12.5 and 25 km of the plant, leaving 9 cases living in more distant areas (11 expected).

The authors also arbitrarily divided the period of study into three: 1968–73, 1974–78 and 1979–84. Four cases (4.6 expected) were observed in the first period, one (4.7 expected) in the second, and ten (4.8 expected) in the third. The authors noted that the combination which gave cause for concern was residence within 12.5 km of Dounreay during the period

1979–84, i.e. the most recent period, with five observed cases compared with 0.5 expected. Four of the cases were aged under 15 years at registration, and this was also true of the one case living between 12.5 and 25 km of the installation. This latter case was also diagnosed between 1979 and 1984. The authors pointed out that no case at all was registered within 25 km of the plant in the period 1968–78. Preliminary examination of cancers of other types in childhood and of leukaemia and certain other types of cancer in adults, and of the occurrence of congenital malformations, were stated not to be significantly increased in the area around Dounreay.

The Committee on Medical Aspects of Radiation in the Environment considered these data in relation to information on radioactive discharges from the site, and concluded that these were too low to account for the excess of leukaemia in young people using conventional dose–risk estimates (COMARE, 1988). The estimated dose equivalents to red bone marrow received by a one-year-old child in Thurso as a result of discharges from Dounreay are between 4 and 400 times less than those received in Seascale as a result of discharges from Sellafield. The Committee observed that although chance could not be entirely dismissed as an explanation of the excess of childhood leukaemia in the vicinity of Dounreay, this was considered less likely than when Sellafield was considered in isolation. These data have been updated to 1991 (Black *et al.*, 1994). In the period 1985–91, four cases of leukaemia and non-Hodgkin lymphoma diagnosed at ages under 25 years were observed in the zone within 25 km of the Dounreay plant, compared with 1.4 expected (*p* = 0.059). This reinforces the earlier concern that the cases were concentrated in the most recent years studied.

A case–control study of young people registered with leukaemia or lymphoma in the Dounreay area, a birth cohort study of young people born to mothers resident in Thurso and a neighbouring area, and a school cohort study of children attending schools near Dounreay were recommended (COMARE, 1988).

A small case–control study of leukaemia and non-Hodgkin lymphoma occurring in children aged under 15 years diagnosed in the period 1970–86 in Caithness, Scotland, was reported by Urquhart *et al.* (1991). The study is described in more detail in the section on parental occupational exposure to ionizing radiation. In contrast to the findings of Gardner *et al.* (1990a), the excess cannot be explained by paternal occupation at Dounreay or by paternal exposure to external ionizing radiation before conception. The authors considered that an apparent positive association with the use of beaches around Dounreay might be an artefact of multiple testing and influenced by recall bias.

A cohort study of 4144 children born in the Dounreay area in the period 1969–88 and 1641 children who attended local schools in the same period but who had been born elsewhere was carried out (Black *et al.*, 1992). Data from the Scottish National Cancer Registration Scheme for the period 1969–88 were linked with birth and school records by computerized record linkage. The data on leukaemia in the 0–24-year age group had been subjected to a validation exercise. Five cancer registrations were traced from the birth cohort, compared with 5.8 expected on the basis of national rates. All five cases were of leukaemia or non-Hodgkin lymphoma (O/E = 2.3, 95% CI 0.7–5.4). All of the cases were resident in the area at the time of diagnosis. Three cancer cases were traced from the school records, all of which were of leukaemia (O/E = 6.7, 95% CI 1.4–19.4). Thus, the incidence of leukaemia and non-Hodgkin lymphoma was raised in both those born in the area and those resident in the area but born elsewhere, in contrast to the studies of Gardner *et al.* (1987a,b) in Seascale. Although the mobility of the population at risk was high, with a fairly constant outward movement before school age of about 30% of children born in the area, the incidence rates of leukaemia and non-Hodgkin lymphoma reported in the earlier geographical studies did not overestimate the risk in the local population.

Kinlen *et al.* (1993a) suggested that the excess of cases near Dounreay beginning in 1979 was due to population mixing linked to the expansion of the oil industry (see Chapter 7 for further comment). The persistence of the excess in the period 1985–91 may be due to specific local aspects of population mixing (Black *et al.*, 1994).

Darby and Doll (1987) considered the excess around Dounreay in relation to exposure to radiation due to discharges from both the Dounreay and Sellafield plants in the context of data on the association between childhood leukaemia and fallout from weapons testing. The lack of any consistent increase in the frequency of childhood leukaemia after the period of peak fallout indicated that current estimates of the risk of leukaemia per unit dose of radiation at low doses and low dose rates, and of the relative biological efficiency of high as compared with low linear energy transfer radiation, were unlikely to be underestimates. A possible explanation was underestimation of doses to the red bone marrow due to discharges at Dounreay relative to the dose from fallout. The authors considered a number of ways in which it might theoretically be possible for a discrepancy to have occurred, but the limited evidence available suggests that these are unlikely. However, the authors noted that the exposure to radionuclides from fallout is mainly from inhalation, whereas that for discharges is mainly from ingestion. Thus, substantial differences might be produced if the assumed proportion of plutonium transferred from the lung into the bloodstream is too high, or the assumed proportion transferred from the digestive tract is too low. Other possible explanations included a misconception of the site of origin of childhood leukaemia, outbreaks of an infectious disease, and exposure to some other unidentified agent, the latter also having been discussed by other authors in relation to the Sellafield excess.

*Nuclear reprocessing plants: La Hague, Normandy*

Data are available in relation to one other specific nuclear reprocessing plant, La Hague in Normandy, France, which has been in operation since 1966, but with significant releases only from 1968 (Dousset, 1989; Viel & Richardson, 1990). The total amount of effluent discharged is stated to have been much lower than that from Sellafield. Sellafield has released 10–160 times more caesium-137 than La Hague, whereas La Hague has released 4 times more antimony-125. In addition to the nuclear reprocessing plant, there are a low-level radioactive waste depository, a nuclear power station 16 km away, and navy dockyards where nuclear fuel for submarines is handled 19 km away (Pobel & Viel, 1997).

Dousset (1989) compared cancer mortality between the Beaumont-Hague canton in which the plant is situated and the entire Département de la Manche. The canton corresponds to a radius of about 10 km around the installation. No death from leukaemia in persons aged under 25 years occurred during the period 1970–82, selected to allow for a two-year latency period, compared with an expected 0.7. Also, no death from other types of cancer in this age group occurred during the period 1975–82, selected to allow for a seven-year latency period, compared with an expected 0.9.

In the study of Viel and Richardson (1990), observed deaths due to childhood leukaemia during the period 1968–78 and 1979–86 were considered in three age groups: 0–4 years, 5–14 years and 15–24 years. All electoral wards having half or more of their area within specified radii — 10 km, 20 km and 35 km — of a nuclear plant were studied. Expected numbers of deaths were estimated by applying the age-specific rates for the Département de la Manche for each period to 1975 and 1982 census populations of the relevant ten electoral boards. Only one death, that of an individual in the oldest age group in the latter period, occurred in the area closest to the installation in the total period 1968–86. Only one standardized mortality ratio was significantly different from one, the ratio for the 5–14-year age group living 10–20 km of the plant during 1968–78 indicating a decreased risk. Overall, 21 deaths were observed, compared to 23.6 expected. No significant trend between the two periods was found. As acknowledged by the authors, the study is limited by being mortality-based.

Viel *et al.* (1993) assessed the incidence of leukaemia in the 0–24-year age group during the period 1978–90 in the same area. Cases of leukaemia among people with a residential address in cantons with at least half of their area within 35 km of La Hague were identified from various sources including a university hospital, a paediatric referral hospital, general practitioners and the Regional Cancer Institute. Since there was no cancer registry in the Département de la Manche, reference rates from the adjacent Département du Calvados were used. The overall SIR for the study area was 1.2 (95% CI 0.7–1.8). Within a radius of 10 km of the plant, the SIR was 2.5 (95% CI 0.5–7.4). The only significant excess was in the 0–4-year age group in a 20–35 km radius (SIR 3.2, 95% CI 1.0–7.4). The authors observed that the workforce of a nuclear power station which began operation in December 1985 is resident in this area. This might be compatible with an effect of population inflow, as postulated by Kinlen (1988).

Subsequently, further analysis was made for the period 1978-92 using data from the same sources (Viel *et al.*, 1995). An excess of childhood leukaemia was observed in the canton which included the reprocessing plant (SIR 2.8, 95% CI 0.8–7.2). Results of a sensitivity analysis involving two further statistical techniques were consistent with this and suggested a decline in risk with increasing distance (up to 8 km) from La Hague. A further sensitivity analysis explored the effects of using different reference rates for the calculation of expected numbers. The observed data were for the Département de la Manche for the period 1979–81; the expected numbers were based on cancer registration data from four départements for the period 1978–82. In each of the four analyses, the maximum cumulative SIR (range 2.7–3.3; $p = 0.05–0.07$) was observed in the canton containing La Hague.

A case–control study of 27 cases of leukaemia diagnosed at ages under 25 years during the period 1978–93 and 192 controls was reported by Pobel and Viel (1997) as described in the section on parental occupational exposure to ionizing radiation. No association with parental occupational exposure to ionizing radiation was found. There were elevated relative risks associated with use of local beaches more than once a month by the mothers during pregnancy and by the index child compared with less often, and with consumption of local fish and shellfish by the index child. All four children who lived in the electoral ward which includes the reprocessing plant played on the beach at least once a month, compared with 13 of the 23 similarly affected children who lived in the remaining area, and 14 of the 33 controls resident in the same electoral ward (Viel, 1997). Therefore, the observed geographical excess might be explained by the association between leukaemia and playing on the beach. However, the possibility that selection bias, recall bias, and as multiple statistical testing was carried out, chance, might account for the results has been debated (Clavel & Hémon, 1997; Law & Roman, 1997; Viel, 1997; Wakeford, 1997).

*Nuclear reprocessing plants: studies of groups of installations*

The results of studies based on data pooled from areas around several nuclear plants, compared with pooled data from control areas, are less likely to be affected by small-area differences in prevalence of exposure to other risk factors than those of studies based on single sites (Cook-Mozaffari *et al.*, 1987). In France, Hill and Laplanche (1990) found no overall excess mortality due to leukaemia in persons aged 0–24 years associated with residential proximity to two nuclear reprocessing plants (Marcoule and La Hague). However, their data overlap with those of Dousset (1989) and Viel and Richardson (1990), although the units of area considered in the analysis differ between the studies. In the USA, Jablon *et al.* (1990) compared cancer mortality between areas around nuclear installations and control areas. These authors considered separately 52 installations whose primary function was to produce electricity, 'electric utilities', and ten whose primary function was other than this, including reprocessing plants, 'Department of Energy' facilities. Within each group, the only notable difference in rates of mortality, due either to leukaemia or to other cancers considered as a group for the 0–9 and 10–19-year age groups, during the periods after start-up of the facilities, was a statistically significant but weak deficit (RR = 0.88) of mortality due to leukaemia in the 10–19-year age group. Before start-up, there was a non-significant excess (RR = 1.45) leukaemia mortality in the 0–9-year age group for Department of Energy facilities, and a deficit for the 10–19-year age group (RR = 0.68). For the other electric utilities, there was a weak statistically significant excess (RR = 1.08) of leukaemia in the 0–9-year age group, and a significant deficit of other cancers (RR = 0.94).

*Nuclear facilities of any type: studies of areas around groups of existing or proposed sites of installations*

Ecological comparisons of cancer incidence or mortality in areas close to nuclear installations and control areas have been carried out in England and Wales, France, Germany and the USA. The basic features of the designs of the studies and results relating to total malignancies and leukaemia in children or young persons are summarized in Table 4.2. In the table, for studies in which more than one measure of exposure based on distance of residential areas from the installation, data for the largest areas have been presented.

In England and Wales during the period 1959–80 (Cook-Mozaffari *et al.*, 1987, Forman *et al.*, 1987), the nuclear installations were considered in two groups. The first was a heterogeneous group concerned with the enrichment, fabrication and reprocessing of nuclear fuel, with the provision of supporting research and development, with radionuclide manufacture and with defence applications, all of which were started up before 1955. Sellafield was excluded from this group. Second were those whose primary function is electricity generation, referred to as CEGB installations. These began operations between 1961 and 1971.

Overall, there was little evidence of a raised risk of total malignancies or of leukaemia in the 0–24-year age group in areas within 16 km of nuclear plants. The relative risks based on incidence data are all slightly higher than those based on mortality data. The authors noted that the ratio of the number of cancer registrations to the number of cancer deaths was higher in areas

around pre-1955 installations than in the corresponding control areas, suggesting more complete ascertainment in areas around such installations. This pattern was particularly pronounced for brain tumours, and the authors commented that initial examination of the material suggested that these tumours were particularly subject to variation in diagnostic standards. Therefore, these investigators considered that conclusions based on mortality data were more reliable.

Four distance zones were considered: (1) areas with at least two thirds of their population within 6 miles (9.6 km) of an installation; (2) areas with at least two thirds of their population within 8 miles (12.8 km) of an installation; (3) areas with at least two thirds of their population within 10 miles (16 km) of an installation; and (4) areas with at least one third of their population within 10 miles of an installation. Forman *et al.* (1987) considered the data not only for the groups of installations but also each installation and all installations, and tabulated relative risks between areas around installations and control areas which were significantly different from unity. Standardized mortality rates for areas in the vicinity of nuclear installations were significantly lower than those in control areas more often than the reverse. The deficit is likely to have been due to socioeconomic or environmental differences between the areas.

No trend of mortality rate with distance from installations was found for either group of nuclear plants for total leukaemia, malignant neoplasm of the brain or other malignant neoplasms. Similarly, no time trend was apparent for these categories. However, increases over time in mortality attributed to lymphomas, non-Hodgkin lymphomas, and all leukaemias and lymphomas were found for pre-1955 installations. In addition, for the years 1968–80, for which data on leukaemia subtypes were available, there was a significant increase in mortality due to lymphoid leukaemia in the innermost zone around the pre-1955 installations. This was consistently found for the four plants with areas in the innermost zone.

By contrast, mortality due to lymphoid leukaemia was elevated in the outer two zones around CEGB installations, with a reported *p* value for trend of 0.015 (Forman *et al.*, 1987). For the CEGB installations, a similar pattern of increasing risk compared with control areas with increase in distance from the plants was found for brain tumours in the 0–24-year age group. Around CEGB installations, mortality rates

## Table 4.2. Summary of studies of cancer incidence or mortality in children in which groups of existing or potential sites of nuclear installations have been considered

| Country, period of study | Exposed areas | Control areas; matching or stratification variables | Outcome, age group | Exposure group | (I)ncidence, (M)ortality | Number of cases exposed | SIR or SRR | Number of cases unexposed | SIR or SRR | RR | Reference |
|---|---|---|---|---|---|---|---|---|---|---|---|
| UK, England and Wales, 1959–80 | Local authority areas with at least one third of the population resident within 16 km of 15 nuclear installations. | Same rural/urban status, approximately same size and, where possible drawn from same cancer registry region as exposed areas. | All malignancies 0–24 | Installations with start-up date prior to 1955 | I / M | 2005 / 1140 | 110.8 / 98.3 | 1921 / 1179 | 102.5 / 98.8 | 1.08 / 0.99 | Cook-Mozaffari et al., 1987 |
| | | | | CEGB installations | I / M | 346 / 230 | 99.1 / 101.6 | 295 / 211 | 86.0 / 93.7 | 1.15 / 1.08 | |
| | | | Leukaemia | Installations with start-up date prior to 1955 | I / M | 442 / 409 | 110.0 / 99.4 | 406 / 447 | 97.9 / 106.0 | 1.12 / 0.94 | |
| | | | | CEGB installations | I / M | 91 / 87 | 115.6 / 111.3 | 73 / 77 | 95.0 / 98.9 | 1.22 / 1.13 | |
| UK, England and Wales, 1969–78 | 70 county districts with 0.1% or more of their population resident within 16 km of 15 nuclear installations. | 330 other districts in the remainder of England and Wales. Adjustment was made for social class, rural/urban status, population size and regional health authority. | All malignancies 0–24 | All installations | M | NS | NS | NS | NS | 1.07* | Cook-Mozaffari et al., 1989a |
| | | | Leukaemia 0–24 | All installations | M | 745 | NS | 3485 | NS | 1.15* | |
| | 20 county districts with 0.1% or more of their population resident within 16 km of potential sites of nuclear installations and which were not within this vicinity of existing sites. | 299 other districts in the remainder of England and Wales. Adjustment was made for social class, rural/urban status, population size and regional health authority. | All malignancies 0–24 | All potential sites | M | 566 | NS | NS | NS | 1.10 | Cook-Mozaffari et al., 1989b |
| | | | Leukaemia 0–24 | All potential sites | M | 189 | NS | NS | NS | 1.14 | |
| UK, England and Wales, 1966–87 | Electoral wards 25 km of 23 nuclear installations. | Expected numbers from national rates. | Leukaemia and non-Hodgkin lymphoma 0–14 | 8 generating stations / 7 other installations which emitted non-negligible quantities of radioactivity during study period. | I / I | 480 / 1269 | 98 / 100 | – / – | – / – | – / – | Bithell et al., 1994 |
| | | Electoral wards within 25 km of 6 control sites that had been investigated for generating stations but suitability never used. | | 8 installations excluded from above two groups either because emissions believed to be small or because operations started too late to affect most of children in study. | I | 1945 | 99 | – | – | – | |
| | | | | 6 control sites | I | 406 | 102 | – | – | – | |

**Table 4.2. (contd) Summary of studies of cancer incidence or mortality in children in which groups of existing or potential sites of nuclear installations have been considered**

| Country, period of study | Exposed areas | Control areas; matching or stratification variables | Outcome, age group | Exposure group | (I)ncidence, (M)ortality | Number of cases exposed | SIR or SRR | Number of cases unexposed | SIR or SRR | RR | Reference |
|---|---|---|---|---|---|---|---|---|---|---|---|
| France, 1968–87 | Communes within 21 km of 6 nuclear installations. | Communes in the same departement having the closest total population figure to the exposed communes. | All malignancies 0–24 | All installations | M | 166 | 97 | 160 | 102 | 0.95 | Hill & Laplanche, 1990 |
|  |  |  | Leukaemia 0–24 | All installations | M | 58 | 87 | 62 | 101 | 0.86 |  |
| USA, 1950–84 | 107 counties in which at least 20% of the area was within 16 km of 62 nuclear installations. | 292 counties matched on ethnic group composition, urban-rural status, employment in manufacturing, education level, mean family income, net migration rate, infant death rate, and population size. | All cancer except leukaemia, 0–9 / 10–19 | All installations | M | 1717 / 1963 | 103 / 101 | 3243 / 3671 | 102 / 98 | 0.99 / 1.03 | Jablon et al., 1990 |
|  |  |  | Leukaemia, 0–9 / 10–19 | All installations | M | 1390 / 996 | 101 / 95 | 2572 / 2063 | 97 / 102 | 1.03 / 0.94 |  |
|  | 5 counties in which at least 20% of the area was within 16 km of 4 nuclear installations. | SEER data for Connecticut and Iowa. | Leukaemia, 0–9 | All installations | I | 81 | NS | NS | NS | 1.36* | Jablon et al., 1991 |
| Federal Republic of Germany 1980–90 | Counties (Landkreis) with at least 1/3 of their area within 15 km of 20 nuclear installations. | Counties matched on social class distribution, population density; referral centres for paediatric oncology and with closest boundary to reference location between 30 and 100 km. | All malignancies 0–14 | All installations | I | 805 | 92 | 611 | 95 | 0.97 | Michaelis et al., 1992 |
|  |  |  | Acute leukaemias 0–14 |  | I | 274 | 93 | 190 | 88 | 1.06 |  |
| Canada, Ontario 1950 | Counties in which nuclear installations located. | Ontario, whole province | Leukaemia, 0–14 | Research facilities | M / I | 17 / 16 | 71 / 70 | – / – | – / – | – / – | Clarke et al., 1991 |
|  |  |  |  | Uranium refining | M / I | 20 / 21 | 114 / 111 | – / – | – / – | – / – |  |
|  |  |  |  | Uranium mining | M / I | 38 / 43 | 138 / 127 | – / – | – / – | – / – |  |
|  |  |  |  | Generating stations No. 1 | M / I | 33 / 75 | 128 / 114 | – / – | – / – | – / – |  |
|  | Zones within 25 km of nuclear facilities. |  |  | No. 2 | M / I | 5 / 9 | 155 / 124 | – / – | – / – | – / – |  |
|  |  |  |  | Research facilities | M | 2 | 33 | – | – | – |  |
|  |  |  |  | Uranium mining, milling and refining | M | 16 | 111 | – | – | – |  |
|  |  |  |  | Generating stations | M | 36 | 140 | – | – | – |  |

NS, Not stated.

* Reported as statistically significant.

attributed to total malignancies and lung cancer in subjects aged 25 years or more increased with increasing distance from the plant in both installation and control areas. The excess was more pronounced in the outer zones after start-up, but the reverse was true when the innermost zones were considered. Thus, the findings in relation to CEGB plants may be attributed to chance and uncontrolled confounding.

An excess of lymphoid leukaemia around installations that started operation before 1955 is, however, supported by other evidence in the study. There was a weak excess (RR = 1.2, $p$ = 0.115) of this type of cancer in coastal areas, which may have been associated with discharges from the Sellafield plant (see above). The excess around pre-1955 plants, the inverse association with distance and the excess in coastal areas are more pronounced when the 0–9-year age group is considered. However, the investigators point out that both for the 0–24 and 0–9-year age groups, the excesses depend on unusually low standardized mortality rates in control areas in the innermost zone.

Subsequently, Cook-Mozaffari *et al.* (1989a) compared mortality from 11 causes of death during the period 1969–78 between 70 county districts around the 15 nuclear installations considered in the earlier study (Cook-Mozaffari *et al.*, 1987) and 330 other districts, adjusting for social class, rural status, population size and health authority region. For the 0–24-year age group, statistically significantly raised relative risks associated with residence near nuclear installations were observed for total malignancies (1.07, $p$ = 0.03), leukaemia (1.15, $p$ = 0.01), lymphoid leukaemia (1.21, $p$ = 0.01) and Hodgkin's disease (1.24, $p$ = 0.05). Mortality rates for lymphoid leukaemia and Hodgkin's disease were not inter-correlated. There was a slight deficit of deaths due to causes other than malignancies (RR = 0.97, $p$ = 0.02). There was a significant deficit of mortality from lymphoid leukaemia in persons aged 25–64 years (RR = 0.86, $p$ = 0.05) that was not correlated inversely with the excess at ages 0–24, either for installations or all districts. No significant trends were observed with an increasing proportion of the population living near to the installations.

Although not entirely independent of the earlier study, the methods were different. First, in the more recent study the control population comprised around 40 million, compared with 2.5 million. Second, larger geographical units were used, so the population defined as exposed comprised about 7.5 million rather than under 3 million. Third, potential confounding by socioeconomic variables was controlled by regression methods rather than by matching. As in the previous study, there was a significant excess of lymphoid leukaemia around installations other than Sellafield with start-up dates before 1955 (RR = 1.21, $p$ = 0.02). An excess of similar size (RR = 1.20) was apparent for the CEGB installations, but was not statistically significant.

The authors acknowledged that mortality due to leukaemia in young persons declined during the period of study, one in which new and more effective treatment was being introduced, and that the treatment in the nuclear installation areas might have been less adequate than the average. However, they considered that as treatment is largely carried out in regional centres, adjustment for health service region and rural status should have accounted for geographical variation in the efficacy of treatment. The authors accepted that definitive studies should be based on incidence, but noted that the available registration data were inadequate.

As the excess of leukaemia was substantially greater than that expected from the annual radiation doses received by children near the installations, the authors considered the possibility that other features of these areas might not have been taken into account. Therefore, in a companion study, they compared mortality rates for the same 11 causes of death in the same 1969–78 period between areas around two sites of nuclear installations which started operation in 1981 and 1983, and six other sites which had been seriously considered for construction of nuclear installations (Cook-Mozaffari *et al.*, 1989b). These eight sites are referred to as potential sites of nuclear installations. Districts in the vicinity of both existing and potential sites were excluded from consideration. Thus 20 county districts near to potential sites only were compared with 299 other districts using the same methods as in the companion study (Cook-Mozaffari *et al.*, 1989a).

In the 0–24-year age group, excesses of similar magnitude to those observed near existing sites were found for total malignancies (RR = 1.10) and leukaemia (RR = 1.14) but these were not statistically significant. In contrast to the companion study, the excess was more pronounced for leukaemia types other than lymphoid. This may reflect sampling variation or inaccuracy of classification of leukaemia types on death certificates. The deficit of lymphoid leukaemia in the 25–64-year age group was more substantial near potential sites (RR = 0.80, $p$ =

0.03). A greater excess of Hodgkin's disease (RR = 1.50, $p$ = 0.05) was found near potential than existing sites. An excess near potential sites in the 25–64-year age group also was apparent (RR = 1.23, $p$ = 0.01), whereas this was not found for existing sites. The authors conclude that there are systematic differences between districts near existing, or potential, sites of installations and other districts.

Using incidence data, Bithell *et al.* (1994) examined the assocation between leukaemia and non-Hodgkin lymphoma diagnosed in the period 1966–87 at ages up to 14 years and residential proximity to 23 nuclear installations in England and Wales. Three groups of installations were considered: (1) eight generating stations; (2) seven other installations which emitted non-negligible quantities of radioactivity during the study period, and (3) eight installations excluded from the above groups either because emissions were believed to be small or because operations started too late to affect most of the children in the study. In addition, six sites which had been investigated for suitability for a nuclear power station but where construction had not taken place were considered. These were considered in the studies of Cook-Mozaffari *et al.* (1987, 1989b). Regions of 25 km radius were investigated, as in previous studies. The size was partly influenced by consideration of what constitutes a reasonable commuting distance for workers at the plants. The observed numbers of cases were compared with expected numbers using a Poisson regression model, with adjustment for socioeconomic variables. In addition, a new test, the linear risk score test, designed to be sensitive to excess incidence in close proximity to a putatiave source of risk, was applied. There was no evidence of an increase in the incidence of leukaemia and non-Hodgkin lymphoma within 25 km of the sites considered, or for a general effect of spatial proximity to the sites as determined by the linear risk score test. The only statistically significant results using this test were for Sellafield (group 2) (which was entirely due to the cases in Seascale), Burghfield (group 3) and one of the control sites.

Sharp *et al.* (1996) investigated the incidence of leukaemia and non-Hodgkin lymphoma diagnosed in children aged under 15 years in the vicinity of all seven nuclear sites in Scotland during the period 1968–93. Three of the seven installations were electricity power generating plants, three were nuclear submarine bases, and the other was the nuclear reprocessing plant at Dounreay. As in other studies, regions of 25 km radius were investigated. The data on leukaemia and non-Hodgkin lymphoma were verified from multiple sources and diagnostic review was carried out for all but a small proportion of cases, whether resident near nuclear sites or elsewhere. There was no evidence of a general increased incidence of childhood leukaemia and non-Hodgkin lymphoma near nuclear sites in Scotland. As observed in other studies, there was a significant excess risk in the zone around the Dounreay nuclear reprocessing plant (O/E 1.99, $p$ value for Stone's maximum likelihood ratio test for raised risk of disease in the vicinity of a point source, 0.03). The result of a linear risk score test for a trend of decreasing risk with distance from the site was not statistically significant, but the power of the study to detect such a trend was low. The excess was only partly accounted for by the sociodemographic characteristics of the study area. The only other excesses observed were around one of the electricity generating plants (O/E 1.08) and one of the submarine bases (O/E 1.02). The results of Stone's maximum likelihood ratio test and of the risk score for trend were not statistically significant.

In France, Hill and Laplanche (1990) compared mortality in the 0–24-year age group between communes within 21 km of six nuclear plants which started operation in 1975 or earlier and control communes. No substantial or significant difference in standardized mortality rates between exposed and control areas was found. Expected numbers of cases were calculated from national rates. In exposed areas, a significantly high SMR (197) was observed for Hodgkin's disease, and a significantly low SMR (41) for malignant brain tumours; these deviations were no longer significant after adjustment for multiple comparisons. For leukaemia, no excess was observed. There was no effect of sex and age or type of installation, and no trend associated with distance from the installation.

In the USA, no association between residence in a county with a nuclear installation and death attributable to cancer of any specific type before the age of 20 years was found (Jablon *et al.*, 1990). Mortality due to 16 cancer-related categories was compared between 107 counties in which at least 20% of the area was within 16 km of 62 nuclear installations and 292 counties matched on a variety of sociodemographic characteristics (Table 4.2). For children under 10 years of age, the only relative risk significantly greater than unity for counties near installations versus control counties after start-up was for cancer of the trachea, bronchus and lung (RR =

2.24, $p < 0.01$, 26 exposed and 19 unexposed cases). However, this excess depended in large part on a low SMR (0.61) in the control countries in the periods before the nuclear plants started operation, significantly lower than that in the same countries after start-up (RR = 0.40). For children aged 10–19 years, the only relative risk significantly greater than unity for the period after start-up was for digestive cancer (RR = 1.30, $p < 0.05$, 105 exposed and 150 unexposed cases). A significant deficit of Hodgkin's disease was observed (RR = 0.69, $p < 0.01$, 115 exposed and 336 unexposed cases) in this age group.

The consistency of relative risks of leukaemia mortality before 10 years of age associated with residence near individual facilities was assessed. Relative risks based on fewer than three deaths in the installation or control areas, or where there were fewer than 10 deaths in installation and control areas combined, were excluded. For the period after start-up, 19 installation areas were associated with relative risks of unity or more compared with 16 areas with relative risks of less than unity. Before start-up, 35 areas were associated with relative risks of unity or greater, compared with 16 areas where these were less than unity. For all cancers other than leukaemia in children aged under 10 years, when the areas near to installations were compared either with the control areas after start-up or themselves before start-up, two thirds of the facilities had relative risks of unity or more, none of which was statistically significant. The largest relative risk (1.24 after start-up) was for installations whose primary function is electricity production and in which operations began in the period 1975–81. The elevation in risk depended on low mortality rates in control areas (SMR = 0.85, compared with 1.02 in the areas near the installations).

Data on incidence were available for five counties in Connecticut and Iowa in the vicinity of four installations, all of whose primary function was electricity generation (Jablon *et al.*, 1990). Since incidence data were not available for all of the control counties, assessment was based on standardized registration ratios (SRR), with expected numbers derived from state-wide registrations, before and after start-up. Before start-up, the SRR for leukaemia under age 10 years in all facilities combined was 1.13 (not significant) whereas after start-up the SRR was 1.36 ($p < 0.01$) (Jablon *et al.*, 1991). The finding largely depended on an excess around one plant in Connecticut. The result may be due to chance in view of the large number of comparisons, and installations other than nuclear plants may be

relevant. For example, in the county in which the excess was found, there is a large naval shipyard.

In Germany, no excess incidence of total malignancies before the age of 15 years diagnosed between 1980 and 1990 was found to be associated with proximity to nuclear installations (Michaelis *et al.*, 1992). Three zones of exposure within the former Federal Republic were considered: counties with at least one third of their area within 15 km, 10 km or 5 km of 20 nuclear installations and 6 potential sites of nuclear installations. Control counties were selected randomly from those matching the exposed ones on social class, population density, paediatric oncology centre, and having their closest boundary to the reference location between 30 and 100 km. Counties closer than 15 km to the sea, to a foreign border, or to the border with the former Democratic Republic were excluded. Age-standardized incidence rates were lower than expected on the basis of national rates in both exposed and control areas. An increased relative risk associated with areas within 15 km of an installation was observed for acute leukaemia diagnosed before 5 years of age (RR = 1.28, $p = 0.037$) and for non-Hodgkin lymphoma before 15 years of age (RR = 1.67, $p = 0.017$). The relative risk of acute leukaemia in the 0–4-year age group within 5 km of the plant was 3.01 ($p = 0.015$), but both this and the finding relating to proximity within 15 km depend on low standardized incidence rates in the control regions. This was also true for non-Hodgkin lymphoma. No excess was observed for Hodgkin's lymphoma. For acute leukaemia, the relative risks were greatest for plants starting operation before 1970 but, again, this was largely due to low rates in the control regions. A trend of decreasing relative risk with increasing distance from the installations was observed in this period, but was reversed for the other periods. The incidence of total childhood cancer in regions in which nuclear power plants had been planned was slightly higher than in regions in which such plants were in operation.

Mortality due to leukaemias in children aged 0–14 years during the period 1950–87 and incidence during the period 1964–86 in Ontario, Canada, has been investigated (Clarke *et al.*, 1991; McLaughlin *et al.*, 1993a). Unlike the UK, Canada has no nuclear fuel reprocessing plants or weapons research and manufacturing facilities. However, there are reactor research establishments in which experimental processes could give rise to a wide range of potential emissions, uranium mines, mills and refineries which potentially could release radioactive dust into the environment, and nuclear power generating stations which may release low levels of radioactive waste. Ontario is the only province with all three types of facility. The primary hypothesis was that there might be an excess of childhood leukaemia in the vicinity of the two nuclear research facilities in Ontario, because some of the emissions might be similar to those of the Sellafield plant. The second hypothesis was that there might be an excess in the vicinity of the two uranium facilities concerned with uranium mining, milling and refining. The analysis of leukaemia frequency in the vicinity of the nuclear power generating stations was exploratory. Residence was classified according to (a) county and (b) zone within 25 km around each of the nuclear facilities. On the basis of the results of studies in the UK, it was postulated that any excess risk would be limited to children who were born in the vicinity of the facilities.

A deficit of both incidence and mortality was observed in the vicinity of the nuclear research facility. Slight and non-statistically significant excesses of both incidence and mortality were observed in areas around the uranium mining and refining plants, and around nuclear power generating stations. Mortality ratios were examined for the periods before and after the opening of one of the nuclear plants. There was no difference between the mortality ratios when residence at death was considered, but when mortality by residence of birth was considered, the mortality ratio in the period after the plant commenced operations was greater than in the period before. The study had sufficient power to detect excess risks of the magnitude observed in Sellafield and Dounreay, but no excess of this magnitude was found.

In a study of 656 cases of childhood leukaemia in Sweden ascertained during the period 1980–90, no evidence of excesses in the vicinity of the four nuclear power facilities in the country was found (Waller *et al.*, 1995). Population counts from the 1982 census were used. There was little difference in the results obtained when counts averaged over the 1976, 1982 and 1988 censuses were considered.

## Other studies of areas around nuclear installations

In the UK and the USA, the frequency of childhood cancer in areas around single installations or a small group of installations, in the latter case motivated by suspicion of excess, has been examined in a number of studies (for reviews, see Cook-Mozaffari *et al.*, 1987; Gardner, 1989; Jablon *et al.*, 1990; MacMahon, 1992a). Elsewhere, there was no excess of leukaemia in

the vicinity of a nuclear plant in the Negev, Israel (Sofer *et al.*, 1991) or of total childhood cancer in the area around the Würgassen plant in Germany (Prindull *et al.*, 1993).

## Background radiation: terrestrial gamma radiation

Kneale and Stewart (1987) and Knox *et al.* (1988) investigated the association between outdoor terrestrial gamma radiation exposure levels, based on measurements for 95% of the 2400 10-km grid squares of Great Britain (time period of measurement unspecified) and deaths due to childhood cancer (*n* = 22 351) during the period 1953–79. The address at the time of death, or birth if this was known to be different, was coded to local authority district; the first level of matching of local authority district and grid square resulted in 911 geographical units, called "demographic districts". There was no association between the death rate due to childhood cancer and degree of outdoor terrestrial gamma radiation exposure at this level of analysis. However, when the analysis was repeated with stratification by 100-km grid squares, to provide some control for broader geographical variation which might be due to social factors, a significant positive association between childhood cancer death and gamma radiation emerged. In an analysis of a subset of 14 759 cases in which data from matched controls were used to characterize the cohorts of births in the 911 demographic districts, there was a weakly significant positive association between the childhood cancer death rate and gamma radiation, independent of positive associations with maternal age and prenatal exposure to X-rays. The authors acknowledged that cases for whom complete data on sociodemographic factors and medical exposures were available may not have represented the totality of cancer deaths. The risk per unit dose from terrestrial gamma radiation was greater than that from prenatal X-rays, which the authors suggested was due to differences in timing of exposure. Prenatal X-ray exposure was concentrated in the third trimester, whereas the terrestrial gamma radiation exposure occurred in all trimesters, including the very sensitive first trimester.

Again in Great Britain, in the fifteen-year period 1969–83, no association between childhood leukaemia and outdoor and indoor gamma radiation levels was found (Muirhead *et al.*, 1991, 1992; Richardson *et al.*, 1995). The geographical units of analysis were the 459 district level local authorities in England and Wales, and regional districts in Scotland. The measurements of outdoor terrestrial gamma radiation exposure levels were the same as those considered in the studies of Kneale and Stewart (1987) and Knox *et al.* (1988).

## Background radiation: radon

In Sweden, there has been concern about residential exposure to radon, in part as a consequence of increased use of building materials based on lightweight concrete containing alum shale, and central heating and energy-saving insulation with attempts to eliminate uncontrolled ventilation, leading to raised indoor concentrations of radon daughters (Stjernfeldt *et al.*, 1987). Concern among parents of children with cancer regarding high radiation levels in their homes led these authors to study the gamma and alpha radiation levels in the homes of a group of children in Östergötland. Cases comprised 28 children with all types of childhood cancer who had been regularly seen at the university paediatric unit between 1980 and 1984. For 15 cases, measurements could be made in all of the dwellings in which the child with cancer had lived from the time of conception to diagnosis. For each of these, a playmate matched on age and sex was chosen as a control. There was no appreciable difference between the groups in gamma radiation or radon daughter exposure. The median cumulative dose to the gonads from gamma radiation was 0.80 mGy for cases and 0.75 mGy for controls. The median cumulative radon daughter exposure for cases was 120 $Bq/m^3$ and 150 $Bq/m^3$ for controls. For the other 13 children with cancer, access to all dwellings in which they had lived was not possible, and measurements were made only at their current residence. On the basis of current residence, the estimated median cumulative gamma radiation dose was 0.55 mGy and the radon daughter exposure was 140 $Bq/m^3$. The annual average radon daughter concentration in each of these three groups is similar to the national average for Sweden.

Wakefield and Kohler (1991) reported a case–control study in which indoor radon concentrations over the same three-month period were assessed in the bedroom and living room of children in the Wessex Health Region. The cases comprised 42 children with cancer diagnosed in a three-year period, 45% of whom had ALL. There were 39 controls, matched with cases on age and area of residence. Cases who had moved house during the year before diagnosis and controls who had moved house in the year before the diagnosis of the matched

case were not recruited. The mean indoor radon concentrations were similar between the groups.

The association between childhood cancer and indoor radon exposure has been assessed in several ecological studies. Henshaw *et al.* (1990) found a correlation between the incidence of total childhood cancer in 13 countries and population-averaged arithmetic mean radon concentrations, weighted according to the number of measurements, of 0.78 ($p < 0.01$). The correlation with indoor gamma radiation measurements determined from a variety of published sources was 0.44; this was not statistically significant. The assumption of the analysis is that national mean radon concentrations apply to areas for which cancer registration data were available. Butland *et al.* (1990) observed that both records of cancer incidence and estimates of average radon exposure were of questionable accuracy for some of the countries included in this analysis, and they reanalysed the data, including only six countries on which more reliable data were available. The correlation coefficient was 0.85 ($p < 0.05$). Thus, the correlation coefficient was not reduced. In early work, it was assumed that radon exposure leads to a negligible dose contribution to the fetus and to red bone marrow. Henshaw *et al.* (1990) postulated a mechanism whereby inhalation of radon and radon daughters might expose bone marrow stem cells to biologically effective doses, but this was subsequently challenged by Mole (1990a).

In England and Wales, Alexander *et al.* (1990c) considered the correlation between ALL in children aged up to 14 years and annual effective dose equivalent exposures to radon gas and gamma rays in households for 22 administrative counties during the period 1984–88. The Spearman rank correlation coefficient between county standardized morbidity ratios and the geometric means of the radiation measures was 0.65 for radon ($p < 0.005$) and –0.13 for gamma rays (not significant). The authors noted that the incidence of leukaemia and lymphoma tends to be high in south-west England and radon levels there are also high, so that the correlations might merely reflect an association between disease risk and some other factor in the south-west. However, after exclusion of the six south-western counties, the correlation between ALL and radon increased to 0.74 ($p < 0.001$). The authors note that the correlation for ALL remained statistically significant even after applying a correction for multiple significance testing. The data were based on location at diagnosis, and previous residences were not taken into account. Potential confounding by socioeconomic variables has been discussed, but its effect is unclear (Lucie, 1991; Wolff, 1991a).

Muirhead *et al.* (1991, 1992) considered data on leukaemia and non-Hodgkin lymphoma in children ascertained from the Childhood Cancer Research Group register during the period 1969–83 in 459 county districts in England and Wales and regional districts in Scotland. Average indoor radon concentrations and gamma dose rates obtained by the UK National Radiological Protection Board were used. With data aggregated into counties, the regression coefficient for indoor radon concentration was positive and that for indoor gamma dose negative when both terms were included simultaneously into a Poisson regression model, both terms being of borderline statistical significance. However, when analysis was made by district within each country, the coefficient for radon was negative and that for indoor gamma dose was positive. This difference between the analyses based on counties and on the smaller districts within them suggests that the between-county analysis was affected by geographical confounding factors. Further analysis of essentially the same database using a Poisson regression approach including environmental co-variates and a hierarchical Bayesian model in which Poisson over-dispersion was modelled showed no consistent evidence of any association with radon levels (Richardson *et al.*, 1995).

In Devon and Cornwall, which are the countries with the highest levels of exposure to radon in England and Wales, the incidence of childhood malignancies of all types was lower in postcode sectors with radon exposures of 100 Bq/m$^3$ or more than in sectors with lower exposure (Thorne *et al.*, 1996). This difference was not statistically significant. When specific types of childhood cancer were considered, the incidence of neuroblastoma was statistically significantly higher in the sectors of higher exposure than in those with lower exposure. This may be a chance finding in view of the multiple significance tests performed. Furthermore, the incidence rate of neuroblastoma in the sectors of higher exposure was similar to that of the rest of the UK (Parker & Craft, 1996).

Collman *et al.* (1991) examined cancer death rates among children aged under 15 years during the period 1950–79 in counties within North Carolina ranked according to average groundwater radon concentration. This concentration was available from surveys of 308 public water supplies in communities with a population of at least 100 people, carried out in 1975 and in 1981–82. The geometric mean radon concentration was calculated for 75 counties where direct measurements were available for one or more water supplies. For the 25 counties for which no such measurements were available, radon concentration was imputed by linear regression based on concentrations in other counties in North Carolina with similar geological characteristics. All counties were subsequently ranked in tertiles of exposure. For total childhood cancer, the relative risks compared with the tertile of low exposure were 1.16 (95% CI 1.05–1.28) for the middle tertile and 1.23 (95% CI 1.11–1.37) for the high tertile. The corresponding relative risks for childhood leukaemia were 1.26 and 1.33. In general, residences in counties with high radon concentrations in groundwater will have higher indoor radon exposures in air and/or water. The authors noted that counties with high radon concentration in groundwater tended to be located in the western and central portions of the state. Thus, it was possible that there was some unknown confounding factor that also had this geographic distribution, but the authors were unable to identify one.

Following local concern about a possible excess of childhood cancer in Ellweiler, a village in the Rheinland-Pfalz state of Germany, in the late 1980s, the incidence of childhood malignancies within radii of 5, 10, 15 and 20 km of a uranium-processing plant during the period 1970–89 was investigated (Hoffmann *et al.*, 1993). The plant was built in 1961 about 1.5 km from the village. There appeared to be an excess of childhood leukaemia (7 cases diagnosed at ages under 20 years observed vs 2.3 expected on the basis of rates for the neighbouring state of Saarland), but not of solid tumours of childhood, within 5 km of the plant. Four of the seven cases occurred in two particular villages, in which about 23% of the population of the area within 5 km of the plant resided. The subsoil of the region within 20 km of the plant contains high concentrations of natural uranium ore, and there are high levels of external gamma radiation and high levels of indoor radon. However, the geographical distribution of these exposures did not appear to account for the distribution of leukaemia cases. Radiation-specific chromosome observations were found in one of two healthy siblings and one father of a leukaemia case as well as in three healthy individuals living in houses with high radon activities (it is not clear whether these observations were made in systematic family studies in the area). It was suggested that the drinking water of the villages in which four of the cases had lived might have become contaminated by radium-226 from dumps of ore from which uranium had been extracted, but no measurements of drinking water contamination were available.

Pobel and Viel (1997), in a case–control study of childhood leukaemia in the vicinity of the nuclear reprocessing plant at La Hague, France, found an increased risk of leukaemia associated with a surrogate for radon exposure. The relative risk per year of residence in homes reported to be made of granite material or built on granite ground was 1.18 (95% CI 1.03–1.42). The presence of granite in the building materials could be verified for the current but not previous residences. No association was observed with the length of residence in homes with double glazing, which might have been expected to lead to concentration of radon gas within the home. (Further details of this study are given in the section on paternal occupational exposure).

## Conclusions regarding the effects of residential exposure to ionizing radiation

The data on the effects of the atomic bomb explosions in Japan do not indicate any substantial increase in the risk of cancer among the offspring conceived by survivors after the explosions. A modest increase in risk was found for children exposed *in utero*, but this was not apparent for leukaemia, which appears to be inconsistent with the findings for prenatal X-ray exposure. With regard to the three reactor accidents whose effects on childhood cancer have been considered, the data are either inadequate or the follow-up is as yet insufficient to evaluate the effects of the most serious, that at Chernobyl. No excess was found in relation to the accident at Three Mile Island, and the predicted excess following the Windscale fire is too small to be detectable.

There is no clear evidence of a relationship between fallout due to weapons testing and childhood leukaemia in studies in the USA, the UK, the Nordic countries or in Kazakstan. A relationship between fallout and thyroid disease was found in a study in Nevada and Utah, but bias in the ascertainment of thyroid disease might have been substantial.

Excesses of childhood leukaemia have been identified in the area around two nuclear processing plants in the UK, at Sellafield and Dounreay. Similar excesses have not been found around nuclear reprocessing plants in France or the USA. Weak excesses of lymphoid leukaemia deaths around installations other than Sellafield with start-up dates before 1955 were found in England and Wales, but not for other categories of nuclear installations. There were also weak excesses near sites either which have been considered for construction of nuclear installations in England and Wales and in Germany or in which start-up of a nuclear installation was after the period of study in England and Wales. No association between leukaemia or total cancer, mortality or incidence, and proximity to nuclear plants was found in studies in Canada, France, Germany or the United States. The discrepancy between observations in the UK and in other countries has led investigators in the UK to consider characteristics of the areas in which nuclear installations, or potential sites of these are located, other than the presence of the installations themselves.

A relationship between markers of indoor radon concentration and total childhood cancer has been found in one international correlation study and in an ecological study in North Carolina, and with leukaemia in two ecological studies at county level in the UK. However, the relationship is not apparent at district level. These analyses do not take potential confounding factors into account. The two available case–control studies do not suggest any relationship between childhood cancer and indoor radon concentrations, but were very small.

## Parental occupational exposure

### Paternal occupational exposure associated with the Sellafield nuclear plant in West Cumbria

Considerable debate followed the reporting of a positive association between leukaemia and non-Hodgkin lymphoma in the under-25s and paternal preconceptional exposure to ionizing radiation in West Cumbria, an area where there has been a prolonged excess of these diseases (Gardner *et al.*, 1990a,b). As described above, the study followed a recommendation of the Black Committee (Independent Advisory Group, 1984).

52 cases of leukaemia and 22 cases of non-Hodgkin lymphoma born and diagnosed in West Cumbria were ascertained from pathology records, hospital records, cancer registries and

death certificates during the period 1950–85. Non-Hodgkin lymphoma was included because this could have been confused with leukaemia in the early years of the study and because of evidence of an association with ionizing radiation. Hodgkin's disease (23 cases) was included but analysed separately. Two groups of eight controls of the same sex as the case were taken from the live birth register in which the case's birth was entered. For one group (area controls), searches were made backwards and forwards until the nearest four births from West Cumbria were found. For the second group (local controls), the parish of residence of the mother was an additional matching criterion, but otherwise the selection procedure was similar to that for the first group. A total of 381 area-only controls, 372 local-only controls and 248 who were both was identified, 1001 in all. Data on parental occupation were obtained from three sources. First, parental (mainly fathers') occupations were abstracted from birth certificates. This information was available for 68 (92%) of fathers of cases with leukaemia and non-Hodgkin lymphoma and 969 (97%) of control fathers, but for only 3 mothers of cases and 17 mothers of controls. Ten fathers of cases had been employed at Sellafield at the time of the child's birth: the relative risk compared with area controls (38 exposed) was 2.0 (95% CI 0.9–4.7) and with local controls (54 exposed) was 1.3 (95% CI 0.5–3.4). Second, occupational histories were obtained by postal questionnaire from 48 fathers of cases (67%) and 386 control fathers (39%). Analysis of these data gave similar results to those obtained from the birth certificate data and when examining employment at conception rather than birth. Third, data on the study were cross-matched with records of the plant and current Sellafield workforce. Agreement as to the fact of employment at Sellafield between this and the other two sources was good. One father of a case of Hodgkin's disease and five control fathers recorded as working at Sellafield on the birth certificate were not recorded in the employer's files. One case and seven controls recorded on the employer's files were not recorded on birth certificates.

For subjects identified as having worked at the plant, dates of employment at the site and annual external whole-body ionizing radiation dosimetric data were supplied by the employer; no details of exposure to internally incorporated nucleotides were available at the time of publication. This cross-check could not be made for 11% of cases and 10% of controls (Gardner & Snee, 1990). Relative risks were higher for fathers with a radiation dosimetry record at conception (10 cases, 32 area controls, 45 local controls) than for those with a dosimetry record at any time before conception or diagnosis. Total doses before conception of 100 mSv or more were accumulated by the fathers of four cases, five area controls and three local controls; the relative risk in the comparison with area controls was 6.4 (95% CI 1.6–26.3) and as compared with local controls 8.3 (95% CI 1.4–50.6). It has been suggested that the six month period before conception is the most sensitive for induction of transmissible genetic damage; doses of 10 mSv or more had been accumulated in this period by the fathers of four cases, eight area controls and five local controls. The relative risks were 4.3 (95% CI 1.2–16.1) and 5.0 (95% CI 1.1–22.2) respectively. Later, both sets of relative risk estimates were revised slightly following revision of the estimates of radiation dose to take account of men whose periods of employment in the year of, or before, their child's conception did not cover complete calendar years (Gardner, 1992). On the basis of data on all controls in the study, about 9% of the workforce had accumulated preconceptional doses of over 100 mSv and about 13% had received doses above 10 mSv during the six months before conception.

These findings were not confounded by associations with maternal abdominal X-rays during pregnancy or with maternal age. No association was found with maternal viral infection during pregnancy, Caesarean delivery, social class, paternal age, or birthweight. However, relative risks of the order of 1.5–2.5 were found for paternal employment in three of the other four main industrial groups in West Cumbria which employed more than 5% of control fathers: iron and steel, farming and chemicals. The relative risks were somewhat higher for local controls than area controls.

No association that remained consistent between the comparisons with area and local controls was apparent for the behavioural habits determined by questionnaire, but the response rates were poor and the effect of the widespread publicity upon responses obtained by questionnaire cannot be assessed. Compared with area controls, the relative risk of residence at birth being more than 5 km from Sellafield was 0.17 (95% CI 0.05–0.53). This association was secondary to the association with paternal employment.

No association with any of the factors considered in relation to leukaemia and non-Hodgkin lymphoma was found in the comparison of 23 cases of Hodgkin's lymphoma with 130 area and 133 local controls. The relative risks associated with paternal employment in Sellafield and for the dosage of ionizing radiation received were stronger for leukaemia alone than for leukaemia and non-Hodgkin lymphoma. Thus, the authors interpreted their results as suggesting that occupational radiation exposure causes a germ-cell mutation, but noted the alternative possibility that occupational exposures at the plant led to contamination of the home environment.

In a subsequent case–control study based largely on the same cases as those included in the study of Gardner *et al.* (1990a,b), but different controls, a statistically significant association between leukaemia and non-Hodgkin lymphoma diagnosed before the age of 25 years and preconceptional external radiation dose of the father was found (Health and Safety Executive, 1993). The controls were randomly selected from the same birth registers and same time period as the case children. In contrast to the study of Gardner *et al.* (1990a,b), in which preconception radiation doses were estimated from annual recorded external dose summaries, the estimated external radiation doses were based on the original dose records. The association was apparent only if the father had been resident in Seascale at the time of birth of the index child. This association also was limited to those who started work at the site before 1965. No association was apparent for other types of cancer, and there was no association between childhood leukaemia and non-Hodgkin lymphoma and the father's preconceptional internal radiation dose to the testes, based on biological monitoring data, potential exposure to neutrons and alpha particles, chemical exposures, or involvement in contamination incidents. There were positive associations with potential paternal occupational exposure to tritium and potential exposure to trichloroethyl-ene, as determined by a job–exposure matrix approach. All the cases with potential tritium exposure also had the highest level of potential exposure to trichlorethylene, so the effects could not be disentangled.

Kinlen (1993) has shown that the excess incidence of leukaemia and non-Hodgkin lymphoma in the 0–24-year age group in Seascale is not restricted to persons who were born there, and that paternal preconceptional exposure to ionizing radiation cannot account for the excess among those born outside Seascale. During the period 1951–91, there were five cases (0.74 expected) born outside the

village. Only two fathers had received precon-ceptional exposure to ionizing radiation; one had received a lifetime preconceptional dose greater than 100 mSv, the other 5.5 mSv. Neither of these was exposed in the six months before conception. Kinlen suggested that the association among subjects born in Seascale reported by Gardner *et al.* (1990a), if not partly due to chance, might be indirect.

Parker *et al.* (1993) studied the geographical distribution of 10 363 births in Cumbria during the period 1950–89 to fathers employed at Sellafield, by total preconceptional radiation dose and the dose received in the six months before conception. The authors postulated that if it were true that preconceptional exposure to ionizing radiation accounted for the excess leukaemia in children born and diagnosed in Seascale (Gardner *et al.*, 1990a), then paternal preconceptional radiation doses would be expected to be concentrated in fathers of children born in Seascale, as they considered that there is no evidence of a general excess of childhood leukaemia in the rest of West Cumbria. Contrary to this hypothesis, overall 7% of the collective total preconceptional dose and 7% of the collective dose for the period six months before conception were associated with children born in Seascale. Of all the children whose fathers worked at Sellafield, 8% were born in Seascale. The mean individual preconception-al doses were lower in Seascale than in the rest of West Cumbria. Regarding a general excess in West Cumbria, high rates of ALL in both children and adults in Cumbria during the period 1984–88 have been reported in a study in which ascertainment was based on central diagnostic laboratories and cancer registries (Cartwright *et al.*, 1990).

Following the identification of excesses of leukaemia diagnosed before the age of 25 years in Egremont North (an electoral ward in West Cumbria) and in Broughton (a ward adjacent to West Cumbria), as well as confirmation of the excess in Seascale by Craft *et al.* (1993; see above), Wakeford and Parker (1996) sought to determine whether these excesses could be accounted for by preconceptional occupational radiation exposure of the father. The area of study comprised the area served by West Cumbria District Health Authority and the adjacent Broughton ward. In contrast to the study of Gardner *et al.* (1990a,b), who estimated preconception radiation doses from annual recorded external dose summaries, the cumulative dose of external whole-body radiation was calculated from original dose records. The overall incidence of leukaemia and non-Hodgkin lymphoma diagnosed at ages 0–24 in West Cumbria during the period 1968–85 excluding Seascale ward was not unusual. Analysis at electoral ward level was made for six diagnostic categories and three age groups. Eight of 50 electoral wards had an incidence rate ratio whose lower 95% confidence limit exceeded unity. Among the fathers of the 27 children with leukaemia or non-Hodgkin lymphoma in these wards, the records of seven were definitely linked to a record of radiation exposure during the preconceptional period, and a possible match was identified for a further five. For five of the seven definitely matched, the offspring were resident in Seascale at the time of diagnosis. None of the fathers of the cases resident in Egremont North at the time of diagnosis was matched, either definitely or possibly. One of the fathers of the three cases resident in Broughton had a possible match. Therefore, the association between leukaemia and non-Hodgkin lymphoma and paternal pre-conceptional exposure to radiation apparent in Seascale is not supported by data from elsewhere in West Cumbria.

McKinney *et al.* (1991) carried out a study of leukaemia and non-Hodgkin lymphoma in children aged up to 14 years diagnosed during the period 1974–88, thus partially overlapping the group studied by Gardner *et al.* (1990a,b). Three areas in which high rates of childhood leukaemia had been identified were included: West Cumbria, North Humberside and Gateshead. Interviews were completed with parents of 109 (89%) of the 123 cases identified who were resident in the same area at diagnosis as at birth. Two controls matching with each case on sex, date and health district of birth, and resident in the same area at the time their matched case was diagnosed, were sought. 206 controls were recruited. The participation rate of the first eligible control families approached was 71%. Occupational data relating to the biological father were available for 101 cases and 178 controls for the preconceptional period, and 100 cases and 169 controls for the periconceptional period and during pregnancy. 25 fathers (15 of cases, 10 of controls) reported exposure to radiation during these periods. This information was checked against records of the National Registry for Radiation Workers and British Nuclear Fuels, Sellafield, Cumbria. Exposures to ionizing radiation were recorded as (1) "certain" when a total external gamma dose was recorded in either source; (2) "possible" for other contract workers on nuclear sites and industrial

radiographers; (3) "unlikely" when exposure to ionizing radiation was reported for occupations such as in education and medicine. Exposure to non-ionizing radiation included work as a radar or radio operator.

Paternal exposure to ionizing or non-ionizing radiation in the preconceptional period was associated with a relative risk of leukaemia and non-Hodgkin lymphoma of 3.2 (95% CI 1.4–7.7); this remained significant after adjusting for possible confounding factors, namely health-related occupations, employment in the energy-supply industry, and a variety of chemical exposures. When the definition was restricted to reported exposure specifically to ionizing radiation, the relative risk was 2.4 (95% CI 0.9–6.2). The relative risk associated with radiation (reported as ionizing or non-ionizing) exposure during the periconceptional period and during pregnancy was 15.1 (95% CI 2.4–338.0, based on eight exposed cases and one exposed control), while that associated with postnatal exposure was 3.1 (95% CI 1.0–10.3), based on nine exposed cases and seven exposed controls. The investigators noted that the small numbers of exposed subjects and the high correlation between exposures made it difficult to identify which period of exposure might be the most important. After adjustment for pre-conceptional and periconceptional exposure, the relative risk associated with postnatal exposure was 0.8 (95% CI 0.1–4.9). After adjustment for postnatal exposure, the risks associated with pre- and periconceptional exposure remained significant.

Stratification showed that there was little difference in the proportions of cases and controls who had received "certain", "probable" or "unlikely" exposures to ionizing radiation before conception only, whereas higher proportions of case fathers had received these exposures prior to conception and in the peri-conceptional and gestational period. One case with "possible" exposure and one control with "certain" exposure in the preconceptional period only, and two cases with "certain" exposure in the pre-, periconceptional and gestational periods had been included in the study of Gardner *et al.* (1990a,b). The raised odds ratio for confirmed paternal exposure to radiation in the periconceptional and gestational period was entirely dependent on cases included in the study by Gardner *et al.* (1990a,b). Smith (1991) commented that it would have been appropriate to exclude these subjects in order to make an independent assessment. This point is recognized by the authors as regards ionizing radiation, but the purpose of the study was to examine associations with parental occupation in general. However, the risk was not confined to West Cumbria and exposed case fathers did not work in the nuclear industry exclusively. Recall bias could not have occurred as a consequence of publicity about the study of Gardner *et al.* (1990a,b) as all interviewing was completed before its publication.

Subsequently, Alexander *et al.* (1992b) cross checked this entire study population against the database of Gardner *et al.* (1990a,b) and carried out an analysis restricted to case–control sets that were discordant for paternal radiation exposure and which were not included in that data base. Confirming the initial report of McKinney *et al.* (1991), there was no evidence of an independent risk associated with paternal postnatal exposure. The significant association between leukaemia and paternal preconceptional exposure persisted (RR = 5.1, 95% CI 1.5–22.0, based on 11 exposed cases and 4 exposed controls). Thus, the evidence for increased risk was not confined to West Cumbria. All of the cases had ALL. When subjects exposed to non-ionizing radiation or considered "unlikely" to have been exposed are excluded, the association is no longer statistically significant (RR = 4.6, 95% CI 0.7–45.6). A stronger effect, but based on smaller numbers, was again observed for peri-conceptional exposure (6 cases, zero controls: 95% CI 2.1–∞). Again, this effect is diluted after excluding the above subjects (3 cases, zero controls: 95% CI 0.8–∞).

## Paternal occupational exposure associated with nuclear plants in Ontario, Canada

In a case–control study of leukaemia in Ontario designed specifically to replicate the finding of Gardner *et al.* (1990a,b), no association between leukaemia and paternal pre-conceptional occupational exposure to ionizing radiation was found (McLaughlin *et al.*, 1992, 1993b). The occupational exposure in Ontario was of interest because the workers do not receive the types of chemical exposures experienced by the workers involved in nuclear fuel reprocessing at Sellafield, which may have introduced some confounding in the study by Gardner *et al.* (1990a,b). In addition, workers at Canadian nuclear reactors receive a substantial proportion (20–40%) of their total radiation exposure as an internal dose, largely due to tritium. In order to make the study as efficient as possible, cases and controls were selected from the population which had at least a small chance of receiving the exposure of primary interest, namely preconceptional occupational exposure to ionizing radiation. Therefore, regions of Ontario were identified from which the labour force for the nuclear facilities was likely to be derived. Six facilities were considered: three power generation plants, a research and development facility, a uranium refinery and a uranium mine and mill. The geographical areas from which subjects were selected were based on the residential distributions of the current labour forces of the facilities. Childhood leukaemia cases were identified from the Ontario Cancer Registry. The case series included children who died from leukaemia during the period 1950–88, or who were diagnosed with the disease between 1964 and 1988. A further eligibility criterion was that the mother was to be resident in the vicinity of an operating nuclear facility in Ontario at the time of the child's birth; this information was obtained from birth certificates. The leukaemia diagnosis was verified by review of pathology reports and other information by the physician and, for cases that were considered doubtful by the physician, all information was reviewed by an oncologist with expertise in the diagnosis of leukaemia. Of 112 cases identified, 87% were confirmed by pathology reports.

Eight controls per case were identified from birth certificates, and were matched according to date of birth and mothers' residence at the time of birth. Six control children were ineligible because they died before the development of leukaemia in the associated cases. Thus, 890 controls were included in the analysis.

Data on the occupational exposure to ionizing radiation of the father were obtained by record linkage with the Canadian National Dose Registry and subsequent verification by comparison with records of the employer. Whole-body external radiation doses, largely due to gamma radiation, were determined. In addition, for reactor workers, tritium dose, the most common type of whole-body internal exposure in this group, was assessed. For uranium miners, internal exposure to the lung due to radon and radon progeny was assessed. Total whole-body dose was calculated for each father by summing the external whole-body dose and the tritium dose. In addition to lifetime and annual radiation doses, dose calculations were made for the most critical periods that were identified by Gardner *et al.* (1990a,b), namely the lifetime cumulative exposure ending at the time of conception, and the total exposure during the six-month period before the child's conception. This approach was more precise than the method employed by Gardner *et al.*, which was to divide an annual dose in half to estimate a six-month dose. McLaughlin *et al.* considered that if there were a leukaemogenic effect of radiation acting via male germ cells, the effect might be greatest for exposures during an interval even shorter than the six-month pre-conceptional period studied by Gardner *et al.* (1990a,b). The duration of the period of spermatogenesis in man has been estimated to be 74 days (Courot *et al.*, 1970), so that the several generations of precursor spermotogonia and the spermatozoon that result in conception would have existed in the testes for approximately three months before conception. Therefore, these authors also considered the radiation dose during the three-month period preceding the child's conception. The authors acknowledge that many factors may have affected the quality and consistency of the radiation dose data. In order to evaluate this, dose data obtained from regional records were used to evaluate the quality of the National Dose Registry data, and the sensitivity of the study results to the dose measurement problems was explored in the analysis.

Potential confounding by maternal age, birth weight, birth order, sex and distance between a child's residence at birth and the nearest nuclear facility, was considered using information available from birth certificates.

No association between the risk of childhood leukaemia and either the period or type of paternal occupational exposure to ionizing radiation was found. For example, the relative risk associated with exposure to radiation during the father's lifetime before the child's conception was 0.87 (95% CI 0.3–2.3, based on the exposure of fathers of six cases and 53 controls). No gradient of effect with increasing radiation dose was found. The doses reported by Gardner *et al.* to be most strongly associated with leukaemia risk were specifically considered. None of the cases had fathers with a lifetime pre-conceptional dose of 100 mSv or more, compared with five controls. Again, none of the cases had fathers exposed to 10 mSv or more in the six months preceding conception, compared with nine controls. The prevalences of exposure to these doses were similar among the fathers of controls in the study in Ontario and the study by Gardner *et al.* (1990a,b). The largest relative risk estimate observed was for uranium miners (RR = 7.27, 95% CI 0.6–88.7) based on five exposed cases and 26 exposed controls. This may

be a chance finding, as statistical significance was not achieved, the majority of radon dose would have been to the lung and, in an ecological study in Canada, no excess of childhood leukaemia was observed in the region in which the mine was located (Clarke *et al.*, 1991; McLaughlin *et al.*, 1993a; see section on residential exposure to ionizing radiation).

## Paternal and maternal occupational exposure associated with the nuclear installation at La Hague, France

A case–control study was carried out on 27 cases of leukaemia diagnosed at ages under 25 years during the period 1978–93 in persons resident within 35 km of the La Hague facility, and 192 controls matched for sex, age, place of birth and residence at the time of diagnosis (Pobel & Viel, 1997). The study area was defined as including a radius of 35 km around the reprocessing plant. Thus, the area also included the contiguous low-level radioactive waste depository, a nuclear power station 16 km away, and naval dockyards where nuclear submarine fuel is handled, 19 km away. Controls were selected through the general practitioners of the area who had delivered care to children with leukaemia. Up to ten adult patients of these general practitioners who had a child of the same sex as the index case and similar age, place of birth and place of residence at time of diagnosis, were identified. Of 235 control parents identified as possibly eligible, 35 were subsequently found to be ineligible, and a further eight either could not be contacted or refused to participate, leaving 192 controls. Data were obtained by home interview in the period 1993–96, and from occupational records for those employed at nuclear establishments. Details of external whole-body exposure to ionizing radiation were obtained for all but three fathers who had been employed at nuclear establishments. According to employment and radiation records, none of the fathers of cases had detectable lifetime doses during the preconceptional period. Nineteen (10%) of the control fathers had been exposed during the preconceptional period, seven to doses of 35 mSv or more, seven to doses in the range of 1–34 mSV, and five to lower doses. These doses were lower than those received by fathers occupationally exposed at Sellafield. Sixteen had been exposed in the six-month period before conception (range 0.03–9.10 mSv) and 15 in the three-month period before conception (range 0.02–4.62 mSv). Two fathers of cases and 17 fathers of controls were exposed during the gestational period, and five fathers of cases and 19 fathers of controls during the lifetime of the index child. No association was apparent in either of these periods. A few mothers reported that they had been exposed to radiation, but no association was apparent with leukaemia in their offspring.

## Paternal occupational exposure associated with nuclear plants in Scotland

In a case–control study of leukaemia and non-Hodgkin lymphoma in Scotland in the period 1958–90 among people aged under 25 years who were born in or after 1958 (the year in which nuclear operations began in Scotland), no association with paternal preconceptional occupational exposure to ionizing radiation was found (Kinlen *et al.*, 1993b). Unlike in the studies in West Cumbria (Gardner *et al.*, 1990a) and Ontario (McLaughlin *et al.*, 1992, 1993b), the study was not restricted to the vicinity of nuclear facilities, but covered the whole of Scotland. Thus, the proportion of fathers of controls who received preconceptional occupational exposure to ionizing radiation was substantially smaller (0.8%) than that in the studies in West Cumbria (15.9%) or Ontario (6.0%).

Cases were identified from the Scottish National Cancer Registration Scheme, supplemented by death registries because of incomplete coverage in the early years of the registration scheme. In addition, children born in Scotland but whose disease was diagnosed elsewhere, and cases in North Cumbria, included because some workers at one Scottish nuclear plant (Chapel Cross) live over the border in that area, were ascertained from records of the Oxford Survey of Childhood Cancer, the Childhood Cancer Research Group, and Northern Young Persons' Malignant Disease Register, and records of deaths in England and Wales. Of 1478 cases diagnosed in Scotland, 1261 (85%) had birth certificates traced in Scotland with an associated paternal name. There were an additional 12 children with malignancies diagnosed outside Scotland, and a further 96 children from northern Cumbria. Thus, a total of 1369 cases was identified, for each of whom three controls matched on sex, year and county of birth were selected randomly from birth registers. Details of fathers were matched against records of the nuclear industry.

Among the 5476 men included in the study, only 41 had received preconceptional occupational exposure to ionizing radiation. Compared with unexposed fathers, the relative risk of leukaemia and non-Hodgkin lymphoma in

the offspring of fathers who had received a lifetime preconceptional exposure of 0.01–49.99 mSv was 1.14 (95% CI 0.5–2.5, based on 9 exposed cases and 24 exposed controls), and that in the offspring of fathers who had received doses of 50 or more mSv was 1.02 (95% CI 0.2–5.1, based on 2 exposed cases and 6 exposed controls). There was no association when analysis was restricted to exposures received in the six-month period preceding conception, or in the three-month period before conception, in which the authors postulated that any effect on germ cells would be most evident. Again, no effect was apparent when the analysis was restricted to leukaemia. When levels of dose the same as those reported in the analysis of Gardner *et al.* (1990a) were considered, the relative risk of leukaemia associated with a lifetime exposure of 100 mSv or more was 0.0 (zero exposed cases, three exposed controls), and that associated with an exposure in the six months before conception of 10 mSv or more was 2.3 (95% CI 0.3–17.2, based on two exposed cases and three exposed controls). Thus, as acknowledged by the authors, the findings cannot entirely exclude an association (Kinlen *et al.*, 1993b).

An excess of leukaemia and non-Hodgkin lymphoma in young people had been reported in the area around the Dounreay nuclear installation in Caithness, Scotland, during the period 1979–84 (COMARE, 1988). The Dounreay and Sellafield installations are the only nuclear reprocessing plants in the UK. One of a series of investigations recommended by COMARE was a case–control study. Urquhart *et al.* (1991) reported an investigation of this type in children aged under 15 years in Caithness during the period 1968–86. The authors recognized that the study would not be able to provide insights into the general etiology of childhood lymphoid malignancies because the numbers were small. Instead, the authors sought to determine how far risk factors identified in previous studies might explain excess incidence of the disease within 25 km of the plant.

The parents of 13 out of 14 registered cases agreed to participate. The participation of four controls for each case, matched on sex, date of birth and area of maternal residence at the time of the child's birth, was sought. 47 control parents gave permission for access to employers' records. All parents included in the study were matched against the occupational records held by the UK Atomic Energy Authority at Dounreay and Harwell and by HMS Vulcan, Caithness, to determine periods of employment at nuclear installations in the UK, annual radiation dose and monthly radiation dose for the two years before the birth of the child. 26 of these parents and 11 of the parents of cases were interviewed. When the parents of fewer than two controls were available for interview, substitute controls were selected — 10 in all. The interview data were used to confirm the information on parental occupation obtained from birth certificates and employers' records, and to obtain data on potentially confounding factors.

Three fathers of cases had been employed at Dounreay at the time of the child's birth, compared with 15 fathers of controls; the associated relative risk is 0.6 (95% CI 0.1–2.6). The three fathers of cases all had been employed at the plant in the periconceptional period. With regard to accumulated external dose before conception, one control father had received a cumulative exposure of more than 100 mSv (Fisher's exact $p$ value = 0.79; cf. Gardner *et al.*, 1990a). No case father had received a dose as high as this; the highest dose received by the father of a case was 40 mSv. One father of a case and one father of a control received a dose of more than 10 mSv in the six months preceding conception (Fisher's exact $p$ value = 0.38). When analysis was restricted to subjects resident within 25 km of Dounreay, the odds ratio associated with paternal employment in the nuclear industry at the time of birth or conception was 0.4 (95% CI 0.1–2.3), and the $p$ values associated with the accumulated doses were similar to those observed in the overall analysis. Thus, the excess risk around the plant could not be explained by paternal occupational exposures.

Gardner (1991) observed that Dounreay became operational later than Sellafield. Annual average doses of external ionizing radiation among workers in the nuclear industry have declined. Whereas some 34% of workers of Sellafield had accumulated a dose of more than 100 mSv by 1983, with a mean exposure of 124 mSv, only 13% of workers at Dounreay had received a dose of over 100 mSv by 1979, with a mean exposure of 47 mSv. Therefore, the results presented by Urquhart *et al.* relate to a working environment with lower exposure than that at Sellafield.

### Paternal and maternal occupational exposure associated with nuclear plants in West Berkshire, Basingstoke and North Hampshire, England

An increased incidence of childhood leukaemia in the West Berkshire and Basingstoke, and North Hampshire District Health Authorities was observed during the period 1972–85 (Roman *et al.*, 1987). The excess was concentrated in children aged under five years who were resident within 10 km of the atomic weapons establishments at Aldermaston and Burghfield (see section on residential exposure to ionizing radiation). Roman *et al.* (1993) carried out a case–control study to investigate whether the excess was related to parental employment in the nuclear industry. Cases comprised children under five years of age in whom leukaemia or non-Hodgkin lymphoma was diagnosed between 1972 and 1989, and whose mothers were resident in the area at the time of birth of the child. Information was obtained on 54 out of 56 eligible cases. Six controls, matched for sex, date of birth to within six months and area of residence at birth and time of diagnosis were selected for each case, four from hospital delivery registers and two from live birth registers maintained by the National Health Service Central Register. Twenty-one controls whose families had emigrated before the study began or whose current family health services authority was either not recorded or incorrectly recorded, were replaced. Data were obtained from four sources: the child's birth certificate, personal interview with the parents, the mother's obstetric notes, and employment and health physics records held by the nuclear industry.

One or both parents of five (9%) of the 54 cases and 14 (4%) of the 324 controls had been employed in the nuclear industry (RR = 2.2, 95% CI 0.6–6.9). Three fathers of cases and two fathers of controls had been monitored by being given film badges before their child was conceived (9.0, 95% CI 1.0–107.8); no mother of either a case or control had been so exposed. No father had accumulated a recorded dose of more than 5 mSv before his child was conceived, and no father had been monitored at any time in the four years before his child was conceived. No dose–response relationship was evident among fathers who had been monitored by film badges. The associations, which may be due to chance, cannot account for the observed excess in the area. In the analysis of Bithell *et al.* (1994), described above, the linear risk score test was statistically significant for Burghfield but not for Aldermaston. As Burghfield has substantially lower levels of radioactive emissions than Aldermaston, such emissions appear not to be a plausible explanation of the excess of leukaemia and non-Hodgkin lymphoma in children.

## Paternal occupational exposure associated with nuclear plants in Germany

In a study in the former West Germany comparing the incidence of childhood cancer between areas around nuclear installations and control areas, Michaelis *et al.* (1992) administered self-completed questionnaires to a subgroup of parents of cases. Among 324 questionnaires returned (63.7% participation rate), 12 parents had worked in nuclear installations. Dosimetry data were obtained for an unspecified number of parents. None of these had received a cumulative dose as high as 100 mSv. Subsequently, Michaelis *et al.* (1994) reported a historical cohort study of 9669 children born to 6897 men employed in nuclear plants in the former West Germany. The study was restricted to employees who were monitored for radiation and took part in annual compulsory medical examinations. The maximum preconceptional dose observed was 0.4 mSv. Only one case of childhood leukaemia was associated with preconceptional exposure of the father (SIR 0.8, 95% CI 0.02–4.2). Four cases of leukaemia were observed in the offspring of fathers who could have been exposed until the date of diagnosis (SIR 1.5, 95% CI 0.4–3.8). The corresponding SIR for all types of childhood cancer combined was 0.5 (95% CI 0.1–1.3).

## Paternal occupational exposure associated with the nuclear plant at Tarapur, India

Cancer mortality in approximately 2700 employers, and their families, who worked in a nuclear complex, including a fuel-reprocessing plant and a waste-management facility, in Tarapur, approximately 100 km from Bombay, was compared with mortality data from the Bombay Cancer Registry (Nambi *et al.*, 1992). One child of a male employee died of leukaemia. The overall death rate in children was much lower than in the reference population, because employees and their families have access to medical facilities that are not available for the reference population.

## Parental occupational exposure to ionizing radiation other than from nuclear plants

The results of studies of associations with paternal occupational exposure to ionizing radiation other than those specifically relating to nuclear plants are summarized in Table 4.3. There is limited evidence of an association

between leukaemia and paternal exposure to ionizing radiation determined by a direct question. Buckley *et al.* (1989b) noted that 17 fathers of cases with acute non-lymphocytic leukaemia and 9 fathers of controls had worked in jobs that required a dosimetry badge to be worn. There was no significant trend with duration of exposure, but the odds ratio for exposures of 1000 days or more compared with non-exposure was 1.9 ($p = 0.22$). A weak elevation in the relative risk of leukaemia associated with paternal exposure during the index pregnancy (RR = 1.4, 95% CI 0.6–3.5) was found by Van Steensel-Moll *et al.* (1985b). In the study of Lowengart *et al.* (1987), it was stated that the relative risk was not statistically significant. Subsequently, in an extension of the study specifically to assess associations with residential exposure to electric and magnetic fields, London *et al.* (1991) reported that there were elevated univariate odds ratios associated with paternal occupational exposure to ionizing radiation before and during the pregnancy leading to the birth of the index case, and during the postnatal period. No association with leukaemia and lymphoma was found in the study in which exposure was inferred from industry and occupation reported in a job history (Hicks *et al.*, 1984).

Information on paternal occupation during or before the index pregnancy was sought for 15 279 children dying from cancer during the period 1953–81 in Great Britain, and for an equal number of matched controls (Sorahan & Roberts, 1993). The authors acknowledged that some improvement in survival rates occurred during the later years of the survey. However, the vast majority of exposed cases and controls arose from pre-1971 birth cohorts, and related to periods when the series of childhood cancer deaths was similar to a series of incident cases. The information on paternal exposure was obtained by parental interview, usually of the mother. The proportion of eligible case–control pairs whose parents were interviewed was 79% for 1953–59, 72% for 1960–69, and 49% for 1970–81. Thus, although participation rates fell during the course of the study, they were relatively high in the period when occupational exposure to ionizing radiation was highest. Controls matched on sex and date of birth were selected from the birth register of the local authority in which the case parents were living at the time of interview. The data on paternal occupation were entered into computer files in text form. A total of nearly 37 000 occupation entries were recorded (case–control ratio 1.03)

## Table 4.3. Summary of associations between childhood cancer and parental occupational exposure to ionizing radiation, other than that considered in studies specifically relating to nuclear plants

| Site | Method of assessing exposure | Exposure Timing | Degree[a] | No. of cases exposed | RR[b] | Reference |
|---|---|---|---|---|---|---|
| **Paternal exposure** | | | | | | |
| Leukaemia and lymphoma | Inferred: industry | Pc | "More" | 8 | 0.8–0.9 | Hicks et al., 1984 |
| | | | "Less" | 37 | 1.0–1.1 | |
| | Inferred: occupation | Pc | "More" | 10 | 0.8–1.1 | |
| | | | "Less" | 18 | 1.2–1.4 | |
| Leukaemia | Direct question | Pg | Any | 13 | 1.4 | Van Steensel-Moll et al., 1985b |
| Leukaemia | Direct question | Pc–Dg | Any | NS | 1.0[c] | Lowengart et al., 1987 |
| | | | | | "elevated" | London et al., 1991 |
| Deaths due to leukaemia | Inferred: industry and occupation | Pc (6 months) | Any external radionuclides | 29 | 1.5 | Sorahan & Roberts, 1993 |
| | | | | 11 | 2.8 | |
| Leukaemia and non-Hodgkin lymphoma | Inferred: membership of College of Radiographers | NS | Any | 2 | 3.3 | Roman et al., 1996 |
| ANLL | Question about whether dosimetry badge worn | NS | 1000 days or more | 17 | 1.9 | Buckley et al., 1989b |
| Nervous system | Inferred: industry | Pc | "Less" | 10 | 1.0–1.1 | Hicks et al., 1984 |
| | : occupation | Pc | | 7 | 1.8–2.1 | |
| Central nervous system | Inferred: industry | B | "More" | 28 | 2.2* | Nasca et al., 1988 |
| | | B | "Less" | 61 | 1.7* | |
| | Inferred: occupation | B | "More" | 19 | 1.0 | |
| | | | "Less" | 31 | 1.1 | |
| | Inferred: industry | Dg | "More" | 24 | 1.8* | |
| | | | "Less" | 52 | 1.6* | |
| | Inferred: occupation | Dg | "More" | 20 | 1.2 | |
| | | | "Less" | 28 | 1.1 | |
| Astrocytoma[d] | Inferred: industry and occupation | Pc | Any | 6 | 2.0 | Nass, 1989 |
| | | | Probable | 5 | 2.5 | |
| | | Pg | Any | 1 | 0.5 | |
| Astrocytoma[d] | Inferred: industry and occupation | Pc | "Less" | 25[e] | 0.9 | Kuijten et al., 1992 |
| | | Pg | | 17[e] | 1.1 | |
| | | B–Dg | | 18[e] | 1.0 | |
| Wilms' tumour | Inferred: industry | Pc | "Less" | 12 | 2.6–2.9* | Hicks et al. 1984 |
| Wilms' tumour | Inferred: industry and occupation | | Any | 15[e] | 2.0 | Bunin et al., 1989b |
| | JEM | | Any | NS | 1.0 | |

| Cancer | Exposure assessment | Timing | Exposure category | Number | Relative risk | Reference |
|---|---|---|---|---|---|---|
| Rhabdomyosarcoma | Inferred: industry and occupation | NS | Health technicians or health diagnosing technicians | NS | 1.2 | Grufferman et al., 1991a |
| Germ cell tumours | Direct question | Pc–Dg | Any | 11 | 1.3 | Shu et al., 1995a |
| Deaths due to all cancers except leukaemia and non-Hodgkin lymphoma | Inferred: industry and occupation | Pc (6 months) | Any external radionuclides | 36 / 16 | 1.3 / 3.2* | Sorahan & Roberts, 1993 |
| All cancers except leukaemia and non-Hodgkin lymphoma | Inferred: membership of College of Radiographers | NS | Any | 3 | 2.5 | Roman et al., 1996 |
| **Maternal exposure** | | | | | | |
| Leukaemia and non-Hodgkin lymphoma | Inferred: membership of College of Radiographers | NS | Any | 5 | 1.3 | Roman et al., 1996 |
| Central nervous system | Inferred: industry | Pg | "More" | 22 | 1.1 | Nasca et al., 1988 |
| | : occupation | Pg | "Less" | 32 | 1.2 | |
| | | | "Less" | 19 | 1.2 | |
| Astrocytoma | Inferred: industry and occupation | Pc | Any | 8 | 1.6 | Nass, 1989 |
| | | | Probable | 5 | 2.5 | |
| | | Pg | Any | 7 | 2.3 | |
| | | | Probable | 3 | ∞ | |
| Rhabdomyosarcoma | Inferred: industry | B–1 | Health technicians or health diagnosing technicians | 9 | 4.5* | Grufferman et al., 1991a |
| Germ cell tumours | Direct question | Pc–Dg | Any | 15 | 1.2 | Shu et al., 1995a |
| All cancers except leukaemia and non-Hodgkin lymphoma | Inferred: membership of College of Radiographers | NS | Any | 6 | 0.8 | Roman et al., 1996 |

* Reported as statistically significant.
JEM, job-exposure matrix.
Pc, preconceptional.
Pg, during pregnancy.
B, at time of birth.
Dg, at time of diagnosis.
NS, not stated.
B–1, during year before child's birth.

[a] "More" or "Less" relate to potential exposure to ionizing radiation, based on classification by Moss et al. (1980) applied in the study of Hicks et al. (1984).
[b] A range is given when comparison was made with more than one control group.
[c] It was stated that the association was not statistically significant. No odds ratio was reported.
[d] Studies overlap.
[e] Discordant pairs.

and from these a dictionary of 13 604 unique job titles was produced. This dictionary was supplied to a medical physicist who selected some 200 job titles as having a potential for occupational exposure to ionizing radiation. Subsequently, the external ionizing radiation dose for the six-month period before conception of the child was estimated. Five matched pairs were excluded because either the case father ($n = 2$) or control father ($n = 3$) had been employed at Sellafield. A further 405 matched pairs were excluded either because the child had been adopted or because the data on occupation of the father were not available.

Following Gardner *et al.* (1990a,b), the estimated doses were categorized as: not exposed; 1–4 mSv; 5–9 mSv; and 10 mSv or more. For leukaemia, the associated relative risks were 1.33, 4.00 and 1.00. For non-Hodgkin lymphoma, there were only two exposed case fathers and two exposed control fathers; when this disease was included with leukaemia, the relative risks became 1.39, 1.33 and 2.00. For all childhood cancers excluding leukaemia and non-Hodgkin lymphoma, the relative risks were 1.25, 4.00 and 0.67 (Sorahan & Roberts, 1993).

The relative risks associated with potential paternal exposure to radionucleotides, i.e. unsealed sources, were: for leukaemia 2.75 (95% CI 0.9–8.6, based on 15 discordant pairs); for leukaemia and non-Hodgkin lymphoma 2.20 (95% CI 0.8–6.3, based on 16 discordant pairs); and for all other types of childhood cancer 3.20 (95% CI 1.2–8.7, based on 21 discordant pairs). Models were considered in which both estimated external exposure and potential exposure to radionuclides were included. For total childhood cancer and for childhood cancer other than leukaemia and non-Hodgkin lymphoma, potential exposure to radionuclides was a better predictor of risk than estimated external dose. The findings were less clear for leukaemia and non-Hodgkin lymphoma, although the highest relative risk was found for potential exposure to radionuclides. After adjustment for potential confounding by social class, maternal or paternal age, sibship position of child and history of obstetric radiography, the relative risks of total childhood cancer associated with external radiation exposure were somewhat reduced, whereas that associated with exposure to radionuclides was somewhat increased (Sorahan & Roberts, 1993). The authors observed that the hypothesis generated by the study of Gardner *et al.* (1990a,b) would predict that children of medical radiologists would have been at considerably increased risk

of childhood cancer. In their study, there were only two radiologists, and both were control fathers.

Roman *et al.* (1996) investigated the occurrence of childhood cancer among the offspring of medical radiographers. Of 892 men who were members of the College of Radiographers in the UK, 662 (78%) returned postal questionnaires about current and past jobs, reproductive history and health of any offspring during the period 1988–90. In a total of 998 liveborn offspring of these men, five cancers were diagnosed in childhood, compared with 1.8 expected on the basis of national rates (O/E = 2.7, 95% CI 0.9–6.5). Two of the cases had leukaemia or non-Hodgkin lymphoma (O/E = 3.3, 95% CI 0.4–12.0). Of 5838 women who were members of the College, 4847 (86%) returned questionnaires reporting a total of 6609 livebirths. Eleven cancers were diagnosed (O/E = 1.0, 95% CI 0.5–1.8).

Data on maternal exposure were obtained in three studies relating to leukaemia: one report stated that no significant association was found, but no further details were given (Lowengart *et al.*, 1987), while in the other two, fewer than five mothers of cases were exposed (Van Steensel-Moll *et al.*, 1985b; Buckley *et al.*, 1989b). McKinney *et al.* (1991), in the study described above, reported that eight mothers of cases of leukaemia and non-Hodgkin lymphoma and 14 mothers of controls reported preconceptional exposure to "radiation", giving a relative risk of 1.1 (95% CI 0.4–2.99; prevalence of exposure in both cases and controls 8%).

Hicks *et al.* (1984) found no association between total childhood cancer and paternal or maternal employment in the year preceding the birth of the index child in occupations or industries potentially involving exposure to ionizing radiation. There was no association between potential exposure to ionizing radiation and leukaemia and lymphoma, or nervous system tumours. Significant positive associations were found between bone cancer (based on four exposed cases) and Wilms' tumour (based on 12 exposed cases) and industries involving potential exposure to moderate amounts of ionizing radiation. The associations were consistent between the comparisons with three control groups: brothers of fathers of the index children; fathers of neighbouring children who did not have cancer; and fathers of children without cancer seen in the same clinic as the cases in the same study period. However, the associations were not apparent for industries with potentially higher exposure to ionizing radiation (one exposed case of each type) or when the occupation of the father only was considered.

In the context of investigating a possible association between leukaemia and military radar exposure (see section on occupational exposure to electromagnetic fields), Hicks *et al.* (1984) observed increased risks of total childhood cancer associated with radiation exposure in aircraft mechanics (four out of six fathers of cases were in the armed services) and in military service. The authors suggested that radiation-exposed military personnel and their families might have had better access to medical care than other study subjects, used it more frequently, and in doing so, may have received more frequent diagnostic radiation. In addition, they commented that their positive findings have to be interpreted in the context of multiple testing, and the data on potential confounders were very limited. In addition, no direct measure of exposure was available.

Nasca *et al.* (1988) observed a positive association between central nervous system tumours and paternal exposure to ionizing radiation, as assessed from industrial codes. No association was apparent when occupational titles were used to define potential exposure. Analysis of a matrix of occupational and industrial codes did not reveal any occupational cluster. No association with maternal exposure using either classification was found.

In a multicentre study of 322 cases of rhabdomyosarcoma and matched controls selected by random-digit dialling, there was an elevated relative risk (4.5, 95% CI 1.0–20.8) associated with maternal employment in the year preceding the child's birth as a "health technician" (physician, dentist etc.) or "health diagnosing technician" (Grufferman *et al.*, 1991a). Six of the nine mothers of cases and one of the two mothers of controls reported occupational exposure to X-ray equipment. The relative risk associated with employment as a nurse was 1.2 (95% CI 0.5–2.9). The occupational risk of ionizing radiation may be consistent with the relative risk of 2.1 (95% CI 1.2–3.7) associated with diagnostic X-ray in pregnancy.

## Conclusions regarding paternal occupational exposure to ionizing radiation

In summary, paternal preconceptional occupational exposure to ionizing radiation has been associated with childhood leukaemia in subjects born and diagnosed in the area around the Sellafield nuclear reprocessing plant, but does not account for the excess observed in subjects born elsewhere. Moreover, no evidence in support of the etiological importance of this exposure has been found in studies in Canada, France, Germany or Scotland, and such an association does not explain the excess around the other nuclear reprocessing plant in the UK at Dounreay or the excess in the West Berkshire and North Hampshire health districts, in which two atomic weapons establishments are located.

Using linear and exponential relative risk models based on estimates of total preconceptional external radiation doses, it has been shown that there is a highly significant inconsistency between the risks of leukaemia and non-Hodgkin lymphoma in the children of the Sellafield workforce born in Seascale and the risks in the children born outside Seascale, those for the offspring of the Ontario and Scottish workforces, as well as the offspring of the survivors of the atomic bomb explosions in Japan (Little, 1993; Little *et al.*, 1994). This inconsistency was independent of the model used. It has been suggested that the Sellafield excess may be attributed to an interaction between paternal preconceptional radiation exposure and a cofactor that is restricted to Seascale (Health and Safety Executive, 1993). Little *et al.* (1994) have shown that if this were true, the interaction would be highly supramultiplicative. If there were interacting factors operating during gestation or early life to increase the probability of predisposition to leukaemia and non-Hodgkin lymphoma, then assuming conventional genetic mechanisms, an implausibly high rate of radiation-induced mutation would have to be invoked to account for the excess (Wakeford *et al.*, 1994; COMARE, 1996). Other genetic changes are thought to occur in germ cells. These are poorly understood (COMARE, 1996). However, it remains difficult to account for the uniqueness of the excess of childhood leukaemia and non-Hodgkin lymphoma in Seascale.

In studies other than those specifically relating to nuclear plants, positive associations which were not statistically significant were found when paternal exposure to ionizing radiation was assessed by a direct question. Although this might be compatible with recall bias, it is interesting that the highest odds ratio was reported when the question was whether a dosimetry badge had been worn, and related to prolonged exposure. Associations between exposures inferred on the basis of industry or occupation of employment and specific types of childhood cancer varied within studies according to the definition adopted. In a large study in the UK, a positive association between childhood cancer of all types and potential paternal occupational exposure to radionuclides in the six months before conception was found, whereas there was no clear association with estimated external dose of ionizing radiation.

It would be relevant to study the association between childhood cancer and occupational exposure of the parents to ionizing radiation in areas such as the region around Oberrothenbach, in the former East Germany. Medical files on about 450 000 workers employed in uranium mining and processing are said to amount to "the world's biggest data collection of low-level radiation and health", including a significant proportion of women who received appreciable exposures (Kahn, 1993).

## Non-occupational exposure

### *Maternal preconceptional exposure to diagnostic or therapeutic ionizing radiation*

Stewart *et al.* (1958) considered maternal X-ray histories before marriage and between marriage and the index conception. There was an excess of abdominal X-ray exposure in the pre-marriage period among mothers of cases with childhood cancer. By contrast, there was a deficit of exposed mothers of cases during the period between marriage and the relevant conception. This was not attributable to control mothers having had more previous children, and hence more occasions for obstetric X-ray exposure. Subsequently, in an analysis of deaths due to childhood cancer in the period 1953–60, the relative risk associated with maternal preconceptional abdominal X-rays was 0.97 (Kneale & Stewart, 1980). In addition, there was no association with maternal preconceptional X-ray of either the chest or extremeties, which the authors postulated would not have affected the offspring.

Shiono *et al.* (1980) carried out a case–control study (40 cases of malignant tumour, 80 controls) nested in the National Collaborative Perinatal Project in the USA, in which the liveborn offspring of pregnant women recruited in 12 hospitals were followed to the age of seven years. There was a positive association between malignant tumours and the mother having received radiological examinations before the index pregnancy (RR = 2.6, 95% CI 1.3–5.9;

Shiono *et al.*, 1980). There was no association in a parallel analysis of benign neoplasms (105 cases, 210 controls). A supplementary analysis of these data was reported by COMARE (1996). The relative risk of leukaemia and non-Hodgkin lymphoma associated with maternal preconceptional exposure was 2.2 ($p$ = 0.33, one-sided, based on nine cases).

In a three-centre study of 319 cases with leukaemia and 884 population-based controls in the USA, Graham *et al.* (1966) reported that maternal preconceptional exposure to diagnostic radiation was associated with a relative risk of leukaemia in the offspring of 1.6 ($p$ = 0.006, two-sided). The relative risk was unchanged when individuals receiving dental radiation were omitted. While the effect was apparent only among second or later pregnancies, it did not appear to be enhanced by prior experience of miscarriage or stillbirth. This suggests that confounding arising from an association of both leukaemia and pregnancy X-rays with prior adverse reproductive outcome does not account for the relationship. No clear dose–response gradient was observed. It was not possible to determine whether the association with preconceptional exposure to ionizing radiation was confounded by intrauterine exposure. However, the authors commented that the risks for preconceptional and intrauterine exposure to radiation together were higher than those for these exposures considered separately. In an analysis of a subset of these data relating to leukaemia in children aged 1–4 years at diagnosis, there was no association with preconceptional, maternal or intrauterine irradiation in isolation; elevated risks were apparent only in conjunction with reproductive wastage and/or viral disease in childhood (Gibson *et al.*, 1968).

In a study of prevalent cases of leukaemia in Boston, USA, almost twice as many mothers of cases as mothers of children with other types of cancer or of patients at an orthopaedic clinic reported having received therapeutic irradiation before or during the index pregnancy (Manning & Carroll, 1957). Most of the mothers had received therapy for dermatological conditions, mainly acne.

Shu *et al.* (1994a) carried out a case–control study of leukaemia diagnosed at ages up to 14 in urban Shanghai during the period 1986–91, and other types of childhood cancer during the period 1981–91. Interviews were completed with the parents of 680 (83%) of the 819 eligible cases identified. Controls were randomly selected from the general population of urban Shanghai by a three-stage sampling scheme, first randomly selecting a local government administrative unit, second randomly selecting two groups (each including 15–20 families), and finally randomly selecting potentially eligible children from the roster identified for the groups. All parents of eligible controls participated. The mother was asked about the number of X-ray examinations received at specific sites, two years, five years and at any time before the conception of the index child. Compared with fewer than five X-rays reported by the mother at any time before the index conception, the relative risk of acute leukaemia associated with 5–9 X-rays was 0.7 (95% CI 0.4–1.3), and that with 10 or more X-rays was 1.5 (95% CI 0.6–3.4); this analysis was based on 166 pairs. Based on 87 pairs, the corresponding relative risks for lymphoma were 1.4 (95% CI 0.6–3.2) and 1.4 (95% CI 0.3–5.9). No associations were apparent for the five-year or two-year period preceding conception.

No association with preconceptional X-ray exposure of the mother was found in other studies of childhood leukaemia (Shu *et al.*, 1988; Magnani *et al.*, 1990; Roman *et al.*, 1993; Shu *et al.*, 1994b). With regard to other types of childhood cancer, no association has been observed between maternal preconceptional exposure and brain tumours (Gold *et al.*, 1979; Shu *et al.*, 1994a), neuroblastoma (Kramer *et al.*, 1987), Wilms' tumour (Bunin *et al.*, 1987), hepatoblastoma (Buckley *et al.*, 1989a) or soft-tissue sarcoma (Magnani *et al.*, 1989).

In Denmark, four cancers developed among 143 children born to 260 women who lived longer than a year after receiving injections of Thorotrast, an alpha-particle emitting contrast medium used for cerebral arteriography, compared with 2.9 cases of cancer expected (Andersson *et al.*, 1994). The standardized mortality/morbidity ratio was 1.4 (95% CI 0.4–3.5). The four cases comprised one case of breast cancer, one case of cancer of the uterine cervix, one case of melanoma of the skin and one case of bilateral retinoblastoma with no family history of the disease.

## *Paternal preconceptional exposure to diagnostic or therapeutic ionizing radiation*

Paternal preconceptional exposure to ionizing radiation for diagnostic or therapeutic purposes has been assessed in a few studies. In data on deaths due to childhood cancer in Great Britain during the period 1956–60 (from the study described above), the relative risk associated with paternal preconceptional abdominal X-ray was 1.1 (Kneale & Stewart, 1980). In addition, there was no association with paternal preconceptional X-ray of the chest or extremeties. In the study in the north-eastern part of the USA already described, the relative risk of leukaemia associated with paternal preconceptional irradiation was 1.3 after adjustment for year of birth of the subject, age of the father at the time of birth of the index case and pregnancy order (Graham *et al.*, 1966). No association between paternal preconceptional exposure to ionizing radiation and leukaemia was found in a hospital-based case–control study in Italy (Magnani *et al.*, 1990).

A statistically significant trend with father's reported X-ray dose was found in a study of childhood leukaemia in Shanghai (Shu *et al.*, 1988). This finding is limited by the fact that cases were recruited over a 12-year period, whereas controls were recruited over a two-year period and, as acknowledged by the authors, it was not possible to validate reports of radiation exposure. Data on paternal exposure were obtained from the mother. Subsequently, in a further case–control study of childhood cancer in urban Shanghai described above, this finding was not confirmed (Shu *et al.*, 1994a). In the later study, cases and controls were contemporaneous. The mothers and the fathers of 92% of cases and 96% of controls were interviewed. The father was asked about the number of X-ray examinations received at specific sites, two years, five years and at any time before the conception of the index child. Analysis restricting paternal X-ray exposures to the abdominal or gonadal regions, based on only a few exposed subjects, showed no increase in any type of childhood cancer. Among children aged two years or less at diagnosis, the relative risk of total cancer associated with one X-ray within the two-year period preceding conception of the index child was 1.7 (95% CI 1.0–2.6), and that associated with two or more X-rays in this period was 1.8 (95% CI 1.0–3.3). Similar elevations in risk were apparent for acute leukaemia, but were not statistically significant. It was not possible to validate the information on X-ray examinations, as most were for routine requirements such as entry to school and jobs, and records of these are not maintained in hospitals. The inconsistency between the two studies in Shanghai may be due to methodological differences, but it is also possible that in the former study the main indication for X-rays was likely to have been disease-related, whereas it was likely to have been a routine requirement in the more recent study. During the earlier study period, the doses were probably higher than during the period of the more recent study.

In Denmark, six cancers developed among 226 offspring of 320 men who lived longer than a year after receiving injections of Thorotrast, compared with 4.5 cases of cancer expected (Andersson *et al.*, 1994). The standardized mortality/morbidity ratio was 1.3 (95% CI 0.5–2.9). There was one case each of Hodgkin's lymphoma, cancer of the lung, testis and thyroid and two cases of melanoma of the skin. The mean accumulated dose to the testis before conception was 941 mSv, substantially higher than what is usually encountered in occupational exposures. No case of leukaemia or non-Hodgkin lymphoma occurred, compared with 0.42 expected (SMR 0.0, 95% CI 0–8.8). Little *et al.* (1996) showed that this risk was statistically incompatible with that for the Seascale-born offspring of the Sellafield workforce, irrespective of whether linear or exponential forms of a relative risk model were used, but statistically compatible with the risks to the offspring of the Sellafield workforce born elsewhere in West Cumbria, with the risks to the offspring of the Ontario and Scottish nuclear installation workforces as well as those in the offspring of Japanese atomic bombing survivors. Thus, it appears unlikely that the Seascale childhood leukaemia cases are attributable to paternal exposure to alpha-particle emitters such as plutonium (COMARE, 1996).

In a multicentre study of leukaemia diagnosed before 18 months of age in the USA and Canada, a positive association with paternal preconceptional X-ray exposure was found (Shu *et al.*, 1994b). The risk increased as the period of exposure considered became closer to conception. In addition, the risk varied with site of exposure and histopathological type, the highest risk being observed for ALL related to two or more exposures of the lower gastrointestinal tract and lower abdomen (RR = 3.8, 95% CI 1.5–9.6, adjusted for paternal age, education and alcohol consumption). Significant trends were observed for ALL and number of paternal X-rays of the lower gastrointestinal tract and lower abdomen (*p* < 0.01), and upper gastrointestinal tract (*p* = 0.04). There was also a suggestion of a trend for X-rays to the chest (*p* = 0.08). There was no association with exposure of the head and neck or limbs. No association was apparent for acute myelogenous leukaemia.

Leukaemia has not been described among the offspring of fathers treated with radiotherapy in the available cohort studies (Narod, 1990).

A non-significant positive association (RR = 1.8, *p* = 0.42) with preconceptional gonadal X-rays of the father was found in a small study of sporadic heritable cases of retinoblastoma (Bunin *et al.*, 1989a). No association between paternal lower abdominal X-ray before conception and Wilms' tumour was found in the one available study (Bunin *et al.*, 1987). In a hospital-based case–control study in Italy, no association between soft-tissue sarcoma and paternal preconceptional exposure to ionizing radiation was found (Magnani *et al.*, 1989).

## Maternal diagnostic exposure during pregnancy

A positive association between intrauterine diagnostic radiation and subsequent childhood cancer was first reported from a large case–control study of childhood cancer deaths in Great Britain (Stewart *et al.*, 1956, 1958). Studies of the associations between childhood cancer and diagnostic intrauterine exposure to ionizing radiation are summarized in Table 4.4. The study of Stewart *et al.* (1956, 1958), known as the Oxford Survey of Childhood Cancers, has been continued, and has contributed about three quarters of the information available worldwide on the effects of intrauterine exposure to diagnostic radiation on the risk of cancer in the offspring (Doll & Wakeford, 1997).

### Cohort studies

In the cohort study of Diamond *et al.* (1973), no association between prenatal exposure to ionizing radiation, as documented from hospital records, and deaths due to childhood cancer of all types combined before the age of ten years was found. There was a positive association with death due to childhood leukaemia in whites but not in blacks. The authors considered the possibility that obstetric factors might account for the difference, but differences between exposed and control groups in maternal age, past obstetric history and characteristics of the index pregnancy and birth were similar for blacks and whites. Adjustment for socioeconomic factors decreased the difference between whites and blacks but did not fully account for the difference. The authors concluded that there was differential susceptibility to the effects of ionizing radiation *in utero* between the groups. The total mortality rate of the white exposed group was higher than the white unexposed group, although this difference was not apparent for blacks. The death rates due to malignant neoplasms and cancer, and congenital malformations were similar as between the unexposed whites and blacks. This suggests that the difference between the groups regarding the association between leukaemia and ionizing radiation is unlikely to be due to differences in the procedure for attributing the cause of death.

No association between deaths due to childhood leukaemia and intrauterine exposure to ionizing radiation was found in a cohort study in Great Britain, but the numbers were too small to be informative (Court-Brown *et al.*, 1960). In addition, Doll and Wakeford (1997) reported that the identification of the irradiated women in this study may have been inadequate.

Doll and Wakeford (1997) carried out a pooled analysis of five small cohorts of children born in various periods between 1943 and 1958. Twelve deaths due to cancer were observed in exposed children, compared with 6.7 expected from the unexposed cohorts. When the data from these five cohort studies were added to those of Diamond *et al.* (1973), the relative risk of cancer death associated with intrauterine exposure to diagnostic radiation was 1.2 (95% CI 0.7–2.0; Doll & Wakeford, 1997).

*Case–control studies*

In many studies, a relative risk of the order of 1.5 was found for leukaemia and brain tumours and for total childhood cancer (Table 4.4). The lack of specificity of association has led many investigators to suspect that some kind of bias may account for the association, particularly in view of the absence of an association between childhood cancer and intrauterine exposure resulting from the atomic bomb explosions in Hiroshima and Nagasaki, and the lack of support from animal data for a particularly high sensitivity of the human fetus to ionizing radiation (Monson & MacMahon, 1984).

In most of the case–control studies, the exposure was determined from medical records. In the Oxford Survey of Childhood Cancers, the exposure was assessed by maternal interview. Knox *et al.* (1987) compared maternal reports of abdominal X-rays during pregnancy with medical records. Of 1179 mothers of cases who reported abdominal X-rays during pregnancy, 63.9% were positively confirmed in medical records, while there was similar confirmation for 63.7% of 986 control mothers. There was clear refutation of the maternal report in 5.1% of both case and control mothers, mostly because the mother appeared to have misunderstood the difference between a chest X-ray and an X-ray of the abdomen or pelvis. The majority of failures to confirm were due to missing case notes or missing X-ray records. In addition, the prevalence of abdominal X-rays in pregnancy in the on-going study of childhood cancer in Great Britain was very similar to that recorded at corresponding periods in national surveys (Mole, 1990b). Thus, there is little evidence for recall bias regarding this particular exposure.

It has been suggested that the underlying association is not with intrauterine exposure to ionizing radiation but with the indications for the procedures (Burch, 1970; Totter & MacPherson, 1981). In data on childhood cancer deaths in Great Britain, Stewart and Kneale (1971) found that the association with intrauterine exposure to X-rays was apparent when stratification was made according to the reason for X-ray. Burch (1971) commented that the stratification was too crude to be informative. In the analysis of an expanded series of data on childhood cancer deaths in Great Britain, Knox *et al.* (1987) showed that the association with prenatal exposure to ionizing radiation persisted after adjustment for reported maternal illness and drug use during pregnancy and a number of sociodemographic factors. In data on childhood leukaemia deaths in the north-eastern region of the USA, Monson and MacMahon (1984) found no evidence of confounding by birth order, the sex of the index child, ethnic group, the type of obstetric care, the birth weight of the index child, maternal age, religion, year of birth, previous fetal death, or abnormality of pregnancy. These authors also noted that causes of death other than cancer after three months of age were not associated with intrauterine exposure to radiation. Thus, the association was specific for childhood cancer.

Mole (1974) suggested that the main indication for prenatal X-ray of twins was knowledge or suspicion of twin pregnancy. Therefore, if the positive association between childhood cancer and intrauterine radiation were the result of selection of the cancer-prone for radiography, the excess cancer rate in X-rayed dizygotic twins would be expected to be much lower than the excess in X-rayed singletons. Contrary to this prediction, in data from Great Britain the relative risk of leukaemias and solid tumours in the first 10 years of life associated with prenatal X-rays in twins from pairs of opposite sex was 1.5, similar to the relative risk observed in singleton births. The estimated excess death rate from leukaemia and solid tumours due to radiation was higher for monozygotic twins than for dizygotic twins. Zygosity was determined by the Weinberg

# Table 4.4. Associations between childhood cancer and diagnostic intrauterine exposure to ionizing radiation

| Area and period of study | Cases: Dead (D) newly incident (I) or prevalent (P) | Cases: Upper age limit | Cases: Number | Controls: Type[a] | Controls: Number | Method of assessing exposure[b] | Period of birth of children | Control mothers who had X-ray examinations during pregnancy: Total % | Type of examination (% of examinations of known type): Abdominal | Routine pelvimetry | RR associated with maternal X-ray during pregnancy, by type: Any | Abdominal | Routine pelvimetry | Reference |
|---|---|---|---|---|---|---|---|---|---|---|---|---|---|---|
| **Lymphatic and haemopoietic tumours** | | | | | | | | | | | | | | |
| Great Britain, 1953–67 | D | 14 | 4771 | P | 8513 | I,MR | 1943–67 | 11.5 | 100.0 | 7.0 | – | 1.5* | – | Bithell & Stewart, 1975 |
| **Leukaemia and lymphoma** | | | | | | | | | | | | | | |
| England: North West, West Midlands and Yorkshire, 1980–83 | I | 14 | 245 | GP,H | 490 | MR | 1966–83 | 17.8 | 65.5 | – | 1.1[c] | 1.3 | – | Hopton et al., 1985 |
| **Leukaemia and non-Hodgkin lymphoma** | | | | | | | | | | | | | | |
| UK, West Cumbria, 1950–85 | I | 24 | 28; 45;47[d] | P | 153;167[d] 143;152[d] | MR Q | 1926–85 | 13.0;15.0[d] 10.5;9.2[d] | 100.0 100.0 | – – | – – | 1.3;1.2[d] 1.1;1.3[d] | – – | Gardner et al., 1990a |
| UK, West Berkshire and North Hampshire 1972–89 | I | 4 | 37 51 | H,P | 196 223 | MR I | 1968–85 | 8.8;13.6[e] 1.4;14.7[e] | 100.0 | – | – | 1.1 2.2 | – | Roman et al., 1993 |
| **Leukaemia** | | | | | | | | | | | | | | |
| Norway, Oslo, 1946–56 | | | 55 | | 55 | | | 14.5 | 100.0 | – | – | 0.6 | – | Kjeldsberg, 1957 |
| USA, California, 1955–56 | D | NS | 150 125 | sibs F | 150 125 | | | 16.0 21.6 | 100.0 100.0 | – – | – – | 1.5 1.3 | – – | Kaplan, 1958 |
| USA, Louisiana, 1951–55 | D | 9 | 78 | DO DCa | 306 74 | MR | 1942–55 | 18.3 28.4 | – – | – – | 1.6 0.9 | – – | – – | Ford et al., 1959 |
| USA, Monroe County, NY, 1940–57 | D | 19 | 65 | DO sibs | 65 93 | I,MR | 1921–57 | 4.6 7.5 | 100.0 100.0 | 33.3 85.7 | – – | 1.0[c] 0.6[c] | 1.5[c] 0.7[c] | Murray et al., 1959 |
| USA, Los Angeles, 1950–57 | I | NS[f] | 251 | H | 251 | Q | NS[f] | 23.1 | – | 100.0 | – | – | 1.2[c] | Polhemus & Koch, 1959 |
| USA, Minnesota, 1953–57 | D | 4 | 112 | sibs N | 105 112 | I,MR I,MR | 1949–57 | 26.7 27.7 | 15.2 14.3 | – – | 1.2 1.1 | 1.2 1.4 | – – | Ager et al., 1965 |
| Great Britain, 1945–58 | D | 14 | 9 | coh | 39 166 | MR | 1945–56 | – | – | – | 0.9 | – | – | Court-Brown et al., 1960 |
| USA, Northeast Region, 1947–67, singletons | D | 19 | 704 | H | 14 294 | MR | 1947–60 | 9.4 | 100.0 | 62.8 | – | 1.5 | 1.6 | Monson & MacMahon, 1984 |
| USA, New York State (excl. city), Baltimore and Minneapolis–St. Paul, 1959–62 | I | 14 | 313 | P | 854 | MR | 1945–62 | 22.4 | 28.1 | 11.2 | 1.6* | 1.4 | 2.0 | Graham et al., 1966 |

| Location | | | | | | | | | | | | | | Reference |
|---|---|---|---|---|---|---|---|---|---|---|---|---|---|---|
| USA, Baltimore, 1961–67, singletons: whites | D | 9 | 10 | coh | 235 904.25[g] | MR | 1946–60 | — | — | — | 2.9 | — | — | Diamond et al., 1973 |
| blacks | | 3 | | | 195 836.75[g] | MR | | — | — | — | 0.0 | — | — | |
| Finland, 1959–68 | I | 14 | 373 | P | 373 | MR | 1945–68 | 49.3 | 9.3 | — | 1.1[h] | 1.9 | — | Salonen & Saxen, 1975 |
| Japan, 1969–77 | I | 14 | 4607 | OC | 5968 | NS | 1955–77 | 10.6 | — | — | 1.6 | — | — | Hirayama, 1979 |
| China, Shanghai, 1974–86 | I,P | 14 | 309 | P | 618 | I | 1960–86 | 7.1 | 20.5 | — | 1.4 | 1.5 | — | Shu et al., 1988 |
| Mexico City | I | NS[j] | 81 | PH | 154 | I | NS | 11.7 | — | — | 1.9[i] | — | — | Fajardo-Gutiérrez et al., 1993a |
| Great Britain, 1945–64 (births), twins | D | 10 | 70 | coh | 353 114 | I | 1945–64 | 55.0 | — | — | 1.5 | — | — | Stewart, 1973; Mole, 1974 |
| USA, Connecticut, 1935–71, twins | I | 14 | 13 | P | 109 | MR | 1930–69 | 25.7 | 100.0 | — | — | 1.6 | — | Harvey et al., 1985 |
| Sweden, 1952–83, twins | I | 15 | 29 | P | 190 | MR | 1936–67 | 36.3 | 56.5 | — | 1.0 | 1.7 | — | Rodvall et al., 1990 |
| USA and Canada, CCG, 1983–88 | I | 18 mo | 302 | RDD | 302 | I | 1981–88 | NS | — | — | 1.1 | 1.3 | — | Shu et al., 1994b |
| UK, Oxford, Cambridge and Reading, 1962–92 | I | 30[k] | 143 | H | 286 | MR | 1955–92 | 25.2 | 15.0 | 4.2 | 0.8 | 0.7 | 1.6 | Roman et al., 1997 |
| **ALL** Great Britain, 1953–67 | D | 14 | 2007 | P | 8513 | I,MR | 1943–67 | 11.5 | 100.0 | 7.0 | — | 1.5* | — | Bithell & Stewart, 1975 |
| The Netherlands, 1973–80 | I | 14 | 517 | P | 509 | Q | 1959–80 | 3.7 | — | — | 2.2* | — | — | Van Steensel-Moll et al., 1985a |
| China, Shanghai, 1974–86 | I,P | 14 | 172 | P | 618 | I | 1960–86 | 7.1 | 20.5 | — | 1.6 | 2.0 | — | Shu et al., 1988 |
| Italy, Turin, 1981–84 | I,P | NS[j] | 142 | H | 307 | I | NS | — | 5.5 | — | — | 1.1 | — | Magnani et al., 1990 |
| China, Shanghai, 1986–91 | I | 14 | 166 | P | 166 | I | 1972–91 | — | — | — | 2.4 | — | — | Shu et al., 1994a |
| USA and Canada, CCG, 1983–88 | I | 18 mo | 203 | RDD | 203 | I | 1981–88 | NS | 2.4 | — | 0.8 | 1.1 | — | Shu et al., 1994b |
| UK, Oxford, Cambridge and Reading, 1962–92 | I | 30[k] | 113 | H | 226 | MR | 1955–92 | 20.7 | 15.9 | 4.4 | 1.1 | 0.8 | 1.6 | Roman et al., 1997 |

## Table 4.4. (contd) Associations between childhood cancer and diagnostic intrauterine exposure to ionizing radiation

| Area and period of study | Cases: Dead (D) newly incident (I) or prevalent (P) | Upper age limit | Number | Controls: Type[a] | Number | Method of assessing exposure[b] | Period of birth of children | Control mothers who had X-ray examinations during pregnancy: Total % | Type of examination (% of examinations of known type): Abdominal | Routine pelvimetry | RR associated with maternal X-ray during pregnancy, by type: Any | Abdominal | Routine pelvimetry | Reference |
|---|---|---|---|---|---|---|---|---|---|---|---|---|---|---|
| **ANLL** | | | | | | | | | | | | | | |
| Great Britain, 1953-64 | D, myeloid | 14 | 866 | P | 8513 | I,MR | 1943-67 | 11.5 | 100.0 | 7.0 | - | 1.5* | - | Bithell & Stewart, 1975 |
| | D, other/ unspec. | | 1179 | | | | | | | | | 1.4* | | |
| China, Shanghai, 1974-86 | I,P | 14 | 92 | P | 618 | I | 1960-86 | 7.1 | 20.5 | - | 1.4 | 0.6 | - | Shu et al., 1988 |
| Italy, Turin, 1981-84 | I,P | NS[j] | 22 | H | 307 | I | NS | 8.5 | - | - | 2.4 | - | - | Magnani et al., 1990 |
| The Netherlands, 1973-79 | I | 14 | 80 | P | 240 | Q | 1969-79 | 3.0 | - | - | 1.7 | - | - | Van Duijn et al., 1994 |
| **AML** | | | | | | | | | | | | | | |
| USA and Canada, CCG, 1983-88 | I | 18 mo | 88 | RDD | 88 | I | 1981-88 | NS | 1.9 | - | 1.6 | 1.5 | - | Shu et al., 1994b |
| **Lymphoma** | | | | | | | | | | | | | | |
| China, Shanghai, 1981-91 | I | 14 | 87 | P | 87 | I | 1967-91 | NS | - | - | 3.6 | - | - | Shu et al., 1994a |
| **Solid tumours** | | | | | | | | | | | | | | |
| UK, North West, West Midlands and Yorkshire, 1980-83 | I | 14 | 310 | GP,H | 620 | MR | 1966-83 | 14.2 | 71.6 | - | 1.2 | 1.1 | - | Hopton et al., 1985 |
| Great Britain, 1945-64 (births) twins | D | 10 | 91 | Coh | 353114 | I | 1945-64 | 55.0 | - | - | 1.5 | - | - | Stewart, 1973; Mole, 1974 |
| USA, Connecticut, 1935-71 | I[m] | 14 | 18 | P | 109 | MR | 1930-69 | 25.7 | 100.0 | - | - | 3.2 | - | Harvey et al., 1985 |
| **Central nervous system tumours** | | | | | | | | | | | | | | |
| Great Britain, 1953-67 | D | 14 | 1332 | P | 8513 | I,MR | 1943-67 | 11.5 | 100.0 | 7.0 | - | 1.4* | - | Bithell & Stewart, 1975 |
| USA, Northeast Region, 1947-67, singletons | D | 19 | 298 | H | 14294 | MR | 1947-60 | 9.4 | 100.0 | 62.8 | - | 1.2 | - | Monson & MacMahon, 1984[n] |
| UK, North West, West Midlands and Yorkshire, 1980-83 | I | 14 | 78 | H,GP | 156 | MR | 1966-83 | NS[o] | - | - | 1.0[o] | - | - | Birch et al., 1990b |
| Sweden, 1952-83, twins | I | 15 | 32 | P | 190 | MR | 1936-67 | 36.3 | 56.5 | - | 1.1 | 1.5 | - | Rodvall et al., 1990 |
| **Brain tumours** | | | | | | | | | | | | | | |
| Finland, 1959-68 | I | 14 | 245 | P | 245 | MR | 1945-68 | 49.3 | 9.3 | - | 0.8[h] | 1.1 | - | Salonen and Saxén, 1975 |

| Location | | | | | | | | | | | | | | Reference |
|---|---|---|---|---|---|---|---|---|---|---|---|---|---|---|
| USA, Los Angeles County 1972–77 | I | 24 | 209 | F,N | 209 | I | 1948–77 | – | 15.0 | – | – | 1.3 | – | Preston-Martin et al., 1982 |
| Canada, Toronto, 1977–83 | I | 19 | 74 | P | 138 | I | 1958–83 | – | 15.2 | – | – | 0.9 | – | Howe et al., 1989 |
| Australia, New South Wales 1985–89 | I | 14 | 82 | P | 164 | I | 1971–89 | 12.8 | – | – | 1.3 | – | – | McCredie et al., 1994a |
| China, Shanghai, 1981–91 | I | 14 | 107 | P | 107 | I | 1967–91 | NS | – | – | 1.3 | – | – | Shu et al., 1994a |
| **Astrocytoma** | | | | | | | | | | | | | | |
| USA, Pennsylvania, New Jersey, Delaware, 1980–86 | I | 14 | 163 | RDD | 163 | I | 1966–86 | NS | – | – | – | 0.9 | – | Kuijten et al., 1990 |
| US and Canada, CCG, 1986–89 | I | 5 | 155 | RDD | 155 | 1 | 1981–9 | – | 3.2 | – | – | 1.1 | – | Bunin et al., 1994b |
| **Primitive neuroectodermal brain tumours** | | | | | | | | | | | | | | |
| USA and Canada, CCG, 1986–89 | I | 5 | 166 | RDD | 166 | 1 | 1981–9 | – | 6.6 | – | – | 0.8 | – | Bunin et al., 1994b |
| **Neuroblastoma** | | | | | | | | | | | | | | |
| Great Britain, 1953–67 | D | 14 | 720 | P | 8513 | I,MR | 1943–67 | 11.5 | 100.0 | 7.0 | – | 1.5* | – | Bithell & Stewart, 1975 |
| USA, Greater Delaware Valley, 1970–79 | I | NS[g] | 104 | RDD | 104 | I | NS | NS | – | – | – | 1.2 | – | Kramer et al., 1987 |
| **Eye tumours** | | | | | | | | | | | | | | |
| Great Britain, 1953–81 | D[f] | 15 | 86 | P | 86 | I,MR | 1943–81 | 15.1 | – | – | 1.4 | – | – | Sorahan & Stewart, 1993 |
| Finland, 1959–68 | I | 14 | 37 | P | 37 | MR | 1945–68 | 49.3 | 9.3 | – | 1.7[h] | 3.0 | – | Salonen & Saxén, 1975 |
| **Wilms' tumour** | | | | | | | | | | | | | | |
| Great Britain, 1953–67 | D | 14 | 590 | P | 8513 | I,MR | 1943–67 | 11.5 | 100.0 | 7.0 | – | 1.6* | – | Bithell & Stewart, 1975 |
| Finland, 1959–68 | I | 14 | 96 | P | 96 | MR | 1945–68 | 49.3 | 9.3 | – | 0.8[h] | 0.4 | – | Salonen & Saxén, 1975 |
| USA, Greater Philadelphia 1970–83 | I | 14 | 88 | RDD | 88 | I | 1954–83 | – | NS | – | – | 1.0 | – | Bunin et al., 1987 |
| USA, multicentre, 1984–6 | I | 15 | 200 | RDD | 233 | I | 1969–86 | NS | – | – | 1.0[i] | – | – | Olshan et al., 1993 |
| **Bone tumours** | | | | | | | | | | | | | | |
| Great Britain, 1953–67 | D | 14 | 244 | P | 8513 | I,MR | 1943–67 | 11.5 | 100.0 | 7.0 | – | 1.1 | – | Bithell & Stewart, 1975 |

139

**Table 4.4. (contd) Associations between childhood cancer and diagnostic intrauterine exposure to ionizing radiation**

| Area and period of study | Cases | | | Controls | | Method of assessing exposure[b] | Period of birth of children | Control mothers who had X-ray examinations during pregnancy | | | RR associated with maternal X-ray during pregnancy, by type | | | Reference |
|---|---|---|---|---|---|---|---|---|---|---|---|---|---|---|
| | Dead (D) newly incident (I) or prevalent (P) | Upper age limit | Number | Type[a] | Number | | | Total % | Type of examination (% of examinations of known type) | | Any | Abdominal | Routine pelvimetry | |
| | | | | | | | | | Abdominal | Routine pelvimetry | | | | |
| Finland, 1959–68 | I | 14 | 56 | P | 56 | MR | 1945–68 | 49.3 | 9.3 | – | 0.7[h] | 0.0 | – | Salonen & Saxén, 1975 |
| UK, North West, West Midlands and Yorkshire, 1980–83 | I | 14 | 30 | GP,H | 60 | I,MR | 1966–83 | NS | – | – | 1.0[t] | – | – | Hartley et al., 1988b |
| **Osteosarcoma** | | | | | | | | | | | | | | |
| USA, Los Angeles County, 1972–82 | I | 24 | 64 | F,N | 124 | I | 1948–82 | 32.0 | 45.5 | – | 1.5 | 2.0 | – | Operskalski et al., 1987 |
| USA, New York State, 1978–88 | I | 24 | 130 | P | 130 | I | 1954–88 | NS | – | – | 1.0[t] | – | – | Gelberg et al., 1997 |
| **Ewing's sarcoma** | | | | | | | | | | | | | | |
| USA, San Francisco Bay Area, 1978–86 | I | 31 | 43 | RDD | 193 | I | NS | 22.8 | – | – | 0.7 | – | – | Holly et al., 1992 |
| USA, multicentre, 1983–85 | I | 22 | 204 / 191 | RDD / Sibs | 204 / 191 | I / I | NS | 27.5 / 17.3 | – / – | – / – | 0.8 / 1.5 | – / – | – / – | Winn et al., 1992 |
| **Soft-tissue sarcoma** | | | | | | | | | | | | | | |
| Italy, Padua and Turin, 1983–84 | I,P | NS[u] | 52 | H | 326 | I | NS | 8.0 | 5.5 | – | – | 1.9 | – | Magnani et al., 1989 |
| UK, North West, West Midlands and Yorkshire, 1980–83 | I | 14 | 43 | GP,H | 86 | I,MR | 1966–83 | NS | – | – | 1.0[t] | – | – | Hartley et al., 1988b |
| **Rhabdomyosarcoma** | | | | | | | | | | | | | | |
| USA, North Carolina, 1967–76 | I | 14 | 33 | P | 99 | I | 1953–76 | 12.0 | – | – | 0.5 | – | – | Grufferman et al., 1982 |
| USA, multicentre, 1982–88 | I | 20 | 322 | RDD | 322 | I | 1962–88 | 7.1 | 67.0 | – | 2.1* | – | – | Grufferman et al., 1993 |
| **Hepatoblastoma** | | | | | | | | | | | | | | |
| USA and Canada, CCSG, 1980–83 | I | NS[v] | 75 | RDD | 75 | I | NS | NS | – | – | 1.0[t] | – | – | Buckley et al., 1989a |
| **Germ cell tumours** | | | | | | | | | | | | | | |
| UK, North West, West Midlands and Yorkshire, 1980–83 | I | 14 | 41 / 41 | GP / H | 41 / 41 | I,MR | 1966–83 | 14.6 / 17.6 | – / – | – / – | 1.4 / 1.2 | – / – | – / – | Johnston et al., 1986 |

| Location | | | | | | | | | | | | | | Reference |
|---|---|---|---|---|---|---|---|---|---|---|---|---|---|---|
| USA and Canada, CCG, 1982–89 | I | 14 | 105 | RDD | 639 | I | 1968–89 | 15.8 | – | – | 0.9 | – | – | Shu et al., 1995a |
| **All sites** | | | | | | | | | | | | | | |
| Great Britain, 1953–55 | D | 10 | 1299 | P | 1299 | I,MR | 1943–55 | 14.1 | 50.5 | 11.4 | 1.6[a,c] | 2.1[a,c] | – | Stewart et al., 1958 |
| Great Britain, 1953–67 | D | 14 | 8513 | P | 8513 | I,MR | 1943–67 | 11.5 | 100.0 | 7.0 | – | 1.5* | 2.5* | Bithell & Stewart, 1975 |
| Great Britain, 1964–79 | D | 15 | 8059 | P | 8059 | I,MR | 1948–78 | 12.2 | 100.0 | – | – | 1.9*[w] | – | Knox et al., 1987 |
| USA Louisiana, 1951–55 | D | 9 | 152 | DO | 306 | MR | 1942–55 | 28.4 | – | – | 1.7* | – | – | Ford et al., 1959 |
| USA Northeast Region, 1947–60, singletons | D | 13 | 556 | H | 7242 | MR | 1947–54 | 10.6 | 100.0 | 67.5 | – | 1.4*[w] | 1.6* | MacMahon, 1962 |
| USA, Baltimore, 1961–67, singletons : whites / blacks | D | 9 | 13 / 10 | coh | 235 904.25[g] / 195 836.75[g] | MR | 1946–60 | – | – | – | 0.9 / 0.7 | – | – | Diamond et al., 1973 |
| USA, National Collaborative Perinatal Project, 1966–72 | I | 7 | 40[x] / 105[z] | H | 80 / 210 | MR | 1959–65 | 16.3[y] / 9.0[y] | – / – | – | 1.1 / 0.9 | – | – | Shiono et al., 1980 |
| Great Britain, 1980 | I | 10 | 33 | P | 99 | MR | 1970 (1 wk) | 15.2 | – | – | 2.8 | – | – | Golding et al., 1990 |
| UK, Bristol, 1971–91 | I | 14 | 111 | H | 558 | MR | 1965–87 | – | NS | – | – | 1.3 | – | Golding et al., 1992a |

NS, Not stated.
* P < 0.05.

a P, population-based; H, hospital; Coh, cohort study; GP, neighbourhood, selected through general practices; DO, deaths from causes other than cancer; N, neighbourhood; DCa, deaths from other types of cancer; OC, other types of cancer; F, friends; RDD, random-digit dialling.

b I, maternal interview; MR, medical records; Q, questionnaire completed by parents.

c Crude unmatched analysis of matched-pairs data.

d Local and area controls respectively, or analyses relating to these.

e Controls selected from birth registers and from hospital delivery registries respectively.

f 84% of the children were aged 8 years or less at the time of diagnosis.

g Person-years.

h Miniature chest X-ray.

i Mean age 8.5 years (SD 4.5).

j The authors state that when comparison was made with community controls only, the relative risk was 3.6 (95% CI 1.1–12.5).

k 92% of the children were aged 14 years or less at the time of diagnosis; the proportion was 94% for ALL.

l Mean age of diagnosis of 142 cases with ALL, 22 of ANLL and 19 of non Hodgkin lymphoma was 6.1 years (SD 3.6).

m Cancers other than leukaemia.

n Extension of study of MacMahon, 1962.

o Subset of study of Hopton et al., 1985.

p The authors state that there was no significant (p>0.2) difference between cases and controls.

q The median age of cases at diagnosis was one year.

r Due to retinoblastoma.

s The authors state that the relative risk was <1.5.

t The authors state that there was no significant difference between cases and controls.

u Mean age at diagnosis 6.8 years (± 4.7).

v All but seven cases were aged ≤4 years.

w Adjusted for a series of potentially confounding variables.

x Malignant.

y High or medium dose radiological examinations.

z Benign.

method. If monozygotic twinning predisposed to developing cancer, high rates of cancer would be expected in those who did not receive X-rays during pregnancy, whereas the rates in unexposed monozygotic twins were lower than in dizygotic twins or in singletons. This adds further weight to the argument that the association is not due to confounding by the reason for X-ray examination.

The positive association between childhood cancer of all types combined and intrauterine X-ray in twins was also found in small studies in the USA and in Sweden (Harvey *et al.*, 1985; Rodvall *et al.*, 1990). However, as observed by MacMahon (1985), the incidence of childhood cancer in twins in these studies was lower than that in singletons (see Chapter 10). If the association between childhood cancer and intrauterine X-ray were causal, an increased incidence would be expected in view of the higher prevalence of exposure. However, the available studies have lacked statistical power to detect such an effect (Doll & Wakeford, 1997). Interpretation is further complicated by changes in X-ray techniques over time. For example, in Sweden X-ray techniques changed around 1960, leading to lower doses. Rodvall *et al.* found that the relative risk associated with intrauterine X-ray was 1.6 for the years 1936–59, compared with 1.1 for the years 1960–67.

Changes in the association between childhood cancer and prenatal X-ray over time in data from the Oxford Survey of Childhood Cancer have been considered (Mole, 1990b; Doll & Wakeford, 1997). A reduction in the fetal radiation dose from obstetric radiography starting in 1957 following concern about hereditary damage was associated with a corresponding reduction in the relative risk of mortality due to childhood cancer for births during the next 8–12 years (Mole, 1990b). Doll and Wakeford (1997) observed that a statistically significant decline over time in the relative risk of childhood cancer associated with radiation exposure *in utero* and those born in the period 1940–76 resembled closely the decline in fetal doses which occurred over the same period. In the north-east region of the USA, an excess risk of leukaemia associated with intrauterine X-ray was observed from 1947–57, but was not apparent for children born between 1958 and 1960; the association between solid tumours and the exposure was noted only for births during the period 1951–54 (Monson & MacMahon, 1984). The authors noted that this clustering of the excess of solid tumours was not limited to specific indications for X-ray. Mole

(1990b) observed that conclusive evidence that diagnostic X-rays caused cancer would be a marked decrease in the incidence of childhood cancer in those born most recently and whose antenatal care involved ultrasound rather than X-rays. However, there is no evidence of such a decrease (see Chapter 2).

Information on a possible dose–response relationship with number of X-ray examinations has been presented only in reports from studies of childhood cancer deaths in Great Britain (Stewart *et al.*, 1958; Bithell & Stewart, 1975; Bithell & Stiller, 1988; Gilman *et al.*, 1988), Louisiana (Ford *et al.*, 1959) and the north-east region of the USA (MacMahon, 1962; Monson & MacMahon, 1984). Significant trends were identified in the early reports from the on-going study in Great Britain in which the measure of dose was the number of films taken (Stewart *et al.*, 1958; Bithell & Stewart, 1975), but not in a more recent report in which account was taken of the timing of exposure during pregnancy (Gilman *et al.*, 1988). The investigators acknowledged that the number of films believed to have been taken by radiologists is an extremely crude index of dose and did not include films discarded by the radiographer (Stewart *et al.*, 1958). In addition, Mole (1990b) observed that the dose per film varied. For example, measurements made in 1958 showed that the fetal dose performed for pelvimetry using a single film was more than twice as high as for pelvimetry using multiple films. Therefore, the data on a possible dose–response relationship are unsatisfactory.

In the study of Ford *et al.* (1959), the trend in the relative risks of childhood cancer deaths was assessed in relation to the number of roentgenograms; there was a statistically significant trend (chi-square = 6.54, $p < 0.025$). In the study in the north-eastern part of the USA, no information was available on the radiation exposure per examination and the number of films taken was usually not known (Monson & MacMahon, 1984). Therefore, these investigators categorized examinations as abdominal X-ray, pelvimetry or involving multiple films. Most abdominal examinations involve only one film and most pelvimetries involve several films. The multiple film category included intravenous pyelogram, gallbladder and gastrointestinal series, and four or more abdominal films. There was no suggestion of a dose–response relationship. Most of the excess X-rays observed among children with leukaemia were pelvimetries, while the excess for children with solid tumours was scattered among the three categories.

In a number of studies, variation in risk according to age at diagnosis has been assessed (Ford *et al.*, 1959; Bross & Natarajan, 1972; Bithell & Stewart, 1975; Monson & MacMahon, 1984; Hopton *et al.*, 1985; Knox *et al.*, 1987; McKinney *et al.*, 1987; Rodvall *et al.*, 1990). While some studies suggested an increased risk among young children (Monson & MacMahon, 1984; Hopton *et al.*, 1985; Knox *et al.*, 1987; McKinney *et al.*, 1987), analysis of the Oxford Survey of Childhood Cancer for the period 1953–79 suggests no noteworthy variation in risk by age (Mole, 1990b).

On the basis of an analysis of data from the Oxford Survey of Childhood Cancer, Gilman *et al.* (1988) concluded that the excess risk due to obstetric X-rays was due to exposure in the first trimester. However, Mole (1990b) showed that this excess risk was confined to the offspring of women analysed for non-obstetric reasons in the early years of the study, when hospital records were less complete. Control mothers may have failed to recall their non-obstetric exposures in sufficient detail for their records to be identified (Doll & Wakeford, 1997). Most of the exposure to obstetric X-rays occurred in the third trimester (Gilman *et al.*, 1988).

Bross and Natarajan (1972) suggested that the association between intrauterine exposure to ionizing radiation and childhood cancer was particularly strong among children with a history of certain allergic or infectious diseases, but this interpretation was criticized because the method of selection of some of the indicators of such a history were not specified (MacMahon, 1972). These findings have not been replicated, and it is noteworthy that significant inverse associations between non-T-cell ALL and measles or measles vaccination and a history of asthma or atopic dermatitis were found in a small study in Japan (Nishi & Miyake, 1989). Hirayama (1979) reported a very high relative risk of leukaemia associated with prenatal radiation exposure and a family history of leukaemia; it is stated that similar results were obtained by comparing with controls with other types of cancer and with non-neoplastic controls.

## Other maternal exposure to ionizing radiation during the index pregnancy

In the study of leukaemia diagnosed before the age of 25 years in the area around the La Hague nuclear facility in Normandy, France, described above, an increased risk was apparent for use of local beaches during pregnancy at least once a month compared with less often (RR = 4.5, 95% CI 1.5–15.2; Pobel & Viel, 1997). This exposure was correlated with the child's use of the local beaches (Viel, 1997). The possibility that selection bias, recall bias and multiple testing may account for the results has been debated (Clavel & Hémon, 1997; Law & Roman, 1997; Viel, 1997; Wakeford, 1997).

## Diagnostic and therapeutic exposure during the lifetime of the index child

Studies of the associations between childhood cancer and postnatal exposure to diagnostic and therapeutic ionizing radiation are summarized in Table 4.5. The effects of postnatal exposure of this type have been less studied than the effects of intrauterine exposure. There have been a number of cohort studies of the effects of therapeutic exposure to ionizing radiation in childhood and subsequent cancer occurrence. These studies are not discussed in detail in this review as in most, the risks of cancer in childhood have not been presented separately. In some studies, exposure to X-rays was classified according to the reason for which it was performed (diagnostic or therapeutic), and in some by the part of the body that was X-rayed.

### Leukaemia

In most studies of leukaemia, there was no association with all types of postnatal exposure combined (Table 4.5). Increased risks of leukaemia associated with postnatal irradiation for therapeutic and other reasons also were reported from early studies in the USA (Murray *et al.*, 1959; Polhemus & Koch, 1959). Polhemus and Koch (1959) observed that more than twice as many cases (39%; 98 of 251) as matched controls (19%; 47 of 251) were reported to have had "X-ray shoe-fitting". However, as most controls were surgical patients admitted for repair of hernia or appendectomy, they were unlikely to have been representative of the source population which gave rise to cases. The study of Murray *et al.* is difficult to interpret as the estimated relative risk differed substantially in the comparison with the two sets of controls. In Great Britain, there was a non-significant excess of leukaemia deaths associated with a history of therapeutic exposure (Stewart *et al.*, 1958). No consistent association between leukaemia and postnatal exposure to diagnostic X-rays is apparent (Table 4.5).

### Brain tumours

In an analysis which was restricted to case–control pairs in which the cases were aged 15 years or more at the time of diagnosis, Preston-Martin *et al.* (1982) found a relative risk of brain tumours of 2.5 associated with a history of having

**Table 4.5. Associations between childhood cancer and postnatal exposure to diagnostic and therapeutic ionizing radiation**

| Area and period of study | Cases Dead (D), newly incident (I) or prevalent (P) | Cases Upper age limit | Cases Number | Controls Type[a] | Controls Number | Method of assessing exposure[b] | Type of exposure[c] | Prevalence of exposure in controls (%) | RR | Reference |
|---|---|---|---|---|---|---|---|---|---|---|
| **Leukaemia** | | | | | | | | | | |
| Great Britain, 1953–55 | D | 10 | 619 | P | 619 | I,MR | D<br>T | 12.9<br>0.2 | 1.2<br>5.0 | Stewart et al., 1958 |
| USA, Monroe county, NY, 1940–57 | D | 19 | 65 | DO<br>sibs | 65<br>93 | I,MR | T | 1.5<br>7.5 | 9.0*[d]<br>1.7[u] | Murray et al., 1959 |
| USA, Los Angeles, 1950–57 | I | NS[e] | 251 | H | 251 | Q | D<br>F<br>T | 41.4<br>3.2<br>3.6 | 2.1*[f]<br>3.5*[f]<br>3.7*[f] | Polhemus & Koch, 1959 |
| USA, Minnesota, 1953–57 | D | 4 | 109 | Sibs<br>N | 102<br>110 | I,MR | Any | 16.7[g]<br>18.2[g] | 1.3[g]<br>1.1[g] | Ager et al., 1965 |
| USA: New York State (excl. city), Baltimore and Minneapolis-St Paul, 1959–62 | I | 14 | 319 | P | 884 | MR | Any<br>>1 site | 36.0[h]<br>7.6[h] | 1.2[h]<br>2.1*[h] | Graham et al., 1966 |
| China, Shanghai, 1974–86 | I,P | 14 | 309 | P | 618 | I | Any | 27.3 | 0.9[i] | Shu et al., 1988 |
| Mexico City, N.S. | I,P | 14 | 79 | P,H | 148 | I | Any | 27.0 | 1.1 | Fajardo-Gutiérrez et al., 1993a |
| **ALL** | | | | | | | | | | |
| China, Shanghai, 1974–86 | I,P | 14 | 172 | P | 618 | I | Any | 27.3 | 0.9[i] | Shu et al., 1988 |
| Japan, Hokkaido, 1986–87[j] | I,P | 14 | 63 | H | 126 | I | Dental[k]<br>Hip joint<br>O[l] | NS<br>NS<br>NS | 1.4*<br>0.3*<br>1.0[i] | Nishi & Miyake, 1989 |
| Italy, Turin, 1981–84 | I,P | NS[m] | 142 | H | 307 | I | D | 45.9 | 0.7 | Magnani et al., 1990 |
| China, Shanghai, 1986–91 | I | 14 | 166 | P | 166 | I | Any | – | 1.6* | Shu et al., 1994a |
| **ANLL** | | | | | | | | | | |
| China, Shanghai, 1974–86 | I,P | 14 | 92 | P | 618 | I | Any | 27.3 | 1.0[i] | Shu et al., 1988 |
| Italy, Turin, 1981–84 | I,P | NS[m] | 22 | H | 307 | I | D | 45.9 | 1.0 | Magnani et al., 1990 |
| **Lymphoma** | | | | | | | | | | |
| China, Shanghai, 1981–91 | I | 14 | 87 | P | 87 | I | Any | – | 1.3 | Shu et al., 1994a |
| **Brain tumours** | | | | | | | | | | |
| USA, Los Angeles County, 1972–77 | I | 24 | 68[n] | E,N | 68[n] | I | Dental[o] | 12.0 | 2.5* | Preston-Martin et al., 1982 |
| Canada, Toronto, 1977–83 | I | 19 | 74 | P | 138 | I | D, chest<br>D, skull | 8.0[p]<br>4.3[p] | 2.1[q]<br>6.7*[j] | Howe et al., 1989 |
| Australia, New South Wales, 1985–89 | I | 14 | 82 | P | 164 | I | Dental<br>D, skull | 9.1<br>2.4 | 0.4<br>2.3 | McCredie et al., 1994b |
| China, Shanghai, 1981–91 | I | 14 | 107 | P | 107 | I | Any | – | 1.5 | Shu et al., 1994a |
| **Astrocytoma** | | | | | | | | | | |
| USA, Pennsylvania, New Jersey, Delaware, 1980–86 | I | 14 | 163 | RDD | 163 | I | Head or neck<br>Dental | NS<br>NS | 1.0<br>0.9 | Kuijten et al., 1990 |
| USA and Canada, CCG, 1986–89 | I | 5 | 155 | RDD | 155 | I | Any head, neck or dental X-ray<br>Dental<br>D, head injury | 13.5<br>9.0<br>3.2 | 1.2<br>1.0<br>1.1 | Bunin et al., 1994b |

| Cancer / Study location, years | Age | No. cases | Controls[a] | No. controls | Method[b] | Type of exposure | % | OR | Reference |
|---|---|---|---|---|---|---|---|---|---|
| **Primitive neuroectodermal brain tumours** | | | | | | | | | |
| USA and Canada, CCG, 1986–89 | 5 | 166 | RDD | 166 | I | Any head, neck or dental X-ray | 12.0 | 1.1 | Bunin et al., 1994b |
| | | | | | | Dental | 8.4 | 0.5 | |
| | | | | | | D, head injury | 4.2 | 0.9 | |
| **Neuroblastoma** | | | | | | | | | |
| USA, North Carolina, 1972–81 | 14 | 104 | H | 208 | MR | Chest X-ray | 33.2 | 0.3* | Greenberg, 1983 |
| | | | OC[c] | 105 | | | 11.7 | 2.0 | |
| | | | H | 208 | | Cranial X-ray | 6.2 | 0.3 | |
| | | | OC[c] | 105 | | | 1.3 | 1.6 | |
| | | | H | 208 | | Abdominal X-ray | 6.7 | 0.4 | |
| | | | OC[c] | 105 | | | 3.9 | 0.8 | |
| **Osteosarcoma** | | | | | | | | | |
| USA, Los Angeles County, 1972–82 | 24 | 59 | F,N | 112 | I | Any except dental | 71.4 | 0.9 | Operskalski et al., 1987 |
| USA, New York State, 1978–88 | 24 | 130 | P | 130 | I | Medical | NS | 1.0[l] | Gelberg et al., 1997 |
| **Ewing's sarcoma** | | | | | | | | | |
| USA, Minnesota, 1975–81 | 20 | 98 | RDD | 98 | I,P | Any | NS | 1.0[o] | Daigle, 1987 |
| | | 95 | Sibs | 95 | | | NS | 1.0[o] | |
| USA, San Francisco Bay Area, 1978–86 | 31 | 43 | RDD | 193 | I | Any except dental | 70.5 | 0.6 | Holly et al., 1992 |
| USA, multicentre, 1983–85 | 22 | 204 | RDD | 204 | I | D | 37.7 | 1.6* | Winn et al., 1992 |
| | | | | | | Dental | 50.0 | 1.2 | |
| | | 191 | Sibs | 191 | | D | 39.8 | 1.6 | |
| | | | | | | Dental | 53.9 | 0.9 | |
| **Soft-tissue sarcoma** | | | | | | | | | |
| Italy, Padua and Turin, 1983–84 | NS[f] | 52 | H | 326 | I | D | 44.8 | 0.8 | Magnani et al., 1989 |
| **Thyroid cancer** | | | | | | | | | |
| USA, Rochester, New York, 1950–87 | 14 | 6 | Coh | –[u] | MR | X-ray treatment for enlarged thymus gland | – | 210[v] | Shore et al., 1993 |
| **All sites** | | | | | | | | | |
| Great Britain, 1953–55 | 10 | 1299 | P | 1299 | I,MR | D | 13.6 | 1.0 | Stewart et al., 1958 |
| | | | | | | T | 0.2 | 2.7 | |
| UK: North West, West Midlands and Yorkshire, 1980–83 | 14 | 535 | GP,H | 1068 | I | ND | 0.3 | 2.0 | Hartley et al., 1988a |
| | | 465 | | 928 | MR | | 1.0 | 1.1 | |
| Canada, Toronto, 1950–85 | 14 | 3 | Coh | 1073 | MR | D | – | 1.4 | McLaughlin et al., 1993c |
| | 14 | 2 | Coh | 293 | MR | D | – | 0.8 | |
| China, Shanghai, 1981–91 | 14 | 642 | P | 642 | I | Any | – | 1.3* | Shu et al., 1994a |

NS, Not stated.
*P < 0.05.

a  P, population; GP, neighbourhood; selected through general practice; H, hospital; F, friends; N, neighbourhood; RDD, selected by random-digit dialling; Coh, cohort study.
b  I, maternal interview; MR, medical records.
c  D, diagnostic; T, therapeutic; F, fluoroscopy; ND, neonatal diagnostic; OD, other diagnostic
d  Crude unmatched analysis of matched-pairs data.
e  84% of the children were aged 8 years or less at the time of diagnosis.
f  Compared with subjects who had not received postnatal irradiation of any type.
g  Exposures in the year preceding death of the cases or the corresponding period in controls were excluded from analysis.
h  Exposure in six months before diagnosis of case or interview of controls excluded from analysis.
i  Crude relative risk.
j  ALL of the non-T cell type.
k  >1 film.
l  The authors state that the odds ratio was not statistically significant.
m  Mean age of diagnosis of 142 cases with ALL, 22 of ANLL and 19 of non-Hodgkin lymphoma was 6.1 years (SD 3.6).
n  Restricted to patients aged 15 years or more at diagnosis.
o  Five or more full-mouth X-rays starting at least 10 years before diagnosis.
p  Exposures during the five-year period before diagnosis of cases, and the corresponding period for controls, excluded from analysis.
q  Chest and skull X-rays included simultaneously in regression model.
r  Wilms' tumour.
s  The author stated that the frequencies of exposure to X-rays were similar for cases and controls.
t  Mean age at diagnosis 6.8 years (+4.7).
u  In the analysis by attained age, comparison was made with age-sex-year-specific rates for New York State.
v  Observed:expected ratio.

had at least five full-mouth dental X-rays starting at least ten years before the diagnosis. Cases and controls were similar in the histories of exposure to therapeutic and other types of diagnostic X-rays. Howe *et al.* (1989) reported independent positive dose–response associations with chest and skull X-rays taken at least five years before the diagnosis. When both exposures were simultaneously included in the regression model as dichotomous variables, the relative risk associated with exposure to chest X-rays was reduced and no longer significant. The relative risk for injuries to the head or neck requiring medical attention was 3.2 (95% CI 1.4–7.1). The reported history of such injuries was not highly correlated with a history of skull X-rays ($r = 0.2$) and the magnitude and significance of these effects were essentially unchanged when both factors were included simultaneously in the regression model. The authors considered that the association with exposure to skull X-rays might be related to symptoms of the eventual development of brain tumours. In the one available study of childhood astrocytoma, no association was found with dental X-rays at least one year before diagnosis and there was no association with X-ray of the head or neck more than a year before diagnosis (Kuijten *et al.*, 1990).

No significant association between brain tumours and postnatal exposure to X-rays was found in other studies (McCredie *et al.*, 1994b; Shu *et al.*, 1994a).

### Osteosarcoma

Of 220 children given radium-224 intravenously as therapy for tuberculosis, 36 developed bone neoplasms, most frequently osteosarcoma (Spiess & Mays, 1970, 1971, 1973). Only two children showed a correlation between sites affected by both diseases (Miller, 1981). No association between postnatal exposure to diagnostic ionizing radiation and osteosarcoma was found in a study of 84 cases and 124 friend and neighbour controls (Operskalski *et al.*, 1987). The statistical power of this study was low.

### Thyroid cancer

Patients who were treated as children for enlarged thymic glands in Rochester, New York, between 1926 and 1957 had a substantially elevated risk of thyroid cancer later in childhood, compared with unirradiated sibs (Shore *et al.*, 1993; see Table 4.5). The median thyroid dose was 0.3 Gy, and the median age of treatment was five weeks. In the 5–14-year age group, the absolute excess risk associated with thymus irradiation was 21 per 10 000 person years per Gy. In Israel, 98 cases of thyroid cancer were diagnosed in 10 834 subjects who received radiotherapy to the scalp for ringworm (Ron *et al.*, 1989). There were 57 cases among 10 834 matched unexposed subjects and 5392 unexposed sibs. The doses were substantially lower than in the series in New York. The relative risk of malignant thyroid tumours associated with a thyroid dose of 0.09 Gy was 4.0 (95% CI 2.3–7.9). Those exposed under the age of five years had a significantly higher relative risk than those exposed later in childhood. The absolute excess risk associated with radiotherapy to the scalp was 13 per 10 000 person years per Gy.

### Other types of childhood cancer

No association between postnatal exposure to radiation and neuroblastoma, Ewing's sarcoma or soft-tissue sarcoma has been found (Table 4.5).

### All types of childhood cancer combined

In a study in Great Britain, no association was found between childhood cancer death and postnatal diagnostic exposure, but there was a non-significant excess of cases with a history of therapeutic exposure (Stewart *et al.*, 1958). The 11 children (8 cases and 3 controls) who had received radiotherapy were all girls treated for naevi. Two of the three cases had already been X-rayed *in utero*. Stewart *et al.* (1958) noted that similar rays were emitted by shoe-shop X-ray machines (pediscope machines) as by diagnostic X-ray sets. Therefore, if medical X-ray examinations had an effect, it would be expected that this also would be seen from pediscope records. No such excess was observed (RR = 0.9, 95% CI 0.7–1.1). Hartley *et al.* (1988a) found that a positive association with diagnostic X-rays carried out in the neonatal period apparent on the basis of interview data was not apparent when data from medical records were considered. A positive association with postnatal X-ray exposure of any type reported by the parents was found in a study in Shanghai (Shu *et al.*, 1994a). The relative risk associated with exposure to three or more X-ray examinations was 1.8 (95% CI 1.2–2.9). Details of X-ray exposure could not be validated from medical records.

McLaughlin *et al.* (1993c) investigated mortality and incidence due to cancer of any type in patients exposed to radiation from diagnostic cardiac catheterization in Toronto, Canada, between 1950 and 1965. As the procedure relies on both fluoroscopy and angiography, the radiation dose received during cardiac catheterization is greater than that of other procedures used in diagnostic radiology. Linkage was made between records of the procedure in a major children's hospital and death certificates and the Ontario cancer registry. A total of seven deaths due to cancer were observed, compared with 5.7 expected on the basis of rates in Ontario (O/E = 1.2, 90% CI 0.6–2.3). There were 13 cases of cancer registered, compared with 17.3 expected (O/E = 0.8, 90% CI 0.4–1.2). Similar results were obtained when follow-up to the age of 14 years only was considered (Table 4.5). The radiation dose could not be estimated directly, because the relevant information was not recorded at the time of catheterization. A slight increase in risk was apparent with increasing number of procedures in the analysis relating to mortality, but this is based on seven cancer deaths only. It was not possible to assess the effect of associated medical conditions, for example, Down's syndrome, which is associated both with leukaemia and with cardiac defects.

## Other postnatal exposure to ionizing radiation of the index child

In the study of leukaemia and non-Hodgkin lymphoma in West Cumbria (UK) described above, there was no association with the child having played on the beach, played on the hills, with fish-eating habits, or with the family having grown their own vegetables or used seaweed as a fertilizer (Gardner *et al.*, 1990b). In the study of leukaemia and non-Hodgkin lymphoma in Caithness (Scotland) already described, all five cases resident within 25 km of the Dounreay plant had played on the beach before diagnosis; none of the controls individually matched with those cases had done so (*p* = 0.04; Urquhart *et al.*, 1991). The authors considered that this finding might be an artefact of multiple testing and influenced by recall bias. Subsequently, no unusual levels of radioactivity were found in measurements in children who had been diagnosed with leukaemia or in unaffected children in the Dounreay area (Watson & Sumner, 1996).

In the study of leukaemia in the area around the La Hague nuclear facility in Normandy (France), described above, the relative risk associated with use of local beaches at least once a month was 2.9 (95% CI 1.1–8.7; Pobel & Viel, 1997). This exposure was highly correlated with maternal use of the beaches during pregnancy (Viel, 1997). The relative risk associated with consumption of local fish and shellfish at least once a week was 2.7 (95% CI 0.9–9.5). Both of these associations exhibited statistically significant dose–response relationships. There was no association with reported consumption of local raw milk, consumption of local vegetables or fruit, or use of seaweed as fertilizer. All four children with leukaemia who lived in the electoral ward in which the reprocessing plant is located and in which an excess of leukaemia was observed in the study of Viel *et al.* (1995) were reported to have played on the beach at least once a month, compared with 13 of 23 similarly affected children who lived elsewhere, and 14 of the 33 controls resident in the same electoral ward (Viel, 1997). The possibility that selection bias, recall bias and multiple testing may account for the results has been debated (Clavel & Hémon 1997; Law & Roman, 1997; Viel, 1997; Wakeford, 1997).

## Conclusions regarding non-occupational exposure to ionizing radiation

In early studies, intrauterine exposure to diagnostic radiation was associated with a modest increased risk of leukaemia and other types of childhood cancer. This association was consistent between studies carried out in different countries, and was not attenuated by adjusting for potential confounding factors. The relative risk has declined over time, which is compatible with a reduction in dose to the fetus. The precise dose–response relationship remains uncertain, but it seems unlikely that the association can be accounted for by non-causal factors. A strong positive association between postnatal exposure of the child to ionizing radiation and thyroid cancer has been observed. No clear association is apparent between postnatal exposure and other types of childhood cancer. The effects of preconceptional exposure of the parents to diagnostic and therapeutic ionizing radiation have been less investigated. No consistent association between maternal or paternal preconceptional exposure is apparent in the available studies. However, an association between paternal preconceptional exposures of this type and leukaemia in young children cannot be excluded.

# Chapter 5
# Electromagnetic fields

In 1979, Wertheimer and Leeper reported a positive association between residential proximity to sources of high current flow, as assessed from wiring configurations, and childhood cancer. Although subsequently criticized (US Congress Office of Technology Assessment, 1989), the report stimulated subsequent studies in a research area that did not previously exist (Poole & Trichopoulos, 1991). Assessment of the health effects of residential exposures to electromagnetic fields is a particularly difficult issue, as some hypotheses suggest that the biological effect may not be a simple dose–response relationship and methods of assessing exposure have not yet been fully developed. Moreover, the scientific studies have been carried out in an atmosphere of considerable political and social pressure (Brodeur, 1989a,b,c).

In this chapter, general methodological considerations are discussed first. Each of the studies of residential exposure is then described. An attempt is made to synthesize the results regarding residential exposure for leukaemia, lymphomas and brain tumours. Finally, studies of occupational exposure are considered. This differs from residential exposure as (1) primarily paternal exposure is considered, and (2) the frequency of many of the electromagnetic fields encountered at work differs from the power frequency fields encountered at home.

Electromagnetic fields comprise time-varying fields with frequencies of up to 300 GHz (NRPB, 1992). These fields lie within the part of the electromagnetic spectrum bounded by static fields and infrared radiation. Even at the highest frequency of 300 GHz, there is insufficient quantum energy to cause ionization in matter, and therefore this part of the spectrum, together with optical frequencies, is referred to as non-ionizing. There are two types of electromagnetic field: (1) those that travel long distances from their source, and (2) those that are confined to the immediate vicinity of their source (US Congress Office of Technology Assessment, 1989). Fields of the latter type, such as those associated with power distribution, where one wavelength is several thousand kilometres, decrease in intensity much more rapidly with distance from the source than fields of shorter wavelength such as radio waves (1–100 metres).

When confined fields are considered, exposure to electric and magnetic fields has to be assessed separately (NRPB, 1992). The human body can be shielded relatively easily from external electric fields, but not easily from magnetic fields. For example, houses attenuate electric fields from nearby power lines by about 90% (US Congress Office of Technology Assessment, 1989). Magnetic fields are shielded only by structures containing large amounts of ferrous or other special metals. Electric fields are also attenuated substantially within the body. The resultant internal electric fields are usually negligible compared with background electric fields in the body generated by thermal fluctuations (ORAU, 1992). By contrast, external magnetic fields penetrate the body without attenuation.

## Residential exposure

A summary of the methods in the available studies of the association between childhood cancer and residential exposure to electromagnetic fields is presented in Table 5.1. Most of these studies relate to power frequency fields (50–60 Hz). Direct measurements in or around the home of magnetic and/or electric fields have been made in only a few studies (Tomenius, 1986; Savitz et al., 1988; London et al., 1991; Feychting & Ahlbom, 1992; Preston-Martin et al., 1996a). The direct measurements were obtained for a limited proportion of eligible subjects. In one of these studies, only a single spot measurement was taken (Tomenius, 1986). In the other studies, spot measurements were taken from several locations in or around the home. In two studies, measurements inside the home were taken under low-power conditions, with lights and selected appliances turned off, and under high-power conditions (Savitz et al., 1988; London et al., 1991). The purpose of taking measurements under low-power conditions was to attempt to isolate the contribution of external power lines (Savitz *et al.*, 1988), while measurements under high-power conditions indicate the combined exposure from outside power lines and wiring in the home. Twenty-four-hour measurements of magnetic and electric fields were taken in the index child's bedroom in the study of London *et al.* (1991) and for a subset of subjects, in both the index child's room and in a second room where the child spent the most time (Preston-Martin *et al.*, 1996a). In the study of Savitz *et al.* (1988), the correlation between averages of spot magnetic flux density measurements made at the centres of multiple rooms of 56 homes in 1985 and 1990 was 0.7. This correlation was similar for homes with high and low current configurations and for measurements made under conditions of high- and low-power use. In the study of London *et al.* (1991), the reproducibility of spot measurements was assessed by taking repeat measures over 5–10 minutes in 55 residences. The ratio of the between- to within-residence coefficients of variation was 2.6. Under conditions of low-power, the correlation between spot measurements in the child's bedroom and mean 24-hour magnetic field measurement was 0.63, and under conditions of normal power 0.67. There was no correlation between spot measurements of electric fields and either 24-hour magnetic field measurements or spot magnetic field measurements.

In four studies, potential magnetic field exposure from power lines and other electricity distribution equipment was estimated using data on load carried by power lines, the configuration of the line, and distance of the home from the installation (Myers *et al.*, 1990; Feychting & Ahlbom, 1992; Olsen *et al.*, 1993b; Verkasalo *et al.*, 1993). The details of the methods of estimation differed between the studies. In the study of Feychting and Ahlbom (1992), the exposure assessments were verified in a number of ways. First, the algorithm used to calculate historical magnetic fields was also used to calculate contemporary fields, and these data were compared with spot measurements. Spot measurements were made according to the procedures used by Savitz *et al.* (1988). There was good agreement between calculated and measured fields (weighted kappa 0.71, 95% CI 0.66–0.77). Most of the differences were due to the spot-measured fields being higher than the calculated ones. Second, the measured fields were compared with the historical calculated fields in order to determine the effect of using measured fields assessed under contemporary conditions as estimates of historical fields. Not

surprisingly, the agreement between these measures was less good (weighted kappa 0.52, 95% CI 0.47–0.57). Again, the vast majority of differences were due to the spot-measured fields being higher than those calculated. The authors note that the agreement between measured and calculated fields was better for one family houses than for apartment houses, the latter being particularly poor as regards the agreement between spot measurements and calculated historical fields. It was concluded that measured contemporary fields would not be accurate as predictors of past fields.

In a number of studies in the USA, proximity of homes to certain types of electrical transmission and distribution wiring configurations has been considered (Wertheimer & Leeper, 1979; Fulton *et al.*, 1980; Savitz *et al.*, 1988; London *et al.*, 1991; Gurney *et al.*, 1996b; Preston-Martin *et al.*, 1996a). The basic approach developed by Wertheimer and Leeper (1979) in the Greater Denver (Colorado) area was applied in the other studies. Wertheimer and Leeper (1979) visited the address of each case of childhood cancer at the time of birth and death, and the address of control infants at the time of death of the matched case. A map of the electrical wires and transformers in the vicinity was drawn. The authors observed that as the Denver area had been growing fast, many new primary wires had been installed to accommodate increased power demands. Many of these new primaries could be easily distinguished from older wires. However, where the more modern wiring was observed, it could not be determined whether this represented a new installation or replacement wiring. Therefore, data on all primary wires seen near homes occupied before 1956 was considered as unreliable, and these homes were coded strictly according to their more stable secondary wire configuration. Homes were defined to have high current configurations if (1) they were less than 40 metres from 13 kV (primary) wires built to take high current (large gauge) or less than this distance from an array of six or more 'thin' primaries; (2) less than 20 metres from an array of 3–5 thin primaries or from high tension (50–230 kV) wires; and (3) less than 15 metres from secondary (240 V) wires which issued directly from the transformer and had not yet lost any current through a service drop occurring beyond the transformer pole (first-span secondaries). All other configurations were considered to be 'low current configurations'. Subsequently, in a study of adult cancers, Wertheimer and Leeper (1982) expanded their wiring classification method to include four

Table 5.1. Summary of methods of studies of childhood cancer and residential exposure to electromagnetic fields

| Area and period of study | Measure of exposure: Type | Method | Timing[a] | Cases: Upper age boundary | Type | No. (% participation) | Controls: Type[b] | No. (% participation) | References | Comment |
|---|---|---|---|---|---|---|---|---|---|---|
| USA, Greater Denver, Colorado, 1950–73 | Wiring configuration | Mapping of electrical wiring and transformers in vicinity of subjects' homes 1976–7 | B | 18 | All | 272 (79) | B | 272 (79) | Wertheimer & Leeper, 1979 | Study based on deceased cases only. Assignment of wiring configurations was not done blindly, but other work shows high level of agreement between blinded and non-blinded assignment. |
| | | | D | | All | 328 (95) | | 328 (95) | | |
| USA, Providence, Rhode Island, 1964–78 | Wiring configuration | Mapping of electrical wiring in vicinity of subjects' homes | B–Dg | 20 | Leukaemia | 198 (95)[y] | B | 225 (94) | Fulton et al., 1980 | All addresses of cases between birth and diagnosis were compared with addresses at time of birth for controls. Re-analysis by Wertheimer and Leeper (1980) attempted to minimize potential bias thereby introduced. |
| | | Wertheimer & Leeper, 1979 | | 8 | Leukaemia | 104[d] | B | 184 | Wertheimer & Leeper, 1980 | |
| Sweden, Stockholm County, 1958–73 | Distance between dwelling and electrical construction | Pacing distance by foot | B–Dg | 18 | All | 1129 (96)[c] | B | 969 (95)[c] | Tomenius, 1986 | Analysis related to dwellings rather than individuals. Benign tumours were included, in contrast to other studies. Magnetic fields were measured outside the front doors, mainly of apartment buildings; these measurements have since been shown to have poor correlation with measurements within apartments (Feychting & Ahlbom 1995). |
| | 50-Hz magnetic field | Outside front door of single family houses; near outside door and individual apartment door of apartment houses | | | | | | | | |
| USA, Denver, Colorado, 1976–83 | Wiring configuration | Wertheimer & Leeper, 1982 | Dg | 14 | All | 320 (90) | RDD | 259 (93) | Savitz et al., 1988 | As cases were selected up to nine years after diagnosis, controls were restricted to those who had lived in the same home at the time of diagnosis of the matched case at the time of selection. Therefore, compared with the source population, the control group would not reflect |
| | | | Dg minus two years | | | 135 (38) | | 148 (53) | | |
| | 60-Hz electric and magnetic fields | Arithmetic mean of measurements taken outside front door, in child's bedroom and in any other room in which child spent at least 1 hour/day | Dg | | All | 128 (36) | | 207 (75) | | |
| | Maternal use of electrical appliances during pregnancy | Interview | Pg | | All | 233 (65) | | 206 (74) | Savitz et al., 1990 | migration out of the study area during the period between case diagnosis (1976–83) and control selection (1984–85). |
| | Index child's use of electrical appliances | Interview with mother | B–Dg | | All | 244 (69) | | 216 (78) | | |

| Location, period | Exposure | Method of assessment | | | | | | | Reference | Comments |
|---|---|---|---|---|---|---|---|---|---|---|
| UK, South London, 1965–80 | Distance between residence and transformers or overhead high-voltage power lines | Geographical grid references | Dg | 17 | Leukaemia | 84f | C | 141f | Coleman *et al.*, 1989 | Cancer controls were used. This may have influenced the relative risk. |
| Taiwan, Taipei | Residence within 50 m of a high-tension (22 kV) power line, transformer or substation | NS | NS | NS | All | 216 | H | 422 | Lin & Lu, 1989 | Reported only in an abstract. |
| UK, Yorkshire Health Region 1970–79 | Estimated magnetic field exposure from overhead power lines, and residential proximity to overhead power lines | Electricity board records and indirect estimates by engineers for conditions of maximum demand and mapping of overhead power lines in vicinity of subjects' homes | B | 14 | All | 374 (89) | B | 588 (90) | Myers *et al.*, 1990 | Only 5% of subjects lived within 50 m of a powerline and only 1 case and 4 controls were exposed to estimated fields of more than 0.1 µT. |
| USA, Los Angeles County 1980–87 | Wiring configuration | Wertheimer & Leeper, 1982 | Pg–Ref^g | 10 | Leukaemia | 219 (66) | E,RDD | 207 (81) | London *et al.*, 1991 | Controls were selected by two different methods at two different times. Possible inadequate adjustment for potential confounders has been noted (NRPB, 1992). |
| | 60-Hz electric and magnetic fields | 24 hour measurement in child's bedroom | | | | 164 (50) | | 144 (56) | | |
| | | Spot measurements at time of interview under conditions of low power and normal power use | | | | 140 (42) | | 109 (42) | | |
| | Maternal use of electrical appliances during pregnancy | Interview | Pg | | | 232 (70) | | 232 (90) | | |
| | Index child's use of electrical appliances | Interview with mother | B-Ref^g | | | 232 (70) | | 232 (90) | | |
| Sweden^h, 1960–85 | Historical magnetic fields | Calculation based on distance of home from power line, line configuration, and records of the load on the line | Dg / Dg minus 1 year / Dg minus 5 years / Dg minus 10 years / B | 16 | All | 141 (99) / 100 (70) / 78 (55) / 55 (39) / 72 (51) | R | 554 (99) / 393 (72) / 315 (57) / 209 (38) / 248 (44) | Feychting & Ahlbom, 1992, 1993 | Spot measurements within residences were not available for 200 of the 626 apartments; measurements in hallways were taken instead. Some cases are likely to have been included in the study of Tomenius (1986). |
| | 50-Hz magnetic fields | Arithmetic mean of room closest to line, furthest from it, and in central room; in apartments, in hall if access to specific apartment not possible, assessed under conditions of low power use | C | 16 | All | 89 (63) | R | 344 (62) | | |
| | Distance between residence and power line | Mapping of position of residence in relation to power line, verified by home visit | C | 16 | All | 141 (99) | R | 554 (99) | | |
| Denmark, 1968–86 | Average annual 50-Hz magnetic field exposure | Calculation based on distance of home from installation, category of line, type of pylons, ordering of phases, current flow | Occ | 14 | Leukaemia, lymphoma and nervous system tumours | 1707 (100) | P | 4788 (100) | Olsen *et al.*, 1993b | |
| | Cumulative 50-Hz magnetic field exposure | Multiplication of number of months exposed by average magnetic field exposure | | | | | | | | |

# Table 5.1. (contd) Summary of methods of studies of childhood cancer and residential exposure to electromagnetic fields

| Area and period of study | Measure of exposure | | Timing[a] | Cases | | | Controls | | Reference | Comment |
|---|---|---|---|---|---|---|---|---|---|---|
| | Type | Method | | Upper age boundary | Type | No. (% participation) | Type[b] | No. (% participation) | | |
| Finland, 1970–89 | Historical 50-Hz magnetic field exposure within 500 m of overhead power lines | Calculation based on distance of home from power line, current flow and location of phase conductors | Any | 19 | All | 140 | Coh | 134 800[i] | Verkasalo et al., 1993 | |
| | Cumulative 50-Hz magnetic field exposure | Sum of products of average exposure per year and duration of such exposure | | | All | 140 | Coh | 134 800[i] | | |
| Greece, Attica and Crete, 1987–92 | Distance between residence and substation or power lines | Telephone interview with parents | Dg | 14 | Leukaemia | 136 (74) | H | 187 (72) | Petridou et al., 1993 | Controls were hospital-based, and were of a higher social class than cases. Childhood leukaemia usually is associated with high socioeconomic status. |
| Mexico City, NS | Distance between residence and transformers, power lines, substations or transmission towers | Interview with father | At time of interview and at any previous time | NS | Leukaemia | 81 (94) | H | 77 (96) | Fajardo-Gutiérrez et al., 1993b | Prevalent cases were included. |
| USA, Seattle, 1984–90 | Wiring configuration | Wertheimer & Leeper, 1982 | Dg | 19 | Brain tumours | 120 (67) | RDD | 240 (76) | Gurney et al., 1996b | |
| | Maternal use of electrical appliances during pregnancy | Interview with mother and postal questionnaire | Pg | | | 92 (51) | | 193 (56) | | |
| | Index child's use of electrical appliances | Interview with mother and postal questionnaire | B-Dg | | | 92 (51) | | 193 (56) | | |
| USA, Los Angeles County, 1984–91 | Wiring configuration | Wertheimer & Leeper, 1982 | Dg, longest and B minus 9 months | 19 | Brain tumours | 281 (64) | RDD | 250 (58) | Preston-Martin et al., 1996a | |
| | Spot measurements taken at front door, around water meter and water pipes, and of static magnetic field | Assessed for first, longest residence, or as time weighted average | Pg-Dg | | | 252[j] (58) | | 203[j] (47) | | |
| | Magnetic field profiles taken over front wall, perimeter | | | | | 233[k] (53) | | 171[k] (39) | | |
| | 60-Hz magnetic fields | 24 hour measurements in child's room and other room in which child spent most time | Dg | | | 110[l] | | 101[l] | | |

| Location, period | Exposure assessed | Description of exposure assessment | Code[a] | Age | Disease | No. of cases (%) | Method[b] | No. of controls (%) | Reference |
|---|---|---|---|---|---|---|---|---|---|
| Norway[m], 1965–89 | Historical magnetic fields | Calculation based on distance of home from power line, height of towers, distance between phases, ordering of phases and records of the load on the line | B-Dg | 14 | All | 500 (94) | P | 2004 (95) | Tynes & Haldorsen, 1997 |
|  | Distance between residence and power line | Obtained from local municipal authorities | Dg |  |  |  |  |  |  |
| Germany, Lower Saxony, 1988–93 | 50-Hz magnetic fields | 24 hour measurements in child's bedroom | Long | 14 | Leukaemia | 129 (59) | P | 328 (54) | Michaelis *et al.*, 1997b |
|  |  | Spot measurements taken every foot (30.4 cm) while walking through the different rooms and floors of the residence | Pg-Dg | 14 | Leukaemia | 141 (64) | P | 357 (58) |  |
| USA, multicentre, 1989–94 | 60-Hz magnetic fields | 24 hour measurements in child's bedroom. Spot measurements in child's bedroom, family room, kitchen | B-Dg | 14 | ALL | 638 (78) | RDD | 620 (63) | Linet *et al.*, 1997 |
|  |  | Spot measurement in room in which mother slept during index pregnancy | Pg |  |  | 257 (31) |  | 239 (24) |  |
|  | Wiring configuration |  | Pg-Dg |  |  | 408 (50) |  | 408 (41) | Wertheimer & Leeper, 1992 and Kaune & Savitz, 1994 |

[a] B, birth; D, death; Dg, diagnosis; Pg, pregnancy; NS, not stated; C, current in homes where cases and controls lived at time of diagnosis of case; Occ, during the time the family occupied the residence; Long, at residence in which child had been living for the longest period before diagnosis.

[b] B, selected from birth certificates; RDD, selected by random-digit dialling; C, children with a solid tumour other than lymphoma; H, children hospitalized for reasons other than cancer; F, friends of cases; R, random sample of individuals resident within 300 m of a power line; P, randomly selected from central population register.

[c] Addresses of patients. In all, 119 eligible cases were identified, of whom 66 had been resident at one address before diagnosis, 34 at two addresses each, and 19 at three or more addresses each. Complete address histories were mapped for 110 (92%) of cases.

[d] Addresses.

[e] Addresses of subjects. 716 cases with cancer of any type and a similar number of matched controls were included. Participation rates were not specified for the under 18s. Overall, information was obtained for 95% of eligible cases and 89% of eligible controls.

[f] The study was of leukaemia in all age groups.

[g] Ref: reference date: diagnosis for children aged 1 year or less; diagnosis minus 6 months for children aged 1–2; diagnosis minus 1 year for children aged 2 or more.

[h] Subjects resident within 300 m of a 220 kV or 400 kV powerline.

[i] 978 100 person-years.

[j] Information on completeness of data for many different spot measurements was presented. These figures relate to fields assessed at the front door, as these are the main results presented.

[k] Front wall.

[l] At least one room. These measurements carried out on a sample of subjects, stratified on case or control status, wiring configuration and exterior static magnetic field of residence.

[m] Subjects resident in census wards crossed by 45 kV+ (urban areas) or 100 kV+ (rural areas) power line in 1960, 1970, 1980, 1985, 1987 or 1989.

categories: 'very high-current configurations', 'ordinary high-current configurations', 'ordinary low-current configurations', and 'end-pole configurations'. This method was employed in modified form by Savitz *et al.* (1988) in Denver, by London *et al.* (1991) in Southern California, by Gurney *et al.* (1996b) in Seattle, and by Preston-Martin *et al.* (1996a) in Los Angeles.

There has been considerable discussion as to whether wiring configuration is an appropriate marker of exposure. Wertheimer and Leeper (1982) justified the use of wiring configuration not only on the grounds that participation rates are likely to be higher than if assessment methods require access to the home, but also because they considered that spot measurements give a poor index of the typical field to be expected from a given residential situation, due to large hourly, seasonal and long-term variations in current use. In addition, they postulated that relatively continuous exposures to magnetic fields are of greater etiological importance than relatively brief but strong exposures. Nevertheless, they observed that ranking of spot measures of magnetic fields corroborated ranking based on wiring configurations. This was also shown in the studies of Savitz *et al.* (1988) and London *et al.* (1991). In a subset of 81 homes of subjects who participated in the study of Savitz *et al.* (1988) in Denver, Colorado, wire codes assigned to homes in 1985 and again in 1990 by two independent groups were in agreement for 90% of the 73 homes (Dovan *et al.*, 1993).

Kaune *et al.* (1987), in a field study of 43 residences in western Washington State, found a statistically significant correlation (coefficient 0.41) between average 24-hour residential magnetic flux density and the Wertheimer and Leeper (1982) wiring code. No correlation was observed between wiring configuration and electric field measurements. Savitz *et al.* (1988) commented that it is not unusual for historical data to be estimated more accurately by surrogate measures of past exposure than by accurate indices of current exposure. For example, cumulative exposure to tobacco smoke is more accurately estimated by taking a smoking history than by determining current urinary cotinine level. Another example is that a food frequency questionnaire provides a better index of long-term dietary intake than a 24-hour dietary recall (Savitz *et al.*, 1989). Preston-Martin *et al.* (1996a) noted that the Wertheimer–Leeper classification discriminated homes with high direct measurements of magnetic and electric fields better in Denver than in Los Angeles. In

Los Angeles, homes with high-current configurations had interior magnetic fields about half those of homes with similar configurations in Denver.

The most simple measurement of electromagnetic field exposure is distance from a power line or other installation. This was assessed in addition to other measures in the studies of Tomenius (1986) and Feychting and Ahlbom (1992). It was the sole measure used in the studies of Coleman *et al.* (1989), Lin and Lu (1989), Myers *et al.* (1990), Lowenthal *et al.* (1991), Fajardo-Gutiérrez *et al.* (1993b) and Petridou *et al.* (1993).

Certain electrical appliances, particularly electric over-blankets and water-bed heaters, may be sources of prolonged power frequency magnetic field exposures (NRPB, 1992). Other appliances used intermittently for short periods of time such as hair dryers and electric razors emit strong magnetic fields. Electric and magnetic fields at higher frequencies are emitted by a variety of appliances or installations such as stereo headphones (about 1 kHz), television sets (about 20 kHz), frequency-modulated (FM) radio and television transmitters (about 100 MHz), and microwave ovens (about 2 GHz). Many of these higher-frequency sources induce more intense currents in the body than those induced by a power-frequency electric field of 3 kV/m (US Congress Office of Technology Assessment, 1989). Appliance use by the mother during the pregnancy leading to the birth of the index child, and by the index child during his/her lifetime, has been considered in four studies (Savitz *et al.*, 1990; London *et al.*, 1991; Gurney, *et al.*, 1996b; Preston-Martin *et al.*, 1996a).

In addition to the debate about methods of exposure assessment, a criticism made of a number of studies concerns control selection (Poole & Trichopoulos, 1991; NRPB, 1992; Jones *et al.*, 1993; Gurney *et al.*, 1995). If individuals of low socioeconomic status are less likely to participate as controls than individuals of high socioeconomic status, and also are more likely to live near power lines and other electricity distribution equipment, the proportion of controls exposed to higher-intensity electromagnetic fields will be lower than the proportion of the source population at risk of developing childhood cancer. If there were no participation bias among cases, the relative risk of childhood cancer associated with higher intensity electromagnetic fields would be overestimated. In a study of the households of 392 women in western Washington state, selected randomly after stratifying on reported income from among

2643 women recruited as controls in four case–control studies by random-digit dialling, there was an inverse association between family income and residence in homes with very high current configurations as defined by the Wertheimer–Leeper method (Gurney *et al.*, 1995). Applying this finding to a hypothetical case–control study in which it was assumed that there was no causal association between wiring configuration and cancer occurrence, the estimated range of biased odds ratios due to differential control participation rates as a function of family income was 1.03–1.24. The upper limit was calculated assuming that all eligible controls in the lowest income group did not participate. One limitation of this study was use of a population of participating controls to evaluate the possible impact of non-participation.

In some of the studies, the main analysis related to all types of childhood cancer (Wertheimer & Leeper, 1979; Tomenius, 1986; Savitz *et al.*, 1988, 1990; Lin & Lu, 1989; Myers *et al.*, 1990; Feychting & Ahlbom 1992; Verkasalo *et al.*, 1993). The statistical power to investigate the association with specific types of childhood cancer was limited in some. In the study of Myers *et al.* (1990), the only categorization made was between non-solid and solid tumours.

## Description of studies which considered all types of childhood cancer

The results of these studies which relate to leukaemia, lymphoma and brain tumours are presented in Tables 5.2, 5.3 and 5.4, respectively.

### *First Denver study (Wertheimer & Leeper, 1979)*

The first case–control study of childhood cancer and electromagnetic fields was carried out in the Denver area (Wertheimer & Leeper, 1979). Cases comprised persons dying of cancer before the age of 19 years during the period 1950–73. Controls were selected from birth certificates. Wiring configurations were determined for birth addresses and for addresses in which cases were resident at the time of death and controls were resident at the time that the matched case died (the reference date), during the years 1976 and 1977. Birth addresses were those listed on the birth certificates. Addresses at the time of death of the case were determined either from city directories or from death certificates.

For total childhood cancer, the relative risk associated with residence in homes with high-current configurations versus those with low-current configurations was in excess of 2, irrespective of whether the birth or death address

was used. The most striking difference was observed for subjects who had only one address from birth to death or reference date. This might be explained by the dilution of the effects of configurations at one address by the effects of configurations at other addresses for subjects who moved. The results were not explained by potential confounding by urban/suburban differences, socioeconomic class, primiparity and maternal age, or proximity to roads with heavy traffic. The relative risks were similar for cancer with onset before six years of age and for cancer with an older age of onset.

### *Second Denver study (Savitz et al., 1988, 1990)*

In a study covering the same geographical area as the study by Wertheimer and Leeper (1979), wiring configurations, direct measurements of electric and magnetic fields, and use of electrical appliances by the mother during pregnancy and by the index child were assessed (Savitz *et al.* 1988, 1990). There was no overlap with the case group included in the earlier study. Cases of childhood cancer diagnosed up to the age of 14 years between 1976 and 1983 were ascertained through the Colorado Cancer Registry and two hospitals in the area providing diagnosis and treatment for childhood malignancy. Controls were selected by random-digit dialling and matched to cases by age, sex and telephone exchange area. Since cases had been diagnosed up to nine years before the time of selection, controls were restricted to those who had lived in their residence at the time the case was diagnosed. As a result, relative to the source population, the control group would not have reflected migration out of the study area during the period between case diagnosis (1976–83) and control selection (1984–85). This would have introduced a bias if the tendency to move were related to magnetic field exposure level and to case control status.

Wiring configurations were obtained for 90% of case residences at the time of diagnosis, and 93% of control residences at the reference date, that is, the date of diagnosis of the corresponding case. Relative to the homes with buried wires, the relative risk associated with homes with very high-current configuration was 2.2 (95% CI 0.9–5.2). There was no clear dose–response association with a five-level wire code at the time of diagnosis. The relative risk for homes for which no wiring configuration could be coded was 1.8 (95% CI 0.9–3.5). To consider a possible latency effect, the authors also examined the association for homes occupied two years before the diagnosis. Wiring configurations for homes

## Table 5.2. Summary of results of studies of childhood leukaemia and residential exposure to electromagnetic fields around the time of diagnosis

*Studies in which spot measurements of magnetic fields were made*

| Reference | Number of cases | Comparison | RR (95% CI) | Consideration of potential confounding | Circumstances of measurement | Prevalence of highest level of exposure in controls (%) |
|---|---|---|---|---|---|---|
| Tomenius, 1986 | 243[a] | ≥0.3 μT vs <0.3 μT | 0.3 (0.1–1.2) | – | – | 4.7 |
| Savitz et al., 1988 | 36 | ≥0.2 μT vs <0.2 μT | 1.9 (0.7–5.6) | The relative risk after adjustment for maternal age, paternal education, family income, maternal smoking during pregnancy and traffic density varied between 1.8 and 2.4 | Lower power use | 7.7 |
| London et al., 1991 | 37 | ≥0.2 μT vs <0.2 μT | 1.4 (0.6–3.5) | | High power use | 14.2 |
| | 140 | ≥0.125 μT vs <0.125 μT | 1.1 (0.5–2.5) | | Low power use | 10.0 |
| Feychting & Ahlbom, 1992 | 24 | ≥0.2 μT vs <0.2 μT | 0.8 (0.3–2.3) | A similar pattern was found when analysis stratified by geographical area and type of residence | Low power use | 20.3 |
| Michaelis et al., 1997b | 129 | ≥0.2 μT vs <0.2 μT | 0.9 (0.2–3.6) | No confounding by socioeconomic status, degree of urbanization, or residential mobility | At residence where child lived longest | 2.1 |
| | 141 | | 0.6 (0.2–3.7) | | Maximum of measurements at all residences where child had lived 1 year + | 3.1 |
| Linet et al., 1997 | 638 | ≥0.2 μT vs <0.065 μT | 1.2 (0.9–1.8) | Adjusted for age at diagnosis (reference date for controls), sex, maternal education and family income | Time weighted average of 24 hour measurement in child's bedroom and spot measurements | 11.3 |

*Calculated historical fields*

| Reference | Number of cases | Comparison | RR (95% CI) | Consideration of potential confounding | Prevalence of highest level of exposure in controls (%) |
|---|---|---|---|---|---|
| Myers et al., 1990 | 180[b] | ≥0.03 μT vs <0.03 μT[c] | 1.6 (0.5–4.7)[d] | No confounding by house type for all tumours combined | 2.2 |
| Feychting & Ahlbom, 1992 | 38 | ≥0.2 μT vs <0.1 μT | 2.7 (1.0–6.3) | Similar pattern when analysis stratified by sex, age and geographical area. When analysis stratified by type of residence, no excess risk apparent for apartments | 8.3 |
| Olsen et al., 1993b | 833 | ≥0.25 μT vs <0.1 μT | 1.5 (0.3–6.7) | Adjusted for sex and age at diagnosis | 0.2 |
| Verkasalo et al., 1993 | 35 | ≥0.2 μT vs general population | 1.6 (0.3–4.5) | Adjusted for sex, age and calendar period | 5.1 |
| Tynes & Haldorsen, 1997 | 148 | ≥0.14 μT vs <0.05 μT | 0.3 (0.0–2.1) | No confounding by socioeconomic status, type of dwelling or number of dwellings | 2.4 |

## Wiring configuration

| Reference | Number of cases | Comparison | RR (95% CI) | Consideration of potential confounding | Prevalence of highest level of exposure in controls (%) |
|---|---|---|---|---|---|
| Wertheimer & Leeper, 1979 | 155 | HCC vs LCC | 3.0 (1.7–5.2) | No confounding by area of residence, socioeconomic status, family pattern, traffic congestion, age and sex for all types of childhood cancer combined | 18.7 |
| Fulton et al., 1980 | 198 | Highest quartile vs lowest quartile | 1.0 (0.4–2.3) | – | 25.0 |
| Wertheimer & Leeper, 1980 | 104 | HCC vs LCC | 1.7 (1.0–2.8) | – | – |
| Savitz et al., 1988 | 97 | high vs low[e] | 1.5 (0.9–2.6) | The relative risks changed little when adjustment was made for maternal age, paternal education, family income, maternal smoking during pregnancy and traffic density | 20.0 |
| | | very high vs buried | 2.8 (0.9–8.0) | | 3.1 |
| London et al., 1991 | 211 | high vs low[e] | 1.7 (1.1–2.5) | – | 11.7 |
| | | very high vs buried | 1.8 (0.7–4.6) | – | |
| | | very high vs buried or very low | 2.2 (1.1–4.3)[f] | Relative risk attenuated to 1.7 (0.8–3.7)[g] after adjustment for reported use of indoor pesticides, hair dryers, black-and-white televisions, father's occupational exposure to spray paint during pregnancy and other chemical exposures post-pregnancy | |
| Linet et al., 1997 | 408 | very high vs buried or very low | 0.9 (0.5–1.6) | Matched analysis adjusted for sex, maternal education and family income | 6.4 |
| | | high vs low[h] | 1.0 (0.7–1.7) | | 11.8 |

## Distance

| Reference | Number of cases | Comparison | RR (95% CI) | Consideration of potential confounding | Prevalence of highest level of exposure in controls (%) |
|---|---|---|---|---|---|
| Coleman et al., 1989 | 84 | <50 m from substation vs ≥50 m | 1.7 (0.8–3.6) | – | 10.6 |
| Myers et al., 1990 | 180[b] | <50 m from powerline vs ≥50 m | 1.1 (0.5–2.5)[d] | No confounding by house type for all tumours combined | 5.4 |
| Feychting & Ahlbom, 1992 | 38 | ≤50 m from powerline vs >50 m | 2.9 (1.2–7.2) | No confounding by area of residence, socioeconomic status or pollution from car exhausts. Association not apparent for those resident in apartment houses or those diagnosed in first part of study period | 6.1 |
| Fajardo-Gutiérrez et al., 1993b | 81 | <20 m from power line vs ≥20 m | 2.1 (0.8–5.9) | No confounding by age at diagnosis, parental age, social class or parental occupation | 10.4 |
| | | <200 m from substations vs ≥200 m | 1.6 (0.3–8.9) | | 3.9 |

## Table 5.2. (contd) Summary of results of studies of childhood leukaemia and residential exposure to electromagnetic fields around the time of diagnosis

### Distance (contd)

| Reference | Number of cases | Comparison | RR (95% CI) | Consideration of potential confounding | Prevalence of highest level of exposure in controls (%) |
|---|---|---|---|---|---|
| Petridou et al., 1993 | 136 | <5 m from powerline vs ≥50 m<br><100 m from substation vs ≥100 m | 1.2 (0.6–2.4)<br>0.4 (0.1–1.1) | Adjusted for sex, age, sibship size, maternal education, birth order, attendance at crèche, and area of residence | 17.6<br>7.0 |
| | | <50 m from powerline vs ≥50 m | 1.0 (0.6–1.6) | – | 70.6 |
| Tynes & Haldorsen, 1997 | 148 | <51 m from powerline vs ≥101 m | 0.6 (0.3–1.3) | No confounding by socioeconomic status, type of dwelling or number of dwellings | 9.5 |

HCC, high current configuration.
LCC, low current configuration.

[a] Addresses of subjects.
[b] Non-solid tumours: 127 of the 180 cases had leukaemia.
[c] At time of birth of index child.
[d] Crude unmatched analysis of matched data.
[e] High = high or very high wire code; low = buried, very low or low wire code.
[f] *p* value for trend across categories 0.008
[g] *p* value for trend across categories 0.017
[h] Classification of Kaune & Savitz (1994)

## Table 5.3. Summary of results of studies of childhood lymphoma and residential exposure to electromagnetic fields around the time of diagnosis

| Reference | Number of cases | Comparison | RR (95% CI) | Consideration of potential confounding | Circumstances of measurement | Prevalence of highest level of exposure in controls (%) |
|---|---|---|---|---|---|---|
| Tomenius, 1986 | 132[a] | ≥0.3 µT vs <0.3 µT | 1.8 (0.2–∞) | – | | 0.9 |
| Savitz et al., 1988 | 13 | ≥0.2 µT vs <0.2 µT | 2.2 (0.4–10.3) | Adjustment for per capita income raised the relative risk to 3.2 | Low power use | 7.7 |
| | 13 | ≥0.2 µT vs <0.2 µT | 1.8 (0.5–6.9) | – | High power use | 14.2 |

### Calculated historical fields

| Reference | Number of cases | Comparison | RR (95% CI) | Consideration of potential confounding | Prevalence of highest level of exposure in controls (%) |
|---|---|---|---|---|---|
| Feychting & Ahlbom, 1993 | 19 | ≥0.2 µT vs <0.1 µT | 1.3 (0.2–5.1) | | 8.3 |
| Olsen et al., 1993b | 250 | ≥0.25 µT vs <0.1 µT | 5.0 (0.3–82.0) | Adjusted for sex and age at diagnosis | 0.1 |
| Verkasalo et al., 1993 | 15 | ≥0.2 µT vs general population | 0.0 (0.0–4.2) | Adjusted for sex, age and calendar period | 5.1 |
| Tynes & Haldorsen, 1997 | 30 | ≥0.14 µT vs <0.05 µT | 2.5 (0.4–15.5) | No confounding by socioeconomic status, type of dwelling or number of dwellings | 2.4 |

### Wiring configuration

| Reference | Number of cases | Comparison | RR (95% CI) | Consideration of potential confounding | Prevalence of highest level of exposure in controls (%) |
|---|---|---|---|---|---|
| Wertheimer & Leeper, 1979 | 44 | HCC vs LCC | 2.1 (0.8–5.1) | No confounding by area of residence, socioeconomic status, family pattern, traffic congestion, age and sex for all types of childhood cancer combined | 25.0 |
| Savitz et al., 1988 | 30 | high vs low[b] | 0.8 (0.3–2.2) | The relative risk changed little when adjustment was made for maternal, age, paternal education, family income, maternal smoking during pregnancy and traffic density | 20.0 |
| | | very high vs buried | 3.3 (0.8–13.7) | | 3.1 |

HCC, high current configurations.
LCC, low current configurations.

[a] Addresses of subjects.
[b] high: high or very high wire code.
low: buried, very low or low wire code.

**Table 5.4. Summary of results of studies of childhood CNS tumours and residential exposure to electromagnetic fields around the time of diagnosis**

*Studies in which spot measurements of magnetic fields were made*

| Reference | Number of cases | Comparison | RR (95% CI) | Consideration of potential confounding | Circumstances of measurement | Prevalence of highest level of exposure in controls (%) |
|---|---|---|---|---|---|---|
| Tornenius, 1986 | 294[a] | ≥0.3 µT vs <0.3 µT | 3.9 (1.2–12.7) | – | – | 1.2 |
| Savitz et al., 1988 | 25 | ≥0.2 µT vs <0.2 µT | 1.0 (0.2–4.8) | No evidence of confounding by maternal age, paternal education, family income, maternal smoking during pregnancy or traffic density | Low power use | 7.7 |
|  | 25 | ≥0.2 µT vs <0.2 µT | 0.8 (0.2–2.9) |  | High power use | 14.2 |
| Feychting & Ahlbom, 1992 | 23 | ≥0.2 µT vs <0.2 µT | 1.1 (0.4–2.9) | A similar pattern was found when analysis was stratified by geographical area and type of residence | Low power use | 20.3 |
| Preston-Martin et al., 1996a | 228 | ≥0.2 µT vs <0.2 µT | 0.7 (0.3–1.5) | – | – | 8.2 |

*Calculated historical fields*

| Reference | Number of cases | Comparison | RR (95% CI) | Consideration of potential confounding | Prevalence of highest level of exposure in controls (%) |
|---|---|---|---|---|---|
| Feychting & Ahlbom, 1993 | 33 | ≥0.2 µT vs <0.1 µT | 0.7 (0.1–2.7) | No association apparent in subgroup analysis by sex, age, geographical area and type of residence | 8.3 |
| Olsen et al., 1993b | 624 | ≥0.25 µT vs <0.1 µT | 1.0 (0.2–5.0) | Adjusted for sex and age at diagnosis | 0.3 |
| Verkasalo et al., 1993 | 39 | ≥0.2 µT vs general population | 2.3 (0.8–5.4) | Adjusted for sex, age and calendar period | 5.1 |
| Tynes & Haldorsen, 1997 | 156 | ≥0.14 µT vs <0.05 µT | 0.7 (0.2–2.1) | No confounding by socioeconomic status, type of dwelling or number of dwellings | 3.6 |

*Wiring configuration*

| Reference | Number of cases | Comparison | RR (95% CI) | Consideration of potential confounding | Prevalence of highest level of exposure in controls (%) |
|---|---|---|---|---|---|
| Wertheimer & Leeper, 1979 | 66 | HCC vs LCC | 2.4 (1.2–5.0) | For all types of childhood cancer combined, no confounding by area of residence, socioeconomic status, family pattern, traffic congestion, age or sex | 25.8 |
| Savitz et al., 1988 | 59<br>59 | high vs low[b]<br>very high vs buried | 2.0 (1.1–3.8)<br>1.9 (0.5–8.0) | The relative risks changed little when adjustment was made for maternal age, paternal education, family income, maternal smoking during pregnancy and traffic density | 20.0<br>3.1 |
| Gurney et al., 1996b | 120<br>120 | high vs low[b]<br>very high vs buried | 0.9 (0.5–1.5)<br>0.5 (0.2–1.6) | No confounding by age, sex, county, reference year, maternal education, family history of brain tumours, passive tobacco smoke exposure, farm residence, history of head trauma, X-ray of head or neck, epilepsy or fits from severe fevers | 21.7<br>6.7 |
| Preston-Martin et al., 1996a | 281<br>281 | high vs low[b]<br>very high vs very low or low | 0.8 (0.5–1.1)<br>1.2 (0.6–2.1) | – | 52.0<br>9.6 |

Unchanged relative risk after adjustment for age, sex, birth year, socioeconomic status and maternal waterbed use

HCC, high current configurations.
LCC, low current configurations.

[a] Addresses of subjects.
[b] high = high or very high wire code.
low = buried, very low or low wire code.

occupied two years before diagnosis were only available for 38% of cases and 53% of controls. Again, no clear dose–response gradient was found, but the relative risk for very high-current configuration homes relative to homes with buried wires was 5.2 (95% CI 1.2–23.1, based on eight exposed cases and two exposed controls). The relative risk for homes for which this could not be determined was 2.2 (95% CI 1.3–3.7).

Potential confounding could only be assessed using the data on subjects for whom parental interviews were completed (71% of cases and 80% of controls). The variables assessed included the child's sex, age, and year of diagnosis; markers of residential stability; maternal and paternal age, ethnic group and education; per capita income of the family; family history of cancer; exposure *in utero* to tobacco smoke, alcohol, X-rays, influenza and medications; and congenital anomalies, birth order, birth weight, medications, illnesses and X-rays. While positive associations were identified with young maternal age, low educational attainment of father, low per capita income, maternal smoking during pregnancy, and traffic density, these did not confound the relationship with wiring codes.

Electric and magnetic field measurements were sought at the time of interviews at those residences which had been occupied before the date of diagnosis. Measurements were taken near the front door, in the child's bedroom, in the parents' bedroom and, in addition, in any room reported in the interview to have been occupied by the child on average at least one hour per day. In an attempt to evaluate the persistent fields produced from outside power lines, magnetic field measurements were taken under low-power conditions. As a measure of the combined exposure from outside power lines and wiring in the home, measurements of both electric and magnetic fields were also taken under high-power conditions (with all lights and selected appliances turned on). Several approaches to summarizing the home value were considered but as the correlations between measures were all above 0.95, the simple arithmetic mean was selected for detailed analysis. These measurements were obtained for 36% of cases and 75% of controls.

In a four-level categorization of exposure, a weak relationship was found between childhood cancer and magnetic fields assessed under conditions of low-power use, with relative risks of 1.3, 1.3 and 1.5 respectively. No association was apparent with magnetic or electric fields assessed under conditions of high-power use. Savitz (1988) presented data stratified on father's education and on family income. The reported effect of an increase in risk of total childhood cancer and of leukaemia was largely confined to the low-income/low-education group. In addition, the relative risk of leukaemia among the offspring of fathers who were college graduates compared with fathers who were less educated was 0.9, while that associated with a family income of $7000 per annum or more compared with lower incomes was 0.5. These observations suggest a deficit of leukaemia associated with high socioeconomic status, contrasting with other reports (see Chapter 2). In conjunction with the positive associations between total childhood cancer and maternal smoking and traffic density, and associations between total childhood cancer and father's education and family income similar to those described for leukaemia, it seems likely that there was a deficit of controls of low socioeconomic status (NRPB, 1992). Jones *et al.* (1993) found that in Columbus, Ohio, the proportion of homes with a high-current configuration was substantially higher if the family had been resident for less than 55 months than if it had been resident for longer periods. The duration of 55 months was chosen to coincide with the average period of residential stability in controls in the study of Savitz *et al.* (1988). Therefore, the association with high current configurations in the study of Savitz *et al.* may be an artefact of selection bias.

Later, information on plumbing conductivity was obtained from water suppliers for the homes of 347 cases and 277 controls, as substantial ground currents are most often found in homes having conductive plumbing (Wertheimer *et al.*, 1995). The relative risk of all types of childhood cancer combined associated with living in a home with conductive plumbing was 1.7 (95% CI 1.0–2.9). When the analysis was restricted to subjects who stayed in one residence from the reference date to the study date, the relative risk was 3.0 (95% CI 1.3–6.8).

Savitz *et al.* (1990) also considered use of electrical appliances. Use of some of these, such as electric blankets, is associated with prolonged exposure and relatively high magnetic fields of 1–2 µT. Others, such as hairdryers, are associated with higher magnetic field strengths, of 5 µT or more, but only brief periods of exposure. Prenatal and postnatal use of electrical appliances was assessed by parental interview, completed for 71% of cases and 80% of controls. Complete data on use of appliances by the mother during pregnancy was available for about 93% of those interviewed, and for use by the index child by about 97% of those interviewed. Primary consideration was given to the mother's and child's use of electric blankets, heated water beds, and bedside electric clocks, all of which were subsequently identified as providing significant exposures to magnetic fields. None of the appliances used during pregnancy was associated with childhood cancer overall. As water beds became more widely used late in the study period, a subgroup analysis was made for children diagnosed before age 2 years; the relative risk was 2.3 (95% CI 0.7–6.3).

Electric blanket use was examined in more detail. Potential confounding by the factors mentioned above was considered. The only variable for which the crude and adjusted relative risk associated with electric blanket use differed markedly was per capita family income; the relative risk of total cancer increased after adjustment for this variable. The relative risk associated with prenatal electric blanket use in children from families with a per capita annual income of $7000 or more was close to unity, compared with 1.5 in lower-income families. It has been suggested that differences in recalling electrical appliance use between parents of cases and controls were greater for low- than for high-income groups (NRPB, 1992). An alternative explanation is that since electrical appliance use would be expected to vary according to income, adjustment for income by a dichotomous variable may not adequately control for income-related differences in both electrical appliance use and in participation of control subjects.

Postnatal exposure of the child to the electric appliances considered was relatively rare. Only 4% of controls had used electric blankets and 6% had used heated water beds. The highest relative risk observed for total cancer was 1.5, for use of electric blankets. The authors considered the possibility that cancer precursors affect behaviour and thereby produce spurious associations with exposure. For example, the early symptoms of cancer such as chills might motivate children to begin using electric blankets. The authors observed a relative risk associated with electric blanket use within one year of diagnosis of 3.0 (95% CI 0.8–9.2), which would be consistent with this hypothesis.

### Stockholm County study (Tomenius, 1986)

Tomenius (1986) considered cases of cancer diagnosed before 19 years of age in Stockholm county during 1958–73. Some 760 cases born and diagnosed in the county, and ascertained from the Swedish Cancer Registry, were included. Benign tumours were included. For each case, an age–sex matched control individual was selected from birth registry records in the same parish as the case. In addition, for the 400 cases who still lived in the parish of birth at the time of diagnosis, controls resident in the same parish at the time of diagnosis were selected.

96% of dwellings at the time of birth and diagnosis were visited; the remaining dwellings had either been demolished or were not occupied. The relative risk of total childhood cancer associated with the dwelling being located within 150 metres of high-voltage wires, transformers, electric railroads or subways was 1.4 (95% CI 1.0–1.9). The results of this study related to dwellings rather than individuals unless otherwise stated, with some individuals contributing more than one home to the analysis. Since the characteristics of the dwellings contributed by each individual may be more similar to one another than with dwellings occupied by other individuals, the statistical significance of the results is likely to have been overstated to a small degree (NRPB, 1992). When the distance was subdivided into 50-metre intervals, the relative risk increased with increasing distance from the installation, from 1.2 for proximity within 50 m, to 1.3 for proximity between 50 and 99 m, to 1.9 for proximity between 100 and 150 m. This effect was largely accounted for by the association with 200 kV wires.

In this investigation, a direct measurement of the magnetic field at the front door of the home was made. The average magnetic field outside the door of the dwellings of cases was 0.069 µT, very similar to that for control dwellings (0.068 µT). A magnetic field of 0.3 µT or more was recorded at 48 dwellings (34 of cases and 14 of controls), giving a relative risk of 2.1 (95% CI 1.1–4.2). However, the reason for dichotomizing the value of magnetic field exposure at this level was not specified and, as mean values were similar in cases and controls, the choice of this value may have affected the estimate of risk obtained (Savitz *et al.*, 1988; Poole & Trichopoulos, 1991; Wartenberg & Savitz, 1993). For dwellings within 150 m of a 200 kV wire, the measured magnetic field was significantly correlated with distance from the wire ($r = 0.45$, $p < 0.01$), and the magnetic field was also significantly correlated with the magnetic field under the wires ($r = 0.43$, $p < 0.01$). However, when analysis was restricted to dwellings within 150 m of 200 kV wires, the relative risk associated with magnetic fields of 0.3 µT or more was 1.1, and that with magnetic fields of < 0.3 µT was 2.6. This was the inverse of what was observed when the data on all dwellings were considered. For analysis based on individuals, the relative risk associated with magnetic fields of 0.3 µT or more was 2.6, irrespective of whether the dwelling at the time of birth or at the time of diagnosis was considered.

## Taipei study (Lin & Lu, 1989)

The study of Lin and Lu (1989) in Taipei, Taiwan, during the period 1950–73 has been reported only in an abstract. No association between childhood cancer and residence within 50 m of a high-tension power line, transformer or substation was found.

## Yorkshire study (Myers et al., 1990)

In a study in the Yorkshire Health Region of the UK, cases diagnosed in the decade 1970–79 were ascertained primarily from the local childhood cancer registry, supplemented by two national sources (Myers *et al.* 1990). Controls were identified as the nearest entries of the same sex in the birth register containing the record of the case child. Birth addresses for which sufficient information about proximity to overhead power lines was available were obtained for 89% of cases and 90% of controls.

There was no significantly raised odds ratio in any 25 m distance band from the nearest overhead line up to 100 m, and there was no evidence of any trend with distance. In addition, there was no evidence for different associations with distance for solid and non-solid tumours.

Magnetic field strengths were estimated from the maximum load current carried by nearby overhead lines in the year of birth, assuming that this was proportional to each child's exposure in that year. Currents for all lines at 33 kV and above were obtained directly from the records of meters at strategic points in the system. For 275 and 400 kV lines, the loads were those recorded at the period of maximum demand on the whole system in a given year. For 11 kV and low-voltage lines, indirect methods of estimating maximum demand were agreed with engineers from the area boards concerned, and the estimates were made by engineers who were not otherwise involved in the study. For the years before 1974, the load data for 1974 were taken to apply. For other years where no record existed for particular lines, the maximum load in the years immediately before and after the relevant year was taken. Less than 4% of cases and controls had exposures estimated to be greater than 0.1 mG, assumed to be the 50 Hz background level on the basis of a field survey of the homes of 44 volunteers who were not involved in the main investigation (Myers *et al.*, 1985).

Different categorizations of estimated magnetic field were used, defined *a priori* on the basis of the results of previous studies. No relative risk estimate was significantly different from unity, and there was no trend with increasing estimated magnetic field. The authors noted a suggestion of highest values at intermediate field strengths. This was apparent for both solid and non-solid tumours. House type was considered as a possible indicator of social class, and cases were slightly more likely than controls to live in terraced housing. The possibility that this might have obscured a relation with distance from overhead lines or from estimated magnetic fields was considered, but no association was apparent either on stratification or by including house type in the conditional logistic regression model.

## Swedish study (Feychting & Ahlbom, 1992, 1993)

Feychting and Ahlbom (1992) reported a study of childhood cancer of all types and of leukaemia and brain tumours in adults in relation to residential exposure to magnetic fields of the type generated by high-voltage power lines. The study base for children comprised those who had lived in a corridor within 300 m of any of the 220 and 400 kV power lines in Sweden during the period 1960–85, as identified from the population registry. As the procedure was very time-consuming, two of the 21 power lines in Stockholm had to be excluded. In addition, the registries of a small number of parishes were organized in such a way that residences could not be accessed. Cases were identified through record linkage with the Swedish Cancer Registry and the mortality registry, and the diagnosis was verified from hospital records. Four controls per case were selected randomly from the study base after matching for year of diagnosis and power line and, where possible, age, sex and parish.

Three assessments of exposure were made. The main method of assessing magnetic field exposure was the calculation of historical fields, taking into account distance of the home from the line, the configuration of the line, and data on load on the line. Data on load were obtained from detailed records about the operation of the line for each hour of the day, every day of the year. The calculations were made for the year of diagnosis, 1, 5 and 10 years before diagnosis, the time of birth and the time of conception. Spot measurements were made according to the procedures used by Savitz *et al.* (1988). The distance between the residence and power line was measured by mapping, and this was verified during the visit to the home when the spot measurements were performed.

There was no association between total childhood cancer and any of the measures of exposure.

## Danish study (Olsen et al. 1993b)

The Danish study was based on a total of 1707 cases of childhood leukaemia, lymphoma and tumours of the central nervous system, newly diagnosed during the period 1968–86 and ascertained from the National Cancer Registry (Olsen *et al.*, 1993b). Controls matched on sex and date of birth were selected from the Danish central population register. The selection was made from among subjects who had survived without cancer until the date of diagnosis of the case. Residential histories were obtained by identifying parents from the central population register and extracting details of addresses from this register and each of the 276 local population registries in Denmark.

Exposure assessment proceeded in two stages. First, homes were classified as being within a potential exposure area, a 'view distant area', or as unexposed on the basis of distance from an installation. This distance varied by type of installation and the voltage. The potential exposure area was one in which exposures from installations of 0.1 µT or more are likely, this being the minimal value that would outweigh the combined exposure to 50 Hz magnetic fields from other sources in and around a house. The 'view distant area' was defined to include exposures from installations of less than 0.1 µT, and corresponded to a distance from an installation greater than that defined for the potential exposure area up to about twice the maximum distance within which an exposure of 0.1 µT or more was likely. For example, the potential exposure area for overhead lines and transformer substations with a voltage of 220–440 kV was up to a distance of 150 m, while the view distant area for these installations was between 151 and 300 m. The second stage involved the calculation of 50 Hz magnetic field exposures based on the distance of the home from the installation, the category of the line, the type of pylons, the ordering of phases and current flow. As the load in the individual installations was not registered systematically in the past, all such information was in the form of estimates. The average magnetic field strength was calculated for each dwelling for the period during which the family was resident. The main results relate to the highest average magnetic field level to which the child was ever exposed.

There was no marked increase in risk of the three types of childhood cancer combined associated with exposure to magnetic fields of 0.1 µT or more (RR = 1.4, 95% CI 0.7–3.0). When the intermediate cut-off point of 0.25 µT, defined *a priori*, was considered, the relative risk was 1.5 (95% CI 0.6–4.1). The authors considered an odds ratio function for stepwise increases in the cut-off point of exposure from 0.1 to 0.8 µT, with adjustment for multiple testing. The odds ratio increased when cut-off points of 0.3–0.4 µT were used. The lowest *p* value was observed when the cut-off point was 0.5 µT ($p = 0.02$, adjusted for multiple testing). The authors selected the cut-off point of 0.4 µT for presentation on the basis of this finding and the fact that the risk for each of three tumour types was raised. However, for each tumour type, only one control was exposed to magnetic fields of 0.4 µT or more. Among the ten cases exposed to an average flux density of 0.1 µT or more, five had received maximal exposure at conception and all but one had been exposed before two years of age. The relative risk of exposure to 0.25 µT or more for children aged less than one year at the time of onset of exposure was 3.4 (95% CI 0.9–13), whereas that for children first exposed at a later age was 0.4 (95% CI 0.0–3.0). There was no variation in risk with latent period or with period free of exposure before diagnosis.

## Finnish study (Verkasalo et al., 1993)

The Finnish study was a cohort study of cancer diagnosed at ages under 20 years in 134 800 children resident at any time in the period 1970–89 within 500 m of overhead power lines of 110, 220 or 400 kV with calculated magnetic fields of 0.01 µT or more (Verkasalo *et al.*, 1993). Residential information was obtained from the central population register. As in the study in Denmark described above, the threshold of 0.01 µT was chosen to include most buildings in Finland likely to have increased magnetic fields from power lines. The magnetic fields were calculated on the basis of the distance of the power line from the central point of a building, current flow and typical locations of phase conductors in power lines. Cumulative exposure also was calculated. Data on cancer was obtained from the National Cancer Registry. Expected numbers of cases were calculated from national rates.

A total of 140 cases of childhood cancer in the exposed cohort was observed, compared with 145 expected. There was no association with having ever lived in a home within 600 m of an overhead power line with a calculated magnetic field of 0.01 µT or more, or with cumulative exposure to such fields.

## Norwegian study (Tynes & Haldorsen, 1997)

Tynes and Haldorsen (1997) identified children who had lived in a census ward in Norway crossed by a high-voltage power line (45 kV or more in urban areas, 100 kV or more in rural areas) during at least one of the years 1960, 1970, 1980, 1985, 1987 or 1989. This cohort was linked with the Norwegian national cancer registry and 532 cases of cancer diagnosed at ages up to 14 in the period 1965–89 were ascertained. For each case, up to five controls matched on sex, year of birth and municipality were selected randomly (*n* = 2112). Complete information on residence was available for 500 cases and 2004 controls. Historical magnetic fields were calculated on the basis of distance from the power line, height of towers, distance between phases, ordering of phases and historical load on the line. Changes of the voltage and configuration of the power lines, and for dwellings within 50 m of a line, the altitude of the home relative to the altitude of the line, were taken into account. In a study of 65 school children living close to a 300 kV power line, the correlation between 24-hour calculated fields and fields measured by personal dosimeters over a 24-hour period, in conjunction with questionnaire information on where the child had spent that time, were highly correlated, indicating that calculated exposure was a good predictor of actual exposure. Electric fields were calculated by a method similar to that used for historical magnetic fields, but as shielding between the residences and power lines was not taken into account, the calculated electric field may not have been representative of the field inside the home.

There was no association between time-weighted average exposure to magnetic fields and cancer at all sites, leukaemia, lymphoma or brain tumours. Cancer at other sites combined showed elevated relative risks for time-weighted average exposures of 0.05 µT or more compared with less than 0.05 µT, for magnetic fields of this magnitude closest in time to diagnosis and also during the first year of life. The relative risk of osteosarcoma associated with magnetic fields closest in time to diagnosis of 0.05 µT or more was 10.9 (95% CI 1.1–107.8). Although based on only 17 cases, this is intriguing in view of the therapeutic use of magnetic fields in bone healing. There was no association between childhood cancer overall or of any specific type and distance from the lines. Electric fields were not associated with childhood cancer.

## Description of studies which considered only leukaemia (Table 5.2)

### Providence study (Fulton et al., 1980)

In Providence, Rhode Island, Fulton *et al.* (1980) mapped power lines within 50 yards of each of 209 residences of 119 patients with leukaemia and the birth addresses of 240 controls. Wiring configurations were assessed and exposure weights were assigned using Wertheimer and Leeper's (1979) median field strength reading for each. No association was found. However, the coding values used in calculating a measure of summary exposure differed from those of Wertheimer and Leeper, but re-analysis using the codes originally used by these workers also did not reveal any association (Wertheimer & Leeper, 1980). Wertheimer and Leeper (1980) pointed out that as a result of all addresses of cases between birth and diagnosis being compared with addresses at the time of birth for controls, a bias was introduced whereby addresses occupied in the 1950s were controls for addresses occupied by teenage cancer cases in the 1970s. During this period, the proportion of the population living in suburban areas increased, and the general pattern was for families to live first in urban areas and then to move to the suburbs. Suburban residence would have been associated with less exposure to high-current configurations. In consequence, a bias towards a null result appears to have been produced. Wertheimer and Leeper (1980) reanalysed the data, considering only addresses occupied by cases aged eight years or less (birth addresses of cases were not available). A weak positive association of borderline statistical significance at the 0.05 level was found (odds ratio for high-current configuration versus low-current configuration 1.7).

### South London study (Coleman et al., 1989)

Coleman *et al.* (1989) carried out a population-based case–control study of leukaemia at all ages in south London. Some 84 cases of leukaemia in patients aged under 18 years were compared with 141 controls with a solid tumour, matched on sex, age (by single year) and year of diagnosis. No details of participation rates by age were presented; overall 95% of eligible cases and 89% of eligible cancer controls were available for analysis. Exposure to electromagnetic fields was assessed indirectly from address at diagnosis, the measures of exposure for childhood leukaemia being the distance and type (overhead power line or substation) of the electricity supply equipment (source) within 100 m of the subject's home. Underground cables were excluded from exposure assessment, as these produce weak fields which decay approximately with the inverse cube of distance. The investigators determining the grid references for the sources and the subjects' homes were kept 'blind' to the status of the subject. Only one case and one control was resident within 100 m of an overhead power line. There was no significant trend in risk associated with distance of residence from a substation. The relative risk associated with residence within 100 m of a substation was 0.9; that associated with residence within 50 m was 1.5 (95% confidence interval 0.7–3.4). The use of cancer controls may have influenced the relative risk. Details of the distribution of cancer type in controls are not presented, but it would be expected that CNS tumours would be the largest single group. If there were a positive association with CNS tumours, the relative risks of leukaemia would have been underestimated.

## Los Angeles leukaemia study (London et al., 1991)

London *et al.* (1991) reported a case–control study of childhood leukaemia and (1) measurement of magnetic fields in subjects' homes over 24 hours or more; (2) spot measurements of both electric and magnetic fields; (3) wiring configuration; and (4) use of electrical appliances by the mother during pregnancy and by the child. The case group comprised children with leukaemia diagnosed between 1980 and 1987 up to the age of 10 years and resident in Los Angeles County, California. In total, 331 cases were eligible. Maternal interview was completed with 232 (70%), 24-hour magnetic field measurements for 164 (50%), spot measurements for 140 (42%), and wiring configurations were assessed for 219 (66%). 139 of the cases and 131 controls had been included in the study of Lowengart *et al.* (1987), and were recontacted. Controls were matched with cases on sex, ethnic group and age and selected mainly by random-digit dialling; about a quarter were drawn from friends of cases. Interviews were completed with 232 control mothers (90% of eligible controls identified), 24-hour measurements of magnetic fields for 56% of the eligible controls, spot measurements for 42%, and wiring configurations for 81%.

To identify residences in which measurements were to be made, the reference period was defined as the interval between the mother's last menstrual period before the birth of the index case up to a date dependent on the age of diagnosis. Only 43% of cases and 34% of controls had lived for the entire reference period in the residences measured. It is possible that stability of residence was associated with control participation (NRPB, 1992). The measurements covered residences occupied for at least half the reference period for 63% of cases and 55% of controls.

Wiring configurations were assessed blindly by the method of Wertheimer and Leeper (1982). Compared with a reference category comprising buried wires and very low-current configurations, the crude relative risk associated with 'ordinary' low-current configurations was 1.0, with 'ordinary' high-current configurations 1.4, and with very high-current configurations 2.2; there was a statistically significant trend ($p = 0.008$).

The data collected on potential confounding factors included demographic information, medical history of the child and parents, use of medications, occupational history of both parents, exposure to environmental chemicals, and use of recreational drugs and incense. Potential confounding was identified for use of indoor pesticides, hairdryers, black and white televisions, and father's occupational exposure to spray paint during pregnancy and to other chemical exposures after the birth of the child. The $p$ value for trend associated with wiring configuration became 0.017 after adjustment for these variables. However, London *et al.* may have underestimated the possible effect of confounding, as the variables in question are unlikely to have been assessed with great accuracy, and may have been surrogates for other variables (NRPB, 1992). Moreover, the contrast between 'ordinary' low-current configurations and 'ordinary' high-current configurations contributed most to the chi-square for trend, yet most 24-hour and spot magnetic field measurements were similar between the categories (NRPB, 1992). The only exception was the percentage of the 24-hour measurement during which the magnetic field was greater than 2.5 mG; this was higher for 'ordinary' low-current configurations (11.6%) than for 'ordinary' high-current configurations (6.4%). Thus, the trends associated with wiring codes may reflect other aspects of housing than magnetic fields, particularly in view of the absence of an association with direct measures of magnetic field.

Spot measurements of electric and magnetic fields were taken in the main living area, the parents' bedroom, the child's sleeping area, and the living area closest to the electrical distribution wiring, unless that room was one of the other three. In addition, outdoor measurements were made in the front and/or backyard areas which the child used and over the waterpipe. These measurements were carried out under both low-power conditions and normal power conditions, for the purposes of comparability with the study of Savitz *et al.* (1988). None of the spot measurements of electric and magnetic fields was associated with the risk of childhood leukaemia. The authors considered the possibility that they might have missed an association with measured electric and magnetic fields as a result of a relationship between unwillingness to have measurements performed with both electromagnetic field exposure and case/control status. However, the magnetic fields predicted from wiring configurations were similar between the homes in which measurements were made and those in which they were not.

No association was found with maternal use during pregnancy of any of five types of electrical appliance. The highest relative risk observed was 1.2 (95% CI, 0.7–2.3), for electric blanket use. For the 13 appliances about which information on use at least once a week by the child was sought, nine relative risks were greater than unity; those associated with use of black and white television (RR = 1.5) and electric hairdryers (RR = 2.8) were statistically significant, but this needs to be considered in the context of multiple significance testing. The highest odds ratios were for the use of electric blankets and curling irons, but the numbers of exposed subjects were very small. The relative risk associated with the use of dial electric clocks was 1.9, contrasting with 1.1 for digital electric clocks; the former generate much higher magnetic and electric fields than the latter. It is unclear what checks for confounding were made in assessing the associations with appliance use. The authors considered that recall bias might be important, and it is difficult to estimate the effect of recontacting subjects who had participated in the earlier investigation.

*Tasmania study (Lowenthal et al., 1991)*

Lowenthal *et al.* (1991) presented a preliminary report of leukaemia and lymphoma in 69 children and acute lymphoblastic leukaemia (ALL) in 7 adults in Tasmania diagnosed between 1972 and 1980. The proximity of the 180 addresses occupied by these subjects to high-tension power lines was assessed. One of the addresses was within 50 m of a high-tension power line. On the basis that about 800 of 170 000 residences in Tasmania lie within 50 m of a high tension power line, the expected number of addresses for the case series was 0.8.

*Greek study (Petridou et al., 1993)*

In a study designed primarily to investigate the association between childhood leukaemia and early attendance at crèches, the proximity of residence at diagnosis from electricity substations and power lines was determined (Petridou *et al.*, 1993). The relative risk associated with residence within 100 m of a substation, compared with greater distances, was 0.4 (95% CI 0.1–1.1). Compared with residence 50 m or more from a power line, the relative risk associated with residence at distances between 5 and 49 m was 1.1 (95% CI 0.5–1.8), and with distances less than 5 m, 1.2 (95% CI 0.6–2.4). Thus, the associations were inconsistent and were not statistically significant. As acknowledged by the authors, the study is limited by the fact that controls were hospital-based and by data not being available for a substantial proportion of subjects (the participation rate of cases was 74% (136 of 183) and that of controls was 72% (187 of 260)). Controls were of higher social class than cases, whereas childhood leukaemia is usually associated with higher socioeconomic status.

*Mexico City study (Fajardo-Gutiérrez et al., 1993b)*

In a study in Mexico City, the proximity of residence at interview of the father of 81 cases with prevalent or incident leukaemia and 77 controls to transformers, high-tension power lines, substations and transmission towers was determined (Fajardo-Gutiérrez *et al.*, 1993b). It is stated that photographs of such installations were used in an attempt to minimize recall bias, but the precise method of assessment of distance from such installations is unclear. The relative risks associated with proximity to each type of installation were all greater than unity. The relative risks were statistically significant for high-tension power lines and transmission towers when no precise distance was specified. However, all of the relative risks were attenuated when a precise distance (less than 20 m for transformers and high-tension power lines, less than 200 m for substations and transmission towers) was specified; none of these was statistically significant. When adjustment was made for reported exposure to insecticides, chemicals, frequency of infections during the first year of life, and prior history of abortions, only the relative risk associated with proximity to power lines remained elevated. The study is limited by the fact that controls were hospital-based. The participation rates were not specified.

### Study in Wessex, England (Coghill et al., 1996)

In a study in the Wessex area of England, 56 cases with ALL diagnosed at ages up to 14 years in the period 1986–95 were ascertained by methods including media advertising, personal introduction and contacting self-help groups (Coghill *et al.*, 1996). Parents of the cases were asked to identify control children of the same age and sex living nearby. Cases and controls were excluded if they had not normally slept for at least a year in the room being assessed before diagnosis, or if major wiring alterations had occurred since diagnosis. Electric and magnetic fields were measured over 24 hours in the bedplaces of study subjects using purpose-built instruments. A random selection of instruments was validated for accuracy of magnetic field measurements. There was no statistically significant difference in the mean magnetic field assessed over 24 hours. The mean electric field strength over 24 hours, and over the period 20:00 h – 08:00 h, differed significantly between cases and controls. The relative risk of ALL associated with an electric field of 20 V m$^{-1}$ or more compared with one of less than 5 V m$^{-1}$ was 4.7 (95% CI 1.2–27.8). As acknowledged by the authors, this study is limited by a number of poor design elements, such as selection bias and lack of standardization of the placing of test instruments. For this reason, it has not been included in Tables 5.1 or 5.2.

### Study in Lower Saxony, Germany (Michaelis et al., 1997b)

In Lower Saxony, Germany, 129 (59% of 219 potentially eligible) cases of leukaemia newly diagnosed at ages up to 14 years during the period 1988–93 were compared with 328 matched controls selected from files of local government offices for registration of residents (Michaelis *et al.*, 1997b). Two controls were matched with each case on gender and date of birth. One control also was matched on registration office and the other was selected from a registration office chosen randomly in Lower Saxony. Magnetic field measurements were made over 24 hours in the child's bedroom at the residence where the child had been living for the longest period before the date of diagnosis, and spot measurements were made throughout all residences where the child had been living for more than one year. The relative risk of leukaemia associated with a median of the 24-hour measurement in the child's bedroom of 0.2 µT or greater compared with lower exposures was 3.2 (95% CI 0.7–14.9). Elevations in risk which were not statistically significant were apparent also when the mean of the 24-hour measurements in the child's bedroom, the median during the night and the mean of the medians in the child's bedroom and in the living room were considered. There was no association with the mean of spot measurements taken at the residence where the child had lived longest or the maximum spot measurements of all residences where the child had lived for at least a year.

### Multicentre study in USA (Linet et al., 1997)

In the USA, 638 children with ALL diagnosed before the age of 15 years in the period 1989–94 and 620 controls selected by random-digit dialling were included in an investigation of the effects of residential exposure to magnetic fields (Linet *et al.*, 1997). The participation rate was 78% for cases and 63% for controls. Magnetic field measurements were made over 24 hours in the child's bedroom, and spot measurements of magnetic fields were made in the child's bedroom, the family room, the kitchen, the room in which the mother had slept during the index pregnancy, and outside the front door. The investigators attempted to make these measurements in all of the homes in which children under the age of five years at diagnosis (or the reference date for controls) had lived for at least six months, and for older children, the homes in which the child had been resident for at least 70% of the five years immediately preceding the reference date. Magnetic field measurements covered more than 90% of the reference period for 83% of the subjects. In contrast to earlier studies, magnetic fields were usually measured within 24 months after the diagnosis of ALL.

The relative risk of ALL associated with a time-weighted average magnetic field exposure of 0.2 µT or more compared with an exposure of less than 0.065 µT was 1.2 (95% CI 0.9–1.8), adjusted for age, sex, maternal education and family income. The relative risk associated with an estimated summary exposure of 0.3 µT or more was 1.7 (95% CI 1.0–2.9). However, there was no trend of increasing risk with increasing magnetic field exposure. Moreover, no association was apparent when analysis was restricted to subjects who lived in a single home during the study period or those who lived for the entire reference period in homes for which 24-hour bedroom measurements were obtained. In addition, the results were similar if only bedroom measurements in the period 16:00 h – 06:00 h or 20:00 h – 06:00 h were considered.

Wiring configurations were determined for 408 case–control pairs in which both subjects had lived in one home for at least 70% of the reference period according to a five-level adaption of the Wertheimer–Leeper code and the modified three-category code (Kaune & Savitz, 1994). There was no association between ALL and wiring configuration using either scheme. Wiring configurations were similar for participating and non-participating controls.

There was no association with measured magnetic field levels of the homes in which the mother had been resident during the index pregnancy, which were determined for 257 cases and 239 controls. As observed in other studies, there was a significant correlation between measured magnetic fields and wire codes. In addition, for the 225 pairs whose mothers' residences during pregnancy had their wiring configurations determined, no association with wire code was found. This was also true when analysis was restricted to ALL diagnosed before the age of three years.

## Description of studies in which only brain tumours were considered (Table 5.4)

### Seattle study (Gurney et al., 1996b)

Gurney *et al.* (1996b) reported a case–control study of childhood brain tumours and wiring configuration and use of electrical appliances or electric heating sources by the mother while pregnant or by the child before diagnosis. The case group comprised subjects with brain tumours diagnosed at ages up to 19 years during the period 1984–90 in the Seattle area. Of a total of 179 eligible cases, maternal interviews were completed with 133 (74%). Controls were selected using random-digit dialling and matched with cases on age, sex and general area of residence. Of 343 potentially eligible controls, interviews were completed with the mothers of 270 (79%). Information on use of electric blankets and heated water beds by the child before the reference date or by the mother during pregnancy, a partial residential history and data on potential confounding factors, was obtained from the interview. Subsequently, a questionnaire was mailed to participating mothers requesting a residential history to include every home in which the child lived during the three-year period up to their reference date and during the mother's pregnancy and

information on the use of a number of other electrical appliances. Questionnaires were returned by 98 (74%) of case mothers and 208 (77%) of control mothers. The wiring configuration of the homes at the reference date was determined for 92 of these cases and 193 controls. No association was found between brain tumours and wiring configuration, either according to the five-level Wertheimer–Leeper code or when exposure was dichotomized. Moreover, no association was apparent in subgroup analysis by sex, age at diagnosis or histological sub-type, and the distribution of the five-level code was similar for study participants and non-participants. No association was observed for use of electric blankets, water beds or electric heating sources either by the mother during pregnancy or by the index child during his/her lifetime. The relative risks associated with the use of electrical appliances by the index child varied between 0.7 and 1.6, being above unity for eight appliances and below unity for four. The relative risks associated between maternal use of four electrical appliances during pregnancy ranged between 0.7 and 1.1.

### Los Angeles brain tumour study (Preston-Martin et al., 1996a)

Preston-Martin *et al.* (1996a) reported a case–control study of brain tumours in children and (1) measurement of magnetic fields in subjects' homes over 24 hours or more; (2) spot measurements of magnetic fields and magnetic field profiles; (3) wiring configuration; and (4) use of electrical appliances by the mother during pregnancy and by the child. A total of 437 eligible cases was diagnosed with brain tumours at ages up to 19 years in Los Angeles County during the period 1984–91. Maternal interviews, including a complete residential history, were obtained for 298 (70%). Age–sex-matched controls were selected by random-digit dialling. Maternal interviews and complete residential histories were obtained for 298 (69%) of 433 controls identified as eligible.

Of a total of 1002 residences occupied by mothers of cases from conception to age at diagnosis, wiring configurations and exterior spot and profile measurements of magnetic fields were obtained for 592 (59%). Of a total of 998 residences occupied by mothers of controls, these measurements were obtained for 539 (54%). The information was not obtained if the address was incomplete (12.4% of residences of cases and 15.0% of residences of controls) or if the residence was outside Los Angeles County (19.6% of cases and 20.3% of controls). A further

9% of residences of cases and 10.6% of residences of controls could not be measured, usually because staff could not locate the residence, e.g. because of demolition, or because the address turned out not to exist.

For a subset of subjects, 24-hour measurements of magnetic fields were taken in the child's room (106 cases, 99 controls) and in a second room where the child spent the most time (99 cases and 91 controls). The reason a higher proportion of controls had no measurements of the magnetic fields is that 16 controls who lived in Los Angeles at the time of selection did not live in the county during the period between conception and the reference date, and thus had no eligible residence. This arose because cases diagnosed up to $4^{1}/_{2}$ years before the start of the interview study were included in order to increase the statistical power of the study. As cases who had moved out of Los Angeles County after diagnosis were eligible for inclusion, it was decided not to exclude controls who had moved into the county since the reference date, because such an exclusion might have resulted in a bias towards greater stability of residence among controls, which was a point of criticism of the study of Savitz *et al.* (1988).

Wiring configurations were assessed blindly by the method of Wertheimer and Leeper (1982). Compared with a reference category comprising very low- and ordinary low-current configurations, the crude relative risk associated with ordinary high-current configuration was 0.8 (95% CI 0.6–1.2), and with very high-current configurations 1.2 (95% CI 0.6–2.1). The relative risk associated with buried wires was 1.9 (95% CI 1.0–3.6). This is thought to be an artefact introduced by the partial non-contemporaneity between cases and controls. No excess risk was apparent in an analysis restricted to the later years of the study when cases and controls were accrued concurrently. Although measured magnetic fields were highest in the highest of the five wire code categories, magnetic field strengths in homes in this category were much lower in Los Angeles than in Denver, where the code was developed.

For the mean, median and 90th percentiles of all 24-hour magnetic field measurements of the child's room and the other room in which the child spent the most time, the relative risk appeared to be elevated in the small subset of children in homes at the 90th percentile and above of each of these variables, compared with those with measurements below the median. These were the only groups of homes where fields were as high as those in Denver homes with high-current configurations. No increase was observed for homes in the 90th percentile of various exterior measurements of magnetic fields, and there was no evidence of a dose–response relationship for internal or external measurements.

The relative risk associated with use of an electric water bed during pregnancy was 2.1 (95% CI 1.0–4.2). No noteworthy association was apparent for any other electrical appliance used during pregnancy. The relative risks for 10 electrical appliances used by the index child ranged between 0.6 and 2.0; none of these was statistically significant.

## Synthesis of results: leukaemia

In six studies, direct measurements of magnetic fields were made (Table 5.2). No consistent association is apparent when the spot measurements, made in all of the studies, but following different protocols, are considered. However, these may not reflect the longer-term exposure of individuals. In one of the studies, 24-hour measurements of magnetic fields in the index child's bedroom were obtained for 50% of cases and 56% of controls (London *et al.*, 1991). The relative risk associated with a magnetic field of 0.268 µT or more versus 0.067 µT or less was 1.5 (95% CI 0.7–3.3). There was no dose–response relationship. None of a variety of summary statistics (arithmetic and geometric means, median, 90th percentile, and percent of time with readings of over 0.025 µT) was associated with risk. In the study of Michaelis *et al.* (1997b), 24-hour measurements were obtained in the bedroom of residence in which the index child had lived for the longest period for 59% of cases and 56% of controls. The relative risk associated with the median of these measurements being 0.2 µT or greater compared with less than 0.2 µT was 3.2 (95% CI 0.7–14.9), based on four exposed cases and three exposed controls. The relative risks were not statistically significantly increased for other characteristics of the magnetic field at varying cut-points. In the study of Linet *et al.* (1997), magnetic field measurements covered more than 90% of the reference period for 83% of the subjects. No association between ALL and measured magnetic fields was apparent, although there was a tendency for the risk to be higher among subjects with summary exposure levels of 0.3 T or more. The number of children with such high levels of exposure was small.

Spot measurements of electric fields were made in the studies of Savitz *et al.* (1988) and London *et al.* (1991). No association with childhood leukaemia was found in either study.

In four of the five studies of childhood leukaemia and calculated historical exposure to magnetic fields, an elevated relative risk was observed (Table 5.2). The studies in Sweden, Denmark and Finland were planned in concert with a view to the possibility of carrying out a combined analysis and although there are differences in design, it has been suggested that these are unlikely to account for the differences in relative risk estimates between the studies (Ahlbom *et al.*, 1993). The combined relative risk of leukaemia associated with the highest level of magnetic field exposure was 2.1 (95% CI 1.1–4.1), based on 13 cases with the highest level of exposure. More recently, in a combined analysis of the Danish and Swedish studies, the relative risk of leukaemia tended to be increased when the cut-off point for high exposure was increased (Feychting *et al.*, 1995). The Norwegian study does not support an association between leukaemia and magnetic fields, but only one case and 14 controls had time-weighted average exposures of 0.14 µT or more, and the highest time-weighted average exposure was 0.19 µT (Tynes & Halderson, 1997).

Three out of five studies in the USA showed a relationship with living in residences inferred to have high-current configurations, with a relative risk for high-current configurations versus low-current configurations of about 2 (Table 5.2). Re-analysis of one of the two studies in which no association was found, in an attempt to resolve a bias identified in the design, changed the odds ratio from unity to 1.7 (95% CI 1.0–2.8). The most recent study, which did not show any relationship between ALL and wiring configuration, was designed to address the weaknesses of earlier studies, and is substantially larger than the others.

No consistency is apparent for the association with distance from electrical installations (Table 5.2). Washburn *et al.* (1994) carried out a meta-analysis of childhood cancer based on a mixture of crude measures of distance, more exact measures, and measures also including other aspects of magnetic field exposure from diverse types of installation. The combined relative risk was elevated, but there was significant heterogeneity between studies, most of which was attributable to the study of Wertheimer and Leeper (1979). After exclusion of this study, the combined relative risk was 1.3 (95% CI 1.0–1.7). Feychting and Ahlbom (1995) noted that the use of the most crude measurement of exposure available may have reduced the heterogeneity between studies, but also may have attenuated the measure of effect.

No consistent association between leukaemia and maternal use of electrical appliances during pregnancy or the use of such appliances by the index child was apparent in the two studies in which this was investigated (Savitz *et al.*, 1990; London *et al.*, 1991). In a study of 27 cases of leukaemia diagnosed at ages under 25 years, and 192 matched controls, in an area within a 35-km radius of the La Hague nuclear waste reprocessing plant in Normandy, France, the relative risk associated with the index subject having ever used an electric hair dryer was 2.3 (95% CI 0.8–6.5; Pobel & Viel, 1997). It was stated that relative risks were around unity for various surrogates of exposure to electromagnetic fields (see Chapter 4 for further details of this study).

Olsen *et al.* (1993b) noted that whereas electricity consumption in Denmark had increased 30-fold since 1945, the incidence of childhood leukaemia had not changed substantially in this period, so the proportion of the disease that might be caused by power-frequency electromagnetic field exposure must be small. Similarly, in the USA, the increase in residential electric consumption has not been accompanied by a substantial increase in the risk of childhood leukaemia (Jackson, 1992). However, although power consumption may have increased over time, magnetic field exposures may have decreased because of increased use of higher-voltage primary distribution lines, changes in the type of wiring and voltage of appliances used in the home, and the increased use of nonconductive elements in the plumbing systems into which electrical power is grounded (Wertheimer & Leeper, 1992). In Canada, during the period 1971–86, childhood leukaemia rates did not change, whereas there was a doubling of residential electricity consumption (Kraut *et al.*, 1994). In New Zealand, trends in childhood leukaemia were not clearly related to changes in household consumption of electricity (Dockerty *et al.*, 1996).

Sahl (1994) suggested that residential proximity to electricity distribution installations might be a surrogate for viral contacts. In the study of Savitz *et al.* (1988), selection of controls was constrained to the residentially stable, whereas this restriction was not applied in the selection of cases. If childhood leukaemia were associated with residential mobility, the different criteria for cases and controls would have produced a bias. Kinlen (1988) postulated that certain patterns of residential mobility may alter the pattern of exposure to relatively common infections in childhood, and leukaemia may be an uncommon response to an atypical pattern of exposure (see

Chapter 7). However, in the study of London *et al.* (1991), the extent of residential mobility appears to have been somewhat greater among controls than among cases, yet a similar association with wiring configurations was identified. In connection with the Kinlen hypothesis, it would be relevant to examine changes in the electricity distribution network associated with the growth of new towns, and in particular to determine whether this differs between relatively isolated and other areas.

### Synthesis of results: lymphoma

In both available studies of lymphoma and spot measurements of magnetic fields, raised relative risks were observed (Table 5.3). However, these results may be attributable to chance, to selection bias and/or incomplete control of confounding. In a pooled analysis of three of the four studies based on calculated historical fields, carried out in Denmark, Finland and Sweden, the relative risk of lymphoma associated with the highest level of magnetic field exposure was 1.0 (95% CI 0.3–3.7; Ahlbom *et al.*, 1993). More recently, in a combined analysis of the Danish and Swedish studies, the relative risk of lymphoma associated with a calculated historical field of 0.2 µT or more was 2.1 (95% CI 0.8–5.5; Feychting *et al.*, 1995). The three cases in this exposure category in the Danish study all had Hodgkin's lymphoma.

The two available studies of wiring configuration and lymphoma are inconsistent when the most comparable categorization is considered (Table 5.2). In the meta-analysis of five studies based on a mixture of measures of exposure already described in relation to leukaemia, the combined relative risk was 1.6 (95% CI 0.9–2.8; Washburn *et al.*, 1994).

### Synthesis of results: brain tumours

The observation of an increased risk of brain tumours associated with spot measurements of magnetic fields at the front door of the home in the Stockholm county study (Tomenius, 1986) has not been replicated in three subsequent studies (Table 5.4). In a combined analysis of the three Nordic studies based on calculated historical fields, the relative risk of nervous system tumours associated with the highest level of magnetic field exposure was 1.5 (95% CI 0.7–3.2; Ahlbom *et al.*, 1993). This was based partly on multiple cancers in one subject in the Finnish study. In that study, an elevated risk was observed for boys only, and this was largely attributable to one boy with neurofibromatosis type 2 disease who developed three primary tumours of the nervous system with different

morphologies and locations. In a recent combined analysis of data from the Danish and Swedish studies, the relative risk of central nervous system tumours associated with a calculated historical magnetic field of 0.5 µT or more was 2.3 (95% CI 0.6–8.0), based on three exposed cases (Feychting *et al.*, 1995).

Positive associations between brain tumours and high-current configurations found in two studies in Denver have not been confirmed in more recent studies in Seattle and Los Angeles. It is unlikely that this inconsistency is due to differences in the power distribution systems of these areas, as the Wertheimer–Leeper code has similar correlations with measured magnetic fields in Seattle and other areas of the USA as in Denver (Gurney *et al.*, 1996b). However, the highest category of the Wertheimer–Leeper code involved higher-intensity magnetic field exposures in Denver than in Los Angeles (Preston-Martin *et al.*, 1996a).

The association between brain tumours and electrical appliance use was considered in four studies. In the study of Savitz *et al.* (1990), no association with prenatal or postnatal exposure to heated water beds, bedside electric clocks or heating pads, or postnatal exposure to electric blankets, was found. However, there was a positive association with prenatal exposure to electric blankets (RR = 2.5, 95% CI 1.1–5.5, after adjustment for family income). The risk was largest for children under five years of age and those exposed during the first trimester of pregnancy. In a study in New South Wales, Australia, non-significant inverse associations were found with regular use of an electric blanket (RR = 0.4, 95% CI 0.2–1.2) and an electrically-heated water bed (RR = 0.2, 95% CI 0.0–1.5; McCredie *et al.* 1994b). In a multicentre study of astrocytoma and primitive neuroectodermal tumours of the brain diagnosed at age five years or less in the USA and Canada, no association with maternal use of electric blankets and heated water beds during pregnancy was found (Bunin *et al.*, 1994b). In the studies in Los Angeles and Seattle, no association with use of a variety of types of electrical appliances was found (Gurney *et al.*, 1996b; Preston-Martin *et al.*, 1996a). In a combined analysis of these two studies together with a study of similar design in the San Francisco–Oakland metropolitan area, no association with prenatal or postnatal use of electric blankets and water bed heaters was found (Preston-Martin *et al.*, 1996b). The relative risks did not vary significantly by age, sex, ethnic group, socioeconomic status or histological category.

Poole (1996) observed that there is a need to integrate appliance-use into one measure, and to combine this with measures of exposure from power lines and other sources, but this remains problematic because of uncertainty over the choice of the appropriate characteristics of electromagnetic fields about which to propose hypotheses (Preston-Martin *et al.*, 1996c).

Most of the possible mechanisms which have been proposed and found in experiments on cells as being responsible for biological effects of electromagnetic fields are based on resonance phenomena which involve both the alternating power-frequency field and the earth's local geomagnetic field (Philips, 1994). In the study of Preston-Martin *et al.* (1996a), brain tumour risk did not relate to whether exterior static fields were in or out of resonance.

## Electromagnetic fields to which the general population is exposed other than from electricity distribution and domestic appliances

Low-level exposure to radio-frequency fields (100 kHz–300 GHz) is ubiquitous (NRPB, 1992). The field strengths associated with low-power radio-frequency transmitters decrease rapidly with distance from the source.

Following concern about an apparent excess of cases of leukaemia and lymphoma in adults near the Sutton Coldfield radio and television transmitter in the West Midlands, England, cancer incidence during the period 1974–86 near radio and television transmitters in Great Britain was investigated (Dolk *et al.*, 1997a,b). The national database of postcoded cancer registrations was used with population and socioeconomic data from the 1981 census. Study areas were defined as circles of 10 km radius around the transmitters, within which 10 bands of increasing distance from the transmitter were defined as a basis for testing for a decline in risk with distance. While an excess of adult leukaemia was confirmed in Sutton Coldfield, with a significant decline in risk with increasing distance from the transmitter, there was no excess of childhood leukaemia or childhood cancer overall (Dolk *et al.*, 1997a). In the analysis of cancer incidence around 21 radio and television transmitters of at least 500 kW effective radiated power for television and 250 kW effective radiated power for frequency-modulated radio transmission, including Sutton Coldfield, the relative risk of childhood leukaemia associated with residence within a 10 km radius of a transmitter was 0.97 (95% CI 0.87–1.08), and that of malignant brain tumours

in children 1.03 (95% CI 0.90–1.18) (Dolk *et al.*, 1997b). There was no significant decline in risk with distance. A limitation of the study is that population figures from the 1981 census may not have given an accurate count of the population of children at risk over the period of the study.

In a study in Sydney, Australia, cancer incidence and mortality during the period 1972–90 was compared between an inner area comprising three municipalities surrounding three television transmission towers (within a radius of approximately 4 km) and an outer area comprising six adjacent municipalities (Hocking *et al.*, 1996). For children and adults combined, the rate ratio for total leukaemia incidence was 1.2 (95% CI 1.1–1.4). For children, the rate ratio for leukaemia incidence was 1.6 (95% CI 1.1–2.3, based on 134 cases) and for mortality 2.3 (95% CI 1.4–4.0, based on 59 deaths). The incidence of, and mortality due to, brain tumours was not increased. The incidence of, and mortality due to, childhood leukaemia and brain tumours was similar between the outer area and New South Wales as a whole.

An excess of acute leukaemia was observed in children in the Waianae Coast, Hawaii, during the period 1979–90 (standardized incidence ratio 2.1, 95% CI 1.1–3.7; Maskarinec *et al.*, 1994). A case–control study (12 cases, 48 controls) was carried out of potential risk factors including parental occupation, X-ray exposure, smoking, family and medical histories, and distance of the residence of the index child from low-frequency radio towers. The relative risk associated with having lived within 4.2 km (2.6 miles) of radio towers before diagnosis was 2.0 (95% CI 0.1–8.3).

Selvin *et al.* (1992) applied three statistical approaches to detect spatial clusters of disease associated with a point source exposure in data on childhood cancer in the city of San Francisco during the period 1973–88. The three measures of clustering were distance on a geopolitical map, distance on a density-equalized map, and relative risk. The point source of exposure was a large microwave tower; it is not clear whether there had been public concern about the potential effects of this. A total of 51 cases of leukaemia, 35 of brain cancer and 37 of lymphatic cancer diagnosed under the age of 21 years in white individuals was ascertained from the SEER cancer registry. As exact geographical information on location was not available, each case was plotted at the centroid of the census tract of residence. No systematic spatial variation with respect to the point source was found for any diagnostic category.

## Parental occupational exposure

The highest levels of occupational magnetic field exposure are likely to be encountered by arc welders and induction furnace workers (NRPB, 1992). For people who work in the electricity supply industry, about 70% of total magnetic field exposure arises at work. All of the studies on childhood cancer and parental occupational exposure to electromagnetic fields have been based on job titles. While the fundamental assumption that electrical workers have higher exposure than non-electrical workers has been confirmed in several studies, data to classify the exposures of specific subgroups of electrical workers other than those in the electricity supply industry are sparse (Savitz *et al.*, 1993).

### Neuroblastoma

The possibility of an association between paternal occupational exposure to electromagnetic fields and childhood cancer was raised by the finding in Texas of a positive association (RR = 3.2, 95% CI 1.1–8.9) between deaths due to neuroblastoma and a group of occupations including electrical, insulation and utility workers, and workers in electric, electronics and printing occupations (Spitz & Johnson, 1985). These authors considered that this finding might be consistent with Wertheimer and Leeper's (1979) report of a positive association between childhood cancer and residential electromagnetic fields, and therefore reclassified together all occupations considered to have electromagnetic field exposure using narrow and broad definitions. For the narrow definition, comprising electricians, electric and electronics workers, linemen, and utility employees and welders, the odds ratio was 2.1. The same odds ratio was observed for the broad definition, which also comprised electrical equipment salesmen and repairmen; this was reported as statistically significant, but such an assessment is inappropriate as this was an *a posteriori* analysis. For electronics workers only, the odds ratio was 11.8 (based on six exposed cases and one exposed control). There were no statistically significant differences in urban versus rural residence at time of birth, sex, ethnic group, parental age, legitimacy or the duration of prenatal care.

Subsequently, in a study based on 104 cases of neuroblastoma ascertained from paediatric tumour registries in Philadelphia, with one matched control for each recruited by random-digit dialling, and in which both parents were interviewed to obtain their occupational histories, the same occupational classifications were applied for preconceptional and gestational exposure (Bunin *et al.* 1990b). The findings of the previous study in relation to paternal occupation were not confirmed; the fathers of four cases and one control had been electrical and electronic products assemblers in the periconceptional period. Two mothers of cases and no control mothers had jobs in the group of occupations for which the elevated risk had been observed in the study of Spitz and Johnson (1985) during the preconceptional period; both of these women had been electrical and electronic products assemblers. The authors acknowledged that the low participation rate of controls (57%, versus 70% for cases) might have produced selection bias, but they observed that slightly more case than control fathers were blue-collar workers, which would have been expected to bias the results in favour of a positive association with jobs with exposure to electromagnetic fields, as most of these were blue-collar jobs.

Wilkins and Hundley (1990) considered 101 cases of neuroblastoma ascertained from a paediatric tumour registry in Ohio, for each of which four matched controls were selected from birth certificates; these were the source of information on paternal occupation. No association was apparent for the group of occupations for which an elevated risk had been observed in the study of Spitz and Johnson (1985). In addition, these authors considered the more restrictive definition of Hoar *et al.* (1980) and broader definitions developed by Lin *et al.* (1985) for a study of brain tumours in adults, and by Deapen and Henderson (1986) for an investigation of the role of potential exposure to electric shock in the etiology of amyotrophic lateral sclerosis. No case father was exposed according to the definition of Hoar *et al.* (1980); five control fathers were exposed. Only one case father and three control fathers were exposed according to Lin *et al.*'s (1985) category of 'definite' exposure to electromagnetic fields. Combination of Lin *et al.*'s categories of 'definite' and 'probable' exposure produced a group comparable with the 'narrow' definition of Spitz and Johnson (1985). The odds ratio was 1.9 (95% CI 0.4–9.7) after adjustment for a number of birth characteristics, parental age and a job-coding ambiguity score. Adjustment for the ambiguity score was intended to take account of a difference in the ease with which occupational data for cases and controls could be coded; 'difficulty' was encountered in coding for 12.9% of cases and 20.8% of controls. The odds ratio was 1.6 (95% CI 0.3–9.1) for the broadly similar definition of Deapen and Henderson (1986). When Lin *et al.*'s category of 'possible' exposure was combined with the categories of 'definite' and 'probable' exposure, the resulting group was roughly comparable with the 'broad' definition of Spitz and Johnson (1985); the odds ratio then became 0.7 (95% CI 0.3–1.5). Thus, the strength and direction of association depended on the definition of exposure; a strict definition produced an inverse association for very small numbers of exposed subjects, a less strict definition a positive association which was not statistically significant, and a broad definition no association.

In a case–control study of neuroblastoma in parts of Germany heavily contaminated with caesium-137 as a result of the Chernobyl accident, no increased risk was observed for the offspring of electricity workers (Michaelis *et al.*, 1996). Data were obtained by a combination of postal questionnaire and telephone interview on 67 cases and 120 controls.

## Tumours of the central nervous system

Parental occupational exposure to electromagnetic fields has also been considered in relation to tumours of the central nervous system (CNS). Nasca *et al.* (1988) applied the 'narrow' and 'broad' definitions of Spitz and Johnson (1985) in a study in New York State of 338 cases of CNS tumour, for each of which two controls were selected from birth certificates. Data on parental occupations were obtained by telephone interview with the mother; participation rates were 85% for cases and 70% for potential controls (control replacement was used). Paternal employment at the time of birth of the child in occupations included in the 'narrow' definition was associated with an odds ratio of 1.7 (95% CI 0.8–3.6) and in occupations included in the 'broad' definition with an odds ratio of 1.6 (95% CI 0.8–3.1). For paternal employment at the time of diagnosis of the case, the odds ratios were 1.3 (95% CI 0.6–2.9) and 1.1 (95% CI 0.5–2.5), respectively. Too few mothers had occupations in these categories to permit meaningful analysis.

In Texas, Johnson and Spitz (1989) investigated associations between CNS tumours and paternal occupations involving use, repair or manufacture of electrical and electronic equipment, using a similar design to their earlier study of neuroblastoma (Spitz & Johnson, 1985). Thus, information was obtained from birth certificates for 499 deaths due to CNS tumours and 998 livebirths frequency-matched on year of birth, sex and ethnic group. The categories of occupation considered were developed with the assistance of an industrial hygienist, and based on the previous study of neuroblastoma; these comprised categories based on industry and on occupation. For all the industry categories involving potential exposure to low-frequency electromagnetic fields combined (25 cases and 31 controls exposed), the odds ratio was 1.6 (95% CI 1.0–2.8). The odds ratios for specific categories defined *a priori* ranged from 0.7 to 4.1. For all of the occupation categories involving potential exposure combined (28 cases and 39 controls exposed), the odds ratio was 1.4 (95% CI 0.9–2.4). The odds ratios for specific categories defined *a priori* ranged from 0.5 to 3.5. That for electricians (3.5) was statistically significant (7 exposed cases, 4 exposed controls); four of the seven cases had brainstem tumours, whereas these generally account for 9–13% of paediatric patients with CNS tumours.

Wilkins and Koutras (1988), in a study in Ohio of similar design (i.e., mortality-based and using information from birth certificates), found a positive association between brain tumours and paternal employment in electrical assembling, installing and repairing occupations in the machinery industry (RR = 2.7, 95% CI 1.2–6.1). This group of occupations was associated with an odds ratio of 1.3 (95% CI 0.6–3.0) in the study of Johnson and Spitz (1989). Subsequently, in a study of cases with brain tumours ascertained from a tumour registry in which information was obtained by interview with both parents, no association was found with the group of occupations which Spitz and Johnson (1985) had found to be associated with an elevated risk of neuroblastoma (Wilkins & Sinks, 1990).

Towards the end of the interviewing period for this study, a mother of a case reported spontaneously in the course of interview that each of three co-workers of her spouse was the parent of a child recently diagnosed with an intracranial neoplasm (Wilkins *et al.*, 1991). These children were not included in the original case–control study, but were later contacted and interviewed. During the course of these interviews, two further children in whom brain tumours had been diagnosed recently were identified. Each child had one parent (two mothers, four fathers) employed by the same company for more than a year before conception, during pregnancy, and for at least six months after birth. Four of the six were still employed by the company at the time of the child's diagnosis. The company was an electronics firm where more than 100 chemical compounds were used in a manufacturing process. About the same time that the connection between the cases was coming to light, a paediatric neurosurgeon contacted the investigators to report what he perceived to be an unusually high number of referrals to treat children with brain tumours from the geographic area in question, a rural county in Ohio.

The six affected children were genetically unrelated and were diagnosed with a primary intracranial tumour within $2^{1}/_{2}$ years of one another. Two cases had astrocytoma, two medulloblastoma, one ependymoma and one an optic nerve glioma. The age at diagnosis ranged from six months to 14 years 10 months. Two mothers reported that they had received dental X-rays in the prenatal period, and three of the index cases were reported to have received dental X-rays. The only non-occupational factor common to all six case families was the use of aerosol insecticides in the home.

As the company is a major employer in a small town in a sparsely populated rural area, the possibility that the cluster was a manifestation of a regional effect was considered. However, no pattern was identified for the 23 counties surrounding the town, and spot maps of case residences did not indicate any pattern of common water supply or proximity to sources of environmental contamination. The authors acknowledged that a diversity of tumour types was observed, but note that astrocytomas, ependymomas and medulloblastomas are all neuroectodermal in origin and that in animal experiments different types of glioma are produced in the offspring after administration of a single dose of carcinogen to the dam. The histological type of tumour may depend on dose and timing of administration.

Kuijten *et al.* (1992) applied the classification of Lin *et al.* (1985) in a study of astrocytoma including 163 case–control pairs. The relative risk associated with 'definite' exposure of the father during the preconceptional period was 1.1 (19 discordant pairs), during pregnancy 0.9 (17 discordant pairs), and postnatally 0.8 (16 discordant pairs). For 'probable' exposure, the relative risks were 1.7, 1.6 and 1.3, respectively; none of these was statistically significant. No association was observed for paternal work in 'electrical assembling, installing and repairing', but a significant positive association, based on nine discordant pairs, was observed for electrical repair only in the preconceptional period.

## Leukaemia

In a study in Los Angeles designed primarily to assess the association between childhood leukaemia and residential exposure to electric and magnetic fields, univariate analysis showed an elevated odds ratio for paternal occupational exposure to 'non-ionizing radiation', and an odds ratio of 4.1 (95% CI 1.1–39.9) for maternal

exposure to 'non-ionizing radiation' during pregnancy (London *et al.*, 1991). No association between acute non-lymphocytic leukaemia and maternal or paternal exposure to 'non-ionizing radiation', including radar and microwave ovens, was found in the multicentre study of Buckley *et al.* (1989b). In a study of ALL in Spain, maternal occupational exposure to 'electricity' during pregnancy was associated with an odds ratio of 0.7, based on five discordant pairs (Infante-Rivard *et al.*, 1991). In view of the association between Down's syndrome and leukaemia, and in view of a reported association between Down's syndrome and military radar exposure (Sigler *et al.*, 1965), Hicks *et al.* (1984) also considered paternal radar-related occupations and military service. No association was found with either of these.

In a study in Spain, Infante-Rivard *et al.* (1991) found a positive association between ALL and the mother having worked at home during pregnancy (RR = 5.8, 95% CI 1.3–26.3, adjusted for birth year, sex, place of residence, household income and the mother's level of schooling). Most of the women were hired by local industries to sew different types of material on a machine. It was suggested that exposure to organic dust and synthetic fibres could have been responsible for the excess risk. Subsequently, it was noted that the electromagnetic field exposures associated with work using factory or home sewing machines are among the highest for any profession, and that this might account for the association observed in the Spanish study (Infante-Rivard, 1995). A limitation of the study of Infante-Rivard *et al.* (1991) is that the residential mobility of cases and controls may have differed. Cases (*n* = 128) were diagnosed during the period 1983–85, whereas controls were selected from the 1981 census. While annual updates of addresses were available if they had been reported by the family, only 67 of the 128 controls for which interview data were obtained were the first potential control selected from census records. About half the unsuccessful attempts to obtain controls were due to the potential control having moved, and about a third were due to no one being at home at the time that the interviewer called. Both of these factors might be related to employment in pregnancy, and therefore the possibility of selection bias cannot be excluded. In a sensitivity analysis in which it was assumed that unlocated controls were 10 times more likely to be working at home than located controls, the relative risk was 2.8, but was still statistically significant.

Infante-Rivard (1995) also suggested that maternal occupational exposure to electromagnetic fields during pregnancy might account for the association between ALL and maternal employment in the textile industry observed in a study in the Netherlands (van Steensel-Moll *et al.*, 1985b). However, no association between leukaemia and maternal work in textile-related occupations was observed in studies in northern England (McKinney *et al.*, 1987) or in Shanghai, China (Shu *et al.*, 1988).

## All types of childhood cancer combined

Bonde *et al.* (1992) investigated the offspring of a cohort of 27 071 Danish men who had been employed for a year or more in Danish steel or mild steel manufacturing companies during the period 1964–84, as identified from records of the national pension fund. A total of 26 529 liveborn children contributing 233 810 person-years of observation was identified from the national population register. Cases of cancer were identified by linkage with the national cancer registry. Two cases (2.6 expected) of childhood cancer were observed among 1774 offspring (17 254 person-years) of fathers verified as having been employed in stainless steel welding before conception, four cases (4.3 expected) among 2764 children (29 077 person-years) whose fathers had been employed in mild steel welding only, and four cases (2.7 expected; RR = 1.5, 95% CI 0.5–3.6) among 1867 children (18 057 person-years) whose fathers were verified as not having been involved in welding. Among the 16 489 offspring (183 866 person-years) whose fathers included metal-workers with unverified job title or department, other production workers, and white-collar workers, the relative risk of childhood cancer was 0.97 (26 observed cases).

## Synthesis of results: parental occupational exposure

No consistent association between inferred paternal occupational exposure to electromagnetic fields and neuroblastoma is apparent. Raised odds ratios have been apparent for some subgroups of paternal occupations in studies of CNS tumours, but the subgroups involved have differed between the studies. It has been suggested

that publication bias may be important as regards the association between CNS tumours and paternal occupational exposure to electromagnetic fields (NRPB, 1992). No direct measures of exposure to magnetic or electric fields have been made in any of the studies. The analysis of Wilkins and Hundley (1990) illustrates the inconsistencies which may be obtained by applying different indirect definitions of exposure. Little information is available on the effects of maternal occupational exposure to electromagnetic fields. Thus, the available evidence is inadequate to assess the role of paternal occupational exposure to electromagnetic fields in the etiology of childhood cancer.

## Conclusions

Childhood leukaemia has been found to be associated with calculated historical exposure to magnetic fields in four out of five studies in which this has been assessed. However, no consistent association is apparent for measured magnetic fields. It has been suggested that the inconsistency between these two sets of findings may be because fields measured near the time of diagnosis are a poor indicator of past exposure. However, in a recent large study, in which measurements were obtained for more than 90% of the reference period for 83% of the study subjects, no association with measured magnetic fields was found, but a small increase in risk among children resident in homes with very high magnetic fields, as suggested in the studies based on calculated historical exposures, could not be excluded. No consistent association between childhood leukaemias and residential proximity to radio and television transmitters has been observed.

Early reports suggesting an association between brain tumours and residential exposure to magnetic fields have not been confirmed. No consistent association between CNS tumours and inferred paternal occupational exposure to electromagnetic fields has been observed. These studies are limited by the lack of direct measurement of occupational exposure.

# Chapter 6

# Exposures to chemicals and dusts

In this chapter, associations between childhood cancer and parental occupational and environmental exposures to chemicals and dusts are considered.

Investigations of associations between childhood cancer and parental occupation have been of two types. The first includes those in which the complete range of occupations of the father, the mother, or both parents, before or during pregnancy, at the time of birth, or after birth, have been considered, i.e., studies in which there was no prior hypothesis. An important difficulty in interpreting the findings of such studies is multiple statistical testing. In addition, it is difficult to compare the results of these studies because of the diversity of methods of grouping job titles and industries. Second, there are those in which a small group of occupations, or a specific occupational exposure, has been examined.

In this chapter, emphasis is given to studies in which specific occupational exposures to chemicals and dusts were investigated, in view of the difficulty of comparing the findings from studies of parental occupations in which there were no prior hypotheses. Studies of parental occupational exposure to ionizing radiation are discussed in Chapter 4, and exposures to electromagnetic fields in Chapter 5.

In virtually all of the studies, paternal occupations were considered. Hypotheses regarding the effects of paternal occupational exposures include: (1) preconceptional occupational exposure of the father may cause childhood cancer through the mechanism of germ-cell mutation; (2) occupational exposure of the father leads to passive exposure of the mother, for example as a result of residual contamination of working clothes, in the preconceptional period, during pregnancy, or during the nursing period (Knishkowy & Baker, 1986); (3) postnatal occupational exposure of the father leads to passive exposure of the child during the lifetime of the child (McDiarmid & Weaver, 1993).

Information on maternal occupation was obtained in about half of the studies. This information could not be obtained in the studies based on birth or death certificates, as in these, usually only the occupation of the father is recorded. As the proportion of women of reproductive age in employment is substantially lower than that of men, the data on associations with maternal occupations tend to be rather limited. Hypotheses regarding the effects of maternal occupational exposures include: (1) toxins resulting from the mother's preconceptional occupational exposure accumulate in her tissues and subsequently have an adverse effect on the developing embryo or fetus; (2) occupational exposure of the mother during pregnancy has an adverse effect on the developing embryo or fetus; (3) cumulative exposure before the birth of the child and/or during the nursing period influences the composition of breast milk, in turn affecting the infant; (4) children of a woman who works may be passively, and possibly actively, exposed to the working environment of the mother.

The studies of parental occupation have been based on: (1) self-reporting; (2) groupings based on job titles and industries; or (3) job–exposure matrices. In some of the studies based on self-report, analyses have been made for more than one period of exposure: preconceptional, during pregnancy, and between birth and a reference date before diagnosis. In such studies, the observations are not independent.

In the largest studies, routine sources of information about parental occupation have been used, such as birth certificates, death certificates, antenatal clinic records, pension fund records and census information. In other studies, data were obtained by interview or postal questionnaire. In a substantial proportion of the studies in which data were obtained by interview, information on paternal occupation was obtained from the mother. Shalat et al. (1987) assessed the accuracy of information on men's occupational exposure to solvents obtained from their wives. The wives of 26 men, who were seen as outpatients for occupational lung disease or chronic obstructive pulmonary disease unrelated to organic solvent exposure, were interviewed by telephone. There were specific questions on the husband's exposure to organic solvents in the workplace, and a complete occupational history was taken. The wives were requested to refrain from discussing the subject of the interview with their husbands, and they were requested not to ask their husbands for information if they were present in the home at the time of the phone call. The same information was obtained from the men subsequently. There was 58% concordance between the husbands' and wives' responses to a simple question regarding solvent exposure; the associated kappa value was 0.18, indicating poor agreement. When solvent exposure status was determined by a modification of the job–exposure matrix approach developed by Hoar *et al.* (1980) and Hsieh *et al.* (1983), the concordance was 81% (kappa = 0.71). The true accuracy of this approach is undefined as the comparison related to recalled work histories and recalled exposures to solvents.

Joffe (1992) compared reports of exposure to eight agents in the present or most recent job with information derived from management in five factories in the printing and plastics industries in England in 1986. The study was carried out in the context of research on the reproductive effects of occupational exposures. The data were obtained by interviewers trained to administer the questionnaire, including an extensive reproductive history section, but apart from this they had no training or experience in occupational hygiene or any related discipline. Values of sensitivity ranged from 24% to 85%, and specificity was at least 67% for seven of the eight agents. The specificity of reported exposure to solvents and degreasing agents was 48%. Exposures which were described in chemically specific terms, for example imidazoline, tended to be reported with higher specificity but lower sensitivity. The author noted that future studies which use employees' reports of exposures would benefit from preparatory work to discover and incorporate the everyday names of agents in use. Subjects who reported a phase of subfertility or at least one miscarriage did not have a higher proportion of false positives than the study group as a whole, indicating an absence of reporting bias.

Shaw *et al.* (1990) compared parental occupation as recorded on birth certificates in California with maternal occupation during first trimester of pregnancy and paternal occupation three months before conception, as determined by interview with the mother between three and

seven years after the birth of the child. For 71% of mothers and 80% of fathers, the occupation on the birth certificate was the same as the occupation determined from the interview. These proportions were similar for cases of severe congenital heart disease and controls. Sensitivity of the birth certificate for determining whether a mother or father was employed in a particular standard occupational category ranged from 50% to 100%. The magnitude of a bias associated with a sensitivity of 75% and a specificity of 80% on the observed odds ratio was considered. In this situation, for a prevalence of exposure of 20% in controls, a true odds ratio of 10 would be observed as an odds ratio of approximately 3. When the prevalence of the exposure is 5%, a true odds ratio of 10 would be observed as an odds ratio of about 2.

In a number of studies in the USA, a system developed by Hoar *et al.* (1980) to link occupations and exposures was used. The linkage system includes an occupation code, an agent list, and links between occupations and agents, with some minimal information on the degree to which workers are exposed to each agent. Occupations were categorized by industry, using the categories defined in the US census of 1970, and by task within the industry, using the United States Dictionary of Occupational Titles. The categorization depends on the level of detail regarding chemical or physical exposure in particular processes. In all, 501 occupational categories were distinguished. The agent list was intended primarily to include known or suspected chemical carcinogens, but was expanded to include some chemicals with other chronic or acute effects. The list was developed by review of the literature published between 1962 and 1977. Some 376 agents were listed. Thus, there are over 15 000 pairs of occupations and agents. A three-level grading of the degree of exposure to an agent which a specific task involves was applied: (1) associated with high degree of exposure to the agent; (2) processing occupations in the same industry as jobs associated with a high degree of exposure to the agent; and (3) engineers, managers, officials, sales persons, production clerks or professionals in the same industry as jobs associated with a high degree of exposure.

Hsieh *et al.* (1983) developed a condensed classification which was applied in several studies of childhood cancer in the USA. First, agents were grouped into 24 categories based on chemical and physical class to form an abridged linkage system. Second, a hierarchical clustering scheme was used to group the occupations linked with each of the 24 categories of agents. Two hundred and forty seven clusters were identified by the statistical procedure, which can themselves be aggregated. Hsieh *et al.* suggested that 30 clusters appeared to provide a manageable cluster scheme.

Wilkins and Sinks (1990) commented that a number of uncertainties remain concerning the validity of the job–exposure matrix developed by Hoar *et al.* (1980), resulting from the focus on known or suspected carcinogens, the lack of validation of the exposure links and the associated estimates of intensity of exposure, and the reliance on review of literature from the 1960s and 1970s. Regarding the last point, volumes 2–10 of the International Agency for Research on Cancer's *Monographs on the Evaluation of Carcinogenic Risks of Chemicals to Man* (1972–76) were used by Hoar *et al.*; as of July 1997, some 69 volumes had been published in this series. Linet *et al.* (1987) found that that the Hoar *et al.* job–exposure matrix demonstrated poor sensitivity but rather high specificity as compared with self-reported occupational exposure to benzene or asbestos. In studies of lung and bladder cancer in adults, analyses using the job–exposure matrix have detected some, but not all, known carcinogens (Bunin *et al.*, 1989b).

In addition to studies of parental occupational exposures, studies of environmental (including household) exposures to chemicals and dusts are considered. These include case–control and ecological studies.

# Leukaemia

## *Pesticides*

Associations between childhood cancer and parental occupational and home exposure to pesticides have been investigated most extensively in relation to childhood leukaemia. Interest in the possible role of pesticides, including insecticides, fungicides and herbicides, in the etiology of childhood leukaemia has been stimulated by the observation of higher incidences in rural than urban areas (see Chapter 2), and by their high biological activity (IARC, 1987). The available studies vary according to the types of leukaemia included, and the specific types and circumstances of exposure considered.

## *Leukaemia of all types combined*

A positive association (RR = 3.5) with maternal occupational exposure to pesticides in pregnancy was found in a study of 309 cases and population-based controls in Shanghai, but was not statistically significant when the analysis

was restricted to women who had reported exposure to a least one of a specified list of agents (Shu *et al.*, 1988). The association appeared to be stronger for acute lymphocytic leukaemia (ALL) than for acute non-lymphocytic leukaemia (ANLL). As already discussed (Chapter 4), a limitation of this study is that controls were not contemporaneous with cases.

In a hospital-based study in Mexico city of 81 cases of leukaemia, 77 community controls matched on age and area of residence, and 77 hospital controls free of neoplastic disease and similarly matched, the relative risk associated with exposure to fertilizers was 4.7 (95% CI 1.1–24.1) and that associated with exposure to insecticides was 1.9 (95% CI 1.1–3.6) (Fajardo-Gutiérrez *et al.*, 1993a). When separate comparisons were made with each control group, the risks were higher in the comparison with hospital than with community controls. It is not clear whether the analysis related to direct postnatal exposure of the child or whether gestational exposure was included.

In a horticultural community in the Netherlands, a four-fold excess of haemato-poietic malignancies in young persons was observed during the period 1980–85 (Mulder *et al.*, 1993, 1994). Subsequently a population-based study was made of the 14 cases diagnosed at ages under 40 years between 1975 and 1989, with four controls per case matched on age and sex selected via local general practitioners. All cases and controls identified participated in the study. There were seven cases of leukaemia (median age six years) and seven of lymphomas (median age 25 years). The relative risk associated with paternal exposure to pesticides of at least three hours per week was 3.2 (95% CI 1.0–10.1), while that associated with the subject's direct exposure of comparable duration was 6.0 (95% CI 0.6–49.3). The corresponding relative risks associated with exposure to petroleum products were 9.0 (95% CI 1.0–66.1) and 8.0 (95% CI 2.2–129.9) respectively. Swimming for at least an hour a week in the local pond was associated with a relative risk of 5.3 (95% CI 1.3–17.4); in the 1970s, the pond had been polluted by accidents with pesticides and petroleum products.

Leiss and Savitz (1995) investigated reported use of home pesticides in a study of childhood cancer in Denver, Colorado (USA) diagnosed in the period 1976–83, in which the primary aim was to investigate associations with electromagnetic fields (see Chapter 5). In the course of interview with the parents, information was sought about use of home pest extermination, treatment of the area around the home with insecticides or herbicides and use of pest strips. Positive associations between use of pest strips and leukaemia were found. The relative risk associated with reported use during the last three months of pregnancy was 3.0 (95% CI 1.6–5.7), that for use in the period from birth until two years before diagnosis 1.7 (95% CI 1.2–2.4) and that for use in the two-year period before diagnosis 2.6 (95% CI 1.7–3.9). The insecticide used in pest strips was dichlorvos, an organophosphate which has been associated with adult onset leukaemia in men (Brown *et al.*, 1990), and exposure to which has been reported in case reports of childhood leukaemia (Reeves *et al.*, 1981). Home pest extermination and insecticide/herbicide treatment of the area around the home were not associated with leukaemia in this study.

In a study in Lower Saxony, Germany, data on 173 cases of childhood leukaemia diagnosed in the period 1988–93 were compared with data from (*a*) local controls, matched with cases on age, sex and area of residence and (*b*) state controls, matched with cases on age and sex only (Meinert *et al.*, 1996). Data were obtained by a combination of postal questionnaire and telephone interview. The participation rates were 77% for parents of cases and 69% for parents of controls. Working as a farmer, gardener or florist was considered to involve potential exposure to pesticides. There was no clear association with either parent having worked for at least one year in one of these occupations within the interval from two years before the birth of the index child until diagnosis. There was no association with reported direct contact with pesticides in the course of such work. In the comparison with local controls, the relative risk associated with pesticide use in gardens or on farms was 2.5 (95% CI 1.1–5.4). No association was apparent in the comparison with state controls, but this may have been the result of a higher proportion of such controls being resident in rural areas. There was no association with reported extermination of insects in the home.

*Acute leukaemia*

A positive association between acute leukaemia and maternal exposure during pregnancy and lactation, and paternal exposure during pregnancy, to household pesticides (RR for use by either parent at least once a week = 3.8, 95% CI 1.4–13.0, 24 discordant pairs) and to garden pesticides or herbicides (RR for use at least once a month = 6.5, 95% CI 1.5–59.3, 15

discordant pairs) was reported by Lowengart *et al.* (1987). These associations appear to be independent of one another and of paternal occupational exposure to chlorinated solvents and employment in the transport-equipment manufacturing industry, but the study is limited by a poor participation rate. Subsequently, in an extension of the study intended primarily to investigate the association with electromagnetic fields, London *et al.* (1991) found a positive association with insecticide use inside the house (RR = 2.5, 95% CI 1.5–4.4), but not out of doors, at any time during a reference period defined as from the date of the last menstrual period to the date of diagnosis minus a variable period depending on the age of the child at diagnosis.

In a study of 201 cases of acute leukaemia and controls hospitalized for other severe disease in Lyon, France, the relative risk associated with the father having worked in a job involving exposure to pesticides was 4.2 (95% CI 1.2–14.0; by unmatched analysis of matched data; Laval & Tuyns, 1988). This finding may be due to selection bias arising from differential referral patterns for cases and controls. In a cohort study of over 240 000 offspring, born in the period 1952–91, of men and women employed in agricultural work in Norway, no association between acute leukaemia (181 cases diagnosed at ages up to 39 years) and pesticide purchase as recorded in the 1969 census was observed (Kristensen *et al.*, 1996). As pesticide purchase is a crude indicator of exposure, and only information on purchases in the year preceding the 1969 census was available, considerable misclassification is likely to have occurred, which would have biased the estimated relative risk towards unity.

*ALL*

No association between ALL and maternal or paternal occupational exposure to "pesticides, herbicides, and insecticides" during pregnancy was found by Van Steensel-Moll *et al.* (1985b) in a study of 519 cases and population-based controls in the Netherlands, or between ALL and maternal occupational exposure to insecticides during pregnancy by Infante-Rivard *et al.* (1991) in Spain, based on 128 cases and population-based controls.

In a multicentre study of 990 cases of ALL and 1636 controls with other types of cancer in the USA and Canada, the relative risk associated with paternal exposure to insecticides was 1.2 ($p > 0.1$) while that associated with exposure of the index child was 1.6 ($p < 0.01$; Buckley *et al.*, 1994). In a comparison between a subset of 404 cases and individually matched controls selected by random-digit dialling, the relative risk associated with paternal exposure was 2.8 (*p* < 0.001) and that with exposure of the child 5.0 (*p* < 0.001). A possible explanation for these inconsistencies is that the cancer control group included diseases that might have a similar etiology to ALL or one of its subtypes. For example, 11% of the subjects in this control group had ANLL, 15% had brain tumours, 14% had neuroblastoma and 10% had Wilms' tumour, and positive associations with pesticides, insecticides or herbicides have been reported for all of these. Analyses by immunophenotype also were carried out. The strongest associations for both paternal exposure and exposure of the index child were apparent for T-cell and common cell leukaemia.

## ANLL

In a multicentre study of 204 cases of ANLL and controls selected by random-digit dialling in the USA and Canada, Buckley *et al.* (1989a) reported positive associations with self-reported maternal occupational exposure to pesticides before (RR = 3.0, 3 exposed cases), during (RR = 6.0, 4 exposed cases) and after (RR = 7.0, 2 exposed cases) pregnancy. Self-reported paternal occupational exposure was associated with relative risks of 1.7–1.9 for the same periods. Paternal occupational exposure inferred by the job–exposure matrix of Hoar *et al.* (1980) was associated with a relative risk of 2.3 (*p* = 0.05). A significant association with duration of exposure was apparent for maternal exposure and a positive association of borderline significance was found for paternal exposure. These associations appeared to be more pronounced for the myelomonocytic (M4) or monocytic (M5) morphology than for the acute myelocytic (M1/M2) morphology. In addition, Buckley *et al.* (1989b) assessed associations with maternal exposure to household fly-sprays, pesticides and garden or agricultural sprays, and treatment of the house by insect exterminators, in the month before the last menstrual period and during the index pregnancy. Similarly, associations were assessed with direct exposure of the child to household pesticides, garden sprays and insect exterminations. There were significant trends of increase in risk with increasing frequency of exposure for both intra-uterine (*p* value for trend 0.05) and postnatal (*p* value for trend 0.04) exposure. These associations appeared to be independent of parental occupational exposure. The authors noted that if there were recall bias arising from

a general perception that pesticides are potentially hazardous to health, this association should have been observed in their other studies relating to childhood cancers, but there was no evidence of this.

## Summary

In most of the available studies, a positive association between leukaemia and pesticide exposure of the index child during his or her lifetime has been observed. The available data are inadequate to assess whether the association is apparent only for certain specific agents. In addition, use of pesticides may be a marker of rural isolation, so the possibility of confounding by patterns of exposure to infection which may be associated with population mixing (see Chapter 7) cannot be excluded. The associations with maternal and paternal occupational exposures are less consistent. No consistent association between leukaemia and employment of the father in agriculture has been found (Fabia & Thuy, 1974; Hemminki *et al.*, 1981; Van Steensel-Moll *et al.*, 1985b; Lowengart *et al.*, 1987; McKinney *et al.*, 1987; Shu *et al.*, 1988; Gardner *et al.*, 1990a; Magnani *et al.*, 1990; Olsen *et al.*, 1991; Roman *et al.*, 1993; Kristensen *et al.*, 1996; Meinert *et al.*, 1996). In two studies, data specifically on ANLL and maternal occupational exposure were presented; the results were inconsistent.

# Agent Orange

Between 1961 and 1971, over 1.7 million hectares of what was then South Viet Nam were sprayed by aircraft with phenoxy herbicides, in an intensive defoliation campaign known as 'Operation Ranch Hand' (Sterling & Arundel, 1986). Agent Orange accounted for 61% of the total volume of herbicides used in the war, and contained peak concentrations of 2,3,7,8-tetra-chlorodibenzo-*para*-dioxin (TCDD) of up to 60 parts per million, with an average of 2 parts per million.

The US Centers for Disease Control undertook a multidimensional assessment of the health of Viet Nam veterans, mandated by Congress, known as the Vietnam Experience Study (Centers for Disease Control Vietnam Experience Study, 1988). A random sample of 48 513 records was drawn from approximately 4.9 million records of personnel who served in the US army during the period of its involvement in Viet Nam. To increase comparability between those who served in Viet Nam and those who served elsewhere, the sample was restricted to those who entered army service during the period

1965–71, served only one term of enlistment, had at least 16 weeks of active service, earned a military occupational speciality other than "trainee" or "duty soldier", and had a pay grade no higher than sergeant when discharged from active service. Application of these criteria reduced the sample size to 18 581, of whom 17 867 were alive on 31 December 1983. Telephone interviews were completed with 7924 (87%) of those who had served in Viet Nam and 7364 (84%) of those who served elsewhere. 25 cancers were reported among children of Viet Nam veterans, and 17 among those of non-Viet Nam veterans. After adjustment for a number of variables relating to army service, maternal age and gravidity, the relative risk was 1.5 (95% CI 0.8–2.8). The main type of childhood cancer observed was leukaemia, with 12 cases among children of Viet Nam veterans and seven amongs children of non-Viet Nam veterans (crude odds ratio 1.6, 95% CI 0.6–4.1). The authors noted that for most reproductive and child health outcomes studied, Viet Nam veterans were more likely to report an adverse event than were non-Viet Nam veterans.

Concern expressed by Viet Nam veterans in the USA about the possibility that exposure to herbicides, notably Agent Orange, might increase the risk of fathering a child with congenital anomalies prompted the Centers for Disease Control to conduct an investigation based on the Metropolitan Atlanta Congenital Defects Program (Erickson *et al.*, 1984). As the investigators were concerned that herbicide exposure assessed by interview would be prone to recall bias, the investigation focused on the fact of service in Viet Nam. A total of 7529 cases of major malformation born during the period 1968–80 were initially identified. After exclusion of births given up for adoption and births which had been included in a pilot study, and the random choice of one birth from sibships in which more than one birth was affected, 7133 births remained eligible for study. The control group comprised live births frequency-matched on ethnic group and year and hospital of birth. 4246 controls were initially identified as eligible. Interviews were carried out during the years 1982 and 1983, and responses about Viet Nam service were verified from army records. Some 56.3% of eligible fathers completed telephone interviews, with most losses reflecting a failure to trace the individual concerned rather than a refusal. Overall, the participation rates were very similar in the case and control groups, and there was little difference in the participation rates of parents of cases by type of anomaly. Eight-seven

cases with "other neoplasms" were included. The odds ratio of this category of anomalies for Viet Nam veterans compared with other men was 1.8 (95% CI 1.0–3.3). Among the offspring of Viet Nam veterans and all other fathers, the neoplasms classified in this group included CNS tumours (5 cases), neuroblastomas (3 cases), Wilms' tumours (3 cases), hepatoblastoma (1 case), rhabdomyosarcoma (1 case), teratomas (14 cases), dermoid and epidermoid cysts (26 cases), lipomas (9 cases), haematomas (5 cases), and miscellaneous benign tumours (24 cases). The observed relative risk should be seen in the context of tests having been performed on 95 categories of congenital anomalies, with only one of which (specified anomalies of the nails) a significant association was found (odds ratio 4.2). Two indices of "exposure opportunity" to Agent Orange were calculated, without knowledge of case or control status. The first was based on occupation, location, and time of service in Viet Nam as recorded in military records. This information was available for 75% of the total of 428 fathers of cases with congenital anomalies of any type, including neoplasms, who had served in Viet Nam, and 67% of the 268 fathers of controls who had served there. The odds ratio for "other neoplasms" associated with the highest level of the score compared with non-Viet Nam service was 2.0; this was not statistically significant. The second score was based on occupation, location and time of service in Viet Nam as determined by interview of Viet Nam veterans. This information was available for 81% of the 428 Viet Nam veteran fathers of cases with anomalies of any type, and 75% of the 268 Viet Nam veteran fathers of control infants. The odds ratio for "other neoplasms" associated with the highest level of the score compared with non-Viet Nam service was 3.7; this was statistically significant. The odds ratios relating to these two "exposure opportunity" indices were stratified by ethnic group and by year and hospital of birth. Further adjustment for maternal age, maternal education, maternal alcohol consumption, the occurrence of congenital anomalies in first-degree relatives of the index birth, and up to 108 additional variables (evaluated for potential confounding), depending on the type of anomaly, gave very similar results.

The final assessment of exposure was based on Viet Nam veterans' reports of exposure to Agent Orange. As recall bias was considered to be potentially a major issue, the analysis was made by internal comparison among parents of infants with major congenital anomalies. About 25% of the Viet Nam veterans interviewed believed that they had been exposed; approximately the same proportion reported that they did not know whether they had been exposed. No significant association for any specific anomaly or group of anomalies was found. The odds ratio for "other neoplasms" was 1.5; this was not statistically significant.

Erickson *et al.* (1984) considered that the nominally significant association between the exposure opportunity index based on interviews and neoplasms could be attributed to unidentified bias or confounding, or chance. Another issue concerns the completeness of ascertainment of neoplasms in a system designed to identify congenital anomalies identified during the first year of life.

In a case–control study of congenital anomalies associated with army service in Viet Nam commissioned by the Australian government, 8517 infants with congenital anomalies, detected at birth or in the first week of life, born in hospitals in New South Wales, Victoria, and the Australian Capital Territory during the period 1966–79, were identified from hospital and cytogenetic laboratory records (Report to the Minister for Veterans' Affairs, 1983; Donovan *et al.*, 1984). Infants with anomalies were matched with liveborn infants without diagnosed anomalies on hospital of birth, maternal age, date of birth and, where possible, the "payment category" for the hospital services. Details of the father were cross-matched with Australian army lists for the period of Australian involvement in Viet Nam (1962–72). There were four cases of "other hamartoses, not elsewhere classified", none of whose fathers had served in the army in the relevant period.

None of 80 births with congenital anomalies of all types in 919 live births to Ranch Hand veterans, almost certainly the group of servicemen most heavily exposed to Agent Orange, was reported to have a congenital neoplasm (Lathrop *et al.*, 1984).

## Hydrocarbons, including benzene

In the course of reviewing a small sample of birth and death certificates of children in Quebec, Fabia and Thuy (1974) observed that a large proportion of fathers of children who had died from cancer appeared to work in petrol-related occupations. The authors proceeded to a formal investigation of the association between deaths due to cancer and paternal occupations involving potential exposure to hydrocarbons at the time of the child's birth. These occupations included motor-vehicle mechanics, machinists,

miners and painters. Data on 386 deaths due to childhood cancer before the age of five years in Quebec in the period 1965–70 were compared with data on 772 controls, selected as the births immediately preceding and immediately following that of the case in the birth registration files. The relative risks of leukaemia and lymphoma ($n = 218$) associated with each of the three occupational categories considered were about two. This finding stimulated investigations into the possible risk of parental occupational exposures in the etiology of childhood cancer.

Associations between childhood leukaemia and paternal occupational exposure to hydrocarbons are summarized in Table 6.1. The original study of Fabia and Thuy (1974) has been excluded from the tabulation as it generated the hypothesis. In most of the studies, exposure was inferred from job title. For purposes of comparison, results relating to the period nearest to the time of birth of the index child have been tabulated.

No consistent association between paternal occupational exposure to hydrocarbons of all types combined and leukaemia of all types or ALL has been observed (Table 6.1). In some studies, more than one reference period of exposure was considered (Gold *et al.*, 1982; Lowengart *et al.*, 1987; Buckley *et al.*, 1989b; McKinney *et al.*, 1991). Within each of these studies, the associations were fairly similar for the different reference periods; the observation that the associations were statistically significant for some reference periods but not others is unlikely to be of importance in view of the probable dependence of exposure between reference periods and the fact that multiple significance testing was performed.

In five studies, paternal exposure to benzene was considered (Shaw *et al.*, 1984; Lowengart *et al.*, 1987; Buckley *et al.*, 1989b; McKinney *et al.*, 1991; Feingold *et al.*, 1992). No consistent association was apparent.

Few studies of maternal occupational exposure to hydrocarbons during pregnancy and childhood leukaemia have been carried out (Table 6.2). With regard to ALL, the two available studies of all types of hydrocarbon combined are inconsistent (Van Steensel-Moll *et al.*, 1985b; Infante-Rivard *et al.*, 1991), and a further study showed no striking association for specific types of hydrocarbon (Shu *et al.*, 1988). In a single study, no clear association with home exposure of either parent to petroleum products during the index pregnancy was found (Lowengart *et al.*, 1987). However, in two out of three studies of ANLL, a positive association with hydrocarbons was apparent. This may be compatible with the observation that benzene is positively associated with ANLL in adults (IARC, 1987). In the study in which no association between childhood ANLL and maternal exposure to hydrocarbons in pregnancy was apparent (Buckley *et al.*, 1989b), there was a significant positive association with reported postnatal exposure of the index child to petroleum products (*p* value for trend = 0.02).

In a number of studies, residential proximity to sources of environmental exposure to hydrocarbons has been considered.

Local concern about the incidence of leukaemia and lymphoma in children and young people in the vicinity of the petrochemical plant at Balgan Bay, South Wales, led to investigation by a television company and a formal investigation (Lyons *et al.*, 1995). Throughout the life of the plant, which opened in 1963, it has produced chain hydrocarbons including ethylene, cyclic hydrocarbons including benzene, polymers such as polyvinyl chloride, and ethanol. The observed numbers of cases of leukaemia and lymphoma diagnosed before the age of 25 years during the period 1974–91 in persons resident within 1.5 and 3.0 km of the plant were compared with those expected on the basis of national rates for Wales. These radii had been chosen by the television company's investigators for unknown reasons. There was no significant excess in any of the comparisons made. In an accompanying paper, Sans *et al.* (1995) analysed the incidence of, and mortality due to, leukaemia in children aged 0–14 years in the area defined by a circle of 7.5 km radius centred on the petrochemical plant during the period 1974–84, using boundary free methods. There was no excess of leukaemia or mortality in the area as a whole compared with regionally adjusted national rates, and there was no evidence of decline in risk with distance.

Knox (1994) sought to validate previously demonstrated spatial clustering of childhood leukaemias (Knox & Gilman, 1992b) by comparing the distances of cluster locations and control locations to a variety of map features. A file of 9406 registrations of childhood leukaemia and non-Hodgkin lymphoma in Great Britain during the period 1966–83 was searched for all pairs whose addresses at diagnosis were within 0.15 km of one another. These pairs were defined to be the clusters. Some of the pairs were components of larger aggregations, and the location of these

was summarized as a single point. A total of 264 cluster locations was identified. Control locations were chosen as the addresses filed alternately 10 000 before and after that of the cluster location in the file of all 1.28 million residential postcodes in Britain. The map features included railways and trunk roads, considered to represent potential sources of pollution; surface water and wooded areas, considered to be possible sources of infection; and churches, considered (in cities) as an indicator of high population density, older houses and less affluent lifestyles. The mean distance between cluster locations and railways was 0.9 km, compared with 1.6 km for control locations. The mean distance between cluster locations and churches was 0.6 km, compared with 0.7 km for control locations. These differences were statistically significant. When the distance from railways was adjusted for distance from churches, the difference remained statistically significant. There was no difference in the pattern according to whether the line was electrified or not, or whether it was used for movement of goods only or for goods and passengers. No significant difference in distance from trunk roads or woodlands was found. The mean distance from cluster locations to surface water was significantly greater for cluster (0.7 km) than for control (0.5 km) locations.

Knox (1994) then carried out a search for industrial facilities served by railways, and investigated their proximity to cluster and control locations. The mean distance between oil and petroleum depots and terminals, petrochemical factories, oil storage and unloading farms, and refineries and cluster locations was 9.9 km, significantly less than the distance between these facilities and control locations (12.7 km). The mean distances from other installations were substantially greater, and did not differ significantly between cluster and control locations. In addition, Knox (1994) compared the distance of all 9406 cases and 9406 control locations selected randomly from the postcode file. The mean distance between cases and oil installations was significantly less than that between control locations and such installations. In both analyses, the distances from non-nuclear power stations, rail yards and steel works were less for cases than for controls, but the magnitude of the difference was less than for the oil installations. Knox (1994) suggested that childhood leukaemia may be associated with exposure to fossil fuels, especially petroleum, as a result of leakage,

185

**Table 6.1. Summary of the studies of the association between childhood leukaemia and lymphoma and paternal occupational exposure to hydrocarbons in the period nearest to the time of birth of the index child**

| Area and period of study | Cases — Deaths (D) or newly incident (I) cases, upper age limit | Cases — N | Controls — Type[a] | Controls — N | Exposure — Source of information (informant)[b] | Exposure — Period of exposure[c] | Exposure — Definition | Exposure — Subgroup | RR (95% CI or p) | Reference |
|---|---|---|---|---|---|---|---|---|---|---|
| **Leukaemia and lymphoma** Finland, 1959–75 | I, 14 | 339 | B | 339 | A (M) | B | Job description (FT)[d] | | 0.5 (0.1–1.9) | Hakulinen et al., 1976 |
| USA, Massachusetts, 1947–57 and 1963–67 (births) | D, 14 | 430 | B | 1372 | B | B | Job classification (FT)[d] | | 1.2 (0.9–1.6) | Kwa and Fine, 1980 |
| USA, Houston, TX, 1976–77 | I, 15 | 142 | H / N / C | 269 / 204 / 359 | I (M,F) | B | Job classification (FT)[d] | | 0.4 (0.2–1.1) / 1.0 (0.3–3.1) / 0.7 (0.3–1.8) | Zack et al., 1980 |
| UK, West Cumbria, North Humberside and Gateshead, 1974–88 | I, 14 | 100 | B | 169 | I (M,F) | Pg | Specific exposures | Xylene / Benzene | 3.2 (0.2–98.2) / 3.0 (0.5–24.2) | McKinney et al., 1991 |
| **Leukaemia** UK, England and Wales, 1959–63 1970–72 | D, 14 | 1771 / 1000 | D | 112840 / 54806 | DC | D | Job classification | | 0.9 (0.8–1.0)[f] / 0.9 (0.8–1.0)[f] | Sanders et al., 1981 |
| USA, Baltimore, 1965–74 | I, 19 | 43 | B / OC | 43 / 43 | I (M) | Pc, Pg | Job classification[f] | Narrow / Broad / Narrow / Broad | 1.0 (ns) / 0.8 (ns) / 2.5 (ns) / 3.0 (ns) | Gold et al., 1982 |
| USA, California, 1975–80 | I, 14 | 255 | B | 510 | B | B | Job classification | Benzene | 1.0 (ns) | Shaw et al., 1984 |
| **Acute leukaemia** USA, New York State (excl. city), 1949–78 | I, 1 | 60 | B | 60[g] | I (M) | Pc, Pg | Job classification | Heavy inferred exposure / Medium inferred exposure | 2.4 (p = 0.032)[g] / 1.3 (p = 0.345)[g] | Vianna et al., 1984 |
| USA, Los Angeles, 1980–84 | I, 10 | 123 | F, RDD | 123 | I (M,F) | Pg | Specific exposures | Oil or coal products / Benzene | 1.0[h] / 1.0[h] | Lowengart et al., 1987 |
| **ALL** The Netherlands, 1973–79 | I, 14 | 519 | R | 507 | Q (M,F) | Pg | Job classification / Specific exposures | Petroleum products, paint or other chemicals / Exhaust gases | 1.0 (0.6–1.7)[j] / 1.2 (0.8–1.7)[j] / 1.3 (0.8–1.9)[j] | Van Steensel-Moll et al., 1985b |
| USA, Denver, CO, 1976–83 | I, 14 | 59 | RDD | 222 | I (M) | Pg | Job-exposure matrix | Benzene | 1.3 (0.6–3.0)[j] / 1.6 (0.5–5.8)[j] | Feingold et al., 1992 |
| **ANLL** USA and Canada, multicentre, 1980–84 | I, 17 | 178 | RDD | 178 | I (M,F) | Pc–Dg | Job-exposure matrix / Specific exposure / >1000 days of exposure | Petroleum products / Petroleum products / Benzene | 1.0[h] / 2.4 (1.3–4.1) / 1.0[h] | Buckley et al., 1989b |

ns, Not statistically significant.
[a] Control type: B, selected from birth certificates; H, children hospitalized for reasons other than cancer; N, neighbourhood; C, cousins; D, selected from death records; OC, children with other types of cancer; F, friends of cases; RDD, selected by random-digit dialling; R, selected from population register.
[b] Source of information: A, parental interview at antenatal clinic visit; B, birth certificates; DC, death certificates; I, parental interview after diagnosis.

Informant: F, information obtained directly from the father for >50% of subjects; M, information obtained from the mother; ± father for <50% of subjects.
[c] Period of exposure: B, birth; Pg, pregnancy; D, death; Pc, pre-conceptional; Dg, diagnosis.
[d] Jobs classified according to method used by Fabia and Thuy (1974).
[e] Proportional mortality ratios.
[f] The narrow definition included factory workers, machinists, drivers, motor vehicle mechanics, service

**Table 6.2. Summary of studies of the association between childhood leukaemia and maternal exposure to hydrocarbons during pregnancy**

| Area and period of study | Cases Upper age limit | Cases N | Controls Type[a] | Controls N | Exposure Source of information[b] | Definition | Subgroup | RR (95% CI) | Reference |
|---|---|---|---|---|---|---|---|---|---|
| **Leukaemia and lymphoma** UK, West Cumbria, North Humberside and Gateshead, 1974–88 | 14 | 105 | B | 186 | I | Specific exposures | Xylene<br>Benzene | 1/0[c]<br>4.0 (0.3–118.0) | McKinney et al., 1991 |
| **Leukaemia** China, Shanghai, 1974–86 | 14 | 309 | R | 618 | I | Specific exposures | Benzene<br>Gasoline<br>Toluene<br>Kerosene<br>Diesel oil | 2.0 (0.9–4.3)[d,e]<br>1.6 (0.8–3.1)[d,e]<br>1.5 (0.6–3.4)[d,e]<br>1.4 (0.6–3.1)[d,e]<br>1.4 (0.6–3.3)[d,e] | Shu et al., 1988 |
| **ALL** The Netherlands, 1973–79 | 14 | 519 | R | 507 | Q | Job classification<br>Specific exposures | Petroleum products, paint and other chemicals<br>Exhaust gases | 2.5 (0.7–9.4)[f]<br>2.4 (1.2–4.6)[f]<br>4/0[c] | Van Steensel-Moll et al., 1985b |
| China, Shanghai, 1974–86 | 14 | 172 | R | 344 | I | Specific exposures | Benzene<br>Gasoline<br>Toluene<br>Kerosene | 1.3 (0.5–3.0)[e]<br>1.7 (1.0–3.0)[e]<br>1.2 (0.5–2.7)[e]<br>1.5 (0.6–3.4)[e] | Shu et al., 1988 |
| Spain, multicentre, 1983–85 | 14 | 128 | R | 128 | I | Specific exposure | Oil, grease or hydrocarbons | 0.5 (0.1–2.7) | Infante-Rivard et al., 1991 |
| **ANLL** China, Shanghai, 1974–86 | 14 | 94 | R | 188 | I | Specific exposures | Benzene<br>Gasoline<br>Toluene<br>Kerosene | 4.0 (1.8–9.3)[e]<br>2.1 (1.1–4.3)[e]<br>2.0 (0.8–5.0)[e]<br>2.3 (0.9–6.3)[e] | Shu et al., 1988 |
| USA and Canada, multicentre, 1980–84 | 17 | 204 | RDD | 204 | I | Job-exposure matrix<br>Specific exposures | Petroleum products<br>Oil or coal products<br>Benzene | 1.0[c]<br>1.0[g]<br>1.0[c] | Buckley et al., 1989b |
| The Netherlands, 1973–79 | 14 | 80 | R | 240 | Q | Job classification and specific exposures | | 3.3 (0.6–18.1)[h] | van Duijn et al., 1994 |

station attendants, miners and lumbermen. The broad definition included painters, dyers and cleaners, in addition to the categories included in the narrow definition.

g Controls were matched with cases by year of birth, sex, ethnic group, county of residence, age of mother and birth order. A second control group was used to assess maternal age and birth order, and matched for all of these factors except maternal age and birth order. Although data were presented on motor vehicle exhaust fumes in the comparison with the second group, these have been excluded from this table as confounding may have occurred.

h The authors stated that there was no association.

i Adjusted for age and sex.

j Adjusted for father's education.

a Control type: B, selected from birth certificates; R, selected from population register; RDD, selected by random-digit dialling.

b Source of information: I, maternal interview; Q, questionnaire.

c Cases exposed/controls exposed.

d Analysis restricted to subjects whose mothers reported at least one occupational exposure during pregnancy.

e Adjusted for age, sex, birthweight, birth order, urban/rural residence, chloramphenicol and syntomycin usage, prenatal and paternal preconceptional X-ray exposure, and mother's age at menarche.

f Adjusted for age and sex.

g The authors stated that there was no association.

h Adjusted for age, sex, social class, alcohol consumption, smoking, medication use, ultrasound, X-rays and viral infections during pregnancy.

evaporation or combustion; or some combination of these. A major limitation of this study was that no child population denominators were available. Control postcodes are likely to have had lower population densities than those of cases, so the associations observed by Knox (1994) may have been secondary to differences in population density (Bithell & Draper, 1995). In addition, control locations sampled from a file of postcodes are unlikely to have been representative of the distribution of the population at risk during the period when cases were diagnosed (1966–83). Movement of population away from the vicinity of the facilities would have compounded the difference in population densities between case and control locations (Bithell & Draper, 1995). In addition, the relationship between the date of diagnosis of cases and the periods of operation of the facilities was not taken into account.

Subsequently, Knox and Gilman (1997) applied a similar approach to the analysis of data on 22 458 deaths from leukaemia and other cancers in children aged up to 15 years in Great Britain during the period 1953–80. The locations of potentially hazardous industrial installations were obtained from business and other directories. The relationship between the birth and death addresses of the cases to these locations and to railway lines and motorways was investigated by counting the numbers of deaths (and births) at successive radial distances and comparing them with expected numbers based on a count of postcodes at similar distances. Relative excesses of leukaemia and solid cancers were found near oil refineries, major oil-storage installations, railside oil distribution terminals and factories making bitumen products. There was no excess around the six major UK benzene refineries. Substantial quantities of volatile organic compounds are discharged during painting of cars. There were excesses of leukaemia and solid cancers around 31 car factories, and in the vicinity of coach-building and body-repair firms. There were no excesses associated with brake or tyre manufacture. Excesses were observed around major users of petroleum products including galvanizing plants, which use solvents for metal-cleaning, spray painting contractors, paint and varnish manufactures, fibreglass fabricators, adhesive makers, factories undertaking powder coating of metals and factories making solvents other than halogenated hydrocarbons. However, there were no excesses associated with electroplating, which involves solvent-based metal cleaning, or

manufacture of chlorinated hydrocarbons. In view of the associations with car manufacture and with galvanizing, proximity to industries involving metal casting and refining was considered. There were positive associations with proximity to aluminium, zinc, iron and steel casting, and steelworks, but not with proximity to lead casting. Excesses were also observed around some other installations involving use of kilns and furnaces – power stations, crematoria, cement works and brickworks. However, there were no excesses around potteries or gasworks. There were associations with proximity to motorways, railways, airfields and harbours. The findings for leukaemias were similar to those for solid tumours. The associations were stronger when the birth addresses of cases were considered than for the addresses at diagnosis. As in the study of Knox (1994), suitable data on child population denominators were not available. A potential concern was that excesses would be secondary to high population densities. However, the population density around some sites was low because the sites were recognized potential hazards, and this also appeared to be the situation around installations which were less segregated, notably paper manufacturers, soap manufacturers, cotton spinners and weavers, brewers, mail-order firms and furniture manufacturers. If such a pattern applied to the other sites, it would dilute any excess observed. However, an important limitation is the lack of information about the relationship between the date of diagnosis of the cases and the period of operation of the installations.

In a multicentre study of ALL in the USA and Canada during the period 1982–91, the relative risk associated with reported exposure of the index child to petroleum products was 1.4 in comparison with controls with other types of cancer, and 1.9 in comparison with controls selected by random-digit dialling; neither of these was statistically significant (Buckley *et al.*, 1994). The association appeared to be confined to the pre-B-cell subtype.

In summary, no consistent association between leukaemia and paternal occupational exposure to hydrocarbons or benzene is apparent. Maternal occupational exposure has been less studied, but it is interesting that in two out of three studies of ANLL, a positive association with maternal occupational exposure to hydrocarbons was found. No clear association with residential proximity to industrial sources of hydrocarbons has been observed.

## Traffic

Savitz and Feingold (1989), in a study whose primary aim was to investigate the risks of childhood cancer associated with residential exposure to electromagnetic fields, found a significant positive association (RR = 2.1, 95% CI 1.1–4.0 based on 17 exposed cases) between leukaemia and the passage of 500 or more vehicles per day through the segment of the street in which the subject lived at the time of diagnosis or interview. This was similar to the relative risk (1.7, 95% CI 1.0–2.8) observed for all types of childhood cancer combined. The association with total childhood cancer was found only for children aged under 5 years at diagnosis, and was much stronger for subjects who lived in the same residence between birth and diagnosis or interview, and for girls than boys. There appears to have been a deficit of controls of low socioeconomic status (NRPB, 1992). Such a deficit might have produced a spurious association with a marker of low socioeconomic status, such as residential traffic density.

Wolff (1990) suggested that an alternative explanation to population mixing (see Chapter 7) for excesses of leukaemia in new towns may be locally higher exposure to benzene from gasoline evaporation and car exhausts caused by sudden local expansion in car ownership and usage. Later, Wolff (1992) suggested that greater use of cars might account for the association of childhood leukaemia with high socioeconomic status. In an analysis at county level of data from a specialist registry of haematopoietic malignancies covering a third of England and Wales during the period 1984–88, Wolff (1992) found a significant geographical correlation between the incidence of ALL and other haematopoietic malignancies diagnosed at all ages (i.e., including adults) and the average number of cars per household recorded in the 1981 census. He postulated that benzene exposure encountered inside cars during travelling and refuelling might account for this. A rapid local expansion in car ownership and usage would not readily explain the excesses associated with increasing proportions of servicemen in rural areas in 1950–53, when petrol rationing was still in force, or why only increases in commuting in, and not commuting out or absolute levels of commuting, were associated with childhood leukaemia (Kinlen & Hudson, 1991; Kinlen *et al.*, 1991; see Chapter 7).

Alexander *et al.* (1996) investigated the distribution of 438 cases of ALL diagnosed in children in the period 1984–89 recorded in the same specialist registry in relation to car ownership as recorded in the 1981 census at electoral ward level. There was no association between ALL and level of car ownership, either overall or for ALL diagnosed at the ages of 1–7 years, defined to include the childhood peak. The relative risk of ALL diagnosed at ages up to 14 years associated with residence in isolated towns and villages compared with built-up areas was 1.8 (95% CI 1.2–2.5), after adjustment for the Carstairs index of deprivation and proportion of households with no car. Thus, levels of car ownership cannot explain the increased rates of ALL observed in isolated areas.

## Solvents

Lowengart *et al.* (1987) reported an increased risk of childhood leukaemia associated with paternal occupational exposure to chlorinated solvents (Table 6.3). The risk was increased for all of the exposure periods considered – one year before pregnancy, during pregnancy, and after delivery. In each of these periods, the reported frequency of exposure of fathers who had ever been exposed was greater for fathers of cases than for fathers of controls. Subsequently, McKinney *et al.* (1991) reported positive associations between paternal occupational exposure to carbon tetrachloride or trichloroethylene (trichloroethene) and childhood leukaemia and non-Hodgkin lymphoma. These associations were apparent in all three reference periods considered, but may have been confounded by other occupational exposures. In a study of leukaemia and non-Hodgkin lymphoma in children and young people born in West Cumbria whose fathers had worked in the Sellafield plant, there was a positive association with potential paternal pre-conceptional exposure to trichloroethylene (RR = 1.8, 95% CI 0.2–17.5 for potential exposure of more than 450.5 days compared with no exposure), as assessed by interviews with personnel who held jobs similar to those of the fathers of cases and controls (Health and Safety Executive, 1993). This association could not be disentangled from an association with potential exposure to tritium. Buckley *et al.* (1989b) reported positive associations between ANLL and paternal occupational solvent exposure, apparent in each of the three reference periods evaluated. In a study of leukaemia in Mexico (Fajardo-Gutiérrez *et al.*, 1993a) and in a multicentre study of ALL in the USA and Canada (Buckley *et al.*, 1996), a positive association with postnatal exposure of the index

## Table 6.3. Summary of studies of the association between childhood leukaemia and exposure to solvents

| Area and period of study | Cases | | Controls | | Exposure | Circumstances | Type of substance | RR (95% CI or *p*) | Reference |
|---|---|---|---|---|---|---|---|---|---|
| | Upper age limit | N | N | Type[a] | Source of information[b] | | | | |
| **Leukaemia and lymphoma** UK, West Cumbria, North Humberside and Gateshead, 1974–88 | 14 | 105 | 186 | B | I | Preconceptional occupational exposure of mother | Carbon tetrachloride Trichloroethene | 3.0 (0.5–24.2) 1.2 (0.1–7.9) | McKinney *et al.*, 1991 |
| | | 100 | 169 | B | I | Periconceptional and gestational occupational exposure of the father | Carbon tetrachloride Trichloroethene | 2.2 (0.5–9.1) 4.4 (1.2–21.0) | |
| **Acute leukaemia** USA, Los Angeles, 1980–84 | 10 | 123 | 123 | F, RDD | I | Occupational exposure of the mother from one year before pregnancy to diagnosis | Solvents or degreasers | 1.0[c] | Lowengart *et al.*, 1987 |
| | | | | | | Occupational exposure of father during pregnancy | Chlorinated solvents | 2.2 (*p* = 0.09) | |
| **Leukaemia** Mexico City, NS | NS[d] | 81 | 154 | H, P | I | Home exposure, timing not specified | Solvents derived from petroleum | 1.9 (0.8–4.6) | Fajardo-Gutiérrez *et al.*, 1993a |
| **ALL,** Spain, multicentre, 1983–85 | 14 | 128 | 128 | R | I | Maternal occupational exposure during pregnancy | Solvents | 0.6 (0.2–1.9) | Infante-Rivard *et al.*, 1991 |
| USA and Canada, multicentre, 1982–91 | NS | 990 404 | 1636 440 | OC RDD | Q | Maternal exposure | Solvents | 1.2 1.6 | Buckley *et al.*, 1994 |
| *By immunophenotype* Pre-B-cell | | 38 36 | 114 72 | OC RDD | | | | 2.1 10.0 (*p* < 0.01) | |
| Null-cell | | 65 61 | 193 61 | OC RDD | | | | 2.4 3.0 | |
| T-cell | | 158 130 | 314 130 | OC RDD | | | | 1.9 1.4 | |
| Common | | 286 177 | 572 177 | OC RDD | | | | 0.9 0.8 | |
| All cases | | 990 404 | 1636 440 | OC RDD | Q | Exposure of index child | Solvents | 1.7 10.5 (*p* < 0.01) | |
| **ANLL** USA and Canada, multicentre, 1980–84 | 17 | 178 | 178 | RDD | I | Paternal occupational exposure during pregnancy | Solvents | 2.1 (*p* < 0.05) | Buckley *et al.*, 1989b |
| | | 204 | 204 | RDD | I | Maternal occupational exposure | Solvents | 1.0[c] | |

NS, Not stated.

[a] Control type: B, selected from birth certificates; F, friends of cases; H, hospitalized children; OC, children with cancers of other types; P, population-based, not otherwise specified; R, selected from population register; RDD, selected by random-digit dialling.

[b] Source of information: I, interview; Q, questionnaire; E, employers' records.

[c] The authors stated that there was no association.

[d] The mean age of cases at the time of interview was 8.5 (S.D. 4.5 years). Both prevalent and incident cases were included.

child to solvents was found. These observations may be consistent with those relating to paternal exposure, as chlorinated solvents have been demonstrated in the exhaled air of workers for many hours after exposure (Lowengart *et al.*, 1987).

No consistent association with maternal exposure to solvents is apparent (Table 6.3).

Painters are commonly exposed to solvents (IARC, 1989b). No consistent association between leukaemia and paternal employment categories including painters has been observed (Fabia & Thuy, 1974; Hakulinen *et al.*, 1976; Kwa & Fine, 1980; Hemminki *et al.*, 1981; Van Steensel-Moll *et al.*, 1985b; McKinney *et al.*, 1987). Lowengart *et al.* (1987) investigated the association between leukaemia and parental occupational and home exposure to paints or pigments before, during and after pregnancy. The specific types of exposure included in the general category "paints or pigments" were spray paints, other paints, dyes or pigments, printing inks, lacquers or stains. Elevated risks were observed for occupational exposure of the fathers to spray paints during the index pregnancy (RR = 2.2, $p = 0.03$), and after delivery (RR = 2.0, $p = 0.02$), and for exposure to dyes and pigments one year before pregnancy (RR = 3.5, $p = 0.06$), during pregnancy (RR = 3.0, $p = 0.09$) and after delivery (RR = 4.5, $p = 0.03$). For each of these exposures, trends of increasing risk with increasing frequency of exposure after the birth of the index child were apparent. Data on maternal occupational exposure were not presented. The relative risk associated with use of paints of lacquers in the home by one or both parents during pregnancy and lactation was 1.4 (95% CI 0.8–2.6).

In a study of ALL in the Netherlands, there was a positive association with reported maternal occupational exposure to "paint, petroleum products or other chemicals" during pregnancy (RR = 2.4, 95% CI 1.2–4.6; Van Steensel-Moll *et al.*, 1985b). In a multicentre study of ANLL in the USA and Canada, parents were asked about occupational exposure to paints or pigments before, during or after pregnancy (Buckley *et al.*, 1989b). The relative risk associated with maternal exposure before pregnancy was 2.3 ($p < 0.08$), during pregnancy 1.5 ($p > 0.1$) and after pregnancy 0.9 ($p > 0.1$). The category included spray paints, other paints, dyes or pigments, printing inks, lacquers or stains, turpentine, paint remover, paint thinner, lacquer thinner, and other paints or pigments. Elevated relative risks were observed for use of spray paints (RR = 3.0 for exposure of

>1000 days, $p$ value for trend 0.03), turpentine (4 mothers of cases exposed, no controls, $p = 0.04$), and paint thinners (RR = 4.0, $p = 0.16$). The latter two associations were no longer apparent when adjustment was made for exposure to spray paints. No data were presented on reported specific paternal exposure to paints or pigments. Based on data from a life-time occupational history, there was a positive association with the father ever having been employed as a painter (7 cases and 1 control father employed; RR = 7.0, $p = 0.02$).

In Woburn, Massachusetts (USA), two of eight municipal wells servicing the community were discovered to be contaminated with several chlorinated organic compounds (Lagakos *et al.*, 1986). On systematic testing in May 1979 for 32 volatile organic compounds, trichloroethylene (267 parts per billion), tetrachloroethylene (21 parts per billion) and chloroform (12 parts per billion) were detected. These wells were then closed. Trichlorofluoroethane (23 parts per billion) and dichloroethylene (28 parts per billion) were also detected in water samples taken several months later. Independently, during site excavations for an industrial complex located near the contaminated wells, large pits of buried animal hides and chemical wastes were discovered. A nearby abandoned lagoon was found to be heavily contaminated with lead, arsenic and other metals.

The closing of the wells and the discovery of the waste sites occurred at about the same time as there was publicity about the possible health effects of another occurrence of environmental contamination (the Love Canal incident), and raised concern among residents of Woburn. In late 1979, a citizens' group produced a list of children diagnosed with leukaemia. Preliminary investigation showed an excess of childhood leukaemia in the period 1969–79; 12 cases were observed, compared with 5.3 expected (O/E 2.3; $p$ given as 0.008, although this is difficult to interpret in view of the local concern). Subsequently, Lagakos *et al.* (1986) obtained information from state and hospital cancer registries on 20 cases of leukaemia diagnosed at the age of 19 years and under between 1964, when the wells began pumping, and 1983. In addition, a telephone sample survey was carried out to obtain information on adverse pregnancy outcomes and childhood disorders between 1960 and 1982 for women resident in Woburn before 1979. It was estimated that the 5010 interviews completed represented 57% of the town's residences with listed telephones. The estimated annual proportion of the household's water from the contaminated wells was compared between cases and non-cases identified by means of the sample survey.

The excess incidence in East Woburn, near the contaminated wells, was confirmed. There was a positive association between childhood leukaemia and inferred exposure to contaminated water, whether analysed as cumulative exposure or any versus none. Comparison between the residential history of cases and the regional distribution of the population gave very similar results. The risk to unexposed individuals was similar between areas of Woburn that never received water from the contaminated wells, and those that received a varying amount of water from the contaminated wells over time. The association with contaminated water, if causal, would have accounted for only about half the excess in Woburn. Apart from the small size of the study, a limitation is that water supply to the house may not be the most appropriate indicator of dose, since a substantial proportion of the water consumed by cases may have been taken at day-care centres or schools (Rogan, 1986).

Lagakos *et al.* (1986) noted that the excess incidence in Woburn continued after 1979, but in West rather than East Woburn. This weakens the evidence for the excess in East Woburn being due to contaminated well water. Kuzmack (1987) noted that there was a marked social difference between East and West Woburn. In East Woburn, many of the families had lived there for several generations; whereas in West Woburn, the residents tended to be of higher socioeconomic status and first-generation residents who moved into newly developed areas. As no information was given about the timing or extent of population growth, it is unclear whether this excess could be accounted for by population mixing, as proposed in the Kinlen hypothesis (see Chapter 7).

## Metal dusts and fumes

A positive association between total reported duration of paternal occupational exposure to lead and ANLL was observed by Buckley *et al.* (1989b). The fathers of 167 cases and 173 controls reported no exposure, those of five cases and five controls reported 1–1000 days of exposure, and those of six cases but no controls reported longer exposures (*p* value for trend = 0.03). A cumulative exposure measure, calculated as a sum of exposure frequency by job duration, did not show a stronger association with the disease than duration alone. Lead exposure was also classified as

being due to direct use of the substance or working in the presence of others using the substance. The trend for direct exposure was not significant. In addition, the trend was not significant when the analysis was restricted to data from interviews completed directly with the father. There was a positive association with maternal occupational exposure to "metal dusts and fumes", the odds ratio for 1–1000 days of exposure being 4.0 (based on four exposed cases and one exposed control), and for longer duration of exposure 6.0 (six exposed cases and one exposed control); the *p* value for trend was 0.02. Controlling paternal lead exposure for maternal exposure to "metal dusts and fumes" had little effect on the strength of association, and vice versa.

Maternal occupational exposure to lead during pregnancy was associated with an increased risk of acute leukaemia (based on five exposed cases) in a study in Shanghai (Shu *et al.*, 1988); 30% of the cases had ANLL, but no details were given as to the type of leukaemia in the offspring of lead-exposed women. In this study, the association with maternal employment in metal refining and processing during pregnancy appeared to be specific to ANLL (odds ratio = 4.6, 95% CI 1.3–17.2, five exposed cases). This would be consistent with Buckley *et al.*'s (1989b) finding of a positive association with maternal exposure to metal dusts and fumes.

In the multicentre study of ALL in the USA and Canada described earlier, raised relative risks associated with maternal exposure to molten metals were observed for the null-cell and T-cell subgroups (Buckley *et al.*, 1994). A raised relative risk associated with paternal exposure was observed for the T-cell subtype.

In the ecological study in Great Britain of Knox and Gilman (1997) described above, there was no association between leukaemia and proximity of residence to industrial facilities in which lead casting was carried out, but there were positive associations with proximity to aluminium, zinc, iron and steel casting and steelworks.

As described in Chapter 2, Alexander *et al.* (1990a) found significant localized clustering of childhood cancer in North Humberside, England, some of which was in an area about which there had been local concern about clustering. The community had suggested various explanations, including attendance at particular schools, emissions from a tin smelter stack, and exposure to dust from a cement works. However, there was no evidence that clustering was confined to this area. Although an excess of childhood leukaemia was found in the catchment area of one of the two schools attendance at which was postulated to increase risk, two of the three cases were in pre-school children. Ratios of observed to expected numbers of cases within circles of various radii located around the tin smelter stack were close to unity for leukaemia. For other malignancies, excesses were apparent both very close to the stack and approximately 7 km from it. The cement works was very close to the tin smelter, so the results of the foregoing analysis were considered to apply equally well to the cement works.

Wulff *et al.* (1996) investigated the incidence of cancer among children born between 1961 and 1990 in the vicinity of a smelter situated in the northern coastal region of Sweden. The smelter emitted lead, arsenic, copper, cadmium and sulfur dioxide. Cancer was diagnosed in 13 children whose mothers lived within a radius of 20 km of the smelter at the time of the child's birth, compared with 6.7 expected on the basis of national rates (standardized incidence ratio (SIR) = 1.95, 95% CI 0.88–3.00). The incidence of childhood cancer was also investigated in parishes more than 20 km from the smelter within the municipality, and in a parish in another municipality which was considered to be a similar area in terms of its geographical and socioeconomic characteristics, but without environmental pollution from the smelter. In these areas, the SIR of childhood cancer was 1.00 (95% CI 0.7–1.3). Mean parental ages and parity did not differ between the groups. Only one parent, a father, of the cases born in the neighbourhood of the smelter had worked there. None of the parents of cases in the reference areas had worked in the smelter. About a third of the cases in the exposed and reference areas had leukaemia.

## Industrial pollutants of all types

Seven cases of ALL occurred between 1983 and 1985 among children who lived in Carbonia, Sardinia (Italy) (Cocco *et al.*, 1996). Concern that this apparent excess might be attributable to pollution from a large industrial complex 10 km from the town led to a study of 9 cases diagnosed in the period 1980–89 and 36 age–sex-matched controls selected from the birth register of Carbonia municipality. No statistically significant associations were found. The industrial area in the vicinity of Carbonia includes a coal- and oil-fired plant, a lead and zinc foundry, an aluminium plant and an aluminium sheet production facility (Cocco *et al.*, 1993). Relative risks of about 4.0 were associated with the presence of a well in the backyard, parental origin outside Carbonia and use of therapeutic drugs in pregnancy. No information was available about possible chemical contamination of local groundwater, but this was thought to be unlikely, as the authorized industrial waste disposal sites were located in a watershed which did not include the town. In addition, none of the study subjects reported that they used the wells as a source of drinking water. A study of the distribution of industrial emissions from the complex suggested that concentrations of industrial pollutants which would have reached the town during the period relevant for the cases diagnosed between 1983 and 1985 would have been negligible.

## Wood dust

In a study of childhood leukaemia and non-Hodgkin lymphoma combined, there was a positive association with maternal occupational exposure to wood dust before the conception of the index child (RR = 3.0, 95% CI 1.0–10.2, based on 14 discordant pairs) (McKinney *et al.*, 1991). Few women were exposed during pregnancy or after the birth of the index child. Relative risks for paternal occupational exposure to wood dust were: in the preconceptional period 2.7 (95% CI 1.4–5.2, 46 discordant pairs), in the periconceptional and gestational period 1.7 (95% CI 0.6–26.9, 30 discordant pairs), and postnatally 1.5 (95% CI 0.8–2.8, 43 discordant pairs).

In the multicentre study of ALL in the USA and Canada already described, the relative risk associated with the index child's exposure to dust was 1.4 (*p* < 0.05) in the comparison with controls with other types of cancer, and 2.3 (*p* < 0.01) in comparison with controls selected by random-digit dialling (Buckley *et al.*, 1994). This excess was apparent for the pre-B-cell and T-cell subtypes. In the latter subgroup, the relevant dust was most commonly recorded as wood dust (seven cases) or talc (three cases).

Buckley *et al.* (1989b) found that six mothers of cases of ANLL and two mothers of controls had reported exposure to sawdust before or during pregnancy.

## Insulation materials

In the multicentre study of ANLL in the USA and Canada already described, an inverse association of borderline statistical significance with maternal occupational exposure to insulation materials was found (Buckley *et al.*, 1989b); this was largely accounted for by five control mothers who reported prolonged exposure to asbestos. No association with paternal exposure was reported. In a study of leukaemia in Los Angeles, there was no association with maternal or paternal exposure to insulation materials (London *et al.*, 1991).

### Bracken spores

Evans and Galpin (1990) suggested that bracken spores might explain the observations of leukaemia clusters in young people near actual or potential sites of nuclear installations, on the grounds that such sites tend to be in remote and uncultivated areas where bracken might be expected to flourish. Cook-Mozaffari *et al.* (1990) divided the 90 districts in England and Wales that had some part within 16 km of such a site according to the degree of cover by vegetation complexes in which bracken is likely to be common (acid grassland, heather moorland, woodland or heath). Only 36 districts were in areas where bracken cover was probably moderate or extensive. Only 25% of the population living in districts near to existing or potential sites of nuclear installations were resident in these 36 districts, a similar proportion to the value for England and Wales as a whole (24%). An additional analysis related to all 400 districts of England and Wales, which were classified according to their probable level of exposure to bracken spores (defined as 'slight', 'some', 'moderate' or 'extensive'). There was no association between probable level of exposure and leukaemia mortality at ages 0–24 years. This absence of a relationship was also evident when the 90 districts adjacent to actual or proposed sites of nuclear installations were excluded from the analysis. Trotter (1990) noted that the validity of the study may have been limited by the use of a measure of potential exposure only and did not take account of prevailing winds which are an important influence on the geographical distribution of the spores. It may be relevant that the highest incidence of childhood leukaemia reported in international data has been from Costa Rica (Linet & Devesa, 1991). In that country, the standardized incidence of gastric and oesophageal cancer is almost three times greater in parts of the country where bracken (and haematuria in cattle) is common than elsewhere, and the authors suggested that carcinogens derived from bracken were consumed in milk (Villalobos-Salazar *et al.*, 1989).

### Lymphoma

In a study of childhood cancer of all types in Denver, Colorado (USA), there was a statistically significant association between lymphomas and treatment of the home by a pest exterminator during the period between birth and two years before diagnosis (RR = 1.8, 95% CI 1.1–2.9; Leiss & Savitz, 1995). There was also a raised relative risk for the period from two years before diagnosis until diagnosis (RR = 1.6, 95% CI 0.9–2.9), but not with treatment of the home in the last three months of pregnancy. No association was found with treatment of the area around the home with insecticides or herbicides, or with use of pest strips.

On the basis of this study, and of studies of lymphoma in adults which suggested a positive association with exposure to phenoxy acids used in grain farming and forestry, Kristensen *et al.* (1996) investigated the offspring of parents engaged in agricultural activities in Norway. There was no association between Hodgkin's disease and residence on a grain farm or on a farm with pesticide spraying equipment as recorded on a census; the relative risk associated with residence on a farm with 2.5 hectares or more given over to forestry was 1.6 (95% CI 0.9–2.6). An unexpected association with chicken farming was observed. There was no association between non-Hodgkin lymphoma and residence on a grain farm or one with at least 2.5 hectares given over to forestry. The relative risk associated with pesticide purchase was 1.7, the risk increasing with higher levels of expenditure (*p* value for trend = 0.04). The increase was largely restricted to farms involved in horticulture, suggesting a relationship with insecticides rather than phenoxy herbicides.

Data specifically on lymphoma and parental occupational exposure have been presented in only two studies (McKinney *et al.*, 1987; Magnani *et al.*, 1990). In the study of McKinney *et al.* (1987), four out of 63 fathers of cases, but no fathers of controls, worked in furnaces, forges or foundries. An elevated relative risk (8.5, 95% CI 1.3–55.1) also was observed for paternal employment in textile work. In the study of Magnani *et al.* (1990), which included 19 cases of non-Hodgkin lymphoma and 307 hospital controls, there were positive associations with paternal employment as a construction worker or lorry driver, and maternal employment as a high-school teacher or baker or confectioner. The relative risks varied according to the period considered (up to child's birth or between birth and diagnosis).

# Central nervous system tumours

## Pesticides

Pesticides (insecticides, fungicides and herbicides) have high biological activities (IARC, 1991). Derivatives of urea and carbonic acid in herbicides and insecticides can react with nitrite in the stomach to form N-nitroso compounds (Inskip *et al.*, 1995). Therefore, exposures to these compounds are of particular interest in relation to the N-nitroso hypothesis (see Chapter 1) for the etiology of brain tumours in children.

In a study of brain tumours in Baltimore, Maryland, Gold *et al.* (1979) reported that insect extermination was more common in the homes of cases of brain tumour between birth and diagnosis than in those of population controls (RR = 2.3, 95% CI 0.9–6.6) but not than in those of controls with other types of cancer (RR = 1.2, 95% CI 0.5–2.8). In six out of eight subsequent studies of brain tumours of all types combined, a raised relative risk associated with intrauterine or postnatal pesticide exposure has been observed (Table 6.4). No association was observed in the three available studies of astrocytoma, or the one study of primitive neuroectodermal tumours of the brain. It is difficult to assess the extent that methodological factors, such as low statistical power to detect an association with an exposure of low prevalence, may account for the inconsistent results, since in some reports only brief details were given.

In a cohort study of offspring of men and women employed in agricultural work in Norway, the relative risk of brain tumours diagnosed at ages up to 14 years associated with pesticide purchase as recorded in the census was 1.7 (95% CI 1.1–2.6), based on 41 exposed cases, and adjusted for year of birth and calendar year (Kristensen *et al.*, 1996). The corresponding relative risk of non-astrocytic neuroepithelial tumours in children was 3.8 (95% CI 1.6–6.9). This increase in risk was not restricted to specific types of farming. As pesticide purchase is a crude indicator of exposure, and only information on purchases in the year preceding the 1969 census was available, considerable misclassification is likely to have occurred. This would have be expected to have biased the relative risks towards unity. In this cohort, the relative risk of brain tumours diagnosed in the offspring at all ages associated with pig farming was 1.6 (95% CI 1.2–2.2), with chicken farming 1.3 (95%CI 0.9–1.9), grain farming 1.3 (95% CI 1.0–1.8) and horticulture 1.3 (95% CI 0.9–1.8). In other studies, no consistent association with paternal employment in agriculture has been observed (Fabia & Thuy, 1974; Hemminki *et al.*, 1981; Wilkins & Koutras, 1988; Wilkins & Sinks, 1990; Kuijten *et al.*, 1992). A positive association between farming and brain tumours in adults has been reported in several studies (Thomas & Waxweiler, 1986; Brownson *et al.*, 1990; Inskip *et al.*, 1995).

The observation in the Norwegian study that associations with indicators of pesticide exposure were stronger for non-astrocytic epithelial tumours than for all brain tumours combined appears to be compatible with the results of the case–control studies, which suggest that the relationship between pesticides and brain tumours is not accounted for by astrocytoma.

## Occupational exposure to N-nitroso compounds

In one study (Wilkins & Sinks, 1990), occupational exposure to nitrosamines, nitrosamides, nitrosatable amino compounds and compounds with a chemical structure similar to that of the N-nitroso group was inferred according to the job–exposure matrix of Hoar *et al.* (1980). The prevalence of inferred moderate to heavy exposure of the father to any such chemical was rarely higher than 4% in the preconceptional period or during pregnancy, and never exceeded 17% in the postnatal period. The prevalence of inferred exposure of the mother to such chemicals was lower still. Relative risks of about 3 or 4 were observed for paternal postnatal inferred exposure to aromatic amino and aromatic nitro compounds. These compounds have not been associated with nervous system tumours in experimental animals (Wilkins & Sinks, 1990).

High-level exposures to exogenous N-nitroso compounds can occur in certain workplaces, notably the rubber, leather, metal and chemical industries, in mining, in pesticide and detergent production, and in fish factories (Preussman, 1984). No consistent association between tumours of the CNS and paternal employment in categories including the rubber and chemical industries has been observed (Johnson *et al.*, 1987; Wilkins & Koutras, 1988; Birch *et al.*, 1990b; Wilkins & Sinks, 1990; Olsen *et al.*, 1991; Kuijten *et al.*, 1992). No clear association with paternal employment categories potentially involving exposure to metals is apparent (Wilkins & Koutras, 1988; Wilkins & Sinks, 1990; Kuijten *et al.*, 1992). In one study, the relative risk of CNS tumours associated with paternal employment in soap factories around

## Table 6.4. Summary of studies of the association between tumours of the central nervous system and exposure to pesticides

| Area and period of study | Cases Upper age limit | N | Controls Type[a] | N | Exposure Source of information[b] | Type | Circumstances | RR (95% CI or p) | Reference |
|---|---|---|---|---|---|---|---|---|---|
| **Brain tumours** | | | | | | | | | |
| USA, Baltimore, MD, 1965–75 | 19 | 84 | B OC | 73 78 | I | Insect extermination | Index child's contact | 2.3 (0.9–6.6) 1.2 (0.5–2.8) | Gold et al., 1979 |
| USA, Los Angeles County, 1972–77 | 24 | 209 | F, N | 209 | I | Home pest extermination Pesticides | During pregnancy | 1.0 (p = 0.59)[c] 1.5 (p = 0.08)[c] | Preston-Martin et al., 1982 |
| | | | | | | Home pest extermination Pesticides | Index child's contact | 0.9 (p=0.29)[c] 1.1 (p=0.44)[c] | |
| USA, Ohio, 1975–82 | 19 | 110 | RDD | 193 | I | Aerosol insecticides Other pesticides | During pregnancy or maternal use before conception | >1 (p<0.05)[d] 1.0[e] | Sinks, 1985; Wilkins & Sinks, 1990 |
| | | | | | | Pesticides | Parental occupational exposure | 1.0[e] | |
| Canada, Southern Ontario, 1977–83 | 19 | 74 | R | 138 | I | Herbicides and insecticides | Index child's contact | 0.9 (0.5–1.9)[f] | Howe et al., 1989 |
| USA, Missouri, 1985–89 | 10 | 45 | F | 85 | I | Pesticides used for nuisance pests | During pregnancy Birth–6 months 7 months–diagnosis | 1.8 (0.9–4.0)[g] 1.9 (0.8–4.3)[g] 3.4 (1.1–10.6)[g] | Davis et al., 1993 |
| | | | OC | 108 | | | During pregnancy Birth–6 months 7 months–diagnosis | 1.2 (0.5–2.9)[g] 1.9 (0.8–4.4)[g] 1.7 (0.5–5.4)[g] | |
| | | | F | 85 | | Insecticides used in the garden or orchard | During pregnancy Birth–6 months 7 months–diagnosis | 1.5 (0.6–3.9)[g] 2.3 (0.7–8.3)[g] 1.6 (0.7–3.6)[g] | |
| | | | OC | 108 | | | During pregnancy Birth–6 months 7 months–diagnosis | 1.2 (0.5–3.0)[g] 1.2 (0.4–3.8)[g] 2.6 (1.1–5.9)[g] | |
| | | | F | 85 | | Herbicides used on the yard | During pregnancy Birth–6 months 7 months–diagnosis | 1.1 (0.5–2.5)[g] 1.7 (0.7–3.9)[g] 2.4 (1.0–5.7)[g] | |
| | | | OC | 108 | | | During pregnancy Birth–6 months 7 months–diagnosis | 1.0 (0.4–2.4)[g] 3.4 (1.2–9.3)[g] 1.7 (0.7–3.9)[g] | |
| France, Ile de France, 1985–87 | 15 | 75 | R | 113 | I | House treated with pesticides | During pregnancy During childhood | 1.8 (0.8–4.1)[h] 2.0 (1.0–4.1)[h] | Cordier et al., 1994 |
| Australia, New South Wales, 1985–89 | 14 | 82 | R | 164 | I | Pesticides | During pregnancy | 2.0 (1.0–3.9)[i] | McCredie et al., 1994a |

| Reference, location | No. of cases | No. of controls | Control type[a] | No. | Source of info[b] | Agent/exposure | Exposure period | Relative risk (95% CI) | Reference |
|---|---|---|---|---|---|---|---|---|---|
| USA, Denver, CO, 1976–83 | 14 | 48 | RDD | 222 | I | Home pest extermination | Last 3 months of pregnancy<br>Birth to 2 years before diagnosis<br>From 2 years before diagnosis to diagnosis | 1.3 (0.7–2.1)[j]<br>1.4 (0.6–2.7)[j]<br>1.1 (0.4–3.0)[j] | Leiss & Savitz, 1995 |
|  |  |  |  |  |  | Use of pest strips | Last 3 months of pregnancy<br>Birth to 2 years before diagnosis<br>From 2 years before diagnosis to diagnosis | 1.5 (0.9–2.4)[j]<br>1.4 (0.7–2.9)[j]<br>1.8 (1.2–2.9)[j] |  |
|  |  |  |  |  |  | Treatment of area around home with insecticides or herbicides | Last 3 months of pregnancy<br>Birth to 2 years before diagnosis<br>From 2 years before diagnosis to diagnosis | 0.6 (0.3–1.1)[j]<br>0.5 (0.2–0.9)[j]<br>0.5 (0.4–0.8)[j] |  |
| Germany, Lower Saxony, 1988–93 | 14 | 75 | R | 433 | Q, I | Work by either parent as a farmer, gardener or florist | 2 years before birth until diagnosis | 1.0[e] | Meinert *et al.*, 1996 |
|  |  |  |  |  |  | Occupational contact with pesticides |  | 1.0[e] |  |
|  |  |  |  |  |  | Pesticides used in gardens or on farms |  | 1.0[e] |  |
| **Astrocytoma**<br>USA, Greater Delaware Valley, 1980–86 | 9 | 96 | RDD | 96 | I | Pesticides | During pregnancy | 1.0[e] | Nass, 1989 |
| USA, Pennsylvania, New Jersey and Delaware, 1980–86 | 14 | 163 | RDD | 163 | I | Insecticides | During pregnancy | 1.2 (0.7–1.9) | Kuijten *et al.*, 1990 |
| USA and Canada, multicentre, 1986–89 | 5 | 155 | RDD | 155 | I | Insect sprays or pesticides | During pregnancy | 1.5 (0.8–2.7)[k] | Bunin *et al.*, 1994b |
|  |  |  |  |  |  | Home pest extermination | During pregnancy | 0.7 (0.4–1.4)[k] |  |
| **Primitive neuroectodermal tumour of the brain**<br>USA and Canada, multicentre, 1986–89 | 5 | 166 | RDD | 166 | I | Insect sprays or pesticides | During pregnancy | 0.7 (0.4–1.4) | Bunin *et al.*, 1994b |
|  |  |  |  |  |  | Home pest extermination | During pregnancy | 1.0 (0.6–1.9) |  |

[a] Control type: B, selected from birth certificates; H, children hospitalized for reasons other than cancer; N, neighbourhood; OC, children with other types of cancer; F, friends of cases; RDD, selected by random-digit dialling; R, selected from population register.
[b] Source of information: I, interview; Q, questionnaire.
[c] One sided *p* value.
[d] The author stated that there was a significant positive association.
[e] The author(s) stated that there was no association.
[f] Adjusted for age at diagnosis.
[g] Adjusted for age at diagnosis, exposure of child to environmental tobacco smoke, family income, education of mother and father, family member in construction industry, and time between diagnosis and interview.
[h] Adjusted for child's age and sex, and for maternal age.
[i] Adjusted for father's schooling.
[j] Adjusted for age at diagnosis, father's education, per capita income, residential stability, maternal age, maternal ethnic group, sex, maternal smoking, wire code and/or year of diagnosis when these factors proved to be confounders.
[k] Adjusted for income level.

the time of conception was 14.1 ($p < 0.01$, based on three exposed cases; Olsen *et al.*, 1991). Thus the available data on paternal occupation do not provide consistent support for the *N*-nitroso hypothesis, but as the data relate to inferred exposure, they do not refute it. The data on maternal occupation are too limited to consider in relation to this hypothesis.

## Paternal employment in the aerospace industry

In a study of 92 cases of brain tumours diagnosed under the age of 10 years compared with a mixture of friend and neighbourhood controls, a positive association with paternal employment in the aircraft industry during pregnancy or at the time of diagnosis (12 exposed cases, 2 exposed controls) was found (Peters *et al.*, 1981). This association was not confounded by maternal pattern of food consumption, drug and alcohol use during pregnancy, or smoking habits. The specific occupations of the father, the exposures reported, and the types of brain tumour observed were diverse. Subsequently, Olshan *et al.* (1986) carried out a study of 51 cases of brain tumour and 142 matched controls selected by random-digit dialling in western Washington State, an area where a relatively high proportion of the workforce is employed in the aerospace industry. Overall, no association was apparent with paternal employment in the industry for at least six months before the diagnosis of the index case. However, for cases diagnosed under 10 years, a relative risk of 2.1 (95% CI 0.8–5.6) was observed, based on eight exposed cases, while for cases aged 10–15 years, the relative risk was 0.1 (95% CI 0.01–1.1), based on one exposed case. A similar pattern was apparent when the definition was restricted to employment in aircraft manufacture. In a study of deaths due to CNS tumours in Texas, no association with paternal employment in the aircraft industry at the time of the child's birth was found (Johnson *et al.*, 1987). In a large study in New York State, no association was found between CNS tumours and paternal employment in the aircraft industry either at the time of the index child's birth or diagnosis (Nasca *et al.*, 1988). However, few fathers of control children had worked in the industry, and therefore the statistical power to detect an association was low.

## Hydrocarbons

No consistent association between brain tumours and paternal occupational exposure to hydrocarbons has been observed (Table 6.5). In the two studies of brain tumours in which maternal exposure during pregnancy was considered, there was no clear evidence of an association with hydrocarbons (Wilkins & Sinks, 1990; Bunin *et al.*, 1994b).

In a study in Denver, Colorado (Savitz & Feingold, 1989), the relative risks of brain tumours associated with exposure to passage of 500 or more vehicles per day through the segment of the street in which the subject lived at the time of diagnosis or interview was 1.7 (95% CI 0.8–3.4). This was similar to the relative risk observed for total childhood cancer. As already discussed, it appears that there was a deficit of controls of low socioeconomic status (NRPB, 1992). Such a deficit might have produced a spurious association with a marker of low socioeconomic status, such as residential traffic density.

## Other associations

Peters *et al.* (1981) reported a positive association between brain tumours in children aged under 10 years and maternal exposures to chemicals during the period from one year before conception until the end of lactation; for skin contact, the relative risk was 3.3 (13 discordant pairs, $p = 0.05$), for inhalation, the relative risk was 3.0 (16 discordant pairs, $p = 0.04$), and for exposure by one or both of these routes, the relative risk was 2.8 (19 discordant pairs, $p = 0.03$). In an extension of this study in which cases between 10 and 24 years old were also included, the relative risk associated with maternal employment during pregnancy in jobs for which they wore protective clothing or equipment was 4.0 (15 discordant pairs, $p = 0.02$; Preston-Martin *et al.*, 1982).

## Neuroblastoma

In two studies of neuroblastoma, paternal occupations involving potential exposure to chemicals and dusts at the time of the index child's birth were investigated (Spitz & Johnson, 1985; Wilkins & Hundley, 1990). No consistent association was identified.

In a cohort study of the offspring of men and women employed in agricultural work in Norway, the relative risk of neuroblastoma diagnosed at ages up to four years associated with growth of field vegetables on the farm at the census closest to the year of birth was 2.5 (95% CI 1.0–6.1), based on seven exposed cases and adjusted for year of birth and calendar year (Kristensen *et al.*, 1996).

In a case–control study primarily intended to investigate an increased incidence of neuroblastoma in parts of the former West

Table 6.5. Summary of studies of the association between tumours of the central nervous system and paternal occupational exposure to hydrocarbons in the period nearest to the time of birth of the index child

| Area and period of study | Cases Deaths (D) or newly incident (I) cases, upper age limit | Cases N | Controls Type[a] | Controls N | Exposure Source of information (informant)[b] | Exposure Period of exposure[c] | Definition | Subgroup | RR (95% CI) | Reference |
|---|---|---|---|---|---|---|---|---|---|---|
| **Central nervous system tumours** | | | | | | | | | | |
| USA, Massachusetts 1947–57 and 1963–67 (births) | D, 14 | 132 | B | 1372 | B | B | Job classification (FT)[d] | | 0.8 (0.4–1.3) | Kwa and Fine, 1980 |
| USA, Houston, TX, 1976–77 | I, 15 | 47 | H N C | 269 204 359 | I (M,F) | B | Job classification (FT)[d] | | 0.5 (0.0–2.0) 1.3 (0.5–5.5) 0.8 (0.0–3.4) | Zack et al., 1980 |
| USA, TX, 1964–80 | D, 15 | 499 | B | 998 | B | B | Job classification (FT)[d] | | 0.7 (0.3–1.5) | Johnson et al., 1987 |
| USA, New York State, (53 counties), 1968–77 | I, 14 | 338 | B | 676 | I (M) | B | Job classification | Narrow Broad | 1.3 (0.7–2.4) 1.4 (0.9–2.2) | Nasca et al., 1988 |
| **Brain tumours** | | | | | | | | | | |
| Finland, 1959–75 | I, 14 | 219 | B | 219 | A (M) | B | Job classification (FT)[d] | | 1.4 (0.5–3.9) | Hakulinen et al., 1976 |
| UK, England and Wales, 1959–63 1970–72 | D, 14 | 1161 760 | D | 112840 54806 | DC | D | Job classification | | 0.9 (0.8–1.0)[e] 0.9 (0.8–1.1)[e] | Sanders et al., 1981 |
| USA, Baltimore, 1965–74 | I, 19 | 70 | B OC | 70 70 | I (M) | Pc, Pg | Job classification | Narrow[f] Broad[g] Narrow[f] Broad[g] | 0.5 (ns) 0.5 (ns) 2.3 (ns) 2.3 (ns) | Gold et al., 1982 |
| USA, Ohio, 1975–82 | I, 19 | 110 | RDD | 193 | I (M,F) | Pg | Job-exposure matrix | Cluster 3[j] Clusters 4 & 5[ij] Clusters 6 & 7[i] Clusters 10–12[j] Clusters 16 & 17[i] Cluster 18[ij] Cluster 20[ik] Clusters 22–24[ik] | 2.0 (0.8–5.1) 0.7 (0.2–2.2) 1.1 (0.4–2.8) 1.6 (0.4–6.0) 0.8 (0.2–2.6) 1.2 (0.3–4.5) 4.7 (1.2–18.7) 1.8 (0.5–6.2) | Wilkins & Sinks, 1990 |
| USA, Denver, CO, 1976–83 | I, 14 | 48 | RDD | 222 | I (M) | 1 year before birth | Job-exposure matrix | | 0.8 (0.3–2.0)[h] | Feingold et al., 1992 |
| **Astrocytoma** | | | | | | | | | | |
| USA, Pennsylvania, New Jersey and Delaware, 1980–86 | I, 14 | 163 | RDD | 163 | I (M,F) | Pg | Job classification Motor vehicle exhaust | Heavy inferred exposure Moderate inferred exposure | 0.7 (0.2–2.6) 0.5 (0.2–1.3) | Kuijten et al., 1992 |

ns, Not statistically significant.
[a] Control type: B, selected from birth certificates; H, children hospitalized for reasons other than cancer; N, neighbourhood; C, cousins; D, selected from death records; OC, children with other types of cancer; E, friends of cases; RDD, selected by random-digit dialling; R, selected from population register.
[b] Source of information: A, parental interview at antenatal clinic visit; B, birth certificates; DC, death certificates; I, parental interview after diagnosis. Informant: F, information obtained directly from the father for >50% of subjects; M, information obtained from the mother; ± father for <50% of subjects.
[c] Period of exposure: B, birth; Pg, pregnancy; D, death; Pc, pre-conceptional; Dg, diagnosis.

[d] Jobs classified according to method used by Fabia and Thuy (1974).
[e] Proportional mortality analysis.
[f] Includes factory workers, machinists, drivers, motor vehicle mechanics, service station attendants, miners, lumbermen.
[g] Includes painters, dyers and cleaners as well as the above.
[h] Adjusted for father's education.
[i] Involves moderate exposure to aromatic hydrocarbons, as defined by Hsieh et al., (1983).
[j] Involves moderate aliphatic hydrocarbons, as defined by Hsieh et al., (1983).
[k] Involves heavy exposure to aromatic hydrocarbons, as defined by Hsieh et al., (1983).

Germany which were highly contaminated by fallout from the Chernobyl accident (see Chapter 4), a positive association with occupational exposure of either parent to insecticides or pesticides was found (RR = 4.2, 95% CI 1.4–12.9; Michaelis *et al.*, 1996). This may have been a chance finding, as there was no *a priori* hypothesis about this exposure and extensive exploratory analysis was carried out. The study was based on postal questionnaires returned by the parents of 67 cases and 120 age–sex-matched controls selected from local population registries; the participation rate of parents of cases was 84% and that of parents of controls 79%.

Neuroblastoma has not consistently been associated with paternal employment in agricultural work (Spitz & Johnson, 1985; Bunin *et al.*, 1990b; Wilkins & Hundley, 1990) or with level of farming activity in the area of residence at the time of diagnosis (Davis *et al.*, 1987).

## Retinoblastoma

### Pesticides

In a multicentre study in the USA and Canada of retinoblastoma, fathers were asked about military service, specifically in Viet Nam, and exposure to herbicides (Bunin *et al.*, 1990a). In the analysis of 67 sporadic heritable cases, defined as having bilateral disease without family history or unilateral disease associated with a 13q deletion but no family history, a significant association with paternal military service was found (RR = 2.8, 95% CI 1.1–8.8). When the timing of military service was known, this occurred with one exception in the preconceptional period; the timing was unknown for three subjects. Seven case and five control fathers had served in south-east Asia. Two case fathers and one control father reported exposure to Agent Orange or other herbicides, while four case fathers and one control father reported taking malaria prophylaxis. No association (RR = 0.6, 95% CI 0.3–1.2) with military service was observed for the non-heritable form of the disease, that is unilateral disease without family history of the disease or a constitutional 13q deletion. Grandpaternal employment in farming (cluster 13 of Hsieh *et al.*, 1983) was associated with the non-heritable form of the disease (RR = 10.0, 95% CI 1.4–433).

In the offspring of men and women employed in agricultural work in Norway born during the period 1952–91, the relative risk of eye cancer associated with growth of field vegetables and pesticide purchase as recorded in the 1969 census was 3.2 (95% CI 0.9–10.9), based on four exposed cases, and adjusted for year of birth and calendar year (Kristensen *et al.*, 1996). Only two of the four cases had retinoblastoma.

### Welding

In the multicentre study of retinoblastoma described already, a positive association between the non-heritable form of retinoblastoma and paternal preconceptional employment in jobs involving welding, machining and paper-processing (cluster 6 of Hsieh *et al.*, 1983) was observed (RR = 4.0, 95% CI 1.1–22.1) (Bunin *et al.*, 1990a). An elevated risk also was observed for the sporadic heritable form of the disease, and for other definitions of occupations involving exposure to metals.

Bonde *et al.* (1992) investigated the offspring of a cohort of 27 071 Danish men who had been employed for a year or more in Danish steel or mild steel manufacturing companies during the period 1964–84, as identified from records of the national pension fund. A total of 26 529 liveborn children contributing 233 810 person-years of observation was identified from the national population register. Cases of cancer were identified by linkage with the national cancer registry. Two cases (2.6 expected) of childhood cancer were observed among 1774 offspring (17 254 person-years) of fathers verified as having been employed in stainless steel welding before conception, four cases (4.3 expected) among 2764 children (29 077 person-years) whose fathers had been employed in mild steel welding only, and four cases (2.7 expected; RR = 1.5, 95% CI = 0.5–3.6) among 1867 children (18 057 person-years) whose fathers were verified as not having been involved in welding. Among the 16 489 offspring (183 866 person-years) whose fathers included metalworkers with unverified job title or department, other production workers, and white-collar workers, the relative risk of childhood cancer was 0.97 (26 expected cases). However, four cases of retinoblastoma occurred (1.15 expected; RR = 3.5, 95% CI 1.1–8.4). These cases were not related to one another.

## Wilms' tumour

### Hydrocarbons

No consistent association between Wilms' tumour and paternal occupational exposure to hydrocarbons has been observed (Table 6.6). In addition, in the one available study of maternal occupational exposure to hydrocarbons of all types combined, no statistically significant association was observed (Bunin *et al.*, 1989b).

**Table 6.6. Summary of studies of the association between Wilms' tumour and paternal occupational exposure to hydrocarbons in the period nearest to the time of birth of the index child**

| Area and period of study | Cases | Controls | | Exposure | | | | | RR (95% CI) | Reference |
|---|---|---|---|---|---|---|---|---|---|---|
| | Deaths (D) or newly incident (I) cases, upper age limit | N | Type[a] | N | Source of information (informant)[b] | Period of exposure[c] | Definition | Subgroup | | |
| USA, Connecticut, 1935–73 | I, 19 | 149 | B | 149 | B | B | Job classification | | 2.7 (1.2–5.7)[d] | Kantor et al., 1979 |
| USA, Massachusetts, 1947–57 and 1963–67 (births) | D, 14 | 34 | B | 1372 | B | B | Job classification (FT)[e] | | 2.6 (1.3–5.4) | Kwa & Fine, 1980 |
| USA, Houston, TX,1976–77 | I, 15 | 26 | H N C | 269 204 359 | I (M,F) | B | Job classification (FT)[e] | | 0.5 (0.0–2.9) 1.1 (0.0–7.4) 0.8 (0.0–4.7) | Zack et al., 1980 |
| UK, England and Wales 1959–63 1970–72 | D, 14 | 270 128 | D | 112840 54806 | DC | D | Job classification | | 1.3 (1.0–1.6)[f] 1.2 (0.8–1.8)[f] | Sanders et al., 1981 |
| USA, Ohio, 1950–81 | I, NS | 62 | B | 124 | B | B | Job classification | Narrow[g] Broad[h] | 1.4 (0.6–3.1) 1.4 (0.7–2.7) | Wilkins & Sinks, 1984b |
| USA, Greater Philadelphia, 1970–83 | I, 14 | 88 | RDD | 88 | I (M,F) | Pg | Job-exposure matrix | Cluster 6[i] Other clusters[j] | 4.3 (1.2–23.7) 1.0[k] | Bunin et al., 1989b |
| USA, multicentre, 1984–86 | I, 15 | 200 | RDD | 200 | Q (M,F) | Pg | Job classification | Narrow[g] Broad[h] Narrow combusted | 1.2 (0.6–2.4) 1.3 (0.5–3.3) 2.3 (0.5–10.0) | Olshan et al., 1990 |
| | | | | | | | Industrial hygienist | All hydrocarbons Combusted hydrocarbons | 1.1 (0.6–1.8) 2.1 (1.1–3.9) | |

NS, Not stated.

a Control type: B, selected from birth certificates; H, children hospitalized for reasons other than cancer; N, neighbourhood; C, cousins; D, selected from death records; RDD, selected by random-digit dialling; Q, questionnaire.

b Source of information: B, birth certificates; DC, death certificates; I, parental interview after diagnosis; M, information obtained from the mother; F, information obtained directly from the father for >50% of subjects; M, information obtained from the mother; ± father for <50% of subjects.

c Period of exposure: B, birth; Pg, pregnancy; D, death.

d Unmatched analysis of matched data.

e Definition of Fabia and Thuy (1974).

f Proportional mortality analysis.

g Included motor vehicle mechanics, service station attendants, drivers/heavy equipment operators, metal workers/machinists.

h As narrow definition, together with lumbermen, miners, painters, printers, leather workers and factory workers (not elsewhere classified).

i Includes moderate exposure to aromatic hydrocarbons, as defined by Hsieh et al. (1983).

j Other job clusters involving inferred exposure to hydrocarbons defined by Hsieh et al. (1983).

k The authors stated that there was no association.

## Lead

Kantor *et al.* (1979) reported a positive association between Wilms' tumour and paternal occupational exposure to lead (RR = 3.4, 95% CI 1.3–8.5; unmatched analysis of matched data). This raised interest in the possible role of occupational exposure to metals in the etiology of Wilms' tumour. In three subsequent studies, the association between paternal exposure to lead and Wilms' tumour was not confirmed (Wilkins & Sinks, 1984a,b; Bunin *et al.*, 1989b; Olshan *et al.*, 1990).

Kristensen and Andersen (1992) investigated the offspring of men who were members of the Oslo unions of printers. 33 (39.2 expected) cases of cancer were ascertained among 12 440 children (193 406 person-years) born in the period 1950–87 and traced by means of linkage with the Norwegian cancer registry during 1965–87. One of the cases had a renal tumour. The standardized incidence ratio associated with paternal exposure to lead for cancer of any type developing in children aged up to 14 years was 0.8 (3 exposed cases, 95% CI 0.2–2.3), while that for children aged over 14 years was 1.4 (9 exposed cases, 95% CI 0.6–2.6). For fathers exposed to lead and solvents, the standardized incidence ratios were 0.3 (one exposed case, 95% CI 0.0–1.4) and 0.6 (five exposed cases, 95% CI 0.2–1.4), respectively.

Positive associations between Wilms' tumour and paternal employment as a welder or in other occupations possibly involving exposure to metals have been reported in a few other studies (Bunin *et al.*, 1989b; Olshan *et al.*, 1990; Olsen *et al.*, 1991; Sharpe *et al.*, 1995). However, in one of these, there was no association between Wilms' tumour and groups of occupations in which there was potential heavy exposure to metals (Bunin *et al.*, 1989b).

## Boron

In a study of 62 cases with Wilms' tumour and 124 controls in which the job–exposure linkage system of Hoar *et al.* (1980) was applied, relative risks of 3.5 or more were observed for 24 of 298 agents which could be evaluated (Wilkins & Sinks, 1984a). The only agent for which the association was statistically significant was boron (7 exposed cases; RR = 3.5, 95% CI 1.02–15.1).

In a multicentre study of Wilms' tumour in the USA (Olshan *et al.*, 1990) a job–exposure matrix, based on a survey of over 4000 workplaces in the USA by a team of engineers (Sieber *et al.*, 1991), was used. The odds ratio for boron exposure during the preconceptional period was 1.4 (95% CI 0.5–3.8; 11 exposed cases), during pregnancy 1.9 (95% CI 0.5–6.7; 6 exposed cases) and postnatally 2.4 (95% CI 0.6–9.6; 6 exposed cases). These were little changed by adjustment for household income, the major confounding factor identified. A limitation of the study is the low participation rates (52% of eligible subjects in case and control groups).

Using the matrix of Hoar *et al.* (1980), Bunin *et al.* (1989b) observed that five of 28 fathers of cases with Wilms' tumour of the 'genetic' type (defined as bilateral disease or associated with nephroblastomatosis) were potentially exposed to boron in the preconceptional, gestational or postnatal periods, whereas no control fathers were exposed; this difference was associated with a *p* value of 0.07. No association was apparent for 42 'non-genetic' cases (defined as unilateral disease without nephroblastomatosis and without a Wilms' tumour-related anomaly); the numbers of prenatally exposed subjects were not specified. As already discussed, the subclassification of cases now appears to be invalid (see Chapter 3).

Thus, there is a consistent association in three studies from the USA between Wilms' tumour and inferred paternal occupational exposure to boron. As no assessment of specific exposure to boron was made in any of the studies, the evidence for an association with boron is weak, particularly as multiple statistical testing was carried out. The association does not appear to have been investigated in other studies.

## Pesticides

In a multicentre study in the USA of 200 cases of Wilms' tumour and 233 matched controls selected by random-digit dialling, the relative risk associated with at least one household extermination for insects or pesticides in the three years preceding diagnosis was 2.2 (95% CI 1.2–3.8; Olshan *et al.*, 1993). The analysis was based on questionnaires obtained for just over 50% of potentially eligible subjects, so the possibility of selection bias cannot be excluded.

High rates of Wilms' tumour have been observed in Brazil (Stiller & Parkin, 1990b). In an investigation intended to explore possible reasons for these high rates, parents of 109 cases of Wilms' tumour admitted to hospitals in four cities in Brazil during the period 1987–89 and 218 age- and sex-matched control children admitted to the same or nearby hospitals for treatment of non-neoplastic diseases were interviewed (Sharpe *et al.*, 1995). The relative risk of Wilms' tumour associated with the father having worked on the farm and having been exposed to pesticides there compared with no farm work was 3.9 (95% CI 1.3–11.1), after adjustment for income and education. The relative risk associated with the father having worked on a farm without pesticide exposure was 1.3 (95% CI 0.6–2.7), again adjusted for income and education; the corresponding relative risk for the mother was 1.2 (95% CI 0.6–2.3). The relative risk, adjusted for income and education, associated with the mother having worked on a farm with exposure to pesticides was 3.1 (95% CI 0.9–10.9). Paternal and maternal exposures to pesticides were correlated. The risk elevations were more pronounced among boys than among girls. The educational level and income of parents of cases was substantially higher than that of controls. Many of the diseases for which controls were undergoing treatment were of types which tend to occur among the poor living in unsanitary, crowded conditions, e.g., pulmonary tuberculosis and amoebic dysentery. Therefore, it is possible that the association with pesticide exposure is, at least in part, an artefact of the source populations of cases and controls being different.

In the offspring of men and women who worked in agriculture in Norway, Wilms' tumour was related to living on a farm with orchards or greenhouses, as recorded at the census closest to the year of birth (RR = 4.8, 95% CI 1.6–14.7), adjusted for year of birth and calendar year (Kristensen *et al.*, 1996). In addition, in the subset of subjects covered in the 1969 census, there was a positive association with residence on a farm with pesticide spraying equipment (RR = 2.5; 95% CI 1.0–6.6; adjusted for year of birth and calendar year). For subjects with both of these exposure indicators, the relative risk was 8.9 (95% CI 2.7–29.5; adjusted for year of birth and calendar year).

Paternal employment in agriculture has not consistently been associated with Wilms' tumour (Kantor *et al.*, 1979; Wilkins & Sinks, 1984b; McDowall, 1985; Olshan *et al.*, 1990).

## Hepatoblastoma

In a study of hepatoblastoma, exposures to chlorinated hydrocarbons were considered because they were thought to be potentially hepatotoxic (Buckley *et al.*, 1989a). The relative risks associated with the mother ever having been exposed to oil or coal products was 3.7 (*p* < 0.05), to paints or pigments also 3.7 (*p* < 0.05),

to a solvent or cleaning agent 1.0, and to plastic materials 1.5. The corresponding relative risks associated with paternal lifetime exposure were 1.9 (0.05 < *p* < 0.1), 1.5, 1.1 and 0.7. In this study, eight case mothers and one control mother reported occupational exposure to metals, welding or soldering (RR = 8.0, 95% CI 1.5–148.4). Most of these exposures occurred before and/or during the index pregnancy. The relative risk associated with paternal exposure to metals was 3.0 (*p* < 0.05); there was no association specifically with welding or soldering. The metals involved in both maternal and paternal exposure were diverse.

## Osteosarcoma

In a case–control study of 130 cases of osteosarcoma diagnosed at ages up to 24 years and a similar number of age–sex-matched controls selected from birth certificates in New York State, no associations were found with parental occupations during the lifetime of the index subject (Gelberg *et al.*, 1997). In a study of 61 cases of osteosarcoma diagnosed at similar ages in Los Angeles and 124 friend and neighbourhood controls, the relative risk associated with the mother having worked in manufacturing industry from the year before pregnancy until the child's birth was 3.8 (95% CI 1.3–11.2; Operskalski *et al.*, 1987). Among the case mothers, 8% reported occupational chemical exposures compared with 5% of the control mothers.

In the offspring of parents engaged in agricultural activities in Norway, osteosarcoma was associated with chicken farming as recorded at the census closest to the year of birth (RR = 2.9, 95% CI 1.4–6.1), adjusted for year of birth and calendar year (Kristensen *et al.*, 1996).

## Ewing's sarcoma

In both of the available studies, a positive association with paternal employment in agriculture was observed (Holly *et al.*, 1992; Winn *et al.*, 1992). In the study of Winn *et al.* (1992), a multicentre investigation in the USA and Canada of 208 cases diagnosed at ages up to 22 years and a similar number of controls selected by random-digit dialling, the relative risk of paternal employment on a farm compared with white-collar work during pregnancy was 2.2 (95% CI 0.7–6.5), and that with the usual employment of the father being in farming was 3.1 (95% CI 0.9–9.5). In the other study, based on 43 cases diagnosed at ages up to 31 years in the San Francisco Bay area and 193 controls selected by random-digit dialling, the relative risk for children whose fathers were engaged in agricultural occupations during the period from six months before conception up to diagnosis was 8.8 (95% CI 1.8–42.7), adjusted for history of poisoning or overdose of medication of the study subject, area of residence, year of birth and family income (Holly *et al.*, 1992). All seven fathers of cases, compared with three of the five fathers of controls who worked in these occupations, reported occupational exposure to herbicides, pesticides or fertilizers (RR = 6.1, 95% CI 1.7–21.9; adjusted as above). Home exposure to pesticides also was considered in this study. The relative risk associated with professional pest extermination in the home during pregnancy was 0.3 (95% CI 0.0–2.1), and that for the corresponding exposure during the lifetime of the index child was 0.6 (95% CI 0.3–1.2).

## Soft-tissue sarcoma

In a study of childhood cancer of all types in Denver, Colorado (USA), there was a positive association (RR about 4) between soft-tissue sarcoma and treatment of the area around the home with insecticides or herbicides during the lifetime of the index child (Leiss & Savitz, 1995). No association was found with use of home pest extermination or pest strips. In a small exploratory study (33 cases, 99 controls selected from birth certificates) of rhabdomyosarcoma in North Carolina, the relative risk associated with childhood exposure to pesticides was 1.5 (95% CI 0.4–6.5) and that associated with exposure to rodenticides was 1.0 (95% CI 0.1–9.9) (Grufferman *et al.*, 1982).

On the basis of the study of Leiss and Savitz (1995), and of studies of soft-tissue sarcoma in adults which suggested a positive association with phenoxy acids used in grain farming and forestry, Kristensen *et al.* (1996) investigated the offspring of men and women engaged in agricultural work in Norway. No association between soft-tissue sarcoma and residence on a grain farm, on a farm with 2.5 hectares or more given over to forestry or on a farm with pesticide spraying equipment as recorded on the census was found. The use of such crude indicators of exposure would have been likely to bias the relative risks towards unity.

In the small study of rhabdomyosarcoma described above, Grufferman *et al.* (1982) reported that residence near a factory that emitted chemical pollution was associated with a relative risk of 3.3 (95% CI 0.5–22). There was no association with reported exposure to fumes, dust or waste. The relative risk associated with exposure during childhood to chemicals other than rodenticides or pesticides was 3.2 (95% CI 1.1–9.2).

## Conclusions

In most studies, a positive association between leukaemia and postnatal exposure of the index child to pesticides has been observed. Positive associations have been observed with maternal and paternal occupational exposure to pesticides in some, but not all, studies. The possibility that these associations may be due to confounding by patterns of infection which may be associated with population mixing cannot be excluded.

No consistent association between leukaemia and paternal occupational exposure to hydrocarbons or benzene is apparent. The effects of maternal occupational exposure have been less studied. In two out of three studies of ANLL, a positive association with maternal occupational exposure to hydrocarbons was observed. No clear association with residential proximity to industrial sources of hydrocarbons, and no consistent association with measures of exposure to vehicle exhaust, has been observed.

In all three studies in which paternal exposure to solvents was investigated, a positive association was found. In two other studies, postnatal exposure of the index child was studied, and again a positive association was found.

In two studies in which data specifically on ANLL were presented, a positive association with reported maternal occupational exposure to metals was found.

In most studies of brain tumours of all types combined, a positive association with intra-uterine or postnatal exposure to pesticides has been observed. No association was observed in three case–control studies of astrocytoma. It is possible that the association is confined to other types of brain tumour. This is suggested by the results of a cohort study in which exposure data were obtained from censuses. In the one available case–control study of primitive neuroectodermal tumours of the brain, no association with household exposure to pesticides was found. The associations with pesticide exposure may be compatible with the hypothesis that childhood brain tumours are caused by exposure to *N*-nitroso compounds.

No clear association with the father working in industries or occupations with high levels of inferred exposure to *N*-nitroso compounds is apparent. No consistent association with paternal occupational exposure to hydrocarbons has been observed.

Two recent studies were suggestive of an association between neuroblastoma and parental occupational exposure to pesticides. This does not appear to be attributable to residence in agricultural areas or paternal employment in agricultural work.

In three studies in which associations between Wilms' tumour and household or parental occupational exposure to pesticides was investigated, a positive association was found. In two of these, selection bias may have occurred, and might have led to overestimation of the relative risks. In the third, the marker of exposure was crude; this would have been expected to bias the relative risk towards unity.

There appears to be a consistent association between Wilms' tumour and paternal employment as a welder or in other occupations possibly involving exposure to metals. An early finding that this was specific to lead was not confirmed in other studies. In the three studies in which inferred paternal exposure to boron was investigated, a positive association was found.

With regard to other types of childhood cancer, two studies suggest a positive association between retinoblastoma and paternal employment in occupations involving welding. In the one available study of hepatoblastoma, there were positive associations with parental occupational exposure to metals, and maternal occupational exposure to oil or coal products, and paints or pigments.

The associations between chemical exposures and lymphomas have been little studied. No consistent association with pesticide exposure or parental occupational exposure has been identified in the few available studies.

In the few available studies, no consistent association between soft-tissue sarcoma and pesticides or other chemicals was found. In both of the available studies of Ewing's sarcoma, there was a positive association with paternal employment in agriculture. In one of these, this appears to be due to pesticides, but there was no association with use of pesticides in the home. No consistent association with maternal occupation was found in the two available studies of osteosarcoma.

Thus, for several types of childhood cancer, positive associations with exposure to pesticides have been reported. In addition, positive associations with parental occupational exposure to metals have been observed for ANLL (maternal exposure), Wilms' tumour (paternal exposure) and retinoblastoma (paternal exposure). These observations require confirmation.

In virtually all of the studies, exposure was assessed on the basis of interview, usually with the mother, or was inferred on the basis of job title. As noted in the introduction, this may have led to substantial misclassification. If this had been non-differential, it would have biased the relative risk towards unity. The studies based on assessing specific exposures by interview may have been affected by recall bias. This might be a concern in relation to pesticides, in view of the fact that associations with this exposure have been observed for several types of childhood cancer. However, the observation of associations for the same types of childhood cancer in a cohort study in Norway as in the case–control studies suggests that this is unlikely.

It would be valuable in future studies to attempt to validate information on occupational exposures from employers' records, and/or where possible, to include biomarkers of exposure. In addition, multicentre collaboration would facilitate assessment of the consistency of association between studies, and potentially increase statistical power, particularly in relation to specific subtypes of childhood cancer.

Virtually all of the specific exposures considered have been of concern also in the study of adult cancer, and in this connection, international collaborative cohort studies are in progress for some occupational exposures, largely in men. Concern has been expressed about the possible teratogenicity of some of the exposures. In particular, relatively little work has been carried out on the possible teratogenic effects of exposures to the father (Taskinen, 1990). Therefore, it would seem worthwhile to explore the possibility of adding an offspring component to on-going collaborative international cohort studies.

# Chapter 7

# Infection

Most investigation of possible relationships between infection and childhood cancer has related to childhood leukaemia and non-Hodgkin lymphoma. Spatial clustering of childhood leukaemia has been observed in Great Britain, Greece and Hong Kong, but not in Sweden or in metropolitan areas of the USA (see Chapter 2). Clusters of childhood leukaemia have been observed around some nuclear sites, and also in areas in which construction of nuclear sites was considered but not initiated (see Chapter 4). This has led to renewed interest in the possibility that there is an infectious etiology of childhood leukaemia. In this chapter, the evidence as to a possible relationship between childhood leukaemia and a potential source of microepidemics of infection, namely population mixing, is discussed. In addition, studies of the associations between infection of the mother during the index pregnancy, and of the index child during his or her lifetime, and childhood leukaemia and other types of cancer are reviewed.

## Leukaemia

### The Kinlen hypothesis: residence in areas with high levels of population mixing

Kinlen (1988) suggested that the excess of leukaemia in young people in the vicinity of the Sellafield and Dounreay nuclear reprocessing plants in the United Kingdom might be due to a rare response to some unidentified mild or subclinical infection, the transmission of which is facilitated by contacts between large numbers of people. An influx of population of diverse origins into a previously isolated area, as has occurred with the construction of new nuclear installations in the UK, would particularly facilitate transmission. Intense exposure would be leukaemogenic, while mild or moderate exposure would be immunizing. Therefore, the incidence of leukaemia would be expected to be higher in areas whose populations had diverse

origins and in which there had been a recent increase to high population density. Thus, an excess of leukaemia in childhood would be expected in isolated areas into which there had been substantial in-migration, and in which there was no nuclear installation. In a first test of this hypothesis (Kinlen, 1988), one area in Scotland, Glenrothes New Town, was identified *a priori* as meeting these criteria. A significant excess of leukaemia deaths below age 25 years was identified during the period 1951–67 (10 deaths observed compared with 3.6 expected on the basis of applying Scottish national mortality rates to the estimated person-years at risk). There was no excess in the period 1968–85, when the community became much less isolated following the opening of the Forth road bridge in 1964. This was the first instance of a particular 'cluster' being found as predicted by a hypothesis specified before the data were collected. The hypothesis has been tested in a number of other situations in Great Britain, France, other parts of Europe and Hong Kong (Table 7.1).

### Areas of population growth (Table 7.1)

In new towns whose populations had the combined features of diverse origins and higher density than that before the area was designated as a 'new town', and also higher density than those in the areas from which most incomers came (referred to as 'rural new towns'), the mortality rate of leukaemia at ages under five years was higher (O/E = 1.9) than that expected on the basis of national rates in the period 1946–85 (Kinlen *et al.*, 1990). The mortality rate was similar to that expected in the 0–4-year age group for new towns built as 'dormitories' for Glasgow and London, which combined the features of little diversity of origin and lower population density than in Glasgow itself or the London boroughs (referred to as 'overspill new towns'). The use of mortality data is a limitation, but the difference between these groups of towns was greater for the first half of the study period (1946–65) than the second. The first half was before improvements in the treatment of childhood leukaemia brought about remarkable declines in mortality (Levi *et al.*, 1995). The reduction of the observed to expected ratio for rural new towns in the second half of the study period, from 2.3 to 1.4, is consistent with a reduction in population mixing, but may be confounded by improvements in treatment.

There were deficits of leukaemia mortality at older ages in both groups of towns; these were statistically significant for the rural new towns. The authors considered that this pattern is consistent with the immunizing effects of the postulated infection. The deficit at older ages was apparent in both halves of the study period in the rural new towns, but only in the second half of the study period in the overspill new towns. This would be consistent with a more severe epidemic in the rural than in the overspill towns. The leukaemia excess in the rural towns was greatest where the population density was highest. The four rural new towns in England and Wales ranked higher than 90% of the 1445 local authority areas outside London for density of children, and two were in the top 5%. By contrast, the density of children in the London overspill towns was lower than in the London boroughs. The excesses were not confined to leukaemia of a single cell type. The authors considered the possibility that the results were produced by the effects of inaccurate population estimates on the calculation of expected numbers of cases. Results were little changed by using different methods of estimating the total number of person-years of exposure, and the effects were still apparent when the analysis was restricted to census years and the years immediately before and after these. In addition, the effects were apparent when local authority districts containing new towns, rather than the new towns themselves, were considered.

Langford and Bentham (1990) noted that new towns were not the only places in the UK in which rapid population growth had been experienced. They compared numbers of observed deaths due to leukaemia in the age range 0–14 years with those expected in all 1366 local authority areas in England and Wales during the period 1969–73, classified by the level of population change between the 1961 and 1971 censuses. The expected numbers of deaths were calculated by applying national rates to the local population at risk as recorded in the 1971 census. In the areas in which the population increase had been by more than 50%, the ratio of observed to expected number of deaths was 1.4 (95% CI 1.1–1.7). The ratio for the 0–4-year age group was 1.3 (95% CI 0.9–1.8), and that for the 5–14-year age group was 1.5 (95% CI 1.1–1.9). None of the observed to expected ratios for areas with lower population growth were markedly different from unity, and none of the departures from unity was statistically significant. There was little effect of excluding the data from the more remote new towns included in the analysis of Kinlen *et al.* (1990). On the basis of Poisson *p*-values calculated for each area compared with the national average, areas of significantly raised leukaemia mortality were concentrated in and around the major conurbations (Langford, 1991).

Laplanche and de Vathaire (1994a) found that leukaemia mortality under the age of 25 years was similar to that expected (44 vs. 42.7) in communes in France in which large and rapid population increases occurred between 1968 and 1990. These communes were defined as those with a population increase exceeding 100% between two consecutive censuses, held in 1968, 1975, 1982 and 1990, and with populations greater than 10 000 inhabitants in 1990. Of a total of 834 communes with greater than 10 000 inhabitants in 1990, 43 had large and rapid population increases; of these 9 had fewer than 1000 inhabitants in 1968, 21 between 1000 and 5000 inhabitants, 11 between 5000 and 10 000 inhabitants, and two had 10 000 or more inhabitants (Laplanche & de Vathaire, 1994b). The study was limited to communes with more than 10 000 inhabitants in order to conform with French legal confidentiality requirements. Person-years were estimated by linear interpolation between censuses. Expected mortality was determined from national rates. There was no difference in leukaemia mortality according to the size of the population increase.

Stiller and Boyle (1996) analysed the effects of migration and diversity of migrant origin on the incidence of acute lymphoblastic leukaemia (ALL) in children aged under 15 years in 403 county districts of England and Wales during the period 1979–85. A total of 2035 cases was ascertained; histological or haematological confirmation of diagnosis was available for 2017 (99%). Information on the proportions of all residents and of children aged under 15 years who had been resident outside the district one year previously were obtained from the 1981 census. There was a positive association between the incidence of ALL at ages 0–4 and 5–9 years and the proportion of children in the district who had recently entered it. This was not found for the 10–14-year age group. There was no association with total migration. In the 0–4-year age group, the incidence of ALL was positively associated with the proportion of economically active men in employment, and in the 5–9-year

## Table 7.1. Summary of studies testing the Kinlen hypothesis: associations between childhood leukaemia and measures of population mixing

*Studies based on comparison of observed numbers of deaths due to leukaemia at ages up to 24 years in exposed and unexposed areas with those expected on the basis of national rates*

| Reference | Area | Period | Exposed area Definition | 0-24 years O | 0-24 years O/E | 0-4 years O | 0-4 years O/E | Unexposed area Definition | 0-24 years O | 0-24 years O/E | 0-4 years O | 0-4 years O/E |
|---|---|---|---|---|---|---|---|---|---|---|---|---|
| Kinlen, 1988 | Scotland | 1951-85 (total) | LAD with population increase of 25% or more between 1951 and 1961, with population >2000 in 1951, not including nuclear installation, furthest from a population centre of 100 000 or more. | 11 | 1.3 | 7 | 2.5 | Other LADs with population increase of 25% or more between 1951 and 1961, not including nuclear power installation | 41 | 0.8 | 12 | 0.8 |
| | | 1951-67 (first half) | | 10 | 2.8 | 7 | 4.7 | | 17 | 0.8 | 7 | 0.8 |
| Kinlen *et al.*, 1990 | Great Britain | 1946-85 (total) | 'Rural' New Town[a] | 39 | 0.9 | 24 | 1.9 | 'Overspill' New Town | 133 | 0.8 | 38 | 0.8 |
| | | 1946-65 (first half) | | 18 | 1.1 | 15 | 2.3 | | 52 | 0.9 | 22 | 1.0 |
| Langford & Bentham, 1990; Langford, 1991 | England and Wales | 1969-73 | Local authority areas with >50% population increase between 1961 and 1971. | 81[b] | 1.4[b] | 30 | 1.3 | Local authority areas with population increase of 50% or less, or no population increase between 1961 and 1971 | 1519[b] | 1.0[b] | 591 | 1.0 |
| Laplanche & de Vathaire, 1994a | France | 1968-89 | 43 communes with population increase of >100% between census years. | 44 | 1.0 | 8 | 0.7 | 791 communes with population increase of ≤100% between census years | 57 | 0.8 | 9 | 0.6 |

*Studies based on comparison of observed numbers of cases or deaths with those expected from national rates in areas with different levels of exposure*

| Reference | Area | Estimation of exposure | Period | Group | Number of cases | Number of levels of exposure | Ratio of O/E in highest vs lowest level | p value (from chi-square for trend if 3 levels of exposure considered) |
|---|---|---|---|---|---|---|---|---|
| Kinlen & Hudson, 1991 | England and Wales | Proportions of servicemen in 1951 census populations in aggregated rural and urban districts. Proportions of servicement in 1951 census populations in LADs. | 1950-53 | Deaths 0-14 | 1329 | 5 | 1.2 | <0.01 |
| | | | | <2 | 168 | 9 | 1.9 | <0.05 |
| | | | | 2-4 | 509 | | 0.9 | NS |
| Kinlen *et al.*, 1991 | England | Extent of increase between 1971 and 1981 in sum of numbers of residents who worked outside a borough and numbers of residents of other areas who worked within the borough in 28 county boroughs/districts whose boundaries did not change between the censuses. | 1972-85 | Incident cases[c] 0-14 | 531 | 10 | 1.5 | <0.001 |
| | | | | 0-4 | 272 | | 1.8 | <0.001 |

| Reference | Location | Description | Period | Case type / age | Number | | Ratio | p |
|---|---|---|---|---|---|---|---|---|
| Petridou *et al.*, 1991 | Greece | Residence at time of death on islands (or groups of islands) with more than 10000 inhabitants. | 1976–89 | Deaths 0–14 | 103 | 1 | 1.1 | ns[g] |
| Kinlen *et al.*, 1993a | Scotland | Ratio of oil workers, as identified from medical records in 1 centre, employer's records in another, and all those who obtained an offshore survival certificate during the period 1976-80, to economically active men in 1981 census, in each postcode sector. | 1974–78 1979–83 1984–88 | Incident cases[c] 0–24 | 400 343 377 | 3 | 1.1 1.2 1.1 | ns <0.01[d] ns |
| | | | 1974–78 1979–83 1984–88 | 0–4 | 130 115 119 | 3 | 0.9 1.6 0.9 | ns <0.01[d] ns |
| Kinlen & John, 1994 | England and Wales: rural districts | Ratio of the number of evacuated people to the number of local children. | 1945–49 | Deaths 0–14 0–4 5–14 | 229 135 144 | 3 | 1.5 1.2 1.9 | 0.020 0.311 0.014 |
| | Urban districts | | | 0–14 0–4 | 574 304 | 3 | 0.9 0.9 | ns ns |
| Kinlen *et al.*, 1995 | Great Britain, rural areas | Residence at time of diagnosis within 10 km of a construction site, or a highland county in Scotland, during the year in which construction began to the year after its completion. | 1946–93 | Incident cases 0–14 0–4 5–14 | 130 63 67 | 1 | 1.4 1.4 1.4 | <0.001 <0.01 <0.05 |
| | | Residence in same areas in five years before start of construction phase. | | 0–14 | 30 | 1 | 1.2 | ns |
| | | Residence in same areas in five years after completion of construction phase. | | 0–14 | 29 | 1 | 0.8 | ns |
| Stiller & Boyle, 1996 | England and Wales, county districts | Child migration. | 1979–85 | Incident cases 0–4 5–9 6–14 | 1039 583 413 | 3 | 1.3 1.6 0.7 | <0.05 <0.05[e] ns |
| | | Total migration. | | 0–4 5–9 10–14 | 1039 583 413 | 3 | 1.3 1.3 1.0 | ns[f] ns ns |
| Alexander *et al.*, 1997 | Hong Kong | Residence at time of diagnosis in groups of small census areas ranked according to population growth during the period 1981–86. | 1984–90 | Incident cases (total) 0–14 0–4 2–6 ALL, 2–6 Common ALL, 2–6 | 30 15 16 15 9 | 1 1 1 1 1 | 1.0[h] 1.1[h] 1.3[h] 1.4[h] 1.8[h] | ns[i] ns[i] ns[i] ns[i] 0.07[i] |

ns, Not statistically significant.
LAD, Local Authority District.
*a* Five in all, including Glenrothes. Figures presented do not include Glenrothes.
*b* 0–14 years.
*c* Leukaemia and non-Hodgkin lymphoma.
*d* In rural areas only.

*e* $p < 0.01$ if child migration analysed as a continuous variable rather than as a categorical variable with three levels.
*f* $p < 0.05$ if total migration analysed as a continuous variable rather than as a categorical variable with three levels.
*g* There was no evidence of heterogeneity in the O/E ratio between the 13 islands or island groups
*h* Comparison was between numbers of cases observed in areas experiencing population growth in the top 10% compared with numbers expected when overall Hong Kong age-sex-specific rates applied to the local population.
*i* $p = 0.014$ or less using Pothoff-Whittinghill method of analysis of spatial clustering.

age group the incidence was positively associated with the proportion of households with a car. Job migration and these measures of socioeconomic status were correlated. Areas of low unemployment attract incoming families, and families of higher social class tend to be more mobile. As population mixing is more likely than socioeconomic status to increase rapidly, and some of the highest incidence rates for leukaemia have been observed in situations of very high increases in the levels of population mixing, it is possible that population mixing may account for some of the association between leukaemia and socioeconomic status.

In 1973 in Hong Kong, a massive programme of building new towns to meet the needs of the expanding population was initiated in the New Territories (Alexander *et al.*, 1997). The population of the New Territories increased over seven-fold by 1979–89. In addition nearly three quarters of a million new housing units were constructed in parts of Hong Kong Island and Kowloon. In areas with the highest deciles of population growth, the incidence of leukaemia was elevated but did not differ significantly from that in other areas. However, within these areas, there was strong evidence of spatial clustering as assessed by the Potthoff–Whittinghill method. This accounted for the overall pattern of spatial clustering observed in Hong Kong during the period 1984–90 (see section on spatial clustering of leukaemia, Chapter 2); there was no significant evidence of clustering in the rest of Hong Kong. The results for spatial clustering were dominated by excess incidence in one small census area. This pattern was accounted for by ALL in young children, and was not observed for sub-groups of childhood leukaemia from which ALL occurring in the childhood peak was excluded.

The series of findings relating to population influx in Great Britain and elsewhere have some similarities with the observation of the cluster of leukaemia in Niles, Illinois, which may have been associated with abrupt changes in patterns of disease associated with rapid expansion of the community (Heath & Hasterlik, 1963; see Chapter 2). Public concern about an increased incidence of childhood leukaemia in south-west Sardinia led to an investigation of incidence in Cagliari province during the period 1974–89 (Cocco *et al.*, 1993). The high incidence in the town of Carbonia during the period 1983–85 was confirmed. The authors noted that this would not be incompatible with population influx, which followed the establishment of new industries in the early 1970s.

Kinlen and Petridou (1995) considered mortality due to childhood leukaemia in 33 countries during the period 1958–87 in relation to the proportion of the economically active population employed in agricultural occupa-tions and qualitative data on rural migration. Countries were classified as 'rural' if the proportion of the economically active population employed in agricultural occupa-tions was at least 30% in 1950 or 20% in 1960. No measure of rural-to-urban migration suitable for international comparisons was available. Internal migration in Greece and Italy was particularly striking, and attempts were made to restrict internal migration in these countries by law. Between 1958 and 1972, Greece had the highest recorded mortality from childhood leukaemia in the world. In the following quinquennium, (1973–77), it had the second highest rate, after which there was a steep decline in mortality from childhood leukaemia. While Kinlen and Petridou (1995) suggested that this may, at least in part, have been accounted for by the decline in internal migration after the early 1970s, it is not possible to separate any possible such effect from that due to improvements in treatment. High rates of mortality attributed to childhood leukaemia also were observed in Italy. However, in Finland, where there was rapid urbanization in the 1950s as a result of the movements of displaced rural inhabitants from Karelia, the childhood leukaemia mortality rate was not particularly high during the quinquenium 1958–62, although the rate was higher during the period 1963–72. In Czechoslovakia, marked rural depopulation occurred in the 1960s, but the rates of childhood leukaemia mortality were not particularly high. In Denmark and Sweden, which were classified as 'urban', high rates of leukaemia mortality were observed but there were no major movements of the rural population. It is possible that the quality of death certification was uniformly high in these countries. Internationally, death rates from leukaemia and ill-defined causes tend to be inversely correlated (West, 1984). In Greece, not only were there higher mortality rates due to childhood leukaemia, but also of deaths from ill-defined causes and of deaths in childhood due to infection. This suggests that the high mortality rate due to leukaemia in Greece may have been real rather than artefactual. In Israel, after large-scale immigration in the 1950s, leukaemia mortality at ages 0–4 years in the period 1956–58 was appreciably higher (5.1 per 100 000) than in 1950–52 (3.2), 1953–55 (3.5), 1959–61 (3.8) and 1962–64 (2.7) (Kinlen, 1994).

An observation which appears to be incompatible with the Kinlen hypothesis is that, according to census data for 1961 and 1971, in districts near sites considered for the construction of nuclear installations the population of young people increased less than in England and Wales as a whole, while the population of adults of working age decreased more (Cook-Mozaffari *et al.*, 1989b). This does not suggest that a leukaemia excess in these areas was brought about by the intermingling of population consequent upon the sudden influx of a new labour force and their families.

*Wartime evacuation*

Wolff (1991b) suggested that if it were true that there is an infective basis for childhood leukaemia, an increase in leukaemia mortality associated with wartime evacuation in Britain might have been expected. As a result of evacuation in Britain during the Second World War, 827 000 unaccompanied children, 524 000 mothers with children under five years old and 13 000 pregnant women migrated from major conurbations into rural areas between 1 and 4 September 1939. However, during the period 1931–50, there was no marked change in the unexplained steady rise in leukaemia mortality in the 0–4-year age group, suggesting that herd mixing may be an inadequate explanation for local increases in the incidence of leukaemia. Wolff acknowledged that extrapolation from overall to local migration trends may be questionable. The evacuation at the beginning of the war was not the sole example of large-scale population movement during the war. For example, before the Normandy landings in 1944, large numbers of troops trained or massed in certain coastal areas of England, but in these areas there had been large-scale evacuation of the local population including adults (Kinlen & Hudson, 1991). Moreover, during the period of compulsory national service after the war, in many areas the numbers of servicemen were larger than had been the case during the war.

Kinlen and John (1994) investigated mortality due to childhood leukaemia during the period 1945–49 in relation to the ratio of government evacuees to local children in September 1941. Information was obtained from a billeting schedule which gave the numbers of unaccompanied and accompanied children, mothers and other evacuated adults present in each local authority area at that time. Data on numbers of evacuees at other times during the war were not available. The numbers of local children in each district in 1941 were estimated

from those recorded in 1947, the only year between 1939 and 1951 for which age-specific populations of children were known for each local authority district. The 476 rural districts were ranked into tertiles according to the evacuee index. (The definition of 'rural' was not explicitly stated.) The relative risk of death due to leukaemia in the districts in the highest tertile of the evacuee index was 1.5 (95% CI 1.1–2.1) compared with those in the lowest tertile, with a significant increasing trend ($p = 0.02$) across the three categories. This trend in part reflected a significantly lower than average death rate from childhood leukaemia in the tertile with the lowest evacuee index. The trend was not apparent for children aged 0–4 years. In view of the absence of any census in the 15 years before 1947, separate calculations were made for the period 1947–49, deriving estimates of the local populations from the national registration records of 1947 and the 1951 census. The excesses were more apparent than in the analysis for the period 1945–49. For each set of areas, leukaemia mortality was also examined in the period 1950–53, in conjunction with denominator data from the 1951 census. No trends were apparent in this period. The numbers of deaths due to leukaemia in urban and rural districts which were evacuated were similar to those expected for both the period 1945–49 and the period 1950–53. No excess or trend was detected in non-evacuated urban areas classified in terms of the ratio of evacuees to local children.

If early and intense exposure to evacuated people in some areas had produced an excess of leukaemia which lasted only 3–4 years – as observed in relation to large concentrations of national servicemen in the early 1950s (Kinlen & Hudson, 1991; see section on National Service below) – this would have been missed. In Devon, which received more evacuees than any other county, four deaths due to leukaemia at the ages 0–4 years were registered among local children, compared with 2.5 expected during the period 1940–44, whereas no deaths at these ages were observed in the period 1945–49, compared with 3.7 expected ($p < 0.05$).

The apparent contradiction between the findings of Wolff (1991b) and those of Kinlen and John (1994) may be explained from the effect that national death rates tend to be insensitive to increases among children living in rural areas, as they represent a small proportion of the total number of children in Great Britain. Increases in the incidence of diphtheria, scarlet fever, measles and whooping cough in reception areas for evacuees were not apparent in national notification rates (Kinlen & John, 1994).

*National service*

Another test of the Kinlen hypothesis involved the determination of whether any excess of childhood leukaemia was associated with the introduction of national service in 1947 (Kinlen & Hudson, 1991). National (military) service was for 12 months on introduction, and was extended to 18 months in 1949, and to two years in 1950. These extensions caused substantial increases in the number of servicemen assigned to different parts of the country. In data from the 1951 census, the only source of details about the distribution of servicemen in England and Wales around that time, in 15 local authority districts, mainly rural, servicemen outnumbered civilian men of working age. The period of study was centred on the 1951 census year, but as no leukaemia data by area were available for 1949, the period of study selected was 1950–53. Rural and urban districts, aggregated by county, were ranked by proportion of servicemen in the population and groups containing similar numbers of children were created. The range in the proportion of servicemen in the highest quintile was 1.5–11.3% for urban areas, and 9.0–27.1% for rural areas. Expected numbers of deaths from leukaemia at ages under one, 1–4, 5–9 and 10–14 years were calculated by applying age-specific death rates from leukaemia in England and Wales during 1950–53. Overall, a significant trend of increase in the mortality due to leukaemia at ages under 15 years was found across the quintiles of proportions of servicemen, with a ratio of observed to expected deaths in the highest quintile for rural and urban areas combined of 1.21. This was mainly due to a more marked excess in rural areas, with a ratio of 1.65 in the highest quintile, again associated with a significant trend. In turn, this reflects excess deaths in rural areas in young children; the ratio for the under-one-year age group was 4.13, and for the 1–4-year age group 1.62.

The authors considered the possibility that this relationship might be indirect, reflecting a high incidence of the disease in groups of counties that happened to include large military encampments. Therefore, a similar analysis was made based on the 1473 individual local authority districts of England and Wales. The population of children was divided into deciles according to the proportion of servicemen in the district. The proportion of servicemen was less than 1% for the first seven deciles, between 0.9%

and 1.5% for the eighth, between 1.5% and 5.2% for the ninth, and ranged up to 69% for the highest. The ratios of observed to expected deaths from leukaemia were expressed relative to the values in the first two deciles combined. As the first analysis had shown a significant trend in rural areas in both the under-one and 1–4-year age groups, the authors considered children aged one together with those aged less than this in this analysis. The ratio of observed to expected numbers of deaths in the category with the highest proportion of servicemen, standardized to the ratio in the two categories with the lowest proportions of servicemen, in the age group under two years, was 1.9, based on 31 observed deaths. This was statistically significant. Although there was a significant trend across the categories, the other ratios were close to unity. The excess was more marked in the aggregation of rural local authority districts than urban districts in the highest category. There was no excess at ages 2–4, 5–9 or 10–14 years. Because the numbers of infants below age one were known to be slightly underestimated in the census, the analysis was repeated using numbers of live births by local authority district from 1950–53 for populations below age one, and in 1949–52 for age one. The findings were not greatly affected and the significance levels were unchanged. Thus, the findings do not appear to be an artefact of the special status of military camps in the census, which may have led to undercounting. The same approach was used for the two succeeding five-year periods (1954–58 and 1959–63). There was no significant excess of leukaemia in any of the four age groups (less than 2, 2–4, 5–9, 10–14 years). In the last period, proportions of servicemen in the 1961 census were also considered, but again there was no excess. In this period, all but 4% of local authority districts showed a decline in the numbers of servicemen. There was one death from leukaemia in children below age one compared with 0.3 expected in the rural area with the greatest increase in the proportion of servicemen, an influx amounting to 31% of the male population of the district in 1961. The lack of persistence of the increase of leukaemia beyond the period 1950–53 would be consistent with the number of susceptible individuals declining to below some critical level, as would happen at the end of an epidemic of any infective disorder.

The excesses of leukaemia affected the very young children of both servicemen and civilians, although the number of cases of leukaemia may have been underestimated among the children of servicemen. Birth certificates of children of servicemen diagnosed with leukaemia at ages of less than two years in urban districts were not traced, so that any father who left the forces during his child's lifetime would have been overlooked. Cases of leukaemia in the children of US servicemen present in rural England during the study period may have been overlooked because of their return to the USA either before the disease was diagnosed or before the child died from the disease. The only population data for children of servicemen in the 1950s were those of births in 1951, and these were used as the basis for examining deaths from leukaemia at the youngest ages in the offspring of servicemen, and were distributed geographically broadly in proportion to the numbers of servicemen. However, as there was a higher than average proportion of 18 and 19-year-old servicemen in rural districts, the number of servicemen with children in these districts is likely to have been overestimated. This means that the excess in rural areas is likely to have been underestimated.

Using the same approach as for leukaemia mortality, available data on deaths attributed to and notifications of childhood infectious diseases were also investigated. At county level, there were excesses both of notifications and of deaths in children aged less than 15 years due to poliomyelitis in the three quintiles with the highest proportions of servicemen. At local authority district level, there were significantly more notifications of this disease among children below aged 15 years in the decile of rural areas with the highest concentrations of servicemen compared with the two with the lowest concentrations. These associations were not apparent for meningococcal infections. In addition, there was no excess of deaths from measles associated with increasing proportions of servicemen at county level, although there was a non-significant excess for deaths due to whooping cough. The authors noted that poliomyelitis resembles the infection they postulated as underlying childhood leukaemia in that only a small proportion of those infected develop an illness.

Kinlen and Hudson (1991) observed that the excess in young children was restricted to those under two years. Leukaemia occurring below the age of two is more commonly myeloid than lymphatic, and when it is lymphatic is more often null- or T-cell in type, than at ages 2–4 years, when there is the characteristic peak in incidence. Analysis by leukaemia sub-type was difficult to interpret because of the small numbers of deaths;

myeloid lymphoid but not monocytic leukaemia was represented in the excess.

As the conditions of military life would have prevented free contact with local people, this was not a typical example of population mixing. However, the authors considered that five features of rural districts might be particularly relevant to the excess of leukaemia found there. First, a greater proportion of the population of these districts would be susceptible to the agent or agents postulated to increase the risk of childhood leukaemia because of their low population density and distance from major population centres. Second, military camps in rural districts held more national servicemen than those in urban districts, and are likely to have been more overcrowded, thus facilitating transmission of infective agents. Third, unlike garrison towns, which were scattered, rural districts in the group with the highest proportion of servicemen often bordered each other, which might have intensified the effects of transmission. Fourth, the authors considered that a large rural military camp probably makes a greater overall impact on the population in its vicinity than would an urban camp. Finally, most Royal Air Force stations were in rural districts, and the relatively high social class of this branch of the national service intake might have implied a higher proportion of people susceptible to infection, increasing the severity of the postulated epidemic in the rural districts.

### Construction work

Another striking example of rural population mixing occurred in northern Scotland as a result of the development of the North Sea oil industry (Kinlen *et al.*, 1993a). The Sullom Voe oil terminal in Shetland was Europe's largest construction site and is sited in Britain's remotest region. Many thousands of men were transported and housed in specially built camps, drawn from diverse areas in Britain. Similar circumstances applied in the construction of the smaller terminal at Flotta in Orkney. In addition, offshore work involves many thousands of men travelling to Aberdeen in north-east Scotland from all over Britain, to be ferried from there to oil platforms by helicopter. Few children live close to these work sites, but the regular home visits of the workers might have brought about indirect exposure of their home communities to the effects of population mixing in the work sites. Kinlen *et al.*, (1993a) therefore investigated leukaemia and non-Hodgkin lymphoma in the 0–24-year age group in the rural home areas of workers at the oil terminal and offshore sites.

Complete records of workers on these sites have not been maintained. Workers at Sullom Voe during its construction phase were identified from records of the medical centre, and are believed to represent a high proportion of all but short-stay workers; information was obtained on more than 17 000 men. Incomplete data were available on 3500 construction workers at Flotta oil terminal. Finally, 10 000 offshore workers were identified from records of issue of an offshore survival certificate required for such work from June 1976, the earliest date for which records have not been destroyed, to 1980. Many of the workers lived outside Scotland, for example more than 40% of the workers at Sullom Voe. The analysis was limited to those resident in Scotland.

The numbers of children were ranked into tertiles according to the ratio of oil workers identified by the above methods to the number of economically active men recorded in the 1981 census in each postcode sector. Three periods were considered: 1974–78, 1979–83 and 1984–88. For the first period, which was considered to be before population mixing began, populations for 1976 were used, estimated as the mean of the relevant age-specific counts from the 1971 and 1981 censuses. For the second period, which immediately followed a substantial increase in terminal and offshore activity in 1977–78 and is therefore regarded as early post-mixing, populations from the 1981 census were used. For the final period, regarded as a later post-mixing period, populations in 1986 were estimated by adjusting the 1981 census figures by proportionate regional changes in the 1986 age-specific estimates of the Registrar General's data. 'Urban' areas were arbitrarily defined as postcode sectors including Aberdeen, Dundee and the central industrial belt extending from Edinburgh to the Firth of Clyde west of Glasgow. The remainder of Scotland was classified as 'rural'. Data on cases of leukaemia and non-Hodgkin lymphoma were obtained from the Scottish National Cancer Registration Scheme.

An excess was apparent only in the period 1979–83, that is shortly after the substantial increase in terminal and offshore activity. The excess was apparent only in rural areas and was almost entirely due to leukaemia, mainly of the acute lymphatic type, in the 0–4-year age group. There was no significant excess in the other two periods in any age group in rural areas, or in any urban group.

When the 0–4-year age group in the highest tertile of oil workers in rural areas was examined by single years of age, there were excesses below age one, at age one, and particularly at age two years. The peak at age two contrasts with that at age three found in other rural areas. In the category of rural areas with the highest tertile of oil workers, the peak was at age three in the earlier period 1974–8. This pattern would be compatible with the spread of an infectious agent in a susceptible area, but the continuation of a peak at age two in these areas in the period 1984–88, when the incidence of leukaemia and non-Hodgkin lymphoma at ages 0–4 years had declined, is not consistent with the end of an epidemic.

Analysis was also made with respect to factors that may influence the prevalence of individuals susceptible to infective agents or the intensity of exposure, namely relative isolation, defined as residence more than 20 km from urban areas; social class, defined as the proportion of the population in classes I and II; density of children, defined as the number of enumeration districts in a postcode sector having a hundred or more children; and increases between 1971 and 1981 in the numbers of men working away from home in the construction and energy industries. The increased incidence at ages 0–4 years was restricted to postcode sectors more than 20 km from urban areas, where it was greater in sectors of higher social class. There was a suggestion of a higher incidence in sectors with a higher child density measure both at ages 0–4 and 5–24 years, irrespective of the distance of the sector from an urban area. In sectors more than 20 km from an urban area only, there was a higher incidence of leukaemia and non-Hodgkin lymphoma at ages 5–24 years in areas with the largest increases of construction workers working away from home between 1971 and 1981.

It is interesting that a severe epidemic of measles among local people in Shetland occurred in 1977–78, to which conditions at Sullom Voe were considered to have contributed. In addition, these conditions are thought to have contributed to unusual outbreaks of whooping cough, scarlet fever and influenza. The authors postulated that the unusual circumstances not only promoted transmission of micro-organisms, but that the population received large doses through repeated exposure to these. The excess of leukaemia and non-Hodgkin lymphoma was not concentrated in the children of oil workers themselves (on the basis of father's occupation in cancer registration and mortality records, and a comparison of the names of all oil workers resident in rural areas with those of the fathers of cases in 1979–83), which is consistent with the excess being due to a community, 'herd', effect, with the relevant agent(s) possibly being transmitted among adults and thence to children.

An unexpected finding of the study was that the Dounreay–Thurso area contained a high proportion of oil workers. In the town of Thurso itself, all of the cases were resident in the west of the town. Most of the residents of this part of the town were nuclear workers not native to the area. Construction workers who came to work at oil terminals just to the north also tended to settle in the western part of the town. Thus, there was a great expansion of construction workers working away from home between 1971 and 1981, and a high child density in the western part of the town. In the eastern part of the town, there was a tradition of men working away from home on construction projects, and the authors consider that there would have been fewer susceptibles there because of prior sporadic exposure to the postulated common infection, which would make them less vulnerable to an epidemic caused by new and sudden population mixing. In this area, the excess involved cases particularly in the 5–24-year age group. In the study as a whole, this particular age group, and not younger children, was affected by the increases of construction workers working away from home in the 1970s. Four of the five individuals who developed leukaemia at ages 5–24 years in Thurso during 1979–88 were incomers; this was also true for the four who were born in the years 1969–74, the birth cohort with the greatest population of incomers. By contrast, all three children with leukaemia at ages 0–4 years in the area within 25 km of Dounreay were born there. The absence of cases in west Thurso older than four years among children born locally may in part reflect the immunity conferred by their recent exposure at earlier ages. The authors considered that the excess in this part of the town in the 5–24-year age group may be due to exposure to infection resulting from the influx of nuclear workers, on which was superimposed further exposure resulting from the influx of workers for the oil industry. Such a double influence was postulated for older children by Alexander (1992), with a recent infection causing childhood leukaemia in young children being superimposed on a persistent infection (see Chapter 2). However, the explanation proposed by Kinlen et al., (1993a) does not appear to be entirely compatible with the observation that the incidence of leukaemia and non-Hodgkin lymphoma was raised in both those born in the Dounray area and those resident in the area but born elsewhere (Black *et al.*, 1992; see Chapter 4).

In the 5–24-year age group in general in Scotland, the absence of an excess in the tertile of postcode sectors with the highest proportions of oil workers conceals a highly significant trend of increase associated with the level of increase of construction workers working away from home in the 1970s, and a deficit of borderline statistical significance in areas with a lower child density or a low increase in the numbers of the construction workers working away from home. This deficit was observed in new towns (Kinlen *et al.*, 1990) and may be attributable to the immunizing effects of a milder epidemic of the underlying infection. There was no discussion of individual types of leukaemia in the study of Kinlen *et al.* (1993a). The results do not appear to be entirely consistent with those found in the national service study. Strict conditions were imposed in the Shetlands to protect both the environment and the local way of life, including restrictions on offsite recreation.

More generally, Kinlen *et al.* (1995) observed that large construction projects in rural districts produce unusual population mixing, as the limited local resources of labour require recruitment of workers from outside. These authors examined the incidence of childhood leukaemia and non-Hodgkin lymphoma associated with rural construction projects outside the North Sea oil and nuclear industries. The sites had to be more than 20 km from a large town (over 70 000 inhabitants), built over at least three successive years, and involve a peak workforce of more than 1000. These projects were mainly power stations, hydro-electric schemes and oil refineries. The time periods selected for study were (*a*) from the year in which construction began to the year after its completion, with different construction phases on the same site separated by two or more years being examined separately; (*b*) parts of this period that overlapped with the operation of the plants; and (*c*) the five-year periods that preceded and followed (*a*). 130 cases diagnosed at ages up to 14 years were observed in the vicinity of the various sites during their construction together with the single following year, compared with 94.8 expected (O/E = 1.4, 95% CI 1.2–1.6). The excess also was significant for the 0–4 and 5–14-year age groups. The excesses were more pronounced in each age group in periods when the operation of the plants overlapped with construction (for all ages combined O/E = 1.7, 95% CI 1.3–2.2). When the social class of the area was taken into account, using census data, the excesses were stronger in areas of higher social class. This was particularly striking during the periods when the operation of the plants overlapped with construction. The excesses were not typical of the areas in question, as they were not present either in the five-year period preceding the start of construction work, or in the five-year period after its completion. The apparent increase in the excess during the period of overlap of the operation of the plants with construction may reflect additional opportunities for contact between outside construction workers and local residents, or because as construction work nears completion, workforce numbers are often maximum and a succession of new workers arrive to perform specialized jobs as others leave, thereby increasing the potential for population mixing.

### Commuting

Population influxes are not the only causes of increased social contact. Kinlen *et al.* (1991) noted that commuting journeys and the area of work itself provide opportunities for new social contact that may be relevant to the transmission of the postulated infection or infections underlying childhood leukaemia. The authors examined the association between leukaemia incidence at ages 0–14 years in the period 1972–85 in relation to changes in commuting levels between the 1971 and 1981 censuses in 28 former county boroughs in England for which such a comparison was possible. Commuting level was defined as the sum of the number of residents who worked outside the borough and the number of residents of other areas who worked within a borough.

When the child-years of residence were divided into tenths by level of commuting increase between the 1971 and 1981 censuses, statistically significant increases in the observed to expected ratio standardized to that in the lowest decile were observed overall, and for the 0–4 and 10–14-year age groups. This pattern remained apparent after exclusion of Reading, which forms part of an area of Berkshire and north Hampshire where an excess of childhood leukaemia had already been recorded that might have been associated with nuclear establishments in west Berkshire (Roman *et al.*, 1987). In order to exclude the possibility that the high incidence of childhood leukaemia in the districts with the highest decile might have been typical of the districts over a longer period, and not related to recent commuting changes, leukaemia incidence in the period 1972–85 was

compared within each district with the rates in the preceding period (1962–71); the magnitude of the excess was increased.

When the effects of changes in the extent of outward commuting were examined separately from those of inward commuting, only the latter was associated with a significant excess of leukaemia. However, this difference is difficult to interpret, since three of the five districts in the highest tenth for change in inward commuting also were included in the highest tenth for total commuting increase. No relationship was found with the absolute levels of commuting, either in 1971 or 1981. None of the districts with the highest commuting levels in either of these years had experienced any marked increase in commuting, suggesting that any increase in the incidence of childhood leukaemia associated with increases with commuting might be temporary, as is the situation for epidemics of most infectious disorders, ending when the number of susceptibles declined below some critical level. Published data on a few infectious diseases were considered; no clear increase in the decile with the highest increase in commuting was observed.

These investigators noted that consideration of the possibility that increases in levels of commuting could explain the excess of childhood leukaemia near nuclear establishments in west Berkshire was complicated by boundary changes. There were population increases in this area of up to 33% during the study period. In the total 28 county boroughs considered, such population changes as occurred did not show a relationship with leukaemia. However, when leukaemia at ages 0–4 years was analysed by change in commuting levels simultaneously with population change, the only category that showed a significant increase was the one with the highest commuting level and the highest level of population change. The authors therefore considered that population changes, which alone may have little effect, may compound the effects of commuting increases. This may be relevant to the situation in west Berkshire.

Roman *et al.* (1994) compared the social contacts of 54 children diagnosed with leukaemia or non-Hodgkin lymphoma before the age of five years during the period 1972–89, born and diagnosed in west Berkshire and north Hampshire, with those of 216 matched controls. There was no association with the level of personal contact of the job of either parent held at birth or at the time of diagnosis, assessed on the basis of job titles. In addition, no increase in risk was apparent when the father reported travelling 20 km or more to work on a daily basis, either at the time of birth or the time of diagnosis of the index child. As acknowledged by the authors, the measures of exposure were somewhat crude and the study lacked statistical power to detect effects of the magnitude observed in other studies.

Stiller and Boyle (1996) investigated the association between commuting and ALL in childhood in 403 county districts of England and Wales during the period 1979–85. Data on commuting in general and on commuting by public transport were obtained from the 1981 census. No statistically significant association of either of these variables was found. While this finding may appear inconsistent with the results of the study of Kinlen *et al.* (1991), districts with a high level of commuting in the study of Stiller and Boyle would have included those where it had been high for a long time. A change in levels of commuting might have a greater effect on herd immunity than a sustained high level throughout.

## Mass tourism

Petridou *et al.* (1991) noted that Greece has more than a hundred inhabited islands that used to be isolated, but where there has been much tourism in the past 30 years. If the Kinlen hypothesis were true, an increase in the rate of childhood leukaemia would be expected, and this might be expected to vary between islands because of the differing times and modes of disturbance of herd immunity from island to island. Preliminary testing of the hypothesis was based on comparison between island groups and the mainland of trends in mortality rates during the period 1976–89. No notable differences were found, but the authors acknowledged that patterns of population mixing arising from tourism are likely to have been different from those associated with, for example, the establishment of rural new towns. Kinlen (1992) observed that Petridou *et al.* (1991) were able only to study childhood leukaemia mortality during a period about 15 years after the start of mass tourism in Greece, whereas excesses in rural new towns and in areas near military encampments associated with post-war national service occurred within a decade of the start of the population mixing involved. Kinlen (1992) pointed out that the recent urbanization of Greece has been more rapid than in most countries at a comparable stage of socio-economic development. Thus, the effects of population mixing might have

applied to the mainland at least as much as to the islands, and could explain the lack of difference in trend between these areas.

## Migration during the index pregnancy or in childhood

In a study in three areas of northern England in which unusual aggregations of cases of childhood leukaemia and non-Hodgkin lymphoma had been observed, 16.5% (18 of 109) mothers of cases were found to have moved during the year before the birth of the child, compared with 7.3% (8 of 109) of mothers of controls; this difference was statistically significant (Alexander *et al.*, 1993). Non-significant differences in the direction of greater mobility of case than control families were found for migration in the period up to two years before diagnosis, concentrated in children aged two years or under, and during the first four years of life. The pre-diagnostic migration differences applied to cases diagnosed during the childhood peak, whereas the other differences applied primarily to cases diagnosed at other ages. The authors acknowledged that the potential for confounding is substantial, although the evidence regarding the associations of the most plausible confounders – infertility, sibship size, parity, maternal age – is inconsistent. An association between childhood leukaemia and infection during pregnancy or soon after birth would be compatible with the results of other studies in Great Britain (Smith *et al.*, 1976; Alexander, 1991).

## Infections during the index pregnancy

The possibility that maternal infection in pregnancy could have carcinogenic effects has been of particular interest in relation to leukaemia, largely because of the observation that leukaemia in cats is caused by a virus transmitted from the mother to the fetus (Knox *et al.*, 1980).

Three cohort studies of maternal infection during pregnancy and subsequent childhood cancer are available. Fine *et al.* (1985) observed 16 cases of cancer with ages of onset between zero and 30 years among 2570 subjects reported to have had intrauterine exposure to viral infection, compared with seven among 2475 unexposed controls matched on sex, date and area of birth. The relative risk of cancer associated with viral infection *in utero* was 2.2 (95% CI 0.9–5.9). In eight of the exposed cases the infection had been with a herpes virus (six with varicella, two with cytomegalovirus). Only one case of cancer was associated with influenza in pregnancy. Fedrick and Alberman (1972) carried out a cohort study of births in Great Britain during the first week of March 1958. Of a total of 16 750 children who survived the neonatal period, the mothers of 1959 reported after the birth that they had had influenza during pregnancy; the proportion exposed was high because there was a pandemic at the end of 1957 and beginning of 1958. Eight of the exposed children developed cancer; the relative risk was 5.0 ($p < 0.001$). Six of the exposed cases had ALL and one had Hodgkin's disease. Of the 12 unexposed cases, six had neoplasms of the lymphatic and haematopoietic tissue. The correlation between the death rate before the age of five years due to these cancers in England and Wales and the rate of new spells of incapacity due to influenza in working women during the period 1955–64 was 0.66 ($p < 0.05$). Vianna and Polan (1976) found three cases of lymphatic leukaemia among 63 pregnancies complicated by varicella identified from two sources in upstate New York, compared with an expected number of much less than one. The study was stimulated by the observation of an association with varicella in an ecological analysis presented in the same paper.

Case–control studies of the most commonly investigated maternal infections during pregnancy and subsequent childhood haematopoietic malignancies or cancer of all types combined are summarized in Table 7.2. With regard to infection in general, relative risks greater than 2 have been observed either when the reported prevalence of exposure during pregnancy was low (Stewart *et al.*, 1958) or when the study was small (Till *et al.*, 1979), and may be attributed to recall bias or to chance. No consistent associations have been found with influenza or varicella infection during pregnancy. In addition, ecological analyses have not shown a consistent relationship between leukaemia and maternal influenza or maternal varicella (Table 7.3).

Knox *et al.* (1980) considered that the emergence of the peak incidence of leukaemia at age 2–4 years, associated with an apparent overall increased incidence of leukaemia, might be a result of a phenomenon analogous to that accounting for increased incidence of congenital rubella syndrome. Using data on deaths due to childhood leukaemia and other tumours in Great Britain during the period 1953–79, these authors investigated indirectly the possibility that an infection with properties similar to rubella might be causal by considering the size of the mother's sibship, age at onset, maternal age at the birth of the index child and the number of older sibs (Knox *et al.*, 1980, 1983). These data were not compatible with this particular form of infectious transmission.

Serum IgG and IgM levels, but not IgA levels, were significantly higher in the mothers of 29 cases of ALL aged 2–10 years in New Delhi, India, than in the mothers of 29 healthy controls from the same community matched for age and sex (Chandra, 1972). The study is limited by the absence of information on methods of recruitment of cases and controls, and participation rates.

## Antibiotic use during the index pregnancy

No association between antibiotic use during pregnancy and leukaemia and related malignancies has been observed (Manning & Carroll, 1957[1]; Van Steensel-Moll *et al.*, 1985a; McKinney *et al.*, 1987; Robison *et al.*, 1989; Gilman *et al.*, 1989; van Duijn *et al.*, 1994; Roman *et al.*, 1997).

In a large study of childhood cancer deaths during the period 1964–79 in Great Britain, the case–control ratio of total childhood cancer associated with the mother's reported use of antibiotics during pregnancy was 1.6 ($p < 0.01$; Gilman *et al.*, 1989). This did not appear to be attributable to any particular type of antibiotic. The case–control ratio for any drug was 1.2 ($p < 0.001$), which suggests that recall bias might account for this association. In a study of twins in Sweden based on linkage of registers of twins, cancer and deaths and medical records relating to the index pregnancy, the relative risks of total childhood cancer associated with "drugs for infection" was 3.5 (95% CI 1.0–12.0; Rodvall *et al.*, 1990). The authors stated that analyses in relation to specific drugs revealed no clear association.

Regarding specific types of antibiotic, sulfonamide use by the mother during or before pregnancy has not been associated with childhood leukaemia (Manning & Carroll, 1957). In two reports of a large study of all types of childhood cancer, no association was found with sulfonamide use during pregnancy (Salonen, 1976; Gilman *et al.*, 1989). Sulfonamides have now largely been supplanted by more effective and less toxic drugs.

---

[1] Maternal preconceptional and gestational use was combined in this study.

## Table 7.2. Summary of case–control studies of associations between childhood haematopoietic malignancies or cancer of all types and maternal infection during pregnancy

| Area and period of study | Cases: Dead (D), newly incident (I) or prevalent (P) | Cases: Upper age limit | Cases: N | Controls: Type[a] | Controls: N | Source of information on maternal infection[b] | Any infection: Prevalence in control mothers (%) | Any infection: RR | Influenza: Prevalence in control mothers (%) | Influenza: RR | Varicella: Prevalence in control mothers (%) | Varicella: RR | Reference |
|---|---|---|---|---|---|---|---|---|---|---|---|---|---|
| **Total childhood cancer** | | | | | | | | | | | | | |
| Great Britain, 1953–55 | D | 10 | 1299 | P | 1299 | I | 0.8 | 13.1[ac] | – | – | – | – | Stewart et al., 1958 |
| Great Britain, 1953–67 | D | 15 | 9074 | P | 9074 | I | – | – | 0.7 | 1.5* | 0.0 | ∞ | Bithell et al., 1973 |
| Great Britain, 1971–76 | D | 15 | 2800 | P | 2800 | I | – | – | – | – | 0.3 | 0.8 | Blot et al., 1980a |
| Great Britain, 1964–79 | D | 15 | 8059 | P | 8059 | I, MR | 1.4 | 1.1 | 2.0 | –[d] | 0.1 | – | Gilman et al., 1989 |
| Sweden, 1952–83 | I, D | 15 | 95 | P | 190 | MR | 42 | 1.6 | – | – | – | – | Rodvall et al., 1990 |
| **Leukaemia and lymphoma** | | | | | | | | | | | | | |
| UK, North West, West Midlands and Yorkshire, 1980–83 | I | 14 | 234 | H, GP | 468 | I, MR | NS | –[e] | NS | –[e] | – | – | McKinney et al., 1987 |
| **Leukaemia** | | | | | | | | | | | | | |
| Mexico City, NS | I, P | 14 | 81 | H, P | 154 | I | – | – | – | – | 0.6 | 3.9 | Fajardo-Gutiérrez et al., 1993a |
| UK, Oxford, Cambridge and Reading, 1962–92 | I | 30[f] | 143 | H | 286 | MR | 0.7[f] | 6.0[ei] | – | – | – | – | Roman et al., 1997 |
| **ALL** | | | | | | | | | | | | | |
| UK, London, 1973–75 | I | 14 | 54 / 84 | F, N / Sibs | 54 / 84 | Q | 3.7 / 7.1 | 4.5[c] / 2.3[c] | 3.7 / 1.2 | 1.5[c] / 4.9[c] | – / – | – | Till et al., 1979 |
| The Netherlands, 1973–80 | I | 14 | 519 | P | 507 | Q | 2.2[f] | 1.4[f] | – | – | – | – | Van Steensel-Moll et al., 1985a |
| Japan, Hokkaido, 1986–87 | I, P | 14 | 63[g] | P | 126 | I | NS | 1.0[h] | – | – | – | – | Nishi & Miyake, 1989 |
| USA and Canada, CCG, 1982–91 | I | NS[j] | 990 / 404 | OC / RDD | 1636 / 440 | Q | – | 0.9 / 1.0 | – | – | – | – | Buckley et al., 1994 |
| *by immunophenotype:* | | | | | | | | | | | | | |
| Pre-B-cell | | | 38 | OC | 114 | | | 1.2 | | | | | |
| Null-cell | | | 65 | OC | 193 | | | 0.5 | | | | | |
| T-cell | | | 158 | OC | 314 | | | 0.8 | | | | | |
| Common | | | 286 | OC | 572 | | | 1.5* | | | | | |
| Unknown | | | 443 | OC | 443 | | | 0.5* | | | | | |
| **ANLL** | | | | | | | | | | | | | |
| UK, Oxford, Cambridge and Reading, 1962–92 | I | 30[f] | 113 | H | 226 | MR | 0.9[f] | 4.0[i] | – | – | – | – | Roman et al., 1997 |
| The Netherlands, 1973–79 | I | 14 | 80 | P | 240 | Q | 1.7[f] | 1.0[f] | – | – | – | – | Van Duijn et al., 1994 |
| **Non-Hodgkin lymphoma** | | | | | | | | | | | | | |
| Sweden, 1973–89 | I | 14 | 168 | P | 840 | MR | 3.2 | 0.7 | – | – | – | – | Adami et al., 1996 |

NS, Not stated.   CCG, Children's Cancer Group.   * $p < 0.05$.

[a] P, population; H, hospital; GP, neighbourhood, selected through general practitioner; F, friends; N, neighbourhood; RDD, selected by random-digit dialling; OC, subjects with other types of cancer; Sibs, siblings.

[b] I, maternal interview; MR, medical records; Q, self-completed questionnaire.

[c] Crude unmatched analysis of matched data.

[d] No relative risk was presented specifically for influenza. The relative risk associated with acute respiratory infection was 1.7 ($p<0.001$) and that associated with acute viral infection was 1.3 ($p < 0.05$). Four cases and no controls reported that they had received immunization against influenza during the first trimester.

[e] The relative risk was <2 and was not statistically significant.

[f] Viral infections.

[g] ALL of non-T-cell type.

[h] The authors state that the odds ratio was not statistically significant and that there was no association.

[i] The percentages of cases aged 15 years or more were, for the pre-B phenotype, 8%; the null-cell phenotype, 14%; the T-cell phenotype, 9%; the common phenotype, 7%; and ALL of unknown phenotype, 5%.

[j] 92% of all leukaemia cases were aged 14 or less at the time of diagnosis. The proportion was 96% for ALL.

## Table 7.3. Ecological studies of maternal infection during pregnancy and childhood leukaemia or all types of childhood cancer combined

| Area and period of birth | Method of assessing exposure to maternal infection | Deaths (D) or newly incident cases (I), upper age limit | Number of cases | Types of infection considered | Result | Reference |
|---|---|---|---|---|---|---|
| **Total childhood cancer** | | | | | | |
| England and Wales, 1955–64 | Spells of incapacity certified as due to influenza | D, 4 | 5190 | Influenza | Highly significant correlation between cancer death rates and prevalence of influenza in preceding winter | Fedrick & Alberman, 1972 |
| UK, Manchester, 1954–68 | Month/year of birth in relation to epidemics defined on basis of sickness benefit claims | I, 14 | 1541 | Influenza | No association | Leck & Steward, 1972 |
| **Leukaemia** | | | | | | |
| Finland, 1953–59 | Absenteeism figures for Helsinki and laboratory records of virus isolations | I, 9 | 179 | Influenza | Positive association with 1957 epidemic of 'Asian' influenza but not with five other epidemics | Hakulinen et al., 1973 |
| USA, Connecticut, 1935–61 | Notifications | I, 9 | 431 | Influenza, rubella, measles, mumps, whooping cough, chickenpox, poliomyelitis | No association | McCrea Curnen et al., 1974 |
| USA, Atlanta GA; Houston, TX, 1957–71 | Month/year of birth in relation to epidemics defined in terms of local excess mortality attributed to pneumonia and influenza | I, 14 | 277 | Influenza | No association[a] | Randolph & Heath, 1974 |
| USA, California, 1950–70 (tumour registry) | Month/year of birth in relation to epidemics defined in terms of school absenteeism, deaths from influenza and pneumonia, and laboratory records of influenza confirmation | I, 14 | 653 | Influenza | Excess, mostly due to 0–4 age group, and to exposure in 1st trimester | Austin et al., 1975 |
| California (pooled data from 3 sources), 1950–72[b] | | | 789 | | | |
| USA, San Francisco, Oakland 1969–73[b] | | | 115 | Influenza | Threefold excess risk for those exposed in 1st trimester; 2.5-fold excess for those exposed in 2nd trimester | |
| USA, upstate New York 1950–61 | Seasonality in epidemic periods defined from mortality data and laboratory viral isolations | I, 9 | 1471 | Influenza | No association | Vianna & Polan, 1976 |
| | Notifications | | | Rubella, rubella and varicella | Seasonal variations in rates of leukaemia and varicella were concordant; annual variation was concordant for the first half of the study period | |

[a] In addition, there was no association when 65 cases of lymphoma were included.
[b] Year of diagnosis.

## Immunizations during the index pregnancy

Salonen and Saxén (1975) found a positive association (RR = 1.8, 98% CI 0.4–11.0, based on 11 exposed cases and 8 exposed controls) between leukaemia and maternal polio vaccination during pregnancy. In a large study in Great Britain, there was a positive association (RR = 1.4, *p* < 0.05) between total childhood cancer deaths and vaccination in pregnancy, largely accounted for by neoplasms of the reticulo-endothelial system (RR = 1.8, *p* < 0.01; Gilman *et al.*, 1989). This was not accounted for by polio vaccination. In a population-based study in the Netherlands, there was no association between vaccination during pregnancy and ALL (Van Steensel-Moll *et al.*, 1985a).

## Infection and related exposures during the lifetime of the index child

Studies of the associations between childhood cancer and postnatal infections of the index child are bedevilled by the difficulty of assessing whether and when the child was exposed. Another difficulty has been in determining whether episodes of infectious disease were a possible cause of the childhood cancer or represented a pre-diagnostic sign of the disease. Some investigators have addressed this issue either by restricting attention to infections during the first year or first six months of life (Van Steensel-Moll *et al.*, 1986; Hartley *et al.*, 1988a; Fajardo-Gutiérrez *et al.*, 1993a), or by considering infections reported only during a specified period before diagnosis in cases and a reference date in controls (Stewart *et al.*, 1958; Ager *et al.*, 1965; Magnani *et al.*, 1989). In most of the studies, only maternally reported infection in the child has been considered. The frequency of reported infections of various types in control children varies substantially between studies, which may be attributed to differences in methodological factors such as the upper age limit of cases, the reference period, and the type of controls selected, as well as to differences in study areas. The available studies are summarized in Table 7.4.

### Serological evidence of infection

Schlehofer *et al.* (1996) investigated the prevalence of antibodies to viruses infecting blood or bone-marrow cells, including Epstein–Barr virus (EBV), human herpes virus type 6 (HHV-6) and parvovirus B19 in the sera of 121 children with leukaemia and 197 controls. 32% of a total of 377 cases aged from six months

to 15 years in paediatric oncology centres and paediatric clinics in Germany participated (Table 7.4). The control group comprised children treated in one of the participating hospitals, frequency-matched for age and sex with the cases. Controls were not eligible for inclusion if the reason for hospitalization involved tumours or infections with EBV or parvoviruses. It is unclear whether excluding subjects who were hospitalized because of infection with EBV as potential controls will have led to an underestimate of the prevalence of EBV infection in the general population. The prevalence of antibodies against EBV in controls (38% in children aged five years and under, 78% in older children) in this study was lower than among children in Belgium (40% in children aged 1–2, 51% in children aged 3–4, 72% in children aged 5–14 years; Lamy *et al.*, 1982) and in children in the Bari area of southern Italy (84% in first six months, dropping to 44% between 1 and 2 years, then rising to over 80% in children aged 5–10 years; Leogrande & Jirillo, 1993). Sera from cases were collected before the confirmation of leukaemia diagnosis and before the start of specific therapy, and from controls during the stay in hospital. There were no significant differences in prevalence of antibody positivity for HHV-6, parvovirus B19 or the adeno-associated virus type 2, which has been found to exhibit tumour-suppressive properties. However, in children aged less than six years, the prevalence of antibodies against EBV in cases was 29.8%, compared with 22.6% in controls; the associated relative risk was 2.1 (95% CI 0.99–4.23). The relative risk in the older age group was 0.5 (95% CI 0.19–1.21). There was no clear association between EBV-positivity and leukaemia immunophenotype. The analysis of data on previous infectious diseases obtained by questionnaire showed that whooping cough, rubella, mumps, measles and herpes labialis were reported less frequently by parents of leukaemia cases than controls. This was also true for vaccination.

A possible explanation for this is that the categories of age used in the logistic regression analysis (6 months–2 years; 3–5 years; 6–9 years; 10–14 years) may have been too broad to adjust for differences in age between cases and controls. If, within each category, controls tended to be older than cases, the probability of a control acquiring one of these infections would have been greater than that of a case. This would tend to bias estimated relative risks to below unity if there were no association with the exposure of interest, and to attenuate positive associations.

## Table 7.4. Associations between haematopoietic malignancies and postnatal infections of the index child

| Area and period of study | Cases — Dead (D), newly incident (I) or prevalent (P), upper age limit | N | Controls Type[a] | N | Method of assessing exposure[b] | Reference period | Type of infection | Frequency in controls (%) | RR | Reference |
|---|---|---|---|---|---|---|---|---|---|---|
| **Leukaemia and lymphoma** | | | | | | | | | | |
| UK, North West, West Midlands and Yorkshire, 1980–83 | I, 14 | 234 | GP, H | 268 | I | <6 months | Viral disease[c] | NS | 4.1* | McKinney et al., 1987 |
| **Leukaemia** | | | | | | | | | | |
| Germany, multicentre, 1990–91 | I, 14 | 121 | H | 197 | Q | Up to time of administration of questionnaire | Whooping cough | 23.4 | 0.5 | Schlehofer et al., 1996 |
| | | | | | | | Rubella | 15.7 | 0.5 | |
| | | | | | | | Mumps | 7.3 | 0.8 | |
| | | | | | | | Measles | 15.7 | 0.9 | |
| | | | | | | | Chickenpox | 42.5 | 1.6 | |
| | | | | | | | Herpes labialis | 14.6 | 0.4* | |
| | | | | | | | Unspecific exanthema | 12.7 | 0.9 | |
| | i, 5 | 99 | H | 59 | SL | In hospital before confirmation of diagnosis | Antibodies against | | | |
| | | | | | | | B-19 | 14.1 | 0.5 | |
| | | | | | | | AAV-2 | 80.8 | 0.7 | |
| | | | | | | | HHV 6 | 42.4 | 1.1 | |
| | | | | | | | EBV | 38.4 | 2.1 | |
| | I, 6–14 | 69 | H | 45 | | | B-19 | 42.0 | 0.7 | |
| | | | | | | | AAV-2 | 89.9 | 0.9 | |
| | | | | | | | HHV 6 | 27.5 | 1.2 | |
| | | | | | | | EBV | 78.3 | 0.5 | |
| Mexico City, NS | I, NS[d] | 154 | P, H | 81 | I | 1st year of life | Any requiring hospitalization | 10.4 | 0.6 | Fajardo-Gutiérrez et al., 1993a |
| | | 153 | | 80 | | Unspecified | Chickenpox | 45.1 | 0.6 | |
| USA, Minnesota, 1953–57 | D, 4 | 112 | N | 112 | MR | Up 1 year before death | Mumps | 6.3 | 1.3[e] | Ager et al., 1965 |
| | | | | | | | Measles | 11.6 | 0.9[e] | |
| | | | | | | | Chickenpox | 17.0 | 0.6[e] | |
| | | | | | | | Whooping cough | 1.8 | 2.6[e] | |
| | | | | | | | Rubella | 6.3 | 1.3[e] | |
| China, Shanghai, 1974–86 | I, P, 14 | 618 | P | 309 | I | Up to age at diagnosis | Chickenpox | 25.4 | 0.9 | Shu et al., 1988 |
| | | | | | | | Mumps | 26.4 | 1.2 | |
| | | | | | | | Rubella | 6.6 | 1.1 | |
| | | | | | | | Dysentery | 0.6 | 2.3 | |
| **ALL** | | | | | | | | | | |
| The Netherlands, 1973–80 | I, 14 | 480 | P | 492 | Q | 1st year of life | Primary infections/ | 5.8 | 0.8 | Van Steensel-Moll et al., 1986 |
| | | | | | | | Any for which the child was hospitalized or received specialist treatment | 12.7 | 0.6 | |
| | | | | | | | Bronchitis | 5.8 | 1.2 | |
| | | | | | | | Otitis | 9.8 | 0.7 | |

| Location and years | Controls[a,b] | Cases (n) | Source | Controls (n) | Method | Timing | Infection | % / value | OR | Reference |
|---|---|---|---|---|---|---|---|---|---|---|
| UK, North West, West Midlands and Yorkshire, 1980–83[c] | I, 14 | 148 | GP, H | 296 | I, MR | <6 months | Hepatitis | 5 | 0.6 | Hartley et al., 1988a |
| | | | | | | | Pneumonia | 8 | 0.7 | |
| | | | | | | | "Strep throat" | 29 | 1.1 | |
| | | | | | | | Otitis media | 32 | 0.9 | |
| | | | | | | | Specific perinatal | 0.3 | 10.3* | |
| UK, London, 1973–75 | I, 14 | 54 | F, N | 121 | I | Up to age at diagnosis | All | 4.1 | 2.9 | Till et al., 1979 |
| China, Shanghai, 1974–86 | I, P, 14 | 172 | P | 618 | I | Up to age at diagnosis | Chickenpox | 25.4 | 1.2 | Shu et al., 1988 |
| | | | | | | | Mumps | 26.4 | 1.3 | |
| | | | | | | | Rubella | 6.6 | 0.9 | |
| | | | | | | | Dysentery | 0.6 | 3.9* | |
| Japan, Hokkaido, 1981–87 | I, P, 14[b] | 63 | H | 126 | I | Up to age at diagnosis | Measles or measles vaccination | NS | 0.2* | Nishi & Miyake, 1989 |
| | | | | | | | Other infections | NS | 1.0 | |
| Italy, Turin, 1981–84 | I, P, NS[j] | 142 | H | 307 | I | Unspecified | Measles | 55.7 | 0.7 | Magnani et al., 1990 |
| | | | | | | | Rubella | 20.2 | 0.7 | |
| | | | | | | | Chickenpox | 39.1 | 0.4* | |
| | | | | | | | Whooping cough | 39.7 | 0.6* | |
| | | | | | | | Parotitis | 29.0 | 0.9 | |
| | | | | | | | Viral | NS | 0.6 | |
| | | | | | | | Bacterial | NS | 0.7 | |
| USA and Canada, CCG, 1982–91 | I, NS | 990 | OC | 1636 | Q | Up to time of administration of questionnaire | Measles | NS | 0.9 | Buckley et al., 1994 |
| | | 404 | RDD | 440 | | | | NS | 0.9 | |
| *by immunophenotype*[k] | | | | | | | | | | |
| Pre-B-cell | | 38 | OC | 114 | | | | NS | 1.7 | |
| Null-cell | | 65 | OC | 193 | | | | NS | 2.6 | |
| | | 61 | RDD | 61 | | | | NS | 9.1* | |
| T-cell | | 158 | OC | 314 | | | | NS | 1.4 | |
| Common | | 286 | OC | 572 | | | | NS | 0.4* | |
| Unknown | | 443 | OC | 443 | | | | NS | 0.6* | |
| **ANLL** China, Shanghai, 1974–86 | I, P, 14 | 92 | P | 618 | I | Up to age at diagnosis | Chickenpox | 25.4 | 0.6 | Shu et al., 1988 |
| | | | | | | | Mumps | 26.4 | 1.1 | |
| | | | | | | | Rubella | 6.6 | 1.6 | |
| | | | | | | | Dysentery | 0.6 | 0.7 | |
| **Non-Hodgkin lymphoma** Sweden, 1973–89 | I, 14 | 168 | P | 840 | MR | In neonatal period | Any | 2.5 | 0.5 | Adami et al., 1996 |

NS, Not stated. CCG Children's Cancer Group.

\* p < 0.05

a P, population-based; GP, neighbourhood, selected through general practice; H, hospital; N, neighbourhood; F, friends; OC, affected with cancer of other types; RDD, selected by random-digit dialling.

b I, maternal interview; MR, medical records; Q, questionnaire; SL, serological.

c Chickenpox, rubella, measles, mumps, viral meningitis, viral influenza. Children with viral disease in the six months before diagnosis were excluded from analysis.

d Mean age 8.5 (S.D. 4.5) years.

e Crude unmatched analysis of matched data.

f Measles, chickenpox, mumps or rubella.

g Subset of data analysed by McKinney et al. (1987).

h ALL of the non-T-cell type.

i The authors state that there was no significant association with varicella, rubella, mumps or other infection.

j Mean age at diagnosis of 142 cases with ALL, 22 of ANLL and 19 of non-Hodgkin lymphoma was 6.1 (S.D. 3.6) years.

k In the original paper, data were presented for two control groups. Here data have been presented for the analysis including the larger number of subjects, except for the null-cell immunophenotype, for which the magnitude of the relative risks differed substantially.

Therefore, it is interesting that a positive association was found with reported history of chickenpox (RR = 1.63, 95% CI 0.91–2.92); this relative risk might be an underestimate.

In contrast to the finding of Schlehofer *et al.* (1996), lower titres of antibodies to EBV were found in 52 children with leukaemia seen at a hospital in Boston than in 115 age-matched Swedish children (Gahrton *et al.*, 1971). This was also true for herpes simplex virus and cytomegalovirus. There was no marked difference in seropositivity for antibodies to the measles and rubella virus. An important limitation of the study is that cases and controls were selected from different populations, although the authors note that the frequency of EBV-positive sera in cases was lower than in other samples of healthy children.

*Infection in early life*

The possible etiological importance of infection in early life has been investigated in some other studies. Memon and Doll (1994) carried out a cohort study of 12 690 infants to investigate the possibility that infants who received blood transfusions shortly after birth or *in utero* might have been infected by some blood-borne oncogenic virus. Infants transfused in the period 1942–70 were identified from the records kept in certain hospitals, blood transfusion centres and maternity homes in Great Britain. Follow-up was carried out using death and cancer registration. Four cases of leukaemia occurred in children aged 1–14 years, compared with 5.4 expected on the basis of national rates. Thus, this study does not support the hypothesis that a blood-borne virus prevalent in adults is able to cause childhood leukaemia. Moreover, in a Swedish record-linkage based study of childhood lymphatic leukaemia, there was no association with exchange transfusion during the neonatal period (Cnattingius *et al.*, 1995a).

In a study of leukaemia and lymphoma in which cases with viral diseases in the six months before diagnosis were excluded, McKinney *et al.* (1987) found a positive association with viral diseases experienced during the first six months of life (RR = 4.1, 95% CI 1.5–11.3) (Table 7.4). The association was particularly apparent for the common null-cell ALL and lymphoma subgroups. The minimum period between viral disease and diagnosis was 2.5 years, whereas it is thought that the period of immunosuppression in the preclinical period is about one year (Stewart, 1980). The authors considered the possibility that recall bias could account for the association. However, while mothers of cases reported at interview more illness in the index children than mothers of controls, this difference was also apparent when medically recorded episodes of illness were examined. In analysis of a data-set on total childhood cancer which includes the data reported by McKinney *et al.* (1987), the relative risk associated with reported viral infections in the first six months was 1.6 (95% CI 0.7–3.7; Hartley *et al.*, 1988a). Thus, the relationship appears to have been specific to leukaemia.

In an investigation of ALL in subjects aged 1–14 years in the Netherlands, the relative risk associated with infection requiring hospitalization or specialist consultation during the first year of life was 0.6 (95% CI 0.4–1.2; Van Steensel-Moll *et al.*, 1986). There was no association with reported primary infections, that is one or more of measles, chickenpox, mumps or rubella, bronchitis, otitis or common colds, or periods of fever, defined as a temperature of more than 38°C for two days or more. In addition, there was no association with the child having been hospitalized or receiving specialist consultation for any reason. Apart from the timing of infection considered, an important difference from other studies is that the data were obtained by postal questionnaire. The response rate of parents of cases was 90%, compared with 70% for first-choice and 68% for second-choice controls. Therefore the possibility cannot be excluded that preferential participation of parents of control children who had infections in early life could have accounted for the observed relative risk being below unity.

In multivariate analysis of a small study of leukaemia (81 cases) in Mexico City in which both community (*n* = 77) and hospital (*n* = 77) controls were included, "a history of infection by chickenpox during the first years" was selected as among the most important variables associated with leukaemia, with a relative risk of 0.5 (95% CI 0.2–0.9; Fajardo-Gutiérrez *et al.*, 1993a). The validity of the multivariate analysis is open to question, as hospitalization with infection during the first year of life also was included in the regression model. The relative risk associated with hospitalization during the first year of life was 0.6 (95% CI 0.2–1.7). When only community controls were considered, the relative risk was 0.5 (95% CI 0.1–1.8).

In a small study, Till *et al.* (1979) found that cases (*n* = 54) with ALL and their sibs had more episodes of infection than control children selected from among the friends and neighbours of the parents of the cases or children with acute myeloid leukaemia (*n* = 28) and their sibs. Much of the difference between cases and control children was accounted for by gastroenteritis during the first year of life and by pyogenic infection.

If infections in early life were of etiological importance, it might be expected that breast feeding would be associated with a reduced risk of leukaemia. However, no consistent association between breast feeding and leukaemia has been observed (see Chapter 8).

In summary, there appears to be no consistency of association between leukaemia and recorded or reported infection in early life.

## Infection up to age of diagnosis

In a large study in Shanghai, China, Shu *et al.* (1988) found no association between leukaemia and a history of chickenpox, mumps or rubella at any stage in childhood (Table 7.4). However, they found a positive association between ALL and dysentery, and positive associations with chloramphenicol and syntomycin, which were mainly used in the treatment of dysentery and fever (see below). The validity of the study is limited by differences in the methods of selection of cases and controls. Cases recruited during a 12-year period were compared with controls recruited during a 2-year period, so the exposures sampled were not contemporaneous and recall bias may have occurred as a consequence of case parents having on average to recall exposures in the reference period over a longer period than control parents.

In a hospital-based study in Turin, Italy, children with ALL were reported to have had a lower frequency of viral and bacterial diseases than controls randomly selected from among children hospitalized in the medical and surgical wards of the same hospital to which cases had been admitted (Magnani *et al.*, 1990). The association persisted when analysis was made using only the subset of controls affected by acute conditions such as severe accidents or appendicitis. As acknowledged by the authors, there were important differences between cases and controls in area of residence and circumstances of interview. In particular, 61% of the total case series were interviewed more than six months after diagnosis, compared with 15% of control subjects.

An inverse association between ALL of the common non-T-cell type and maternally reported measles or measles vaccination in the child before diagnosis was observed in a study in Japan (Nishi & Miyake, 1989). Control children were identified at visits for routine health examinations at health centres and hospitals located in the areas in which the index cases were resident; these approximate to population controls, as 80–90% of children in Japan are taken for health examinations. No association was observed with other infections.

In a study of 228 cases of leukaemia diagnosed before the age of 10 years in the Midlands of England during the period 1953–60, 10 pairs of cases diagnosed within 15 months of one another, and resident within 0.5 km at that time were identified by the Knox method (Morris, 1990). Data relating to infectious diseases were available for 18 of the 20 children in these pairs. Information on matched controls for these children had been obtained during the on-going Oxford Survey of Childhood Cancers. During the 2–3 years before the onset of leukaemia, measles was reported to have occurred more frequently in the cases than in the matched controls ($p = 0.06$, based on five discordant pairs). No such association was apparent when a similar analysis was carried out for cases who were not members of close pairs and their matched controls; data were available for 176 (85%) of the 208 case–control pairs.

In a study of ALL classified by immunophenotype in the USA and Canada, there was a positive association between leukaemia of the null-cell phenotype, which accounted for 11% (66 of 576) of the cases of known immunophenotype, and measles reported up to the age of diagnosis (Buckley *et al.*, 1994). No other noteworthy association with a history of childhood infections was observed.

In a study of leukaemia deaths before the age of five years in Minnesota, no noteworthy association with medically recorded episodes of mumps, measles, chickenpox, pertussis or rubella was found (Ager *et al.*, 1965). Neighbourhood controls were used, which may have resulted in overmatching. As might be expected, no association was apparent in comparison with sibling controls.

It has been suggested that bovine leukaemia virus may be involved in the etiology of leukaemia in humans, in part because it is related to the HTLV family of viruses, and in part because of reports of an increased risk of adult leukaemia in dairy farmers (Bender *et al.*, 1988). In addition, lymphoma has several features in common between humans, cows and other animals. However, in a study based on 131 cases of ALL and 26 cases of non-Hodgkin lymphoma in children in which DNA hybridization techniques were used, none of the cases or 136 control DNA samples demonstrated the presence of bovine leukaemia virus (Bender *et al.*, 1988).

As the tonsils are lymphoid tissue, they may be important in protection against a variety of antigens. For this reason, the association between cancer and tonsillectomy has been investigated (Cassimos *et al.*, 1973). No association between tonsillectomy and childhood leukaemia has been observed (Freeman *et al.*, 1971; Till *et al.*, 1979).

In summary, these studies do not provide clear support for an etiological role for the commonest symptomatic infections of childhood. However, the validity of all of the studies is limited by one or more of the following issues: possible selection bias, crude assessment of exposure or small sample size.

*Chloramphenicol*

In the study of leukaemia in Shanghai, China, described above, there was a positive association with use of chloramphenicol (doses of 30–50 mg/kg per day), a broad spectrum antibiotic, and syntomycin (doses of 60–100 mg/kg per day), a racemic mixture containing 50% laevorotatory and 50% dextrorotatory chloramphenicol and having pharmacological effects similar to those of chloramphenicol (Shu *et al.*, 1987, 1988). The relative risk associated with having ever used chloramphenicol was 2.3 (95% CI 1.7–3.2), and that associated with use of syntomycin was 1.9 (95% CI 1.1–3.2). There were marked increases in risk with increasing total number of reported days of use of chloramphenicol, with relative risks of 1.7 (95% CI 1.2–2.5) for one to five days' treatment, 2.8 (95% CI 1.5–5.1) for six to ten days' treatment, and 9.7 (95% CI 3.9–24.1) for more than ten days' treatment. The corresponding relative risks for syntomycin were 1.5 (95% CI 0.7–2.9), 1.6 (95% CI 0.6–4.4) and 6.8 (95% CI 1.4–33.3). It is not clear to what extent children received both drugs. The elevated risk associated with chloramphenicol persisted after adjustment for a history of anaemia and when analyses were restricted to either first or latest use of this antibiotic more than two years before diagnosis. This makes it unlikely that the association could be explained by an undiagnosed pre-leukaemic condition predisposing to infections which would subsequently be treated by one or other drug. The associations persisted after adjustment for the symptoms associated with use of the drugs (diarrhoea, dysentery and fever). In addition to a number of specified drugs apart from these antibiotics about which information was sought, respondents were asked if the child had been treated with any other drugs, as an open-ended question. The relative risk associated with any report in this category was 0.4 (95% CI 0.3–0.7); the authors state that most of the drugs named were other antibiotics such as penicillin and streptomycin. This suggests that the associations with chloramphenicol and syntomycin cannot be attributed to a systematic difference in recall of drug use between parents of cases and controls.

Chloramphenicol can induce bone marrow depression. The associations with chloramphenicol and syntomycin were somewhat stronger for ANLL than for ALL. Shu *et al.* (1987) observed that this is consistent with a predominance of ANLL in previous reports of chloramphenicol-associated leukaemia. However, the observation of an association for both cell types, as acknowledged by the authors, raises the question as to whether bias could explain the result. There was a long interval between diagnosis (1974–86) and interview (1985–86) for cases, whereas controls were recruited in the two-year period 1985–86. It is interesting that in a study of adult leukaemia in Shanghai during the period 1987–89 by the same group (Zheng *et al.*, 1993), no association was found between chloramphenicol/syntomycin and ANLL or other forms of adult leukaemia.

*Other antibiotics*

Stewart *et al.* (1958) investigated the association between childhood cancer deaths and treatment with sulfonamides and antibiotics first because, then being new drugs, they might have contributed to the increase in leukaemia mortality in Great Britain observed in the 1950s, and secondly because intensive treatment with sulfonamides occasionally causes aplastic anaemia. When children who had a pulmonary infection within two years of the date of diagnosis were excluded, no clear association with either group of drugs was apparent.

## Index child's contact with animals

Around 1970, there was considerable publicity about a possible relationship between human and animal leukaemia (Penrose, 1970). With regard to childhood leukaemia, there was interest in the possible role of feline leukaemia virus (FeLV), because of similarities between human and feline ALL in clinical findings, laboratory data and response to treatment (Malone *et al.*, 1983). In a study in specified areas of New York, Maryland and Minnesota during the period 1959–62, the relative risks of leukaemia associated with reported exposure to

15 types of animal ranged from 0.8 to 1.8 (Bross & Gibson, 1970). The only significant association was with exposure to cats (RR = 1.4, $p$ = 0.04). Compared with children reported never to have been exposed to cats, the age-adjusted relative risk associated with exposure to cats not reported to be ill or to have died was 1.3 (95% CI 0.9–1.7), and that with exposure to cats reported to have been ill or to have died was 2.2 (95% CI 1.2–4.1). All but one of the sick cats was reported to have died. No details of the length of exposure were presented, or whether exposure resulted from living in the same household as the animal or from other contact.

Penrose (1970) reported that cats were kept in 11 of the households of 28 children with leukaemia or lymphoma, compared with 5 in the households of matched healthy controls. The study was described only in the form of a letter. McKinney *et al.* (1987) reported that the relative risk of leukaemia or lymphoma associated with exposure to cats was less than 2 and was not statistically significant.

In a multicentre study of 990 cases of ALL and 1636 controls with other types of cancer in the USA and Canada, the relative risks associated with maternal exposure to farm animals was 1.3 ($p$ < 0.05), that with paternal exposure was again 1.3 ($p$ < 0.05), and that with the index child's exposure was 1.4 ($p$ < 0.01; Buckley *et al.*, 1994). Similar relative risks were observed when a subgroup of 404 cases was compared with individually matched controls selected by random-digit dialling. Analyses stratified by immunophenotype also were carried out. Significantly elevated risks were observed for the pre-B-cell subgroup. The exposure was fairly equally divided over a wide range of farm animals. No overall association with cat ownership was apparent. However, for the pre-B-cell subgroup, an elevation in risk was apparent in comparison with both cancer controls (RR = 2.0, $p$ < 0.1) and with controls selected by random-digit dialling (RR = 4.5, $p$ < 0.01).

In a study in adults in the same geographical area as that in children reported by Bross and Gibson (1970), significant elevations in the relative risk of ALL and chronic lymphocytic Leukaemia associated with exposure to sick cats were reported (Bross *et al.*, 1972). Reports of sick cats were not validated, and other studies have not shown an association between FeLV in cats and leukaemia in subjects living with, or otherwise in close contact with, the infected cats (Linet, 1985).

## Immunizations

Investigations of associations between immunizations and childhood cancers were stimulated by the observation that in a hospital series in Brisbane, Australia, fewer immunizations against diphtheria, whooping cough and tetanus had been withheld from 59 children with leukaemia than from 343 patients without leukaemia admitted in the same period (Innis, 1965). This study was subsequently criticized on the grounds of selection bias and method of statistical analysis (Lancaster & Clements, 1965).

In an analysis of deaths due to childhood cancer before the age of 10 years in Great Britain during the period 1956–60, leukaemia cases and cases with other types of childhood cancer had in general received fewer immunizations of specific types than matched controls (Stewart & Hewitt, 1965). In an extension of this study, including 12 281 deaths due to childhood cancer under the age of 16 years during the period 1953–77, Kneale *et al.* (1986) found significant deficits of immunized cases of childhood cancer deaths of all types as compared to matched controls. The effects were strongest for immunizations over 10 years of age, for the oldest cases (10–15 years), and were stronger for solid tumours than for leukaemia (which would be consistent with the age patterns for leukaemia and solid tumours).

In a multicentre study in the USA and Canada in which analysis of ALL stratified by immunophenotype was made, there was a positive association between pre-B-cell ALL and reported measles/mumps/rubella vaccination (Buckley *et al.*, 1994). Pre-B-cell ALL accounted for under 7% of the cases of known phenotype.

Therefore, no consistent association between leukaemia and immunization has been identified.

## Haematopoietic malignancies and BCG vaccination

Evidence that tubercule bacilli of the Calmette–Guérin strain (BCG) can prevent or suppress challenge from leukaemia or tumour grafts in laboratory animals led to investigations as to whether BCG vaccination might reduce the incidence of cancer in humans, and of leukaemia in particular (Hoover, 1976). The most important evidence is from three controlled trials, details of which are summarized in Table 7.5. In the first trial, in Georgia and Alabama, USA, the mortality due to leukaemia and lymphoma did not differ substantially between vaccinated subjects and controls (Comstock *et al.*, 1971). The mortality rate due

Table 7.5. Incidence of, or mortality due to, cancer in subjects participating in controlled trials of BCG vaccination in childhood

| Area and period of study | Minimum age at assessment of eligibility for vaccination | Cancer incidence (I) or mortality (M) assessed | Length of follow-up (years) | Number of participants | | | | Type of cancer | V | | N- | | N+ | | Reference |
|---|---|---|---|---|---|---|---|---|---|---|---|---|---|---|---|
| | | | | Vaccinated (V) | Non-vaccinated, tuberculin negative (N-) | Non-vaccinated, tuberculin positive (N+) | Refused vaccination | | Number of cases | Rate[a] | Number of cases | Rate[a] | Number of cases | Rate[a] | |
| USA, Georgia and Alabama, 1950 | 5 | M | 21 | 16913 | 17854 | 29369 | – | Leukaemia and lymphoma | 14 | 82.8[b] | 16 | 89.6[b] | 30 | 102.1[b] | Comstock et al., 1971 |
| England, 1950–52 | 14 | M | 15 | 13598 | 12867 | 15704[c] | – | Lymphatic and haematopoietic | 6 | 2.9 | 8 | 4.1 | 9[c] | 3.8[c] | Medical Research Council, 1972 |
| | | | | | | | | Other | 7 | 3.4 | 4 | 2.1 | 17[c] | 7.2[c] | |
| Puerto Rico, 1949–51 | 1 | I | 23 | 50634 | 27338 | 82269 | 31856 | Total | 150 | 12.7 | 77 | 12.1 | – | – | Snider et al., 1978 |

[a] Incidence or mortality per 100 000 per annum, unless otherwise specified.
[b] Mortality rate per 100 000 initial population.
[c] To 3 tuberculin units. A further 6253 subjects were positive only to 100 tuberculin units and were not vaccinated.
There were five deaths due to lymphatic and haematopoietic neoplasms (rate 5.3) and 5 due to other malignant neoplasms.

to these malignancies was higher among those who were initially tuberculin-positive than among those who were initially tuberculin-negative. Tuberculin-negative subjects born in alternate years were assigned to receive vaccination, the remainder being left as controls. A similar method of assignment was used in the trial in Puerto Rico, whereby those born in the middle year of each trio of years of birth were left unvaccinated as controls (Comstock *et al.*, 1975; Snider *et al.*, 1978). This study was based on cancer incidence rather than mortality. In the first report of the Puerto Rico trial, in which the average length of follow-up was 18.8 years, the vaccinated group had a slight deficiency of leukaemia cases and an excess of lymphosarcoma and Hodgkin's disease (Comstock *et al.*, 1975). The excess of lymphosarcoma and Hodgkin's disease was also apparent in the second report, in which the average follow-up was 23.3 years (Snider *et al.*, 1978). The excess was concentrated among subjects who were aged 7–15 years at entry into the study. In the third trial, assignment to receive vaccination among the tuberculin-negative subjects was random. The mortality due to neoplasms of the lymphatic and haematopoietic tissues was lower in the group receiving BCG vaccination than in the unvaccinated tuberculin-negative group, but the converse was the case for other neoplasms (Medical Research Council, 1972). Neither difference was statistically significant. The mortality from all malignant neoplasms was greater among those who were initially tuberculin-positive than among those who were initially tuberculin-negative.

In cohort studies in Quebec and Chicago, a significant inverse association between BCG vaccination and mortality due to leukaemia was reported (Davignon *et al.*, 1970; Rosenthal *et al.*, 1972; Crispen & Rosenthal, 1976). Two major criticisms were made of these studies (Hoover, 1976). First, death certificates were matched only with a register of vaccinated children. Therefore, failure to match because of factors such as migration, change of name, adoption or misspelling could have resulted in a vaccinated child being included in the non-vaccinated group. Second, analysis was not made by person-years at risk. Hoover (1976) re-analysed the study of Rosenthal *et al.* (1972), with calculation of an appropriate denominator. The apparent reduction in mortality due to leukaemia and total cancers was 50% for each, in contrast to 80% and 85% respectively in the initial report. Although the effect of matching death certificates only with a register of vaccinated children cannot be assessed, the studies are interesting in that, in contrast to the trials, in Quebec a substantial proportion of children (Davignon *et al.*, 1971), and in Chicago all children, were vaccinated in the neonatal period. It has been speculated that maximal protection would be conferred only by vaccination in the neonatal period (Hoover, 1976).

In a case–control study in Finland of childhood cancer during the period 1959–68, the BCG vaccination status of the infant was established from the maternity health centre record which includes details of the index pregnancy and perinatal health of the baby (Salonen, 1976). Routine vaccination at the maternity hospital began in the 1950s. As of the 1970s, about 99% of newborns were vaccinated in hospital, infants weighing under 3000 g being vaccinated later. BCG vaccination status could be assessed for 76.5% of cases and controls. In controls, who were the births immediately preceding that of a cancer case in the same maternity health centre, 90% were vaccinated. The relative risk of leukaemia was 0.8 (95% CI 0.3–2.1, based on 373 cases). No association was observed for total childhood cancer and the relative risks of specific tumour types other than leukaemia were in the range of 1.0–1.3 for all except eye tumours (0.3, 95% CI 0.0–6.1, based on 37 cases). The total incidence of childhood cancer did not differ substantially from that in counties with a much lower BCG vaccination rate (Salonen & Saxén, 1975).

In a study of 63 cases of non-T-cell ALL in Hokkaido, Japan, each of whom was matched with two healthy controls on age, sex and residence, the relative risk associated with BCG vaccination was 0.3 (95% CI 0.1–0.8; Nishi & Miyake, 1989). The proportion of controls vaccinated was 94% (118 of 126) compared with 83% (52 of 63) cases. The association was apparent only in children aged less than 7 years at diagnosis. In Japan, BCG vaccination is usually given first at the health examination at 3–4 months of age. It is given again compulsorily to tuberculin-negative reactors at the age of 6 or 7 years, that is at entrance to elementary school. An inverse association was also found for X-ray of the hip joint, a procedure usually carried out at the 3–4 month health examination. Performance of this examination and of the BCG vaccination were more closely related with one another in controls than in cases, and the authors suggest that cases may have received BCG vaccination later than controls.

BCG vaccination was introduced in New Zealand in 1951 (Skegg, 1978). It was offered to children entering secondary school, usually at age 13 years. The school vaccination programme has continued in the North Island, in which about two thirds of the population reside, but was gradually withdrawn in the South Island during 1961 and 1962. Skegg (1978) compared incidence and mortality rates of leukaemia and lymphoma among non-Maori children in the two islands, before and after vaccination was stopped in the South Island. The population at risk before vaccination was stopped comprised children who attained the age of 13 during the period 1955–59; 54% of the children resident in the North Island were vaccinated and 50% of children in the South Island. The mortality rates for leukaemia and lymphoma were similar. The registration rate for leukaemia on the North Island (21.2 per million person years) was significantly lower than that in the South Island (37.7 per million person years), whereas the registration rates of both Hodgkin's and non-Hodgkin lymphomas did not differ greatly. However, registration may have been incomplete in the North Island because there were fewer registrations than deaths attributed to leukaemia. The population at risk after vaccination was stopped in the South Island comprised children who attained the age of 13 during the period 1963–73; 78% of the children resident in the North Island were vaccinated, compared with 1% of children in the South Island. The leukaemia registration rates were similar for the North and South Island, although the mortality rate was higher in the North than in the South Island; this difference was not statistically significant. Mortality and incidence rates for Hodgkin's disease were similar between the two islands. The death rate due to non-Hodgkin lymphoma was four times higher on the North than on the South Island, but the difference between incidence rates, although in the same direction, was small and not statistically significant. Comparison of age-standardized mortality rates for non-Hodgkin lymphoma showed that the death rate in the North Island increased with the proportion of children vaccinated, while in the South Island the rate declined after vaccination was withdrawn.

Since 1945, newborn children have received BCG vaccination in Sweden, school entrants (age 7 years) in Denmark and school leavers (age 13–14 years) in Norway (Waaler, 1970). Waaler (1970) compared age-specific mortality rates for leukaemia between these countries in the mid 1960s. The mortality rate in the 0–4-year age group was lower in Sweden, in the 5–9-year age group in Denmark and in the 10–14-year age group in Norway than in the other countries. While this pattern may be consistent with a protective effect of BCG vaccination, it is also possible that these differences represent chance fluctuations.

BCG vaccination was introduced in the 1950s in the United Kingdom for 13-year-old schoolchildren. In England and Wales, the population vaccinated increased from 7% in 1954 to 65% in 1967 (Hems & Stuart, 1971). For males, in England and Wales and in Scotland, leukaemia mortality rates in the 15–19-year age group declined from the end of the 1950s, and in the 20–24-year age group from the mid 1960s. The trend in the 15–19-year age group was also apparent in females, but there was no decline in the 20–24-year age group. The authors acknowledged that other factors could account for the observed decline, and that the apparent absence of a decline in women aged 20–24 years is not consistent with a protective effect of BCG vaccination.

Kinlen and Pike (1971) observed that in Canada, substantial proportions of infants received BCG vaccination only in Quebec and Newfoundland, and in Scotland, only in Glasgow. These authors compared leukaemia mortality in Quebec with that in Canada excluding this province and Newfoundland (for which the data were incomplete), and in Glasgow with that in the rest of Scotland. For each of the age groups examined (0–4, 5–9, 10–14 and 15–19 years), mortality due to leukaemia in Quebec was no lower than in the rest of Canada. In Glasgow, mortality was lower in the 5–9 and 10–14-year age groups than in the rest of Scotland (O/E ratios 0.6 and 0.7 respectively in period 1951–69), but this was most striking in the period 1955–59, when a negligible proportion of children could have been vaccinated. In subsequent years, as the proportion of vaccinated children increased, the ratio of observed to expected numbers of deaths attributed to leukaemia increased. Subsequently, it was reported that deaths due to cancers other than leukaemia showed similar patterns (Hoover, 1976).

BCG vaccination of newborns was introduced in Austria in 1949 (Ambrosch *et al.* 1986). During the period 1964–75, an inverse association between the time trend in the BCG vaccination rate and that in the leukaemia mortality rate for the 0–5-year age group was found (based on four points, representing triennia). Similarly, there was an inverse geographical association when the five largest provinces were compared during the period 1966–75. This analysis is very limited. It would have been relevant to assess other age groups and mortality due to other types of cancer.

In summary, there is no consistent relationship between BCG vaccination and the subsequent risk of leukaemia and other haematopoietic malignancies.

## Sibship size

Sibship size might be expected to be crude marker of probability of exposure to common childhood infections. A weak inverse association with increasing sibship size reported in a study of ALL in the Netherlands (Van Steensel-Moll *et al.*, 1986) was not confirmed in a study in Minnesota (Kaye *et al.*, 1991) or in a multicentre study in the USA and Canada (Buckley *et al.*, 1994). In a study in Denmark, an inverse association between sibship size when the index child was one year old and the risk of ALL diagnosed at age 1–4 years was observed (RR = 0.9, 95% CI 0.8–1.0; Westergaard *et al.*, 1997). No association between ALL and sibship size at the age of two, three or five years was found. In the same study, there was a positive association between AML and sibship size. This was most pronounced when the sibship size at the time when the index child was aged two or three years was considered. The relative risk of acute myeloid leukaemia (AML) for a sibship size of two or more when the index child was two years old was 2.5 (95% CI 1.5–4.4), compared with being an only child at that age, and the relative risk associated with each extra child in the sibship was 1.5 (95% CI 1.1–1.9). Similar relative risks were observed when the sibship size at age three years was considered.

In the two studies of ALL in which the age interval to the nearest older sib was considered, no consistent association was found (Kaye *et al.*, 1991; Westergaard *et al.*, 1997).

In children aged 0–4 years in the vicinity of two nuclear establishments in southern England, there was no association between sibship size and leukaemia and non-Hodgkin lymphoma (Roman *et al.*, 1994). No noteworthy relationship was reported in a study of leukaemia and lymphoma in the Midlands and northern England (McKinney *et al.*, 1987) or in a hospital-based study in Turin, Italy (Magnani *et al.*, 1990). These studies were smaller, and therefore had lower statistical power, than those relating specifically to ALL. In early studies of deaths due to leukaemia in childhood, a weak inverse relationship was found with increasing birth order (see Chapter 9). The relationship is not apparent in more recent studies, including those based on newly incident cases.

Thus, there is no consistent association between ALL and sibship size. No association was found in studies of leukaemia and lymphoma combined, but these had low statistical power to detect an effect.

## Daycare

Alexander (1993) noted that daycare of the index child and of the siblings is probably the best available proxy measure of exposure to infections. In a hospital-based study of childhood leukaemia in Athens and its surrounding region and in Crete, an inverse association was found with attendance at a crèche (RR = 0.7, 95% CI 0.4–1.1; Petridou *et al.*, 1993). For attendance for a period of three months or more during the first two years of life, the relative risk was 0.3 (95% CI 0.1–0.9). The control series comprised children attending outpatient clinics of the hospitals in which the children with leukaemia were treated, because of "general paediatric problems" (53.5%; 100 of 187), surgical and orthopaedic problems (27.3%; $n = 51$), otolaryngological problems (12.3%; $n = 23$) and ophthalmic problems (7.0%; $n = 13$). The authors stated that the results were not appreciably affected by considering only control children with general paediatric problems. In addition, changing the definition of attendance at a crèche early in life, or restricting analysis to children aged five years or more at diagnosis, did not substantially alter the results. The participation rate of cases was 74% (136 of 183) and of controls 72% (187 of 260), but the authors observed that the control parents who refused to participate were mainly of lower social class. Social class, as assessed by years of education of the mother was not strongly associated with the child attending a crèche. As it is possible that referral for "general paediatric problems" is associated with crèche attendance, selection bias cannot be excluded as a potential explanation for the finding.

In a study of children aged 0–4 years in the vicinity of nuclear establishments in southern England, the relative risk of leukaemia and non-Hodgkin lymphoma associated with the index child having attended a preschool playgroup for three months or more in the year before diagnosis was 0.7 (95% CI 0.3–1.9; Roman *et al.*, 1994). The controls were selected from hospital delivery registers and matched with the cases by sex, date of birth, maternal age, and area of residence at birth and at the time of diagnosis.

Thus, in both available studies, the relative risk of leukaemia associated with daycare was less than one.

## The lymphomas

### Burkitt's lymphoma and postnatal infection with Epstein–Barr virus

In reviewing the association between Burkitt's lymphoma and Epstein–Barr virus (EBV), it is helpful to distinguish studies carried out (1) in areas where Burkitt's lymphoma is endemic, in which childhood lymphomas account for up to 80% of all cancers of children; (2) in non-endemic areas which include the industrialized countries where Burkitt's lymphoma accounts for about 3% of childhood tumours; and (3) in areas of intermediate incidence of Burkitt's lymphoma, such as North Africa, where the tumour accounts for up to 15% of childhood cancer (de-Thé, 1985; see Chapter 2). This distinction suggests that there is a background incidence of Burkitt's lymphoma which is not related to EBV, superimposed on which EBV and perhaps hyperendemic malaria appear to have a prominent role in increasing the incidence of these tumours.

### Studies in areas where Burkitt's lymphoma is endemic

The association between Burkitt's lymphoma and EBV is based on sero-epidemiologic studies and the demonstration of EBV genomes in the majority of tumours from endemic areas. Studies carried out in the late 1960s showed that patients with Burkitt's lymphoma consistently had much higher antibody titres to EBV viral capsid antigen and EBV early antigen than did controls (de-Thé, 1985). In a prospective cohort study in the West Nile district of Uganda, approximately 32 000 serum samples were collected from children aged up to 8 years old living in five selected counties of the district during the period 1972–74 (de-Thé, 1978; Geser *et al.*, 1982). Follow-up of this cohort was continued until March 1979, when civil disturbances in Uganda reached the district and all project activities had to cease. A total of 16 confirmed cases of Burkitt's lymphoma was identified in the cohort. The relative risk increased multiplicatively by a factor of 5 for each standard deviation by which the viral capsid antigen titre was above the average in controls matched for age and sex. The level of other anti-EBV antibody titres did not differ between cases and their matched controls

selected from the cohort. Thus, the elevation of EBV antibody levels before the manifestation of Burkitt's lymphoma was limited to the viral capsid antigen specifically. Comparison of antibody levels in prediagnostic serum samples and postdiagnostic samples showed that the clinical development of Burkitt's lymphoma did not increase the high viral capsid antigen antibody titres observed 1–5 years before disease onset. This indicates that the high viral capsid antigen antibody titres consistently observed in Burkitt's lymphoma cases from endemic areas were not secondary to the development of the disease. Nucleic acid hybridization studies demonstrated EBV DNA within the great majority of Burkitt's lymphoma cases from endemic areas (de-Thé, 1985).

When the Ugandan prospective study was initiated, one hypothesis was that Burkitt's lymphoma developed in those who had a later than average infection with EBV (Smith, 1985). The results failed to support this hypothesis, but did not establish that early infection was a risk factor. Nearly all of the cases and the matched controls selected from the cohort had already been infected with EBV. While one of the 16 cases was bled at three months of age and had a very high antibody titre, two of the four controls for this patient also had high antibody titres at three months. The risk factors for persistently high antibody titres have not been determined. The association of the disease with EBV infection does not explain the descriptive epidemiology of Burkitt's lymphoma – the geographical distribution, the relationship with age, the observation that in general it is the males that are predominantly affected. This suggests that the major epidemiological features of the disease must be due some other exposure or exposures. The factor most discussed in this respect is persistent and heavy malarial infection (Smith, 1985).

Analysis of the coding region of the *EBNA-2* gene in endemic Burkitt's lymphoma has revealed a high prevalence of both EBV type A and type B (Young *et al.*, 1987). This reflects the high prevalence of both types of EBV in the general population in equatorial Africa, and may be indicative of the presence of some immunodeficiency, as there is an increased frequency of type B EBV in various immuno-compromised groups, such as those with AIDS (Sculley *et al.*, 1990).

The geographical distributions of holo-endemic malaria and Burkitt's lymphoma are similar (Booth *et al.*, 1967; Burkitt, 1969; Kafuko & Burkitt, 1970). However, the incidence of

Burkitt's lymphoma is low in certain parts of Latin America and south-east Asia where there are high rates of malaria parasite infection. A possible explanation for this inconsistency is that there are considerable differences in transmission intensity of malaria that can support high levels of parasitaemia by *Plasmodium falciparum* (Morrow, 1985). The transmission intensity may be 10 to 100 times greater in tropical Africa than in parts of Latin America and south-east Asia, and this shows a closer association with Burkitt's lymphoma than the simple occurrence of falciparum malaria. There is a close correlation between the age at which maximum anti-malarial immunoglobulin is acquired and the age of onset of Burkitt's lymphoma (O'Conor, 1970). This suggests that the intensity of host response to malaria is more important in the relationship to Burkitt's lymphoma than infection with malaria itself. Little difference in levels of malaria antibodies has been found between patients with Burkitt's lymphoma and controls, but in most studies, by the time the diagnoses of Burkitt's lymphoma have been made, most patients had received one or more courses of anti-malarial drugs, whereas controls were less likely to have received these drugs (Morrow, 1985). In a study in Ghana, no association between levels of antibodies to EBV and malaria was found (Biggar *et al.*, 1981), indicating that if malaria is involved in the etiology of Burkitt's lymphoma, this is independent of EBV. In studies in Papua New Guinea and the Gambia, malaria was found to reduce the T-cell-mediated control of EBV immortalized cells, suggesting that malaria may promote Burkitt's lymphoma by suppressing cell-mediated immunity (Moss *et al.*, 1983; Whittle *et al.*, 1984). If severe malaria were to play a critical role in the etiology of Burkitt's lymphoma, the sickle-cell trait, which protects against malaria, should also have a protective affect against Burkitt's lymphoma. However, no clear relationship between the two conditions has been identified (Morrow, 1985).

Geser *et al.* (1989) carried out a malaria suppression trial in North Mara district, Tanzania, to determine whether the incidence of Burkitt's lymphoma could be lowered by reducing the level of malarial infection in a child population below 10 years of age by means of chloroquine distribution. Immediately after the initiation of the trial, the prevalence of malaria declined in children in the area, but it rose again in spite of continued distribution of chloroquine. This was due to inefficiency of the peripheral drug distribution and not to chloroquine resistance, which did not develop in the area until 1982. The trend in the incidence of Burkitt's lymphoma in the area appeared to run parallel to the trend in malaria prevalence, with a lag time of two years. However, the possibility could not be excluded that the decline in the incidence of Burkitt's lymphoma in North Mara might have started in 1972, five years before the chloroquine trial was initiated. In the Mengo districts of Uganda, there was a marked decline in the incidence of Burkitt's lymphoma during the 1960s, when case ascertainment was improving (Morrow, 1985). While no specific malaria vector control procedures were in operation during the period, the amount of chloroquine distributed increased greatly, and there was a substantial decline in infant mortality. Decreases in the incidence of Burkitt's lymphoma in Natal and New Guinea as well as in Uganda appear to have occurred as a result of an increase in programmes of malaria eradication (Miller, 1990). This may also account for the low incidence of Burkitt's lymphoma on the islands of Zanzibar and Pemba, which lie just 20 miles off the coast of Tanzania, where the tumour is endemic.

*Euphorbia tirucalli* has a similar distribution to endemic Burkitt's lymphoma in Africa. This plant contains diterpene esters which activate latent EBV within a cell and enhance the production of complete virions (Ito, 1985). In a study in Malawi, patients with Burkitt's lymphoma and age–sex-matched controls were visited and plants growing or present immediately around the house were recorded, using a scoring system for the number of plants and their distance from the home (van den Bosch *et al.*, 1993b). Of four plants with known EBV-promoting capacity, two (*E. tirucalli* and *Jatropha curcas*) were found significantly more often in the vicinity of the homes of cases than of controls. Significant positive associations between the disease and the presence of other plants in the *Euphorbia* family, tobacco and plants used commonly as traditional medicines were found, but not with plants used for building or other purposes. There was no significant association with the score for the number of plants and their distance from the home. For each case, one hospital control and two control children resident in the same village as the case, but not immediate neighbours, were selected. Similar results were obtained when comparison was made with each group of controls separately. An extract of *E. tirucalli* has been shown to induce continuous mitosis and chromosomal rearrangements in EBV-infected B-lymphocytes *in vitro* (Aya *et al.*, 1991). Approximately 10% of the chromosomal rearrangements were the characteristic 8:14 translocation seen in Burkitt's lymphoma, involving activation of the c-*myc* oncogene. The chromosomal changes induced by the *E. tirucalli* extracts were observed only in the presence of EBV infection.

### Burkitt's lymphoma in areas of low and intermediate incidence

In studies in developed countries, the proportion of Burkitt's lymphoma cases found to be associated with EBV, either serologically or by testing for the presence of EBV DNA, has been 30% or less (de-Thé, 1985; Shiramizu *et al.*, 1991; Hummel *et al.*, 1995). In South America, where the incidence of Burkitt's lymphoma appears to be intermediate between that in tropical Africa and in developed countries, the proportion of Burkitt's lymphomas positive for EBV has been found to range from 25 to about 70% (Gutierrez *et al.*, 1992; Drut *et al.*, 1994; Bacchi *et al.*, 1996). In contrast to Burkitt's lymphoma in areas where there is a high prevalence of EBV of both types A and B, in Brazil a high proportion of cases was associated with type A but not type B (Chen *et al.*, 1996). This pattern has also been observed in Egypt and Turkey (Cavdar *et al.*, 1994; Anwar *et al.*, 1995).

### Hodgkin's disease and postnatal infection with Epstein–Barr virus

EBV has been detected in high proportions of tumour samples of paediatric cases of Hodgkin's disease (Armstrong *et al.*, 1993; Weinreb *et al.*, 1996). In a study of 55 cases diagnosed under the age of 15 years in Brazil, Saudi Arabia and the UK, the tumours of children under 10 years of age were particularly likely to be EBV-associated (24 of the 27 cases; Armstrong *et al.*, 1993). Weinreb *et al.* (1996) investigated a series of 277 archival tissue samples from children diagnosed with Hodgkin's disease before 16 years of age in ten countries: Australia, Costa Rica, Egypt, Greece, Iran, Jordan, Kenya, South Africa, the United Arab Emirates and the UK. The proportion of cases positive for EBV latent membrane protein 1 (LMP1) varied between 50% and 100%. Compared with samples from the UK, the proportions positive for LMP1 were significantly elevated for samples from Greece, Costa Rica and Kenya. Using a polymerase chain reaction based typing technique, EBV strain type 1 was predominant in childhood Hodgkin's disease samples from Australia, Greece, South Africa and the UK, while type 2 was predominant

in Egypt, and was found in cases from Costa Rica and Kenya also. Cases with dual infections of type 1 and type 2 were observed in Costa Rica (48%; 13/27), Kenya (36%; 9/25) and the UK (20%; 2/10). While infection with one strain of EBV might be expected to confer immunity to the other strain, the high levels of dual infection in Costa Rica and Kenya suggests that an underlying immune deficiency might account for the high proportion of cases positive for LMP1 observed in these countries. Limitations of the study include the lack of specification of how the archival specimens were sampled, and the small number of specimens analysed in some of the countries.

### Lymphoma and HIV infection of the index child

HIV infection may become an important cause of childhood cancer. In the USA in 1989, an estimated 1.5 per 1000 women giving birth were infected with HIV, and the perinatal transmission rate is of the order of 30% (Gwinn *et al.*, 1991). Among 1321 children enrolled in the Italian Register for HIV Infection in Children as of 30 March 1990, seven had developed malignant tumours (Aricò *et al.*, 1991). There was one case of Kaposi's sarcoma in a haemophiliac child aged 11 years. Among the other six cases born to HIV-positive mothers, four developed non-Hodgkin B-cell lymphomas at ages between five months and four years, one developed an acute B-cell lymphoblastic leukaemia at 18 months, and one was diagnosed with hepatoblastoma at 4.9 years.

Rabkin *et al.* (1992) studied the incidence of non-Hodgkin lymphoma and other cancers in relation to HIV seropositivity in a cohort of 1701 patients with haemophilia and related clotting disorders. The relative risk of non-Hodgkin lymphoma in HIV-positive subjects compared with the general population was 38 in subjects aged 10–39 years, and 12 in older subjects. In the total cohort, the relative risk of Kaposi's sarcoma in HIV-positive subjects compared with the general population was 200 (based on two exposed cases). The incidence of the types of cancer was not increased in the HIV-positive subjects, and HIV-negative subjects with haemophilia had no significant increase in cancer incidence.

### Non-Hodgkin lymphoma and postnatal infection

As discussed in relation to childhood leukaemia, blood transfusion is a potential route whereby infants may be exposed to blood-borne infections. In a few studies, the relationship between childhood cancer and exchange transfusions recorded in medical records or reported retrospectively by the parents has been investigated. No association has been observed with childhood non-Hodgkin lymphoma (Adami *et al.*, 1996). In the study of Memon and Doll (1994) described above, one case of childhood non-Hodgkin lymphoma was observed, compared with 1.08 expected (RR = 0.93, 95% CI 0.02–5.16). However, at ages 15–49 years, the relative risk of non-Hodgkin lymphoma was 2.2 (95% CI 0.6–5.5), similar to that seen in a study of Iowa women (Cerhan *et al.*, 1993).

# Brain tumours

## Maternal infection during pregnancy

In the two available studies, no consistent association between brain tumours and reported maternal infection during pregnancy was apparent (Birch *et al.*, 1990b; Bunin *et al.*, 1994b).

## Maternal polio vaccination during pregnancy

An increased registration rate of brain tumours in children was observed in Connecticut during the late 1950s and early 1960s, principally among children born in the period 1955–60 (Farwell *et al.*, 1979). The polio vaccine used in Connecticut between 1955 and 1961 was subsequently found to contain the virus SV40, which has produced tumours of the CNS in experimental animals. Farwell *et al.* (1979) identified 120 children born during the period 1956–62 who were diagnosed with brain tumours under the age of 20 years from records of the Connecticut Tumour Registry. One third of these cases were chosen randomly for study, together with two controls for each case matched on sex, date and town of birth, selected from birth certificates. A questionnaire was sent to the obstetrician who delivered the index child, enquiring whether the mother had received polio vaccination during pregnancy. The relevant information was returned for 38 cases (95%) and 52 controls (65%). It was stated that 8 of 23 (35%) of glioma patients and 10 of 15 (67%) of medulloblastoma patients had been exposed to SV40, compared with 21% of controls. In a study of 245 case–control pairs in Finland, in which data on vaccination were obtained prospectively during antenatal clinic visits, there was an inverse association between maternal polio vaccination during pregnancy and brain tumours (RR = 0.3, 98% CI 0.0–1.9; Salonen & Saxén, 1975). As the proportion of control mothers who received polio vaccination was only 3%, this study had limited power to detect an association. Moreover, the study was not designed to investigate the possible risk of SV40 contamination.

## Maternal contact with animals during the index pregnancy

In view of an observation that more children with brain tumours than normal controls were reported to have lived on farms and to have been exposed to farm animals early in childhood (Gold *et al.*, 1979; see below), Kuijten *et al.* (1990) considered the association between astrocytoma and maternal contact with pets or farm-related animals during pregnancy. The odds ratio was 1.1 (95% CI 0.6–2.1, based on 53 discordant pairs). In New South Wales, Australia, no significant association was found with the mother having lived or worked on a farm in the month before or during pregnancy, or with the mother having been in contact with cats during this period (McCredie *et al.*, 1994a). In a study based on a similar protocol in the Paris area of France, the relative risk of brain tumours associated with maternal farm residence during pregnancy was 2.5 (95% CI 0.4–16.1; Cordier *et al.*, 1994). The relative risk associated with presence of a cat in the home during pregnancy was 1.6 (95% CI 0.8–3.3); more mothers of cases than mothers of controls reported that they had been scratched by a cat (RR = 5.1, 95% CI 1.2–21.6).

In a multicentre study in the USA and Canada, there was no association between astrocytoma or primitive neuroectodermal tumours of the brain and cat ownership, or the mother having changed the litter box, during pregnancy (Bunin *et al.*, 1994b).

## Contact of the index child with animals

The observations of Bross and Gibson (1970), together with evidence that brain tumours could be induced in a variety of species by known animal oncogenic viruses, stimulated Gold *et al.* (1979) to investigate the association between childhood brain tumours and the index child's exposure to animals. The relative risk associated with residence on a farm was 4.0 (*p* = 0.04, based on 15 discordant pairs) in comparison with controls selected from birth certificate files; no association was found in comparison with controls with other types of cancer. Compared with birth certificate controls, the relative risk associated with exposure to sick pets was 4.5 (*p* = 0.07, based on 11 discordant pairs), whereas compared with children with other types of cancer, no association was apparent (RR = 1.3). No association with sick pets was found in a subsequent study in Toronto, Canada (RR = 1.1, 95% CI 0.5–2.4; Howe *et al.*, 1989), and there was no association with the child having been in contact with animals in a study in New South Wales, Australia (McCredie *et al.*, 1994b). In a study in France based on a similar protocol to that of the study in New South Wales, an elevated relative risk (RR = 6.7, 95% CI 1.2–38) of brain tumours associated with farm residence of the index child was observed (Cordier *et al.*, 1994). This did not appear to be accounted for by reported contact with any particular type of animal.

## Postnatal infection

In a record-linkage based study of 570 childhood brain tumours and 2850 controls in Sweden, treatment by exchange transfusion was associated with a two-fold excess risk (Linet *et al.*, 1996). Two of the three cases treated by exchange transfusion developed plexus papillomas. No association was found in small studies of brain tumours, in which there would have been low statistical power to detect an association (Cordier *et al.*, 1994; McCredie *et al.*, 1994b). No association between neonatal or intrauterine transfusion and solid tumours of childhood was found in the study of Memon and Doll (1994).

In the Swedish record-linkage based study, a positive association between brain tumours and neonatal infections was observed (RR = 2.4, 95% CI 1.5–4.0; Linet *et al.*, 1996; Table 7.6). This did not appear to be specific to any particular type of brain tumour. A number of other indicators of neonatal distress were associated with brain tumours in this study (see Chapter 10). In substantially smaller studies, no association between brain tumours and postnatal infection (Gold *et al.*, 1979) or meningitis (Cordier *et al.*, 1994; McCredie *et al.*, 1994b) was observed.

As the tonsils are lymphoid tissue and therefore may be important in the protection against a variety of antigens, a number of investigators have studied the association between cancer and tonsillectomy (Cassimos *et al.*, 1973). However, no association between tonsillectomy and brain tumours (Gold *et al.*, 1979; Preston-Martin *et al.*, 1982) has been observed.

# Other types of childhood cancer

## Neuroblastoma

In a single study, there was a positive association between neuroblastoma and acute vaginal infections and treatment for them during pregnancy (Michalek *et al.*, 1996). In a study in North Carolina, no clear association with immunization history as recorded in hospital records was found (Greenberg, 1983; Table 7.6).

## Retinoblastoma and postnatal infection

The retinoblastoma gene product (p-105 RB) has been shown to form stable protein complexes with the oncoproteins of three DNA tumour viruses (DeCaprio *et al.*, 1988; Whyte *et al.*, 1988; Dyson *et al.*, 1989). It has been postulated that these oncoproteins inactivate the product of the retinoblastoma gene, which is thought to have a suppressor effect (Matsunaga *et al.*, 1990). The viral hypothesis for the etiology of nonheritable retinoblastoma has not been tested directly in epidemiological studies and patients have not been screened for antiviral antibodies.

## Wilms' tumour and maternal infection during pregnancy

Olshan *et al.* (1993) found a relative risk of Wilms' tumour associated with maternal use of antibiotics during pregnancy of 2.0 (95% CI 1.0–3.7). There was no association with infections of any type except 'other', mostly yeast, and the authors noted that both antibiotic use and yeast infection were found to be over-reported by mothers of children with malformations in a validation study (Werler *et al.*, 1989). In the study of Bunin *et al.* (1987), exploratory analysis showed a positive association with vaginal infection during pregnancy (RR = 5.5, 95% CI 1.0–71.9, based on 13 discordant pairs). The relative risk for use of a vaginal cream or suppository was 5.0 (not statistically significant, based on six discordant pairs).

## Hepatoblastoma

In the one available study, there was no association between hepatoblastoma and maternal influenza or varicella infection during pregnancy, or use of antibiotics during the index pregnancy or the year before it (Buckley *et al.*, 1989a).

## Ewing's sarcoma and postnatal infection

In view of immunohistochemical similarities between blastoma and Ewing's sarcoma, and a

236

case report of a patient with persistent polyclonal B-lymphocytosis, EBV antibodies and subsequent malignant pulmonary blastoma, EBV-specific genome sequences were sought in material from seven patients with Ewing's sarcoma (Daugaard *et al.*, 1991). EBV could not be demonstrated in these tumours by a polymerase chain reaction method.

In a case-control study in the USA of Ewing's sarcoma diagnosed up to the age of 31 years, no noteworthy association with postnatal chickenpox, measles, rubella or infectious mononucleosis was found (Holly *et al.*, 1992).

## Osteosarcoma

In a case–control study of osteosarcoma diagnosed at ages up to 24 years, there was no association with reported maternal exposure during pregnancy to polio, rubella, measles, mumps, chickenpox or influenza (Operskalski *et al.*, 1987).

## Soft-tissue sarcoma and postnatal infection and immunization

In a small exploratory study, a positive association between rhabdomyosarcoma and whooping cough was observed (Grufferman *et al.*, 1982). No other associations were apparent in the two available studies, both of which were small (Table 7.6). In a study of total childhood cancer in northern England in which nine groups of drugs were considered, only one significant difference emerged from a total of 675 comparisons (Hartley *et al.* 1988a). This was a positive association between soft-tissue sarcomas and medically recorded antibiotic use during the neonatal period (RR = 6.8, 95% CI 1.1–71.2), which was mainly accounted for by children with rhabdomyosarcoma (Hartley *et al.*, 1988b).

In the study of Grufferman *et al.* (1982), cases with rhabdomyosarcoma had received substantially fewer routine childhood immunizations than controls. The relative risk associated with smallpox vaccination was 0.2 (95% CI 0.1–0.6), with measles/mumps/rubella immunization 0.3 (95% CI 0.1–1.5) and with diphtheria/tetanus/pertussis immunization 0.7 (95% CI 0.1–7.6). All 33 cases and 96 of 98 controls had received poliomyelitis immunization.

No association of sibship size with soft-tissue sarcoma was found in a study in Italy (Magnani *et al.*, 1989), or with rhabdomyosarcoma in a small study in North Carolina (Grufferman *et al.*, 1982). In the study in North Carolina, no association between rhabdomyosarcoma and exposure of the index child to cats or dogs was found (Grufferman *et al.*, 1982).

## Germ-cell tumours and maternal infection during pregnancy

Two case–control studies of germ-cell tumours of all types and maternal infection during pregnancy are available, one based on 41 cases (25 malignant, 16 benign) in northern England (Johnston *et al.*, 1986), the other based on a multicentre study of 105 cases with malignant germ-cell tumours in the USA and Canada (Shu *et al.*, 1995a). In the study of Shu *et al.* (1995a), there was a positive association with reported maternal urinary infection during pregnancy (RR = 3.1, 95% CI 1.5–6.6). There was no association with other infections. No association with maternal infection of any type was seen in the study of Johnston *et al.* (1986).

## Germ-cell tumours and postnatal exposures related to infection

In the multicentre study of malignant germ-cell tumours in children the USA and Canada, no association with antibiotics taken by the index child with any infections or any viral infections within six months of birth, or with mumps up to the age of diagnosis, was found (Shu *et al.*, 1995a). The relative risk of germ-cell tumours associated with blood transfusion within six months of birth as reported by the parents was 3.5 (95% CI 0.8–15.9). The relative risk associated with smallpox vaccination was 0.5 (95% CI 0.3–0.9). The relative risks associated with other types of vaccination were in the range 0.7–2.4; none was statistically significant. No association with tonsillectomy, of possible interest as the tonsils may be important in the protection against a variety of antigens (Cassimos *et al.*, 1973), was found.

## All types of childhood cancer combined and immunization of the index child

In a study in northern England, children who were reported by their mothers never to have received one of the standard immunizations (against tetanus, diphtheria, whooping cough, poliomyelitis, measles, smallpox or rubella) were found to have a significantly higher risk of developing childhood cancer compared with children who had received one or more of the standard vaccines (RR = 3.6, 95% CI 1.6–8.2; Hartley *et al.*, 1988a). Children under two years of age at diagnosis were excluded from the analysis because, in this age group, symptoms preceding the onset of the tumour may have led to immunization not being carried out. The authors observed that where an explanation for non-immunization had been given at interview, no consistent reason was specified. The

## Table 7.6. Associations between non-haematopoietic malignancies in childhood, or total childhood cancer, and postnatal infections of the index child

| Area and period of study | Cases: Dead (D), newly incident (I) or prevalent (P), upper age limit | Controls: N | Controls: Type[a] | Method of assessing exposure[b] | Reference period | Type of infection | Frequency in controls (%) | RR | Reference |
|---|---|---|---|---|---|---|---|---|---|
| **Brain tumours** Sweden, 1973–89 | I, 14[c] | 570 | P | 2850 MR | In neonatal period | Any Urinary tract | 1.8 0.1 | 2.4* 3.8 | Linet *et al.*, 1996 |
| **Astrocytoma** Sweden, 1973–89 | I, 14 | 263 | P | 1315 MR | In neonatal period | Any Urinary tract | 1.7 0.2 | 3.1[d] 5.0[d] | Linet *et al.*, 1996 |
| **Neuroblastoma** USA, North Carolina, 1972–81 | I, 14 | 104 | H | 208 MR | Unspecified | Pneumonia Other serious infections | 13.2 5.1 | 0.7 0.2 | Greenberg, 1983 |
| **Ewing's sarcoma** USA, San Francisco Bay Area, 1978–86 | I, 31 | 43 | RDD | 193 I | Up to age at diagnosis | Chickenpox Measles Rubella Infectious mononucleosis | 78.8 11.4 20.7 2.6 | 1.2 0.8 0.9[e] 1.5 | Holly *et al.*, 1992 |
| **Soft-tissue sarcoma** Italy, Padua and Turin, 1983–84 | I, P, NS[f] | 52 | H | 326 I | Up to one year before diagnosis | Viral disease Bacterial disease | 69.0 42.0 | 1.2 0.9 | Magnani *et al.*, 1989 |
| **Rhabdomyosarcoma** USA, North Carolina, 1967–76 | I, 14 | 33 | P | 99 I | Unspecified | Measles Mumps Rubella Pertussis Chickenpox Scarlet fever Hepatitis Pneumonia "Strep throat" Otitis media | 27 34 23 4 73 6 5 8 29 32 | 2.0 1.3 0.6 4.1* 0.9 0.5 0.6 0.7 1.1 0.9 | Grufferman *et al.*, 1982 |
| **Germ-cell tumours** USA and Canada, CCG, 1982–89 | I, 14 | 105 | RDD | 639 Q | Within 6 months of birth Up to diagnosis | Any Any viral Mumps | 8.3 57.3 3.2 | 0.7 0.8 1.5 | Shu *et al.*, 1995a |

238

| Study site, period | Type, no. | Cases | Control source | Controls | Method | Exposure | Timing | | | Reference |
|---|---|---|---|---|---|---|---|---|---|---|
| Total childhood cancer Great Britain, 1953–55 | D, 9 | 1299 | P | 1299 | I | Measles | Up to two years before onset | 16.9 | 1.1[g] | Stewart et al., 1958 |
| | | | | | | Chickenpox | | 7.9 | 1.2[g] | |
| | | | | | | Whooping cough | | 12.2 | 1.0[g] | |
| | | | | | | Mumps | | 2.9 | 1.2[g] | |
| | | | | | | Rubella | | 2.6 | 1.0[g] | |
| | | | | | | Scarlet fever | | 1.2 | 1.3[g] | |
| | | | | | | Bronchitis | | 1.5 | 1.0[g] | |
| | | | | | | Bronchopneumonia | | 2.5 | 1.2[g] | |
| | | | | | | Acute tonsillitis | | 0.9 | 1.2[g] | |
| | | | | | | Acute otitis media | | 0.7 | 1.7[g] | |
| | | | | | | All | | 52.7 | 1.1[g] | |
| UK, North West, West Midlands and Yorkshire, 1980–83 | I, 14 | 555 | GP, H | 1110 | I, MR | Specific perinatal | <6 months | NS | 1.0 | Hartley et al., 1988a |
| | | | | | MR | Acute upper respiratory tract[h] | >6 months | 1.4 | 2.3* | |

NS, Not stated.   CCG, Children's Cancer Group
* p < 0.05

a  P, population-based; GP, neighbourhood, selected through general practice; H, hospital; RDD, selected by random-digit dialling.
b  I, maternal interview; MR, medical records; Q, questionnaire.
c  Ten children born in 1973–74 were diagnosed at age 15–17 years.

a  Crude unmatched analysis of matched data.
c  Adjusted for agricultural occupation of the father, poison or overdose of medication, area of residence, year of child's birth and income. The crude relative risk was 1.9 (95% CI 0.9–4.3).
f  Mean age at diagnosis 6.8 (±4.7) years.
g  Case–control ratio.
h  This was the only statistically significant association for medically confirmed conditions when ICD9 illness chapters, groups or specific illnesses were considered.

unimmunized case children were not confined to any diagnostic group.

In a study of 74 deaths due to childhood cancer in Baden-Wurttemberg, Germany, in the period 1972–73, there was a significant inverse association with having received immunization against diphtheria (RR = 0.3, 95% CI 0.1–0.8; Neumann, 1980). There were no marked differences for other immunizations; cases had less tetanus (RR = 0.5, 95% CI 0.1–1.6), poliomyelitis (RR = 0.8, 95% CI 0.2–2.4), and BCG (RR = 0.7, 95% CI 0.3–1.5) immunization but more smallpox vaccination (RR = 1.3, 95% CI 0.6–2.7) than controls.

## All types of childhood cancer combined and postnatal exposures related to infection

In a study of 1299 deaths from childhood cancer in Great Britain during 1953-55, no association with reported infection in the index child with measles, chickenpox, whooping cough, mumps, rubella or scarlet fever was found (Stewart *et al.*, 1958).

## Conclusions

In Great Britain, a variety of measures of population mixing appear to be associated with excesses of childhood leukaemia, particularly in young children. Population mixing also has been associated with excesses of childhood leukaemia in Hong Kong. The association could potentially explain excesses observed in the areas near the nuclear installations at Sellafield and Dounreay and in west Berkshire, although it is not clear that it can explain excesses observed in districts near sites considered for the construction of nuclear installations. A potential limitation of these analyses is that estimates of the population of children at risk of leukaemia may have been inaccurate in areas such as new towns, the reception areas for wartime evacuees, and the areas in which national servicemen were posted. In some analyses, the results were shown to be similar when different estimates of the denominator population were applied (Kinlen *et al.*, 1990; Kinlen & Hudson, 1991; Kinlen & John, 1994).

It is noteworthy that in the studies in which the incidence of, or mortality due to, leukaemia was compared between different levels of exposure (proportion of child migrants, proportions of evacuated people during the Second World War, proportions of servicemen, ratio of oil workers to total economically active men, extent of increase in commuting),

although the trend statistic was significant in certain analyses, inspection of the observed to expected ratios at each level did not always show a steady trend. Kinlen *et al.* (1991, 1993a) noted that absence of a steady trend is typical of many infectious diseases in which outbreaks or epidemics only occur when the density, or the numbers, of infected and susceptible individuals in a population reaches some critical point specific for the agent in question.

It would be relevant to determine whether population mixing can explain the clusters detected in the analysis of Openshaw and Craft (1991), most of which were not in the vicinity of actual or potential sites of nuclear installations, or which were not in the vicinity of new towns (see Chapter 2). High rates of childhood leukaemia mortality in Greece and Italy between the 1950s and 1970s may be attributable to mass migration from rural areas. Excesses of mortality due to leukaemia in childhood have not been associated with rapid population influx in France, or population mixing inferred to have occurred as a result of the growth of tourism in parts of Greece.

The associations between reported maternal infection during pregnancy of any types, or specifically with influenza or varicella, and childhood leukaemia are not consistent. With regard to studies of reported history of infection or serological markers of infection in the index child, no consistent association between leukaemia and infection in early life is apparent. These studies do not provide clear support for an etiological role for the commonest symptomatic infections of childhood. However, the validity of all of these studies is limited by possible selection bias, crude assessment of exposure or small study size. In a single study in Shanghai, a positive association between childhood leukaemia and chloramphenicol and syntomycin was found. This appeared to be stronger for ANLL than ALL. It would seem important to attempt to replicate this finding in studies in developing countries. There is no consistent association between BCG vaccination and the subsequent risk of leukaemia and other haematopoietic malignancies. In relation to less direct measures of exposure to infection, no consistent association between ALL and sibship size has been observed. In the available studies of leukaemia and lymphoma combined, no association was found with sibship size, but these had low statistical power to detect an effect. In both available studies, an inverse association between leukaemia and daycare was observed, but in one of these selection bias cannot be excluded as accounting for the result, and in the other, chance may account for the result.

Alexander (1993) suggested that the data on clustering and clusters in Great Britain are consistent with the hypothesis that ALL commonly arises as a rare outcome of exposure to a common virus or viruses and either (1) gestational or neonatal exposure leading to persistent infection or (2) primary infection at an older age in children whose immune system has been protected from early challenge. Alexander (1993) further argued that the epidemiological characteristics of the herpes viruses could be consistent with such a model in that they can occur in epidemic form in young children, they can infect the fetus, asymptomatic reactivation and re-infection may occur, and that they can induce cell-mediated depression of immunity. In the one available study, no significant difference in the prevalences of antibody-positivity for human herpes virus type 6 was found between cases of leukaemia and hospital controls, and herpes labialis was reported less frequently by parents of leukaemia cases than controls.

On the basis of studies in endemic areas, Burkitt's lymphoma is associated with Epstein–Barr virus. However, this association does not explain the geographical distribution of Burkitt's lymphoma, its relationship with age, or the observation that, in general, predominantly boys are affected. The factor most discussed in relation to these features is persistent and heavy infection with malaria, as the geographical distributions of holoendemic malaria and Burkitt's lymphoma are similar. If true, this may depend on the vectorial capacity, rather than the simple occurrence of falciparum malaria. The proportion of cases of Burkitt's lymphoma associated with Epstein–Barr virus is lower in areas of low and intermediate incidence of the lymphoma than in endemic areas, and the subtypes of the virus involved may differ.

Epstein–Barr virus has been detected in high proportions of tumour samples from paediatric cases of Hodgkin's disease.

Non-Hodgkin lymphoma has been reported in children infected with HIV. HIV may become an important cause of childhood cancer.

The associations between infections and other types of childhood cancer have been little investigated. In a large record-linkage based study in Sweden, a positive association between brain tumours and neonatal infection was observed. There is a need to investigate this in other studies. In one study, a positive association between brain tumours and contact of the index child with animals, and sick pets in particular, was reported, but this has not been observed in other relatively small studies. In two studies of Wilms' tumour, a positive association with maternal infection during pregnancy was found.

# Chapter 8
# Lifestyle

Maternal lifestyle during pregnancy is known to have effects on embryonic and fetal development, and it might be expected that there might be effects on the subsequent risk of cancer in the offspring. Aspects of maternal lifestyle during pregnancy that have been investigated in relation to childhood cancer include diet and vitamin supplement use, smoking, consumption of alcohol and 'recreational' drugs, and use of cosmetics, and these are considered in this chapter. Further aspects of maternal lifestyle that have been investigated are contact with animals during the index pregnancy, discussed in the chapter on infections (Chapter 7), and use of beaches with possible exposure to radioactive deposits (discussed in Chapter 4). Paternal lifestyle in the pre-conceptional period might be postulated to have effects on the risk of germ-cell mutation. Aspects of paternal lifestyle that have been investigated in relation to childhood cancer include smoking, alcohol consumption and use of 'recreational' drugs. In the particular instance of smoking, paternal habits might affect the offspring also by means of passive exposure of the mother during pregnancy or passive exposure of the child during his or her lifetime. The lifestyle of the child might have a direct impact on his/her health. Aspects of the lifestyle of the index child investigated in relation to childhood cancer include diet and vitamin supplement use, passive exposure to tobacco smoke and use of dummies (pacifiers). Further aspects of the lifestyle of the child that have been investigated include contact with animals and social contact (both discussed in Chapter 7) and play on beaches on which there may be radioactive deposits (discussed in Chapter 4).

## Leukaemia

### Maternal diet and vitamin supplement use during pregnancy

In a study of non-T-cell acute lymphoblastic leukaemia (ALL) in Hokkaido, Japan, an inverse association was found with the mother having drunk milk during pregnancy at least one day per week (RR = 0.3, 95% CI 0.1–0.8; Nishi & Miyake, 1989). The association did not persist after adjustment for a variety of postnatal exposures of the child. The reason for collecting information on maternal milk consumption was not specified, and it is not clear whether other aspects of maternal diet during pregnancy were investigated.

In a study designed primarily to assess the relationship between childhood cancer and residential exposure to electromagnetic fields in Denver, Colorado (USA), no association between ALL (56 cases) and maternal consumption of cured meats during pregnancy was found (Sarasua & Savitz, 1994).

A subset of mothers of infants with leukaemia diagnosed at one year of age or less, and controls selected by random-digit dialling included in three multicentre case–control studies of childhood leukaemia in the USA (Buckley et al., 1989b; Robison et al., 1989, 1995; Shu et al., 1994b) was re-approached and supplemental information on maternal diet during the index pregnancy was sought (Ross et al., 1996b). Nearly 80% of cases with infant leukaemia present with a specific genetic abnormality involving the *MLL* gene on chromosome band 11q23 (Ross et al., 1994b). Abnormalities involving 11q23 also have been observed in secondary acute myeloid leukaemias following treatment with epipodophyllotoxins, which inhibit the enzyme DNA topoisomerase II. Therefore, it was postulated that 11q23 infant leukaemias may be associated with naturally occurring agents which inhibit DNA topoisomerase II. These agents include caffeine and are found in a number of dietary sources including a variety of fruit and vegetables, in medications used to treat urinary tract infections and possibly podophyllin resin, which is commonly used in the treatment of genital warts. Based on data from a food-frequency questionnaire assessing consumption of 26 food items during the index pregnancy, there was no association between total estimated dietary intake of topoisomerase II inhibitors and leukaemia of all types combined or ALL (53 cases). However, there was a statistically significant positive association for acute myeloid leukaemia (AML) with increasing maternal consumption of dietary topoisomerase II inhibitors (RR for highest vs lowest tertile 10.2, 95% CI 1.1–96.4, *p*-value for trend = 0.04, based on 29 cases).

In the three available studies of childhood leukaemia and maternal consumption of vitamin supplements of any type in pregnancy, no association was apparent (Table 8.1).

## Breast-feeding

Data on the association between breast-feeding and subsequent leukaemia in the child are relevant to hypotheses about the etiological role of infections, in view of the evidence that breast-fed infants are less severely affected by infections in infancy than are artificially fed infants (Davis *et al.*, 1988). In a case–control study of childhood cancer in Denver, Colorado, designed primarily to investigate the relationship with residential exposure to electromagnetic fields (Savitz *et al.*, 1988; see Chapter 5), the relative risk of ALL associated with artificial feeding only compared with breast-feeding for more than six months was 1.5 (95% CI 0.7–3.1) and that with breast-feeding for periods of six months or less was 2.0 (95% CI 0.9–4.4). This is similar to the pattern observed for childhood cancer of all types combined, for which the relative risk associated with artificial feeding only was 1.8 (95% CI 1.1–2.8) and that associated with breast-feeding for less than six months was 1.9 (95% CI 1.1–3.2). Cases diagnosed before the age of 18 months and their matched controls were excluded from analysis to avoid the possibility that infant feeding practice could be affected by cancer arising in very young children. In other studies, no association was found between breast-feeding and leukaemia and lymphoma combined (McKinney *et al.*, 1987; Magnani *et al.*, 1990) or with ALL (Van Steensel-Moll *et al.*, 1986; Shu *et al.*, 1995b). No association between breast-feeding and all types of childhood cancer combined was observed in a study of 555 cases and 1110 controls selected from hospitals and from general practitioners' lists in northern England (Hartley *et al.*, 1988a), or in a study of 99 cases and 90 hospital controls in northern India (Mathur *et al.*, 1993).

## Postnatal diet of the index child and use of vitamin supplements

Peters *et al.* (1994) investigated the association between the intake of certain food items thought to be precursors or inhibitors of *N*-nitroso compounds and the risk of leukaemia in children aged 10 years and under in Los Angeles County, California. A total of 331 cases were eligible, among whom maternal interview and matching with a control was completed for 232 (70%). 139 of the cases and 131 of the controls had been contacted by Lowengart *et al.* (1987). Sixty-two controls were selected from among the friends of cases, the remainder by random-digit dialling. Twelve questions were asked about the usual frequency of intake of certain food items of the mother, who was then asked to estimate the frequency of consumption by the child during a reference period dependent on the age of diagnosis. In univariate analysis, there were significant trends of increase in risk with increasing intake of ham, bacon and sausage, and hot dogs, and a trend of borderline significance with increasing intakes of bologna, pastrami, corned beef, salami or some combination of these. There was no association with reported intake of fruit or fruit drinks. Only the association with hot dogs persisted after adjustment for use of indoor pesticides, use of a hairdryer by the child, paternal occupational exposure to spray paint and other chemicals, wiring configuration, breast-feeding, identified in earlier analyses of these data (Lowengart *et al.*, 1987; London *et al.*, 1991), and consumption of hot dogs by the father, the only significant association to be identified with estimated intake by either parent. Distributions of measures of socioeconomic status were similar among cases and controls, and adjustment for socioeconomic status did not influence the relative risk associated with consumption of hot dogs.

In a study in Denver, Colorado, the relative risk of ALL associated with consumption of hamburgers by the index child at least once a week compared with less often was 2.0 (95% CI 0.9–4.6; Sarasua & Savitz, 1994). The relative risk associated with consumption of hot dogs and other cured meats, and charcoal broiled foods, was not elevated (Table 8.2).

In Shanghai, China, Shu *et al.* (1988) found a protective effect of at least one year of postnatal use of cod liver oil for both ALL (RR = 0.4, CI 0.2–0.9) and acute non-lymphocytic leukaemia (ANLL) (RR = 0.3, 95% CI 0.1–1.0). A protective effect of vitamins A and D would be consistent with experimental data. As already discussed, the study is limited by the non-contemporaneity of cases and controls, and differences in length of recall associated with this.

In a multicentre study of 990 cases of ALL and 1636 controls with other types of cancer in the

**Table 8.1. Association between childhood leukaemia and maternal consumption of vitamin supplements during pregnancy**

| Area and period of study | Cases[a] Upper age limit | N | Controls Type[b] | N | Source of information on supplement use[c] | Type of supplement | Prevalence of use in mothers of controls (%) | RR (95% CI) | Reference |
|---|---|---|---|---|---|---|---|---|---|
| Leukaemia Finland, 1959–68 | 14 | 373 | P | 373 | AN | Vitamins | 24.5[d] | 1.0 (0.6–1.7)[e] | Salonen & Saxén, 1975 |
| ALL USA, Denver, CO, 1976–83 | 14 | 56 | RDD | 205 | I | Vitamins | 90.2 | 0.5 (0.2–1.1)[f] | Sarasua & Savitz, 1994 |
| ANLL USA and Canada, CCSG, 1990–94 | 17 | 204 | RDD | 204 | I | Vitamins/iron | 87.3 | 1.0 (0.5–2.0) | Robison et al., 1989 |

CCSG, Childhood Cancer Study Group.
[a] These were newly incident in all three studies.
[b] P, population-based; RDD, selected by random-digit dialling.
[c] AN, antenatal clinic records; I, maternal interview.
[d] In total series of 972 controls, matched with cases with any type of childhood cancer.
[e] 98% CI.
[f] Crude unmatched analysis of matched data.

**Table 8.2. Association between childhood leukaemia and reported diet of the index child**

| Area and period of study | Cases[a] Upper age limit | N | Controls Type[b] | N | Period of consumption considered | Cured meats Type | Categorization[c] | RR (95% CI) for highest category | p value for trend | Fruit, fruit drinks, vitamins Type | Categorization[c] | RR (95% CI) for highest category | p value for trend | Reference |
|---|---|---|---|---|---|---|---|---|---|---|---|---|---|---|
| Leukaemia USA, Los Angeles County 1980–87 | 10 | 232 | F RDD | 232 | Pre-diagnostic[d] | Ham, bacon and sausage | To | 2.7 (1.4–5.8) | 0.02 | Orange/orange juice | To | 1.1 (0.0–1.9) | 0.7 | Peters, 1994 |
| | | | | | | Hot dogs | | 5.8 (2.1–10.2) | 0.001 | Apple/apple juice | | 1.6 (0.9–2.9) | 0.5 | |
| | | | | | | Lunch meats | | 1.8 (1.0–2.8) | 0.08 | | | | | |
| | | | | | | Hamburgers | | 2.3 (1.0–5.2) | 0.4 | | | | | |
| | | | | | | Charbroiled meats | | 1.0 (0.4–2.7) | 0.4 | | | | | |
| ALL USA, Denver, CO, 1976–83 | 14 | 56 | RDD | 206 | Pre-diagnostic | Ham, bacon and sausage | 1+/week vs <1/week | 1.2 (0.6–2.3) | – | Vitamins | Any vs. none | 0.6 (0.2–1.3) | – | Sarasua & Savitz, 1994 |
| | | | | | | Hot dogs | | 1.3 (0.5–3.2) | – | | | | | |
| | | | | | | Lunch meats | | 1.1 (0.5–2.3) | – | | | | | |
| | | | | | | Hamburgers | | 2.0 (0.9–4.6) | – | | | | | |
| | | | | | | Charcoal-broiled foods | Any vs none | 1.0 (0.5–2.1) | – | | | | | |

[a] Both studies were based on newly incident cases
[b] F, friends; RDD, selected by random-digit dialling
[c] To, tertiles, with non-consumers in separate group
[d] To intervals before diagnosis depending on the age of the child at diagnosis

USA and Canada, a positive association with vitamin use by the index child was found (RR = 1.7, $p < 0.0001$; Buckley *et al.*, 1994). However, no association was apparent when a subgroup of 404 cases was compared with individually matched controls selected by random-digit dialling. A possible explanation for the inconsistency may be that vitamin use by the index child protects against other types of childhood cancer, thereby lowering the proportion of vitamin users among controls. In a stratified analysis by immunophenotype, the association apparent in the comparison with cancer controls did not appear to be confined to any particular subgroup.

In the study of leukaemia and lymphoma in West Cumbria (UK) in which an association with paternal occupational exposure to ionizing radiation was observed (Gardner *et al.*, 1990a), no clear relationship with fish-eating habits was found. There was no association with the family growing its own vegetables or using seaweed as a fertilizer.

In a study of childhood cancer deaths before the age of 10 years in Great Britain, no association was found with consumption of dried milk, fruit juice or "tinned sieved vegetables" from the third day, first month and fourth month respectively, or with consumption of "other tinned vegetables", "highly coloured cakes or fruit drinks", "coloured sweets" or "shop-fried fish and chips" from the age of 12 months (Stewart *et al.*, 1958).

In a multicentre study in France, Malvy *et al.* (1993) observed inverse associations between newly diagnosed childhood malignancy and levels of β-carotene, retinol and α-tocopherol in serum. The authors attributed these associations to secondary metabolic effects of the tumours. Blood samples were taken before treatment from 418 cases, and from 632 age–sex-matched controls either recruited by the school health service in the same towns in which the cases were recruited, or who were undergoing routine health examination in departments of general paediatrics.

## Tobacco smoking by the mother

In the majority of studies in which the association between smoking and childhood cancer has been considered, attention has been focused on maternal smoking during the pregnancy leading to the birth of the index child. The available studies are summarized in Table 8.3. No consistent association between maternal smoking during pregnancy and leukaemia has been found.

## Tobacco smoking by the father

In most studies of childhood cancer and smoking habits of the father, the period of exposure considered has been up to the birth of the index child (Table 8.4). There is no consistent association between paternal smoking and all types of leukaemia combined or AML.

In four out of the five available studies of ALL, a positive association with paternal smoking was apparent, and was statistically significant in three. The study of Sorahan *et al.* (1995a) related to deaths due to all types of childhood cancer. A positive association with cigarette smoking by the father was found for all types of childhood cancer combined, and was apparent not only for ALL, but also for lymphomas, central nervous system tumours and benign tumours. In view of the lack of specificity of effect, in conjunction with the fact that matched pair interview data were obtained for only 49% of potentially eligible cases, the possibility that selection bias may account for the association cannot be excluded. The study of Shu *et al.* (1996b) related to leukaemia diagnosed up to 18 months of age. While the relative risks of ALL associated with paternal smoking in the month before pregnancy (RR = 1.6, 95% CI 1.0–2.4, adjusted for sex, paternal age, education and maternal alcohol consumption during pregnancy) and during the index pregnancy (RR = 1.5, 95% CI 1.0–2.2) were elevated, there was no dose–response relationship with the number of cigarettes smoked. As a substantial proportion of the information on paternal smoking was obtained by telephone interview with proxy respondents, additional analysis restricted to direct respondents was carried out. There were no appreciable changes in the observed relative risks. The study of Ji *et al.* (1997) was carried out in Shanghai, China, where the prevalence of smoking is high in men but extremely low in women. Information was obtained by direct interview independently with each parent of study subjects. The relative risk of ALL associated with paternal pre-conceptional smoking for more than five pack years was 3.8 (95% CI 1.3–12.3), after adjustment for birth weight, income, paternal age, education and alcohol consumption. There was a statistically significant trend ($p = 0.01$). There was no association with postnatal exposure to paternal smoking. In a study designed primarily to investigate the relationship between childhood cancer and exposure to electromagnetic fields in Denver, Colorado, the relative risk of ALL associated with paternal smoking during the year preceding the birth of the index child was 1.4 (95% CI 0.6–3.1), after adjustment for father's

## Table 8.3. Summary of studies of childhood leukaemia and childhood cancer of all types combined with maternal smoking during pregnancy

| Area and period of study | Cases | | Control type[a] | Prevalence of smoking during pregnancy in control mothers (%) | RR associated with any smoking during pregnancy | Trend[b] | Reference |
|---|---|---|---|---|---|---|---|
| | Upper age limit | Number | | | | | |
| **Lymphatic and haematopoietic tumours** | | | | | | | |
| Sweden, 1978–81 | 16 | 185 | HD | 29.7 | 1.6 | p < 0.01 | Stjernfeldt et al., 1986a |
| Sweden, 1982–87 | 5 | 72 | Coh | 30.0 | 1.0 | No | Pershagen et al., 1992 |
| **Leukaemia and non-Hodgkin's lymphoma** | | | | | | | |
| UK, Caithness, 1970–86 | 14 | 11 | B | 45.7 | 1.0 | | Urquhart et al., 1991 |
| UK, West Berkshire and North Hampshire 1972–89 | 4 | 54 | B | 26.9[c] 20.4[c] | 0.5[c] 0.9[c] | | Roman et al., 1993 |
| **Leukaemia** | | | | | | | |
| Canada, Ontario, 1959–68 and England and Wales, 1965 (1 week) | 10 7 | 22 | Coh | 40.0 | 1.8 | No | Neutel & Buck, 1971 |
| UK: North West, West Midlands, Yorkshire, 1980–83 | 14 | 171 | H, GP | NS | 1.0[d] | No | McKinney & Stiller, 1986; McKinney et al., 1987 |
| Mexico City, NS | 14 | 80 | H | 5.8 | 0.9 | | Fajardo-Gutiérrez et al., 1993a |
| USA, Canada and Australia, CCG, 1983–88 | 18 months | 302 | RDD | NS | 0.7 | No | Shu et al., 1996 |
| USA, multicentre, 1959–66 births | 7 | 17 | Coh | 52.0 | 0.8 | | Klebanoff et al., 1996 |
| **ALL** | | | | | | | |
| The Netherlands, 1973–80 | 14 | 517 | P | 32.2 | 1.0 | | Van Steensel-Moll et al., 1985a |
| Sweden, 1978–81 | 16 | 132 | HD | 29.7 | 1.8 | p < 0.01 | Stjernfeldt et al., 1986a |
| USA and Canada, CCSG, 1983–86 | NS | 742 | RDD | NS | 1.0[d] | No | Buckley et al., 1986 |
| Japan, Hokkaido, 1981–87 | 14 | 63[e] | H | NS | 1.0[d] | No | Nishi & Miyake, 1989 |
| Italy, Turin, 1981–84 | NS[f] | 142 | H | 33.2 | 0.7 | | Magnani et al., 1990 |
| USA, Colorado, Denver, 1976–83 | 14 | 73[g] | RDD | 22.4 | 1.9[h] | Suggestive | John et al., 1991 |
| Sweden, 1982–89 | 7 | NS | P | NS | 0.7 | | Cnattingius et al., 1995a |
| UK, England and Wales, 1977–81 (deaths) | 15 | 400 | B | 41.4[i] | 0.9[j] | No | Sorahan et al., 1995a |
| USA, Canada and Australia, CCG, 1983–88 | 18 months | 203 | RDD | NS | 0.8 | No | Shu et al., 1996 |
| **Acute myeloid leukaemia** | | | | | | | |
| USA and Canada, CCSG, 1980–84 | 17 | 187 | RDD | NS | 1.2 | | Severson et al., 1993 |
| Sweden, 1982–89 | 16 | NS | P | 7.8 | 1.8 | | Cnattingius et al., 1995b |

| Reference | Country, years | Age | No. cases | Controls | % | RR | Significance |
|---|---|---|---|---|---|---|---|
| Sorahan *et al.*, 1995a | UK, England and Wales, 1977–81 (deaths) | 15 | 151 | B | 41.4[j] | 0.9[i] | No |
| Shu *et al.*, 1996 | USA, Canada and Australia, CCG, 1983–88 | 18 months | 88 | RDD | NS | 0.5* | No |
| **ANLL** | | | | | | | |
| Magnani *et al.*, 1990 | Italy, Turin, 1981–84 | NS[f] | 22 | H | 33.2[k] | 2.0 | |
| Van Duijn *et al.*, 1994 | The Netherlands, 1973–79 | 14 | 80 | P | 31 | 0.6 | |
| **All sites combined** | | | | | | | |
| Neutel & Buck, 1971 | Canada, Ontario, 1959–68 and England and Wales, 1965 (1 week) | 10 / 7 | 64 | Coh | 40.0 | 1.3 | No |
| Stjernfeldt *et al.*, 1986a | Sweden, 1978–81 | 16 | 280 | HD | 29.7 | 1.4 | p < 0.05 |
| McKinney & Stiller, 1986 | UK: North West, West Midlands, Yorkshire, 1980–83 | 14 | 555 | H, GP | NS | 1.0[l] | No |
| Buckley *et al.*, 1986 | USA and Canada, CCSG, 1983–86 | NS | 1814 | RDD | NS | 1.0[d] | No |
| Forsberg & Källén, 1990 | Sweden, 1973–84 (birth) | 11 | 69 | B | 29.5 | 1.1 | |
| Golding *et al.*, 1990 | Great Britain, 1980 (1 week) | 10 | 33 | Coh | 38.4[l] | 2.5* | |
| John *et al.*, 1991 | USA, Colorado, Denver, 1976–83 | 14 | 223 | RDD | 22.4 | 1.3[h] | Suggestive |
| Golding *et al.*, 1992a | UK, Bristol, 1971–91 | 14 | 111 | H | NS | 1.2 | |
| Pershagen *et al.*, 1992 | Sweden, 1982–87 | 5 | 327 | Coh | 30.0 | 1.0 | No |
| Sorahan *et al.*, 1995a | UK, England and Wales, 1977–81 (deaths) | 15 | 1641 | B | 41.4[j] | 1.1[m] | No |
| Klebanoff *et al.*, 1996 | USA, multicentre, 1959–66 births | 7 | 51 | Coh | 52.0 | 0.7 | No |

NS, Not stated.
* p < 0.05.
CCG, Children's Cancer Group; CCSG, Childhood Cancer Study Group.

[a] HD, children hospitalized with diabetes; Coh, cohort study; B, from birth records; H, hospital controls; GP, neighbourhood controls selected through general practitioners; P, population-based; RDD, selected by random-digit dialling.

[b] If column is blank, no data enabling a trend to be assessed were presented. 'No', trend assessed but not found.

[c] Data were obtained from two sources. The prevalence of smoking was 26.9% and the odds ratio 0.5 based on interview data. Interviews were completed with 51 (94%) mothers of cases, and 223 (73%) mothers of controls. Based on obstetric records, the prevalence of smoking was 20.4% and the odds ratio was 0.9. Obstetric records were abstracted for 37 (88%) mothers of cases, and 196 (88%) mothers of controls. The authors stated that there was no statistically significant association.

[d] No relative risk was presented.

[e] The study was restricted to ALL of the non-T-cell type.

[f] Mean age at diagnosis of 142 cases of ALL, 22 of ANLL and 19 of non-Hodgkin lymphoma was 6.1 (S.D. 3.6).

[g] Number of cases whose parents interviewed – number on whom information on smoking available may have been somewhat lower.

[h] Comparison was between subjects exposed to mother's cigarette smoking during the first trimester versus subjects who were not exposed to smoking by parents and other household members before and after birth.

[i] Smoking before the index pregnancy.

[j] Reference category comprised never smokers. RR for categories of <10 cigarettes per day (cpd), 10–19 cpd, 20–29 cpd, 30–39 cpd and 40 or more cpd, with these categories treated as a continuous variable.

[k] Smoking at any time up to the child's birth.

[l] Comparison was between mothers smoking five cigarettes or more per day during pregnancy with those not smoking or smoking four cigarettes or less per day.

[m] Odds ratio calculated by unmatched analysis. No trend was apparent in the matched odds ratios presented.

## Table 8.4. Summary of studies of childhood leukaemia and childhood cancer of all types combined and paternal smoking habits

| Area and period of study | Cases Upper age limit | Cases Number | Proportion of interviews at which father present | Period of exposure considered | Prevalence of smoking during this period in control fathers | RR | Reference |
|---|---|---|---|---|---|---|---|
| **Leukaemia and lymphoma** | | | | | | | |
| UK: North West, West Midlands, Yorkshire, 1980–83 | 14 | 234 | 53.2[a] | Any | NS | 1.0[b] | McKinney et al., 1987 |
| **Leukaemia** | | | | | | | |
| China, Shanghai, 1974–86 | 14 | 309 | 8.3 | Any | 55.7 | 0.9 | Shu et al., 1988 |
| Mexico City, NS | 14 | 79 | NS | Any | 44.4 | 1.2 | Fajardo-Gutiérrez et al., 1993a |
| USA, Canada and Australia, CCG, 1983–88 | 18 months | 280 | 68.5 | Pc / P | NS / NS | 1.3 / 1.2 | Shu et al., 1996 |
| **Acute leukaemia** | | | | | | | |
| China, Shanghai, 1985–91 | 14 | 166 | 100 | Any / Pc / Pn | 66 / 16[c] / 18[c] | 1.3 / 2.4** / 1.0[c] | Ji et al., 1997 |
| **ALL** | | | | | | | |
| Italy, Turin, 1981–84 | NS[d] | 142 | 23.7 | B– | 74.3 | 0.9 | Magnani et al., 1990 |
| USA, Colorado, Denver, 1976–83 | 14 | 73[e] | NS[f] | B–1 | 50.0 | 1.4[g] | John et al., 1991 |
| UK, England and Wales, 1977–81 (deaths) | 15 | 371 | NS | Pc | 52.6 | 1.2[h] | Sorahan et al., 1995a |
| USA, Canada and Australia, CCG, 1983–88 | 18 months | 191 | 68.5 | Pc / P | NS / NS | 1.6* / 1.5 | Shu et al., 1996 |
| China, Shanghai, 1985–91 | 14 | 114 | 100 | Pc / Pn | 16[c] / 18[c] | 3.8* / 1.8 | Ji et al., 1997 |
| **Acute myeloid leukaemia** | | | | | | | |
| USA and Canada, CCSG, 1980–84 | 17 | 187 | NS | Any, Pc–1 mth, P, current | NS | 1.0[b] | Severson et al., 1993 |
| UK, England and Wales, 1977–81 (deaths) | 15 | 147 | NS | Pc | 52.6 | 1.0[h] | Sorahan et al., 1995a |
| USA, Canada and Australia, CCG, 1983–88 | 18 months | 79 | 68.5 | Pc / P | NS / NS | 0.8 / 0.8 | Shu et al., 1996 |
| China, Shanghai, 1985–91 | 14 | 52 | 100 | Pc / Pn | 16[c] / 18[c] | 2.3 / 0.5 | Ji et al., 1997 |
| **ANLL** | | | | | | | |
| Italy, Turin, 1981–84 | NS[d] | 22 | 23.7 | B– | 74.3 | 0.9 | Magnani et al., 1990 |
| **All sites** | | | | | | | |
| UK, England and Wales, 1953–55 (deaths) | 9 | 1299 | 0.0 | Any | 80.9 | 1.1[h] | Stewart et al., 1958 |
| USA, Colorado, Denver, 1976–83 | 14 | 223 | NS[f] | B–1 | 50.0 | 1.2[g] | John et al., 1991 |
| UK, England and Wales, 1977–81 (deaths) | 15 | 1641 | NS | Pc | 52.6 | 1.2[h]* | Sorahan et al., 1995a |
| China, Shanghai, 1985–91 | 14 | 642 | 100 | Pc / Any / Pn | 16[c] / 59 / 1.8 | 1.7* / 1.3* / 1.1 | Ji et al., 1997 |

NS, Not stated.
\* $p < 0.05$.

Period of exposure: B–1, during year preceding the birth of index child; Any, ever exposed before interview; B, ever exposed before the birth of index child; P, during pregnancy; Pc, pre-conceptional; Pn, postnatal.

a Figure is for total childhood cancer, from Birch et al. (1985).
b No odds ratio was presented. The authors stated that there was no statistically significant association.
c Associated with >5 pack-years smoking.

d Mean age at diagnosis of 142 cases with ALL, 22 of ANLL and 19 of non-Hodgkin lymphoma was 6.1 (S.D. 3.6).
e Number of cases whose parents interviewed – number on whom information on smoking was available may have been somewhat lower.
f Information was usually obtained from the child's mother.
g Comparison is between subjects exposed to father's tobacco smoking (cigarettes, cigars or pipe) during the 12 months prior to birth and subjects who were not exposed to smoking by parents or other household members before or after birth.
h Reference category comprised never smokers. RR for categories of <10 cigarettes per day (cpd), 10–19 cpd, 20–29 cpd, 30–39 cpd and 40 or more cpd, with these categories treated as a continuous variable.

education (John *et al.*, 1991). No dose–response relationship was apparent. There appears to have been a deficit of low socioeconomic status in this study (NRPB, 1992; see Chapter 5 for further comment). Such a deficit might have produced a spurious association with smoking by either parent. In a hospital-based study in Turin, Italy, the relative risk of ALL associated with paternal smoking before the birth of the child was 0.9 (95% CI 0.6–1.5) (Magnani *et al.*, 1990). Thus, the difference from the other studies may be due to chance and/or the nature of the control group. In these studies, controls of higher socioeconomic status might have been more likely to participate than controls of lower socioeconomic status. This would be expected to reduce the proportion of fathers who smoked, compared with the general population of fathers of children at risk of ALL, leading to overestimation of the relative risk. However, such a phenomenon would also be expected to have affected the association between ALL and maternal smoking, and the studies of AML, for which no consistent association with paternal smoking is apparent.

### Exposure of the child to tobacco smoke after birth

The possible effects on childhood leukaemia of exposure to cigarette smoking after birth have been assessed specifically in only one study. This was carried out in southern California (USA), and was designed specifically to assess the association between leukaemia and residential exposure to electric and magnetic fields. No relationship was found with exposure to cigarettes between the date of the last menstrual period preceding the birth of the case up to a reference date keyed to the date of diagnosis (maximum 10 years) of leukaemia (London *et al.*, 1991).

Moreover, it is unlikely that passive smoking during childhood strongly affects the risk of developing childhood leukaemia. No consistent association between leukaemia and maternal smoking during pregnancy has been found (Table 8.3). As mothers who smoke during pregnancy would be expected to continue to smoke after delivery, this suggests that an association with maternal smoking during the postnatal period is unlikely. In some studies of ALL, a positive association with smoking by the father was apparent, but exposure of the child to tobacco smoke other than from the mother seems unlikely to have a strong effect on the risk of leukaemia, as smoking by the mother contributes much more to passive smoking in the early years of life than does smoking by other adults (Woodward & McMichael, 1991).

### Smoking of marijuana and use of other 'recreational' drugs

A strong association (RR = 11.0, $p$ = 0.003, based on 11 exposed cases and 1 exposed control) has been reported between acute non-lymphoblastic leukaemia and reported use of mind-altering drugs by the mother in the year before or during the index pregnancy (Robison *et al.*, 1989). Marijuana use was reported by a total of ten mothers of cases, and was the only mind-altering drug reported by nine. There was no significant association with paternal use of marijuana in the year before conception of the index child (RR = 1.5, $p$ = 0.32, based on 24 exposed cases and 17 exposed controls). The study was based on cases seen in a total of 101 institutions in the USA and Canada. Of a total of 331 cases identified, 262 were eligible. Parents of some 204 of these cases (77.9%) were interviewed. Out of 260 controls identified as eligible through random-digit dialling, 78% were interviewed. The authors were concerned that the finding could be due to recall bias. In a combined analysis of studies of Ewing's sarcoma and hepatoblastoma in the same group of institutions, together with studies of neuroblastoma in the Greater Delaware Valley (Kramer *et al.*, 1987) and Wilms' tumour in Philadelphia (Bunin *et al.*, 1987), in each of which the methodology used was identical to that used in the study of ANLL, there was no association with reported maternal use of mind-altering drugs during the index pregnancy or in the preceding year. This finding also suggests that it is unlikely that the result is an artefact of the selection of controls by random-digit dialling.

Robison *et al.* (1989) reported that cases whose mothers had used marijuana were younger at the time of diagnosis of ANLL, with a median age of 19 months compared with 93 months for cases whose mothers did not use the drug. Exposed mothers of cases were significantly younger at the delivery of the index child than unexposed mothers of cases (mean 21 years compared with 26 years, $p$ = 0.004). In addition, there is some evidence as to specificity of association for a particular subtype of the disease. Seven of the ten exposed cases were of monocytic or myelomonocytic morphology, compared with 31% of the remaining 194 cases. In contrast, only one of the exposed cases was of the myelocytic morphology, compared with 58% of the other cases. A total review of karyotypes identified 66 cases for whom cytogenetic analysis was considered to be adequate (Buckley *et al.*, 1989b), of which seven had been exposed. A translocation involving either the long or short arm of chromosome 11 was observed only for exposed cases ($n = 4$), while 3 out of 11 cases with trisomy 8 were exposed. The association with marijuana exposure was independent of associations with occupational and household pesticide exposure, paternal occupational exposure to solvents, plastics, petroleum products or lead and maternal occupational exposure to paints and pigments, metal dusts and sawdust. These analyses also suggest that it is unlikely that differential reporting could account for the association with marijuana use.

## Alcohol

The associations between childhood leukaemia and alcohol consumption of the parents has been less studied than those with tobacco smoking by either parent. The majority of available studies related solely to alcohol consumption of the mother and only to consumption during the pregnancy leading to the birth of the index child. No consistent association has been found between maternal alcohol consumption before or during the index pregnancy and leukaemia of all types combined or ALL (Table 8.5).

However, in the three available studies of AML, a positive association with maternal alcohol consumption was found (Table 8.5). First, Severson *et al.* (1993) reported an increased risk of AML diagnosed at or before two years of age for mothers who reported that they had drunk alcoholic beverages during pregnancy (RR = 3.0, 95% CI 1.2–8.4). The increased risk was observed for alcohol consumption in each trimester of pregnancy, and for each type of beverage. There was a suggestion of a dose–response relationship, but the test for trend was not significant. The association appeared to be especially pronounced when the disease had a monocytic component (M4/M5); the relative risk was 9.0 (95% CI 1.3–394.5, based on 12 discordant pairs). It seems unlikely that recall bias or selection bias arising from the random-digit dialling method of selecting controls can explain the finding, as raised risks are not apparent for other subtypes of AML. Second, in a comparison of 80 cases with ANLL with 240 age–sex-matched population controls in the Netherlands, the relative risk associated with reported maternal use of alcohol during pregnancy was 2.6 (95% CI 1.4–4.6; Van Duijn *et al.*, 1994). This was apparent in the 0–4- and 5–9-year subgroups, but not in the subgroup aged 10–14 years at diagnosis. A similar relative risk was found in comparison with 517 cases of ALL from the same study base. There was no statistically significant elevation in risk for use of

alcohol in the year preceding pregnancy by either parent. Third, in a study of 88 cases of AML diagnosed in children aged up to 18 months and matched controls selected by random-digit dialling in the USA, Canada and Australia, the relative risk associated with maternal alcohol consumption during the index pregnancy was 2.6 (95% CI 1.4–5.0; Shu *et al.*, 1996). There was a dose–response relation-ship ($p < 0.01$); the relative risk, adjusted for sex, maternal education and maternal smoking during pregnancy, associated with 1–20 drinks during pregnancy compared with none was 2.4 (95% CI 1.1–5.0), and that associated with more than 20 drinks was 3.1 (95% CI 1.2–8.1). These risks were not attenuated by further adjustment for maternal marijuana use. In contrast to the study of Severson *et al.* (1993), the relative risk was higher for the subgroup with the M2/M2 morphology (RR = 7.6, 95% CI 2.0–28.6) than for the subgroup with the M4/M5 morphology (RR = 1.7, 95% CI 0.7–4.2).

No association between paternal alcohol consumption and childhood leukaemia has been found (Shu *et al.*, 1988; Severson *et al.*, 1993; Shu *et al.*, 1996).

## Lymphoma

### Breast-feeding

In the study of Davis *et al.* (1988), relating to childhood cancer of all types (see above), the relative risk of lymphoma associated with artificial feeding only was 5.6 (95% CI 1.4–22.4), and that associated with breast-feeding for a period of six months or less was 8.2 (95% CI 2.1–31.9). The reference category comprised subjects who were breast-fed for more than six months. It seems likely that there was a deficit of controls of low socioeconomic status in this study (NRPB, 1992). Such a deficit might have produced a spurious association with patterns of infant feeding. It may be noted that the particularly strong association for lymphomas was weakened after adjustment for the number of years of education completed by the mother.

No association with non-Hodgkin lymphoma (19 cases) in children was found in a hospital-based study in Turin (relative risk associated with breast-feeding 1.0, 95% CI 0.4–2.5; Magnani *et al.*, 1990). In a study of 19 cases with lymphoma and 90 hospital controls in northern India, the duration of breast-feeding was significantly shorter for cases than controls (Mathur *et al.*, 1993). In a comparison of 82 cases of lymphoma and age–sex-matched community controls in Shanghai, China, the relative risk of lymphoma

## Table 8.5. Summary of studies of childhood leukaemia and maternal alcohol consumption

| Area and period of study | Cases | | Period of exposure considered (B=birth; P=pregnancy; Pc=pre-conceptional) | Prevalence of alcohol consumption during this period in control mothers | RR | Reference |
|---|---|---|---|---|---|---|
| | Upper age limit | Number | | | | |
| **Leukaemia and lymphoma** | | | | | | |
| UK: Yorkshire, West Midlands, North West, 1980–83 | 14 | 234 | P | NS | 1.0[e] | McKinney et al., 1987 |
| UK: West Berkshire and North Hampshire, 1972–89 | 4 | 54 | P | 5.1–56.5[b] | 1.1–1.8[b] | Roman et al., 1993 |
| **Leukaemia** | | | | | | |
| China, Shanghai, 1974–86 | 14 | 309 | Any | 0.0 | U[c] | Shu et al., 1988 |
| Mexico City, NS | 14 | 81 | P | 4.5 | 0.5 | Fajardo-Gutiérrez et al., 1993a |
| USA, Canada and Australia, CCG, 1983–88 | 18 months | 302 | P–1 month / P | NS / 31.0 | 1.3 / 1.6* | Shu et al. 1996 |
| **ALL** | | | | | | |
| The Netherlands, 1973–80 | 14 | 517 | P–1 year / P | 58.5 / 36.5 | 1.2 / 1.0 | Van Steensel-Moll et al., 1985a |
| Japan, Hokkaido, 1981–87 | 14 | 63[d] | P | NS | 1.0[e] | Nishi & Miyake, 1989 |
| USA, Canada and Australia, CCG, 1983–88 | 18 months | 203 | P–1 month / P | NS / 31.0 | 1.1 / 1.4* | Shu et al., 1996 |
| **Acute myeloid leukaemia** | | | | | | |
| USA and Canada, CCSG, 1980–84 | 17 | 187 | P | NS | 1.4 | Severson et al., 1993 |
| USA, Canada and Australia, CCG, 1983–88 | 18 months | 88 | P–1 month / P | NS / 31.0 | 1.8 / 2.6* | Shu et al. 1996 |
| **ANLL** | | | | | | |
| The Netherlands, 1973–79 | 14 | 80 | P / P–1 year | 35 / NS | 2.6* / 1.2 | Van Duijn et al., 1994 |
| **All sites** | | | | | | |
| UK: England and Wales, 1977–81 (deaths) | 15 | 1641 | Pc | 64.4 | 0.8* | Sorahan et al. 1995 |
| USA, Canada and Australia, CCG, 1983–88 | 18 months | 88 | P–1 month / P | NS / 31.0 | 1.8 / 2.6* | Shu et al. 1996 |

NS, Not stated.
* $p < 0.05$.
CCG, Children's Cancer Group; CCSG, Childhood Cancer Study Group.

[a] No odds ratio presented. The authors stated that there was "no major positive association" with this exposure.

[b] Data were obtained from two sources. The prevalence of alcohol consumption during pregnancy was 56.5% and the odds ratio 1.1 based on interview data. Interviews were completed with 51 (94%) mothers of cases, and 223 (73%) mothers of controls. Based on obstetric records, the prevalence of alcohol consumption was 5.1% and the odds ratio 1.8. Obstetric records were abstracted for 37 (88%) mothers of cases, and 196 (88%) mothers of controls.
[c] Odds ratio undefined; no mother of a case or a control drank.
[d] The study was restricted to ALL of the non-T-cell type.
[e] No odds ratio was presented. The authors stated that there was no statistically significant association.

associated with having been breast-fed in infancy was 0.7 (95% CI 0.3–1.7; Shu *et al.*, 1995b). The inverse association was observed primarily for Hodgkin's disease (RR = 0.2, 95% CI 0.0–4.0, based on 14 cases).

The possible inverse association between lymphoma and breast-feeding is interesting in view of reports of positive associations between non-Hodgkin lymphoma in adults and milk consumption (Franceschi *et al.*, 1989; Ursin *et al.*, 1990), and with an index of vitamin A intake calculated largely on the basis of milk and vegetable consumption (Middleton *et al.*, 1986). It has been suggested that milk may be a source of the bovine leukaemia virus (Ursin *et al.*, 1990) but in a study of non-Hodgkin lymphoma and ALL in children, the presence of the virus was detected in none of the DNA samples obtained from cases or controls (Bender *et al.*, 1988).

## Tobacco smoking by the mother

No consistent association between maternal smoking during pregnancy and lymphoma or non-Hodgkin lymphoma has been found (Table 8.6). In the one available report in which data on Hodgkin's disease in children were presented, no association was found (Stjernfeldt *et al.*, 1986a).

## Tobacco smoking by the father

In a study in Italy, the relative risk of non-Hodgkin lymphoma associated with paternal smoking before the child's birth, based on 19 cases and 307 controls, was 6.7 (95% CI 1.0–43.4) after adjustment for socioeconomic status (Magnani *et al.*, 1990). The authors observed that exclusion of 40 control children affected by respiratory diseases did not substantially alter the odds ratios observed. Nevertheless, the possibility that selection bias affected the result cannot be excluded, as hospital controls were used. No dose–response relationship was evident. Prevalent cases were included. In an overall analysis which also included cases of leukaemia, the odds ratio associated with paternal smoking was 0.5 (95% CI 0.3–1.3) for incident cases and 1.0 (95% CI 0.4–2.2) for prevalent cases.

No consistent association has been found for lymphoma of all types combined (Table 8.7).

# Brain tumours

## Maternal diet and vitamin supplement use during pregnancy

Maternal diet during pregnancy has been of particular interest in the context of the hypothesis that exposure to substances containing *N*-nitroso compounds or precursors to these compounds are of importance in the etiology of brain tumours in children. Cured meat and fish products contain preformed nitrosamines, nitrates and nitrites (Kuijten & Bunin, 1993). The levels of these substances differ considerably between samples of the same type of food, but the highest levels are consistently found in bacon (Gray, 1981). The available studies of brain tumours and maternal consumption of cured meats in pregnancy are summarized in Table 8.8.

The first study to assess the association between childhood brain tumours and maternal diet during pregnancy was that of Preston-Martin *et al.* (1982). There was a significant positive association between brain tumours and frequency of consumption of ham by the mother, and a non-significant trend of increase in risk with increasing consumption of hot dogs. No clear trend was apparent for fried bacon, sausage, salami and "other lunch meats". The authors derived a score for consumption of all types of cured meat, although it is not stated whether the grouping had been defined *a priori*; a significant positive dose–response relationship was found. There was no association between brain tumours and maternal consumption during pregnancy of vegetables which usually contain high levels of nitrate, that is spinach, collards or turnip greens, aubergines, beets and radishes. Similar results were obtained when the data were analysed separately by type of control (friend or neighbour), by tumour type or by age of the patient at diagnosis.

In a study of 100 cases and 180 controls selected by random-digit dialling in Ohio, described only in an abstract, there was a positive association between brain tumours and high intakes of nitrite and dimethylnitrosamine and an inverse association with reported intake of ascorbic acid (Wilkins *et al.*, 1993).

A multicentre case–control study of brain tumours in children in which a common protocol was used is currently being analysed. In the Australian component of the study, carried out in New South Wales, 82 cases and 164 controls were investigated (McCredie *et al.*, 1994a). There was a positive association between brain tumours and maternal consumption of cured meats during pregnancy; the relative risk for the highest quartile of intake was 2.5 (95% CI 1.1–5.7; *p* value for trend 0.01). There was an inverse relation with consumption of vegetables (relative risk for the highest quartile of intake 0.4, 95% CI 0.1–1.0, *p* value for trend 0.06), but no association with consumption of fruit. These

**Table 8.6. Summary of studies of childhood lymphoma and maternal smoking during pregnancy**

| Area and period of study | Cases | | Control type[a] | Prevalence of smoking during pregnancy in control mothers (%) | RR associated with any smoking during pregnancy | Trend[b] | Reference |
|---|---|---|---|---|---|---|---|
| | Upper age limit | Number | | | | | |
| **Lymphomas** | | | | | | | |
| UK, North West, West Midlands, Yorkshire, 1980–83 | 14 | 74 | H, GP | NS | 1.0[c] | No | McKinney & Stiller, 1986 |
| USA, Colorado, Denver 1976–83 | 14 | 26[d] | RDD | 22.4 | 2.3[e] | No | John et al., 1991 |
| Sweden, 1982–87 | 5 | 30[f] | Coh | 30.0 | 1.7–2.0[g] | No | Pershagen et al., 1992 |
| UK, England and Wales, 1977–81 (deaths) | 15 | 139 | B | 41.4[h] | 1.0[c] | No | Sorahan et al., 1995a |
| **Non-Hodgkin lymphoma** | | | | | | | |
| Sweden, 1978–81 | 16 | 16 | HD | 29.7 | 1.8 | No | Stjernfeldt et al., 1986a |
| USA and Canada, CCSG, 1983–86 | NS | 169 | RDD | NS | 1.0[c] | No | Buckley et al., 1986 |
| Italy, Turin, 1981–84 | NS[j] | 19 | H | 33.2 | 1.7 | Yes | Magnani et al., 1990 |
| Sweden, 1982–89 | 7 | NS[k] | B | NS | 1.6 | | Adami et al., 1996 |
| **Hodgkin's disease** | | | | | | | |
| Sweden, 1978–81 | 16 | 15 | HD | 29.7 | 0.6 | No | Stjernfeldt et al., 1986a |

NS, Not stated.
CCSG, Childhood Cancer Study Group.

a HD, children hospitalized with diabetes; Coh, cohort study; B, from birth records; H, hospital controls; GP, neighbourhood controls selected through general practitioners; RDD, selected by random-digit dialling.

b If column is blank, no data enabling a trend to be assessed were presented. 'No', trend assessed but not found.

c No relative risk was presented. The authors stated that there was no statistically significant association.

d Number of cases whose parents interviewed – number on whom information on smoking was available may have been somewhat lower.

e Comparison was between subjects exposed to mother's cigarette smoking during the first trimester versus subjects who were not exposed to smoking by parents and other household members before and after birth.

f Cohort study; all other studies are of a case–control design.

g 16 cases had reticulosis; the associated RR was 1.7 (95% CI 0.6–5.0); 14 cases had "other haematopoietic and lymphatic" tumours; the associated RR was 2.0 (95% CI 0.7–5.5).

h Smoking before the index pregnancy.

i Reference category comprised never smokers. RR for categories of <10 cigarettes per day (cpd), 10–19 cpd, 20–29 cpd, 30–39 cpd and 40 or more cpd, with these categories treated as a continuous variable.

j Mean age at diagnosis of 142 cases of ALL, 22 of ANLL and 19 of non-Hodgkin lymphoma was 6.1 (S.D. 3.6).

k A total of 168 cases was ascertained during the period 1973–89. Smoking data were available only for those born from 1982 onwards.

# Table 8.7. Summary of studies of childhood lymphoma and paternal smoking habits

| Area and period of study | Cases | | Proportion of interviews at which father present | Period of exposure considered | Prevalence of smoking during this period in control fathers | RR | Reference |
|---|---|---|---|---|---|---|---|
| | Upper age limit | Number | | | | | |
| **Lymphomas** | | | | | | | |
| USA, Colorado, Denver, 1976–83 | 14 | 26[a] | NS[b] | B–1 | 50.0 | 1.6[c] | John *et al.*, 1991 |
| UK, England and Wales, 1977–81 (deaths) | 15 | 139 | NS | Pc | 52.6 | 1.1[d] | Sorahan *et al.*, 1995a |
| China, Shanghai, 1981–91 | 14 | 87 | 100 | Pc | 16[e] | 4.5** | Ji *et al.*, 1997 |
| | | | | Any | 59 | 4.0* | |
| | | | | Pn | 18[e] | 5.0** | |
| **Non-Hodgkin lymphoma** | | | | | | | |
| Italy, Turin, 1981–84 | NS[f] | 19 | 23.7 | B– | 74.3 | 6.7* | Magnani *et al.*, 1990 |

NS, Not stated.
* $p < 0.05$.

Period of exposure: B–1, during year preceding birth of index child; Any, ever exposed before interview; Pc, pre-conceptional; B–, ever exposed before birth of index child; Pn, postnatal.

[a] Number of cases whose parents interviewed – number on whom information on smoking available may have been somewhat lower.

[b] Information was usually obtained from the child's mother.

[c] Comparison is between subjects exposed to father's tobacco smoking (cigarettes, cigars or pipe) during the 12 months preceding birth and subjects who were not exposed to smoking by parents or other household members before or after birth.

[d] Reference category comprised never smokers. RR for categories of <10 cigarettes per day (cpd), 10–19 cpd, 20–29 cpd, 30–39 cpd and 40 or more cpd, with these categories treated as a continuous variable.

[e] Associated >5 pack-years of smoking.

[f] Mean age at diagnosis of 142 cases with ALL, 22 of ANLL and 19 of non-Hodgkin lymphoma was 6.1 (S.D. 3.6).

relative risks were adjusted for age, sex, maternal education and the mother's body mass index at the start of the pregnancy. A limitation of the study is that the participation rate of potential controls was relatively low (60%). Women who were interviewed were found to be of slightly higher social class, as ranked by their occupation, than those who refused to participate. In the French component of the study, carried out in the Paris region (Cordier *et al.*, 1994), 75 cases and 113 controls were interviewed. There was no association with maternal consumption of cured meat, most types of vegetables or fruit during pregnancy. No statistically significant association was found with intake of nitrate, nitrite, vitamin C or vitamin E. In the US West Coast component of this study, carried out in Los Angeles County, the San Francisco–Oakland metropolitan area and western Washington state, 540 cases and 801 controls were investigated (Preston-Martin *et al.*, 1996d). The risk of brain tumours increased with reported maternal intake of cured meat during pregnancy, assessed either as an average daily intake (RR for highest vs. lowest quartile 1.7, *p* value for trend 0.002; Table 8.8) or frequency of consumption (RR for more than daily consumption compared with non-consumption 2.1, value for trend 0.003). These relative risks were similar for astrocytoma, primitive neuroectodermal tumours of the brain, and other histological types. With regard to specific types of cured meat, there were positive associations with reported consumption of bacon, hot dogs and sausage, but not ham, lunch meat or "other cured meats" (Table 8.8). While an increase in risk with increasing estimated intake of nitrite from cured meats was observed, no association was found with nitrite from all foods, or with nitrate (which is reduced to nitrite in the mouth) from vegetables. If the *N*-nitroso hypothesis were true, it would be expected that increasing maternal consumption of vitamin C and vitamin E during pregnancy would be associated with a decreased risk of brain tumours in the offspring. As a high proportion of mothers used multivitamin supplements, intakes of micronutrients were highly correlated with each other and with multivitamin intake. There was an inverse association between brain tumours and intake of each of the four micronutrients evaluated, that is vitamins C, E and A, and folate. The relative risk of brain tumours in the offspring of women whose estimated intake of nitrite from cured meats was at least 3 mg per day and who did not take a vitamin supplement compared with vitamin users with a nitrite intake of less than 3 mg per day was 2.2 (95% CI

1.4–3.6). The corresponding relative risk for vitamin users with a nitrite intake of at least 3 mg per day was 1.3 (95% CI 1.0–1.7). However, there was no statistically significant interaction between vitamin supplement use and estimated intake of nitrite from cured meats or reported frequency of consumption of cured meats. A possible limitation of the study is selection bias arising from selection of the controls by random-digit dialling, which may have resulted in the controls being of higher socioeconomic status than the source population of children at risk of developing brain tumours (Greenberg, 1990). Among participating mothers, those of lower socioeconomic status tended to eat somewhat more cured meats than other mothers. Another possible limitation is that only intake of 47 food items relevant to the *N*-nitroso hypothesis was assessed. If an assessment of total dietary intake had been made, it would have been possible to consider the extent to which the observed results might have been accounted for by variation in tendencies to over- or under-estimate total dietary intakes (Willett, 1990).

In a study designed primarily to assess the relationship between childhood cancer and residential exposure to electromagnetic fields in Denver, Colorado, there was a positive association between brain tumours (45 cases) and maternal consumption of hot dogs during pregnancy (RR = 2.3, 95% CI 1.0–5.4; Sarasua & Savitz, 1994). However, there was no association with maternal consumption of ham, bacon and sausage, hamburgers, or charcoal broiled foods, and an inverse association with consumption of lunch meats (relative risk associated with consumption at least once a week compared with less frequently 0.4, 95% CI 0.2–0.8). As already discussed, there appears to have been selection bias in this study which produced a deficit of controls of low socioeconomic status.

In a study in upstate New York so far described only in abstract form, data on maternal diet during pregnancy were obtained on 338 cases of brain tumours and 676 controls matched on year of birth, gender and ethnic group, selected from birth certificate files (Schymura *et al.*, 1996). The relative risk of brain tumours associated with hot dog consumption once per week during pregnancy compared with less often was 1.3 (95% CI 1.0–1.8), and that associated with consumption two or three times per week was 2.0 (95% CI 1.1–3.7). The relative risk associated with consumption of "other" cured meats once per week was 6.0 (95% CI 1.9–19.3). There was no statistically significant association with reported consumption of tea and coffee.

## Table 8.8. Association between tumours of the central nervous system in children and maternal consumption of cured meats during pregnancy

| Area and period of study | Cases Upper age limit | Cases N | Controls N | Controls Type[a] | Type of cured meat | Categorization[b] | Cured meats RR (95% CI) for highest category | p value for trend | Reference |
|---|---|---|---|---|---|---|---|---|---|
| **Brain tumours** | | | | | | | | | |
| USA, Los Angeles County 1972–77 | 24 | 209 | 209 | F, N | Ham<br>Hot dogs<br>Fried bacon<br>Sausage<br>Salami<br>Other lunch meats<br>All | 2+/week vs 1+/week vs <1/month<br><br><br><br><br><br>Score: high/medium/low | 1.9<br>1.7<br>1.1<br>1.4<br>1.3<br>1.1<br>2.3 | 0.008<br>0.08<br>0.39<br>0.07<br>0.09<br>0.38<br>0.008 | Preston-Martin et al., 1982 |
| France, Ile de France, 1985–87 | 15 | 75 | 113 | P | Ham<br>Sausage<br>Salami<br>Paté | 1+/week vs <1/week | 1.0 (0.4–2.7)<br>0.6 (0.2–1.8)<br>0.6 (0.3–1.4)<br>0.6 (0.3–1.4) | | Cordier et al., 1994 |
| Australia, New South Wales, 1985–89 | 14 | 82 | 164 | P | All | Q | 2.5 (1.1–5.7) | 0.01 | McCredie et al., 1994a |
| USA, Denver, CO, 1976–83 | 14 | 45 | 206 | RDD | Ham, bacon and sausage<br>Hamburgers<br>Lunch meats<br>Hot dogs<br>Charcoal-broiled foods | 1+/week vs <1/week<br><br><br>Any vs none | 1.0 (0.5–2.1)<br>0.7 (0.3–1.6)<br>0.4 (0.2–0.8)<br>2.3 (1.0–5.4)<br>0.6 (0.3–1.2) | | Sarasua & Savitz, 1994 |
| USA, West Coast[c], 1984–91 | 19 | 540 | 801 | RDD | Ham<br>Bacon<br>Hot dogs<br>Sausage<br>Lunch meat<br>Other<br>Any<br>All | 1+/week vs never<br><br><br><br><br><br>1+/day vs 4–7x/week vs 2–3x/week vs <1/week vs never<br>Q | 1.0 (0.7–1.3)<br>1.6 (1.2–2.1)<br>1.4 (1.1–2.0)<br>1.6 (1.1–2.3)<br>1.1 (0.9–1.4)<br>1.9 (1.0–3.8)<br>2.1 (1.3–3.2)<br>1.7 (1.2–2.3) | 0.97<br>0.001<br>0.007<br>0.006<br>0.39<br>0.40<br>0.003<br>0.002 | Preston-Martin et al., 1996d |
| USA, upstate New York | NS | 338 | 676 | B | Hot dogs<br>Other cured meats | 1+/week vs <1/week | 1.3 (1.0–1.8)<br>6.0 (1.9–19.3) | | Schymura et al., 1996 |
| **Astrocytoma** | | | | | | | | | |
| USA, PA, NJ & Delaware Valley | 14 | 163 | 163 | RDD | All | 9+/week vs none | 2.0 | 0.04 | Kuijten et al., 1990 |
| USA and Canada, CCG, 1986–89 | 5 | 155 | 155 | RDD | Hot dogs<br>All | 1+/week vs <1/week<br>Q | 1.9 (1.0–3.7)<br>1.7 (0.8–3.4) | 0.10 | Bunin et al., 1994a |
| **Primitive neuroectodermal brain tumours** | | | | | | | | | |
| USA and Canada, CCG, 1986–89 | 5 | 166 | 166 | RDD | Bacon<br>Sausage<br>Hot dogs<br>Ham<br>Lunch meats<br>All | 1+/week vs <1/week<br><br><br><br><br>Q | 1.7 (1.0–2.9)<br>1.4 (0.8–2.6)<br>1.0 (0.6–1.7)<br>0.8 (0.4–1.4)<br>0.9 (0.6–1.5)<br>1.1 (0.6–2.0) | 0.77 | Bunin et al., 1993 |

CCG, Children's Cancer Group.
[a] RDD, selected by random-digit dialling; F, friends; N, neighbourhood; P, population-based; B, selected from birth certificate files.
[b] Q, quartiles.
[c] Los Angeles County, San Francisco–Oakland metropolitan area, and western Washington state.

Kuijten *et al.* (1990) reported a significant positive trend of increase in the risk of astrocytoma with increasing consumption of cured meats during pregnancy; the relative risk associated with consumption nine or more times per week was 2.0 (*p* = 0.04). The effect was only apparent when the mother had had more than a high school education. The authors considered that it was possible that a food item more popular among less educated women might have been omitted from the food frequency questionnaire.

In an analysis of a subset of these data relating to cases diagnosed before the age of 10 years in the Greater Delaware Valley, a positive association was found with maternal consumption of nitrite-processed luncheon meats (e.g., bologna, ham or salami) during the index pregnancy (Nass, 1989). The relative risk associated with consumption at least once a week was in the range of 2.5–2.8, depending on the covariates included in the regression model. However, there was no association with consumption of "processed breakfast meats", e.g. bacon, ham or sausage, or with consumption of citrus fruit.

Bunin *et al.* (1994a) found a weak positive association between astrocytoma in children aged five years or under (*n* = 155 case–control pairs) and reported consumption of cured meats during pregnancy (relative risk for highest quartile of intake compared with lowest 1.7, 95% CI 0.8–3.4; *p* value for trend 0.10). No trend was apparent with reported consumption of nitrate, nitrite, dimethylnitrosamine, vitamin C or vitamin E. In contrast to the finding of Kuijten *et al.* (1990), positive associations with intake of bacon and cured meats were apparent only among subjects whose mothers had no more than a high school education, and from families with a low income. There was a significant inverse association with consumption of iron supplements (RR = 0.5, 95% CI 0.3–0.8); this effect was apparent only in families with high income. No interactions between food groups or nutrients and income were found in a parallel study of primitive neuroectodermal brain tumours (Bunin *et al.*, 1993; see below). There was no association with maternal consumption of caffeinated beverages during pregnancy.

The study was restricted to children aged five years or under at the time of diagnosis, as the authors considered that the effects of gestational exposures would be expected to be manifest early in life. A total of 155 (participation rate 65%) mothers of cases diagnosed between 1986 and 1989 in several centres in North America were interviewed. Control children were selected by random-digit dialling; sufficient information to determine eligibility was obtained from 89% of the residences contacted, and 73% of the controls were the first eligible ones identified. Matching was made not only according to area code and the next five digits of the telephone number, but also date of birth and ethnic group. Mothers were interviewed an average of 5.0 years after the birth of the index child. The data on dietary intake were obtained by a food frequency questionnaire with 53 food items chosen primarily to assess dietary components relevant to the *N*-nitroso hypothesis.

In a parallel study of primitive neuroectodermal brain tumours (166 case–control pairs), there was a significant positive association with maternal consumption of bacon during pregnancy, a weak association with sausage consumption, and no association with consumption of hot dogs, ham or lunch meat (Bunin *et al.*, 1993). Very few mothers ate smoked fish, pickled fish or salted fish. Three food groups were analysed according to quartile of intake. There was no association with consumption of cured meats, while there were significant inverse associations with consumption of fruits and fruit juice and of vegetables. As in the study of astrocytoma, five nutrients relevant to the nitrosamine hypothesis were considered: nitrate, nitrite, dimethylnitrosamine, vitamin C and vitamin E. There were statistically significant inverse associations with intake of nitrate and of vitamin C. There was a non-significant trend of increase in risk with increasing consumption of dimethylnitrosamine. No association with estimated intake of nitrite or of vitamin E was found. In addition to these nutrients, intakes of vitamin A, β-carotene and retinol were considered because of the evidence that vitamin A or β-carotene may be protective against some cancers in adults, and folate was considered because it has been found to prevent the recurrence, and almost certainly the occurrence, of neural tube defects. This observation may be relevant in view of the fact that the neural tube is lined with neuroepithelial cells, which are the precursor cells of primitive neuroectodermal tumours. There were significant inverse associations with intake of vitamin A, β-carotene and folate.

Nearly all (92%) mothers of cases and controls reported that they had taken multivitamins during their pregnancy, and no overall association with primitive neuroectodermal tumours was found. However, the odds ratio associated with multivitamin use in the first six weeks after the last menstrual period was 0.56 (95% CI 0.32–0.96). There were significant inverse associations with reported use of iron supplements, calcium supplements and vitamin C supplements. The apparent protective effects of dietary folate and vitamin C, and calcium supplements, were stronger in those who did not take multivitamins early in pregnancy than in those who did.

There was significant intercorrelation between most of the dietary variables. In multivariate analysis, including seven dietary nutrients and four supplements, the effect of folate became stronger, the effect of nitrate was reduced, and the effects of vitamin A and vitamin C did not persist. The effect of use of multivitamin supplements in early pregnancy was unchanged, but the associations with supplemental iron, calcium and vitamin C were somewhat weaker and no longer statistically significant. The regression model also included dietary vitamin E, nitrite and nitrosamine, even though no trend had been found in the univariate analysis, because of their central importance to the nitrosamine hypothesis. While there was no marked change in the odds ratio observed for nitrite and nitrosamine, a significant positive association became apparent with vitamin E. This raises a concern about the goodness of fit of the model, which was not reported. In analyses in which a series of potentially confounding variables was considered, the effects of dietary folate, use of multivitamin supplements in early pregnancies and dietary vitamin E persisted.

In the parallel study of astrocytoma (Bunin *et al.*, 1994a; see above), there was no association with folate and no protective effect of multivitamin use in the first weeks of pregnancy.

The authors acknowledged that the repeatability of dietary questionnaire was not investigated and that the food frequency questionnaire was not designed to assess folate intake; only about 55% of the intake of this nutrient was assessed. The selection of controls by random-digit dialling has been reported to lead to the control group tending to be of higher socioeconomic status relative to the source population (Greenberg, 1990). If dietary intake of folate and use of multivitamins during pregnancy were related to social class, as has been reported (Elwood *et al.*, 1992), the relationship with intake of certain nutrients and supplements might be an artefact of the method of control selection. On the other hand, Bunin *et al.* (1993) reported that there were no differences between case and control mothers in

health-related behaviours such as smoking, breast-feeding and seeing a doctor early in pregnancy, and cases and controls were similar in demographic characteristics including household income, educational level, type of housing, and number of residences since the index pregnancy. Recall bias is unlikely to explain the association between primitive neuroectodermal tumours and dietary folate intake and multivitamin use, as this association was not apparent for astrocytoma. If it were true that a factor related to neural tube closure also affected the risk of primitive neuroectodermal tumours, it would be expected that children with spina bifida might have an increased risk of developing a primitive neuroectodermal tumour later in life. While an association between brain tumours and spina bifida has been reported (Narod *et al.*, 1997), the possibility that this was a spurious association cannot be excluded (see Chapter 10 for further comment), and the association was not specific to medulloblastoma.

Trends in the incidence of medulloblastoma in parts of the UK have been assessed for the period 1976–91 (Foreman & Pearson, 1993; Thorne *et al.*, 1994). In the southwestern and northern regions combined, the incidence declined from 5.4 cases per million childhood-years in the period 1976–84 to 2.7 in the period 1985–91. In one county in which the trend was more marked (incidence rates 9.4 and 1.6 per million respectively), the pathological findings of all posterior fossa tumours were reviewed for changes in diagnostic criteria; none was found. The authors considered that this change may be compatible with increased use of multivitamin supplementation to prevent neural tube defects, although this appears to have been used primarily to prevent recurrence rather than first occurrence (Elwood *et al.*, 1992).

The associations between childhood brain tumours and maternal consumption of vitamin supplements during pregnancy are summarized in Table 8.9. In addition to the inverse association with primitive neuroectodermal brain tumours already discussed, a non-significant inverse association between astrocytoma and multivitamin supplements was found in a companion investigation (Bunin *et al.*, 1994a). Inverse associations between brain tumours of all types combined and vitamin supplements were observed in studies in the west coast states of the USA (Preston-Martin *et al.*, 1982, 1996d) and Denver (Sarasua & Savitz, 1994). No association with brain tumours was apparent in data from Finland (Salonen &

Table 8.9. Association between tumours of the central nervous system in children and maternal consumption of vitamin supplements during pregnancy

| Area and period of study | Cases[a] | | Controls | | Source of information on supplement use[c] | Type of supplement | Prevalence of use in mothers of controls (%) | RR (95% CI) | Reference |
|---|---|---|---|---|---|---|---|---|---|
| | Upper age limit | N | Type[b] | N | | | | | |
| **Brain tumours** | | | | | | | | | |
| Finland, 1959–68 | 14 | 245 | P | 245 | AN | Vitamins | 24.5[d] | 0.9 (0.5–1.6)[e] | Salonen & Saxén, 1975 |
| USA, Los Angeles County, 1972–77 | 24 | 209 | E, N | 209 | I | Vitamins | 11.0 | 0.6 (p = 0.12) | Preston-Martin et al., 1982 |
| USA, Denver, CO, 1976–83 | 14 | 45 | RDD | 205 | I | Vitamins | 90.2 | 0.7 (0.3–1.8) | Sarasua & Savitz, 1994 |
| USA, West Coast, 1984–91 | 19 | 540 | RDD | 801 | I | Multivitamin | 85.0 | 0.5 (0.4–0.7)[f] | Preston-Martin et al., 1996d |
| **Astrocytoma** | | | | | | | | | |
| USA and Canada, CCSG, 1986–89 | 5 | 155 | RDD | 155 | I | Multivitamin | NS | 0.6 (0.2–1.5) | Bunin et al., 1994a |
| **Primitive neuroectodermal brain tumours** | | | | | | | | | |
| USA and Canada, CCSG, 1986–89 | 5 | 166 | RDD | 166 | I | Multivitamin[g] Vitamin C | NS NS | 0.6 (0.3–1.0) 0.4 (0.1–0.9) | Bunin et al., 1993 |

CCSG, Childhood Cancer Study Group.

a These were newly incident in all studies.
b P, population-based; RDD, selected by random-digit dialling.
c AN, antenatal clinic records; I, maternal interview.
d In total series of 972 controls, matched with cases with any type of childhood cancer.
e 98% CI.
f Unadjusted. In analysis adjusted for gender, year of birth, reference age and geographical area, the RR associated with daily use of prenatal vitamins throughout pregnancy was 0.54 (95% CI 0.39–0.75).
g In first six weeks after the last menstrual period.

Saxén, 1975). In that study, cases and controls were matched on Maternity Welfare District, and this may have led to matching on prescribing habit, which might have biased any association with vitamin supplement use towards the null.

In the US West Coast study (described above), there was a trend of decreasing risk of brain tumours with increasing duration of daily use during pregnancy (Preston-Martin *et al.*, 1996d). Compared with women who either never used multivitamin supplements or who used them only occasionally or sporadically, the relative risk associated with less than two trimesters of daily use was 0.7 (95% CI 0.4–1.1), with two trimesters of use 0.6 (95% CI 0.4–0.8) and with three trimesters of use 0.5 (95% CI 0.4–0.8; *p* value for trend 0.004). This persisted after adjustment for potential confounding factors including maternal age, ethnicity, socio-economic status and ingestion of nitrite from cured meat. The pattern was similar between astrocytoma, primitive neuroectodermal brain tumours and other histological types. As in the study of Bunin *et al.* (1993), the possibility cannot be excluded that the result was an artefact of control selection by random-digit dialling. In contrast to the study of Bunin *et al.* (1993), cases had lower socioeconomic status than controls, but the association with vitamin supplement use persisted after adjustment for socioeconomic status.

Olney *et al.* (1996) suggested that the apparent increase in the incidence of brain tumours at all ages in the USA coincided with the introduction of aspartame into foodstuffs in the early 1980s. Data on maternal consumption of aspartame during the index pregnancy and lactation were available for a subset of subjects (49 cases, 90 controls) in the Los Angeles and San Francisco componenets of the US West Coast study already described (Gurney *et al.*, 1997). No association was apparent either with consumption of aspartame from all sources or with consumption of diet drinks only.

### Breast-feeding

In the study of Davis *et al.* (1988) described above, the relative risk of brain tumours associated with artificial feeding only, compared with breast-feeding for a period of more than six months was 1.8 (95% CI 0.8–4.3), and that associated with breast-feeding for period of six months or less was 1.7 (95% CI 0.6–4.4). No association between breast-feeding and central nervous system tumours was found in a study in northern England (Birch *et al.*, 1990b).

### Postnatal diet of the index child and use of vitamin supplements

Investigations of diet in childhood and brain tumours are summarized in Table 8.10. Preston-Martin *et al.* (1982) found that the relative risk associated with moderate consumption of cured meats compared with low consumption was 1.3, and that associated with high consumption was 2.3 (*p* value for trend 0.01). However, the child's consumption of cured meats was highly correlated with maternal consumption during pregnancy, and the association did not persist after adjustment for maternal consumption. No association with cured meat consumption was found by Howe *et al.* (1989). These authors observed an inverse association with consumption of fruit juices (relative risk associated with consumption of more than one glass per week compared with smaller or no intake 0.2, 95% CI 0.05–0.6). On the other hand, although fruit juice is a major source of vitamin C in children's diets, there was no association with use of vitamin supplements, or specifically with the use of vitamin C supplements. The association with fruit juice may have reflected the apparent preferential participation of control mothers of higher social class identified by the investigators. McCredie *et al.* (1994b) found no clear association between brain tumours and the reported frequency of consumption during the first year of life of eight food items: cured meat; powdered milk formula; dehydrated baby food; vitamin supplements; vitamin syrups; orange juice, apple juice; and blended or solid fruit. Sarasua and Savitz (1994) found no significant association between brain tumours and reported frequency of consumption up to the age of diagnosis of five food items: ham, bacon or sausage; hot dogs, hamburgers; lunch meats; charcoal-broiled foods. As was the case for maternal consumption during pregnancy, there was an elevated relative risk associated with the child's reported consumption of hot dogs (RR = 2.1, 95% CI 0.7–6.1). There were statistically significant increased risks associated with consumption of hot dogs, ham, bacon, sausages and lunch meats when the child was reported not to take vitamin supplements. A similar pattern was observed for ALL, suggesting that selection bias cannot be excluded as a possible explanation for the results (NRPB, 1992). In addition, it is unclear whether these relationships were confounded by maternal consumption during pregnancy. In a study of primitive neuroectodermal tumours with which associations with maternal diet during

## Table 8.10. Association between brain tumours in children and reported diet of the index child

| Area and period of study | Cases[a] Upper age limit | N | Controls Type[b] | N | Period of consumption considered | Cured meats Type | Categorization[c] | RR (95% CI) for highest category | p value for trend | Fruit, fruit drinks, vitamins Type | Categorization[c] | RR (95% CI) for highest category | p value for trend | Reference |
|---|---|---|---|---|---|---|---|---|---|---|---|---|---|---|
| USA, Los Angeles County, 1972–77 | 24 | 209 | F, N | 209 | Up to 1 year before diagnosis | All | T | 2.3 (NS) | 0.01 | – | – | – | – | Preston-Martin et al., 1982 |
| Canada, Toronto, 1977–83 | 18 | 74 | P | 138 | Pre-diagnostic | All | Per serving per day | 1.1 (0.7–1.8) | – | Fruit juices | >1 glass/week vs ≤1 glass/week | 0.2 (0.0–0.6) | – | Howe et al., 1989 |
| | | | | | | | | | | | per glass per day | 0.9 (0.6–1.2) | 0.37 | |
| Australia, New South Wales, 1985–89 | 14 | 82 | P | 164 | First year of life | All | $M_O$ | 2.0 (0.5–7.1) | ns | Orange juice | $T_O$ | 1.8 (0.7–4.6) | ns | McCredie et al., 1994b |
| | | | | | | | | | | Apple juice | $M_O$ | 0.3 (0.0–1.1) | ns | |
| | | | | | | | | | | Blended/ solid fruit | $T_O$ | 0.4 (0.0–1.1) | ns | |
| | | | | | | | | | | Vitamin supplements | $T_O$ | 0.9 (0.3–2.5) | ns | |
| | | | | | | | | | | Vitamin syrups | $T_O$ | 0.5 (0.2–1.4) | ns | |
| France, Ile de France, 1985–87 | 15 | 75 | P | 113 | Pre-diagnostic | All | Any vs. none | 0.7 (0.2–3.0) | – | Orange juice | Any vs none | 0.5 (0.1–2.0) | – | Cordier et al., 1994 |
| | | | | | | Ham | | 0.9 (0.2–3.4) | – | Fresh fruit | | 0.6 (0.1–3.0) | – | |
| | | | | | | Other than ham | | 0.7 (0.3–1.6) | – | Vitamin supplements | | 0.2 (0.1–0.7) | – | |
| USA, Denver, CO, 1976–83 | 14 | 45 | RDD | 206 | Pre-diagnostic | Ham, bacon and sausage | 1+/week vs. <1/week | 1.4 (0.6–3.1) | – | Vitamins | Any vs none | 0.4 (0.2–1.1) | – | Sarasua & Savitz, 1994 |
| | | | | | | Hot dogs | | 2.1 (0.7–6.1) | – | | | | | |
| | | | | | | Lunch meats | | 0.6 (0.3–1.4) | – | | | | | |
| | | | | | | Hamburgers | | 1.2 (0.5–3.0) | – | | | | | |
| | | | | | | Charcoal-broiled foods | Any vs. none | 0.8 (0.4–1.7) | – | | | | | |

ns, Not statistically significant.

[a] All of the studies were based on newly incident cases.

[b] F, friends; RDD, selected by random-digit dialling; N, neighbourhood; P, population-based.

[c] T, tertiles; $T_O$, tertiles; $M_O$, above or below median, with non-consumers in separate group.

pregnancy were the main focus of attention, three factors related to the child's diet approached significance in an analysis which included maternal dietary factors (Bunin *et al.*, 1993). There was an inverse association with consumption of multivitamin supplements (RR = 0.5, *p* = 0.07), a positive association with no consumption of fruit (RR = 3.9, *p* = 0.09) and a positive association with frequent consumption of apple juice (RR = 2.8, *p* = 0.08). In the parallel study of astrocytoma, no significant or noteworthy associations were observed for the child's intake of 11 foods and vitamin supplements during the first year of life (Bunin *et al.*, 1994a).

With regard to the possible causal role of aspartame postulated by Olney *et al.* (1996; see above), analysis of data for a subset of subjects (56 cases, 94 controls) participating in a case–control study of brain tumours in Los Angeles and San Francisco showed no association with the child's reported consumption of foods containing aspartame (Gurney *et al.*, 1997).

## Tobacco smoking by the mother

No consistent association has been found between maternal smoking in pregnancy and tumours of the nervous system in total, tumours of the central nervous system, brain tumours or specific types of brain tumour (Table 8.11). No dose–response relationship was found in any of the studies in which a trend in relative risk associated with amount smoked by the mother during pregnancy was assessed.

## Tobacco smoking by the father

Preston-Martin *et al.* (1982) reported a positive association between brain tumours and the mother having lived in a household with someone else who smoked (RR = 1.5, one-sided *p* value 0.03). In subsequent studies, no consistent association has been found between brain tumours and smoking by the father during pregnancy or before conception (Table 8.12). In most of the studies in which a possible dose–response relationship was investigated, none was found.

## Exposure of the child to tobacco smoke after birth

The association between brain tumours and exposure of the index child to passive smoking between birth and diagnosis has been investigated in only four studies. In a multicentre study in the USA, based on 361 cases and 1083 controls selected by random-digit dialling, there was no association with the average amount smoked by either the mother or the father during the period between birth and diagnosis (Gold *et al.*, 1993). In a study in the areas around Los Angeles, San Francisco and Seattle in the USA, based on 540 cases and 801 controls, the relative risk associated with the child having lived for six months or more with a smoker in their household was 0.9 (95% CI 0.7–1.2; Norman *et al.*, 1996). In a study in New South Wales, Australia, based on 82 cases and 164 controls, no association was found with exposure of the child to tobacco smoke from another member of the household (McCredie *et al.*, 1994b). Finally, in a study in the Paris area in France, based on 75 cases and 113 controls, the relative risk of exposure of the child to tobacco smoke in his/her lifetime was 2.3 (95% CI 1.1–4.6; Cordier *et al.*, 1994). This association remained statistically significant after taking maternal smoking during pregnancy into account; there was no dose–response relationship with the number of persons smoking in the presence of the child. Thus, no consistent association is apparent in the few available studies.

## 'Recreational' drug use by the mother during pregnancy

In the study of astrocytoma in Pennsylvania, New Jersey and Delaware (described above), the relative risk associated with maternal use of marijuana during pregnancy or in the month preceding pregnancy was 2.8 (*p* = 0.07) (Kuijten *et al.*, 1990). The relative risk associated with use specifically during pregnancy was 4.0 (*p* = 0.11). In a multicentre study in the USA and Canada of astrocytoma and primitive neuroectodermal tumours of the brain diagnosed at the age of five years or under, there was no association with maternal use of recreational drugs during pregnancy (Bunin *et al.*, 1994b).

## Incense exposure during pregnancy

Exposure to incense during pregnancy has been considered in studies of brain tumours because incense contains nitrosamines. A significant positive association (RR = 3.3, *p* = 0.005, based on 26 discordant pairs) with brain tumours was found in the study of Preston-Martin *et al.* (1982). No association was found in a study of brain tumours in New South Wales, Australia (RR = 1.3, 95% CI 0.4–4.1; McCredie *et al.*, 1994a), in a study of astrocytoma in Pennsylvania, New Jersey and Delaware (Kuijten *et al.*, 1990) or in a multicentre study of astrocytoma and primitive neuroectodermal tumours of the brain (Bunin *et al.*, 1994b).

## Table 8.11. Summary of studies of tumours of the central nervous system and maternal smoking during pregnancy

| Area and period of study | Cases | | Controls | | Prevalence of smoking during pregnancy in control mothers (%) | RR (95% CI) associated with any smoking during pregnancy | Trend[b] | Reference |
|---|---|---|---|---|---|---|---|---|
| | Upper age limit | Number | Type[a] | Number | | | | |
| **Nervous system tumours** | | | | | | | | |
| Canada, Ontario, 1959–68 and England and Wales, 1965 (1 week) | 10 7 | 20 | Coh | 89 302 | 40.0 | 0.8 | No | Neutel & Buck, 1971 |
| Sweden, 1978–81 | 16 | 43 | H | 340 | 29.7 | 0.9 | No | Stjernfeldt et al., 1986a |
| Sweden, 1982–87 | 5 | 81 | Coh | 497 051 | 30.0 | 1.0 | No | Pershagen et al., 1992 |
| **Central nervous system tumours** | | | | | | | | |
| UK, North West, West Midlands, Yorkshire, 1980–83 | 14 | 78 | GP, H | 7878 | NS | 1.0[c] | No | McKinney & Stiller, 1986 |
| UK, England and Wales, 1977–81 (deaths) | 15 | 312 | P | 312 | 41.4[d] | 1.1[e] | No | Sorahan et al., 1995a |
| **Brain tumours** | | | | | | | | |
| USA, Maryland, Baltimore, 1965–75 | 19 | 84 | P, H | 7378 | 20.5 | 5.0–∞[f] | | Gold et al., 1979 |
| USA, Los Angeles County, 1972–77 | 24 | 209 | F, N | 209 | 38.0 | 1.1 | | Preston-Martin et al., 1982 |
| Canada, Toronto, 1977–83 | 19 | 74 | P | 138 | 23.2 | 1.4 | | Howe et al., 1989 |
| USA, Ohio, 1975–82 | 19 | 110 | RDD | 193 | NS | 1.0[c] | | Wilkins & Sinks, 1990 |
| USA, Colorado, Denver, 1976–83 | 14 | 48[g] | RDD | 196 | 22.4 | 0.7[h] | | John et al., 1991 |
| USA, SEER, 1977–81 | 17 | 361 | RDD | 1083 | 38.0 | 1.1 | No | Gold et al., 1993 |
| France, Ile de France, 1985–87 | 14 | 75 | P | 113 | 20.4 | 1.6 | No | Cordier et al., 1994 |
| Italy, Milan, Varese & Como, 1985–88 | 14 | 91 | P | 321 | 20.8 | 1.6[i] | No | Filippini et al., 1994 |
| Australia, New South Wales, 1985–89 | 14 | 82 | P | 164 | 20.7 | 0.9 | | McCredie et al., 1994a |
| Sweden, 1983–89 | 6 | 96 | P | 484 | 27.1 | 1.2 | No | Linet et al., 1996 |
| USA, Los Angeles, San Francisco and Seattle, 1989–91 | 19 | 540 | RDD | 801 | 19.0 | 1.0 | No | Norman et al., 1996 |
| **Astrocytoma** | | | | | | | | |
| USA, Greater Delaware Valley, 1980–86 | 9 | 96 | RDD | 96 | NS | 1.0[c] | | Nass, 1989 |
| USA, Pennsylvania, New Jersey, Delaware, 1980–86 | 14 | 163 | RDD | 163 | NS | 1.0 | | Kuijten et al., 1990 |
| USA, SEER, 1977–81 | 17 | 148 | | | 38.0 | 1.0[i] | No | Gold et al., 1993 |
| USA and Canada, CCG, 1986–89 | 5 | 155 | RDD | 155 | 40.6 | 1.0 | | Bunin et al., 1994b |
| Sweden, 1983–89 | 6 | 41 | P | 209 | 25.8 | 0.9 | No | Linet et al., 1996 |
| USA, Los Angeles, San Francisco and Seattle, 1984–91 | 19 | 275 | RDD | 801 | 19.0 | 0.8 | No | Norman et al., 1996 |

| | | | | | | | | |
|---|---|---|---|---|---|---|---|---|
| **Primitive neuroectodermal tumour of the brain** USA and Canada, CCG, 1986–89 | 5 | 166 | RDD | 166 | 34.9 | 1.0 | | Bunin et al., 1994b |
| USA, Los Angeles, San Francisco and Seattle, 1984–91 | 19 | 99 | RDD | 801 | 19.0 | 1.0 | No | Norman et al., 1996 |
| **Medulloblastoma** Sweden, 1983–89 | 6 | 17 | P | 81 | 33.3 | 1.1 | No | Linet et al., 1996 |
| **Ependymoma** Sweden, 1983–89 | 6 | 14 | P | 69 | 30.4 | 1.3 | No | Linet et al., 1996 |

NS, Not stated.
CCG, Children's Cancer Group.

[a] Coh, cohort; H, hospitalized children; GP, neighbourhood controls selected through general practices; P, population-based; F, friends; N, neighbourhood controls; RDD, selected by random-digit dialling.

[b] If column is blank, no data enabling a trend to be assessed were presented. 'No', trend assessed but not found.

[c] No relative risk was presented. It was stated that there was no association.

[d] Smoking before the index pregnancy.

[e] Reference category comprised never smokers. RR for categories of <10 cigarettes per day (cpd), 10–19 cpd, 20–29 cpd, 30–39 cpd and 40 or more cpd, with these categories treated as a continuous variable.

[f] Comparison is between mothers who continued to smoke during pregnancy and those who had smoked before pregnancy but had not continued during the index pregnancy. There was no difference between cases and controls in the proportion of mothers who smoked before the index pregnancy.

[g] Number of cases whose parents were interviewed – number on whom information on smoking available may have been somewhat lower.

[h] Comparison is between subjects exposed to mother's cigarette smoking during the first trimester versus subjects who were not exposed to smoking by parents and other household members before and after birth.

[i] Reference category comprises mothers who had never smoked or had stopped smoking before conception and who were not exposed to passive smoking.

[j] Odds ratio calculated by unmatched analysis. No trend was apparent in the matched odds ratios presented.

# Table 8.12. Summary of studies of tumours of the central nervous system in children and paternal smoking habits

| Area and period of study | Cases | | Proportion of interviews at which father present | Period of exposure considered | Prevalence of smoking during this period in control fathers | RR (95%CI or p value) | Trend[a] | Reference |
|---|---|---|---|---|---|---|---|---|
| | Upper age limit | Number | | | | | | |
| **Central nervous system tumours** | | | | | | | | |
| England, North West, West Midlands, Yorkshire, 1980–83 | 14 | 78 | 53.2[b] | P<br>Pc | NS<br>NS | 1.0[c]<br>1.0[c] | | Birch et al., 1990b |
| UK, England and Wales, 1977–81 (deaths) | 15 | 299 | NS | Pc | 52.6 | 1.1[d] (1.0–1.2) | Yes | Sorahan et al., 1995a |
| **Brain tumours** | | | | | | | | |
| USA, Los Angeles County, 1972–77 | 24 | 209 | 0.0 | P | 55.0[e] | 1.5 (p=0.03[e]) | | Preston-Martin et al., 1982 |
| Canada, Toronto, 1977–83 | 19 | 74 | 34.0 | P | 42.0 | 1.1 (0.6–2.1) | | Howe et al., 1989 |
| USA, Colorado, Denver, 1976–83 | 14 | 48[f] | NS[g] | B-1 | 50.0 | 1.6[h] (0.3–3.5) | | John et al., 1991 |
| USA, SEER, 1977–81 | 17 | 361 | 71.0 | B<br>B-2 | 53.0<br>53.0 | 1.0[i] (0.8–1.3)<br>1.1[i] (0.8–1.4) | No | Gold et al., 1993 |
| Australia, New South Wales, 1985–89 | 14 | 82 | 36.6 | Pc - 3 mths<br>P | 34.1<br>29.9 | 2.0 (1.0–4.1)<br>2.2 (1.2–3.8) | No | McCredie et al., 1994a |
| France, Ile de France, 1985–87 | 14 | 75 | 1.1 | P | 61.9[c] | 1.5 (0.8–2.8)[c] | No | Cordier et al., 1994 |
| Italy, Milan, Varese & Como, 1985–88 | 14 | 91 | 35.0 | Any<br>Pc - 3 mths | 70.0<br>61.0 | 1.3 (0.8–2.3)<br>1.4 (0.9–2.4) | Yes[j] | Filippini et al., 1994 |
| China, Shanghai, 1981–91 | 14 | 107 | 100 | Pc<br>Any<br>Pn | 16[k]<br>55<br>18[k] | 2.7 (0.8–9.9)[k]<br>1.4 (0.6–3.2)<br>1.0 (0.3–3.3) | p=0.14<br>No | Ji et al., 1997 |
| USA, Los Angeles, San Francisco and Seattle, 1984–91 | 19 | 540 | 77.3 | Pc<br>P | 47.6<br>38.1 | 1.1 (0.8–1.3)<br>1.2 (0.9–1.5) | | Norman et al., 1996 |
| **Astrocytoma** | | | | | | | | |
| USA, Pennsylvania, New Jersey, Delaware, 1980–86 | 14 | 163 | NS | P | NS | 0.8 (0.5–1.3) | | Kuijten et al., 1990 |
| USA, Los Angeles, San Francisco and Seattle, 1984–89 | 19 | 275 | 77.3 | P | 38.1 | 1.1 (0.8–1.5) | | Norman et al., 1996 |
| USA and Canada, CCG, 1986–89 | 5 | 155 | 78.2 | Any<br>P | 52.9<br>40.6 | 1.1 (0.7–18.0)<br>1.0 (0.6–1.7) | No[j] | Bunin et al., 1994b |
| **Primitive neuroectodermal tumour of the brain** | | | | | | | | |
| USA and Canada, CCG, 1986–89 | 5 | 166 | 83.9 | Any<br>P | 53.0<br>34.9 | 0.9 (0.6–1.5)<br>1.0 (0.6–1.7) | No[j] | Bunin et al., 1994b |
| USA, Los Angeles, San Francisco and Seattle, 1984–91 | 19 | 99 | 77.3 | P | 38.1 | 1.1 (0.7–1.9) | | Norman et al., 1996 |

NS, not stated
CCG, Children's Cancer Group
Period of exposure:  B–1, during year preceding the birth of the index child; Any, ever exposed before interview; B–, ever exposed before birth of index child; P, during pregnancy; Pc, pre-conceptional; Pn, postnatal

[a] If column is blank, no data enabling a trend to be assessed were presented. 'No', trend assessed but not found.
[b] Figure is for total childhood cancer, from Birch et al. (1985).
[c] No odds ratio was presented. The authors stated that there was no statistically significant association.
[d] Reference category comprises never smokers. RR for categories of <10 cigarettes per day (cpd), 10–19 cpd, 20–29 cpd, 30–39 cpd and 40 or more cpd, with these categories treated as a continuous variable.
[e] Mother living with smoker (Preston-Martin et al., 1982) or exposed to tobacco smoke from other family members or at work.
[f] Number of cases whose parents were interviewed – number on whom information on smoking available may have been somewhat lower.

[g] Information was usually obtained from the child's mother.
[h] Comparison is between subjects exposed to father's tobacco smoking (cigarettes, cigars or pipe) during the 12 months before birth and subjects who were not exposed to smoking by parents or other household members before or after birth.
[i] Odds ratios calculated by crude unmatched analysis of matched data.
[j] When mother was a non-smoker and passively exposed in the three months before pregnancy, the relative risk associated with exposures of up to two hours per day relative to no exposure was 1.5 (95% CI 0.6–3.3) and with longer exposure 1.8 (95% CI 0.8–3.8); the p value for trend was 0.10. For passive exposures of the mother during pregnancy similarly defined, the relative risks were respectively 1.7 (95% CI 0.8–3.6) and 2.2 (95% CI 1.1–4.5); the p value for trend was 0.02.
[k] Associated with >5 pack years of smoking.
[l] Daily duration of passive smoking.

## Table 8.13. Summary of studies of tumours of the central nervous system in children and maternal alcohol consumption

| Area and period of study | Cases | | Period of exposure considered (P, pregnancy) | Type of alcohol | Prevalence of consumption by mothers of controls (%) | RR | Reference |
|---|---|---|---|---|---|---|---|
| | Upper age limit | Number | | | | | |
| **Central nervous system tumours** | | | | | | | |
| UK, North West, West Midlands, Yorkshire, 1980–83 | 14 | 78 | P | Any | 58.3 | 0.8 | Birch et al., 1990b |
| **Brain tumours** | | | | | | | |
| USA, Los Angeles County, 1972–77 | 24 | 209 | P | Beer | 25.0 | 1.0 | Preston-Martin et al., 1982 |
| Canada, Toronto, 1977–83 | 19 | 74 | P | Beer | 7.2 | 3.5* | Howe et al., 1989 |
| **Astrocytoma** | | | | | | | |
| USA, Greater Delaware Valley, 1980–86c | 9 | 96 | P<br>Pre-pregnancy | Any | NS | 1.9<br>1.0 | Nass, 1989 |
| USA, Pennsylvania, New Jersey, Delaware, 1980–86c | 14 | 163 | P | Any | NS | 1.4 | Kuijten et al., 1990 |
| USA and Canada, CCG, 1986–89 | 5 | 155 | P | Beer | 7.1 | 1.4 | Bunin et al., 1994b |
| **Primitive neuroectodermal tumours of the brain** | | | | | | | |
| USA and Canada, CCG, 1986–89 | 5 | 166 | P | Beer | 1.8 | 4.0* | Bunin et al., 1994b |

NS, Not stated.
* p < 0.05.
CCG, Children's Cancer Group.

## Alcohol consumption by the mother during pregnancy

The associations between tumours of the central nervous system and maternal consumption of alcohol and beer are summarized in Table 8.13. No consistent association with consumption of alcohol from all sources has been identified.

In view of the observation that certain brands of beer contain nitrosamines (Mangino *et al.*, 1981), beer consumption during pregnancy has been assessed in some studies. Howe *et al.* (1989) reported a relative risk of 3.5 (95% CI 1.2–10.8) associated with any consumption of beer during the index pregnancy. This was thought to reflect participation bias, with control mothers of higher socioeconomic status agreeing preferentially to participate. Beer consumption tended to be lower in those of high socioeconomic status than in those of low socioeconomic status. No association with beer consumption was found in the study of Preston-Martin *et al.* (1982). Bunin *et al.* (1993) reported that five mothers of cases with primitive neuroectodermal tumours reported drinking beer at least once a week during pregnancy, as compared with one control mother; this association was not statistically significant.

## Maternal use of hair colourants during pregnancy

Hair colourants contain aromatic amines, and therefore may be relevant to the hypothesis that exposure to *N*-nitroso compounds increases risk. Personal use may differ from occupational exposure in that consumers at home may use any of the three types of hair colourant, that is, permanent (primarily aromatic amines and aminophenols with hydrogen peroxide), semi-permanent (nitro-substituted aromatic amines, aminophenols, aminoanthraquinones and azo dyes) and temporary (high molecular weight or insoluble complexes and metal salts, such as lead acetate; IARC, 1993). Occupational exposure generally involves only the permanent and semi-permanent hair colourants.

No association between personal use of hair dyes and brain tumours has been found (Table 8.14). In the study of Bunin *et al.* (1994b), maternal use of hairspray and hair permanent products was assessed. No association was found for either astrocytoma or primitive neuroectodermal tumours of the brain.

## Use of other cosmetics during pregnancy

Face make-up has been considered in studies of brain tumours because the preparations used have been reported to contain nitrosamines (Preston-Martin *et al.*, 1982; Kuijten *et al.*, 1990).

Preston-Martin *et al.* (1982) reported an odds ratio of brain tumours of 1.6 (*p* = 0.02) when the mother reported that she had often used face make-up during pregnancy. By contrast, in a study in New South Wales, Australia, an inverse relation between brain tumours and the mother having used foundation cream or liquid on her face in the month before or during pregnancy, was found (RR = 0.4, 95% CI 0.2–0.7; McCredie *et al.* 1994a). No association between maternal use of make-up during pregnancy and astrocytoma (Kuijten *et al.*, 1990; Bunin *et al.*, 1994b) or primitive neuroectodermal tumours (Bunin *et al.*, 1994b) has been found.

## Use of dummies

Use of dummies (pacifiers) has been investigated in some studies of brain tumours in children as part of the evaluation of the role of *N*-nitroso compounds. Until recently, dummies and teats for babies bottles were made of rubber, which is known to contain *N*-nitroso compounds, and these have been found to migrate readily into liquid infant formula, orange juice and simulated human saliva (Havery & Fazio, 1983; Sen *et al.*, 1984), making sucking a likely route of exposure. In a study in New South Wales, Australia, any reported use of a dummy was associated with an increased risk of childhood brain tumours (RR = 2.9, 95% CI 1.6–5.4), but no increase in risk with increasing level of reported use was found (McCredie *et al.*, 1994b). The relative risk associated with bottle feeding daily for at least one month compared with less often was 1.8 (95% CI 0.8–3.9). No association was found between tumours of the central nervous system and method of infant feeding in a study in northern England (Birch *et al.*, 1990b). In a multicentre study in the USA and Canada, use of a pacifier or bottle-feeding were not associated with either astrocytoma or primitive neuroectodermal tumours of the brain diagnosed at the age of five years or less (Bunin *et al.*, 1994b).

# Neuroblastoma

## Maternal vitamin supplement use during pregnancy

In a study of 183 cases of neuroblastoma diagnosed at ages up to 14 years and 372 controls selected from live birth certificates in New York State (excluding New York City), the relative risk associated with maternal vitamin use in pregnancy was 0.5 (95% CI 0.3–0.7; Michalek *et al.*, 1996). The data on vitamin use were based on responses to an open-ended question in which mothers were asked whether their doctor had prescribed medications other than those to which the primary hypotheses of the study had related. It has been suggested that recall bias is more likely to occur if information is sought by open-ended questions than by closed-ended questions (Mitchell *et al.*, 1986). In addition, multiple comparisons were carried out, so the result may be a chance observation. No association between neuroblastoma diagnosed at ages up to eight years and maternal use of either prescribed or non-prescribed vitamins was observed in a hospital-based study in Memphis, Tennessee (USA), in which the control group comprised children with other types of cancer (Schwartzbaum, 1992).

## Maternal consumption of caffeinated beverages

In a study in the Greater Delaware Valley (USA), there was no association between neuroblastoma and coffee consumption during pregnancy when assessed as a dichotomous variable (Kramer *et al.*, 1987). However, mothers of cases reported drinking greater amounts of coffee per day than mothers of controls (mean difference 1.4 cups per day, $p = 0.02$). There was no association with tea consumption.

## Tobacco smoking by the mother or father

No consistent association between neuroblastoma and maternal smoking during pregnancy or paternal smoking has been observed (Table 8.15).

## 'Recreational' drug use by the mother during pregnancy

In the study of Schwartzbaum (1992) described above, there was no association with hard drugs or hallucinogens used by the mother during the year preceding the birth of the index child.

## Maternal alcohol consumption during pregnancy

Concern about the possible role of alcohol in the etiology of neuroblastoma was raised by case reports of neuroblastoma in association with fetal alcohol syndrome (Hornstein, 1977; Seeler *et al.*, 1979). The results of the two available case–control studies, both from the United States, are inconsistent. Kramer *et al.* (1987) found that the relative risk for drinking any amount of alcohol during pregnancy was of borderline statistical significance (RR = 1.4, one-sided $p$ value 0.08, based on 61 discordant pairs). Substantially higher relative risks of between 6

and 12 were associated with all three methods of defining "moderate to heavy" drinking (frequent, binge, either frequent or binge). As acknowledged by the authors, the study is limited by the low participation rate in controls, who were selected by random-digit dialling. Therefore, it is possible that the association is due to a selection bias whereby more affluent control subjects, who might be expected to include a higher proportion of moderate or non-drinkers than the general population, were preferentially included. In the other study (Schwartzbaum, 1992), in which the control series comprised children newly diagnosed with other forms of childhood cancer, there was a non-significant inverse association with maternal alcohol consumption during pregnancy. The inverse relation was consistent for beer, wine and hard liquor and decreased with increasing amounts of alcohol consumption. The inverse association was also found when separate analyses were performed to compare cases with controls diagnosed with ALL only and with controls with other diagnoses. The author acknowledged that participation rates were low (64% for cases and 68% for controls).

## Maternal use of hair colourants during pregnancy

In an exploratory analysis of data on 101 cases and their matched controls selected by random-digit dialling, the relative risk associated with use of hair dye was 3.0 (90% CI 1.6–5.5, one sided $p$ value 0.002, based on 36 discordant pairs; Kramer *et al.*, 1987). In the comparison of 86 cases with sibs, the relative risk was 2.2 (90% CI 0.9–5.2, one sided $p$ value 0.07, based on 16 discordant pairs).

## Retinoblastoma

Bunin *et al.* (1989a) reported an inverse association between retinoblastoma and maternal use of multivitamins during pregnancy. The analysis was reported for two subgroups: (1) 'nonheritable', defined to include unilateral cases without a family history of the disease and without a constitutional 13q deletion ($n = 115$); (2) 'sporadic heritable', defined to include bilateral cases without a family history of the disease, and unilateral cases with a constitutional 13q deletion ($n = 67$). It was postulated that the risk of the former type would be associated with post-conceptional exposures, while the risk of the latter type would be associated with pre-conceptional exposures of either parent. The relative risk of the nonheritable form of the disease associated with maternal use of multivitamins during pregnancy was 0.7 (95% CI

**Table 8.14. Association between tumours of the central nervous system in children and maternal use of hair colourants during pregnancy**

| Area and period of study | Cases | | Controls | | Prevalence of use in mothers of control (%) | RR[b] | Reference |
|---|---|---|---|---|---|---|---|
| | Upper age | Number | Type[a] | Number | | | |
| **Brain tumours** | | | | | | | |
| USA, Los Angeles county, 1972–77 | 24 | 209 | F, N | 209 | 17.0 | 1.3 | Preston-Martin et al., 1982 |
| Australia, New South Wales, 1985–89 | 14 | 82 | P | 164 | 23.8 | 0.8 | McCredie et al., 1994a |
| **Astrocytoma** | | | | | | | |
| USA, Greater Delaware Valley, 1980–86[c] | 9 | 96 | RDD | 96 | NS | 0.5[d] | Nass, 1989 |
| USA, Pennsylvania, New Jersey and Delaware 1980–86[c] | 14 | 163 | RDD | 163 | NS | 0.9 | Kuijten et al., 1990 |
| USA and Canada, CCG, 1986–89 | 5 | 155 | RDD | 155 | 11.6 | 0.7 | Bunin et al., 1994b |
| **Primitive neuroectodermal tumour of the brain** | | | | | | | |
| USA and Canada, CCG, 1984–89 | 5 | 166 | RDD | 166 | 9.0 | 1.1 | Bunin et al., 1994b |

NS, Not stated.
CCG, Children's Cancer Group.

[a] F, friends; N, neighbourhood; RDD, selected by random-digit dialling,
[b] None was significantly different from unity at or below the p = 0.05 level.
[c] Studies overlap.
[d] The RR associated with hair dye use before the index pregnancy was 0.9.

**Table 8.15. Association between neuroblastoma and smoking by either parent**

| Area and period of study | Cases | | Controls | | Maternal smoking during pregnancy | | | Paternal smoking | | | Reference |
|---|---|---|---|---|---|---|---|---|---|---|---|
| | Upper age limit | N | Type[a] | N | Prevalence in control mothers | RR[b] | Trend | Period | Proportion of control fathers who smoked | RR[b] | |
| UK, North West, West Midlands, Yorkshire, 1980–83 | 14 | 35 | GP; H | 70 | NS | 1.0[c] | No | B– | NS | 1.3 | McKinney & Stiller, 1986 |
| USA, Greater Delaware Valley, 1970–79 | NS[d] | 104 | RDD | 104 | NS | 1.3 | – | B-2 | NS | 1.6 | Kramer et al., 1987 |
| USA, Memphis, Tennessee, 1979–86 | 8 | 101 | OC | 690 | 26.2 | 1.9 | Suggestive | – | – | – | Schwartzbaum, 1992 |
| UK, England and Wales, 1977–81 (deaths) | 15 | 93 | P | 93 | 41.4[e] | 1.0[f] | No | Pc | 52.6 | 1.0[d] | Sorahan et al., 1995 |
| Germany, 1988–92[g] | 4 | 67 | P | 120 | NS | 1.2 | – | – | – | – | Michaelis et al., 1996 |

NS, Not stated.
Period of exposure: B–, ever exposed before the birth of the index child; B-2, during the two-year period preceding the birth of the index child; Pc, pre-conceptional.

[a] GP, neighbourhood controls selected through general practices; H, hospital controls; RDD, selected by random-digit dialling; OC, children with other types of cancer; P, population-based controls.
[b] None of the relative risks was statistically significant at or below the p = 0.05 level.
[c] The authors stated that there was no association.
[d] Median age was 1 year.
[e] Smoking before the index pregnancy.
[f] RR refers to a change of one category for "daily cigarette consumption" (non-smokers, <10 cigarettes per day, 10–19, 20–29, 30–39 and 40+).
[g] Areas in the former West Germany which were contaminated with more than 6000 Bq/m² caesium-137 from the Chernobyl accident.

0.3–2.0, based on 19 discordant pairs). The relative risk associated with use in the first trimester was 0.4 (95% CI 0.2–0.9). For the sporadic heritable form of the disease, the relative risks were 0.2 (95% CI 0.02–0.7, based on 14 discordant pairs) and 0.3 (95% CI 0.1–0.9) respectively. The reported use of multivitamins during pregnancy did not correlate with that before pregnancy – the relative risk associated with use before pregnancy was close to unity. Thus, the inverse association apparent for the sporadic heritable form of the disease was not consistent with the prior expectation that associations would be apparent only with pre-conceptional exposures. The possibility cannot be excluded that the results may be explained by bias arising from selection of controls by random-digit dialling, or by chance; multiple statistical testing was performed.

In a small study (37 cases and their matched controls) in Finland, no association with maternal use of vitamins during pregnancy was found (Salonen & Saxén, 1975).

In the study of Bunin *et al.* (1989a), there was no association between the nonheritable form of the disease and maternal consumption of tobacco and alcohol during pregnancy, or paternal consumption of tobacco during pregnancy or of alcohol during the preceding month. There was no association between the sporadic heritable form of the disease and maternal or paternal alcohol consumption. The relative risk of the sporadic heritable form associated with maternal smoking during pregnancy was 2.0 (95% CI 0.7–6.5), and that associated with paternal smoking in the month before pregnancy was 2.3 (95% CI 0.8–7.0). In a cohort study in Sweden in which 28 cases of retinoblastoma occurred, no association with maternal smoking during pregnancy was found (Pershagen *et al.*, 1992).

In the study of Bunin *et al.* (1989a), the relative risks associated with the father's use of 'recreational' drugs during the year before pregnancy were 2.2 (95% CI 0.8–6.9) for the nonheritable form of the disease and 1.7 (95% CI 0.3–10.7) for the sporadic heritable form.

# Wilms' tumour

## Maternal vitamin supplement use during pregnancy

No association with maternal use of vitamins during pregnancy was observed in either of two studies (Salonen & Saxén, 1975; Olshan *et al.*, 1993).

## Maternal consumption of caffeinated beverages during pregnancy

In a study of 23 children diagnosed at Cincinnati Children's Hospital with Wilms' tumour associated with nephroblastomatosis, born during the period 1951–75, and pair-matched with neighbourhood controls nominated by the parents of the cases, a positive association with frequent tea or coffee consumption during pregnancy was found (LeMasters & Bove, 1980). The associations with each beverage separately were not presented. In a subsequent study in Philadelphia, the relative risk of Wilms' tumour associated with maternal tea consumption during pregnancy was 2.2 (95% CI 1.0–4.7, based on 41 discordant pairs; Bunin *et al.*, 1987). Subgroup analysis was performed according to whether the cases were to be considered of 'genetic' etiology or not. However the classification used does not appear to be appropriate, according to current understanding of the genetic basis of Wilms' tumour (see Chapter 3). The mean interval between pregnancy and interview was 10 years (range 2–24 years). The association with consumption was apparent both for subjects for whom the interval between interview and the index pregnancy was between 2 and 10 years, and those for whom the interval was 11 years or more. In a multicentre study in the USA, no association between Wilms' tumour and maternal regular consumption of coffee or tea during pregnancy was found (Olshan *et al.*, 1993). Regular coffee and tea consumption was not differentiated. There was no association with maternal consumption of decaffeinated coffee. A limitation of this study is that the participation rate was relatively low (61% for cases and 52% for controls).

## Tobacco smoking by the mother or father

No consistent association between maternal smoking during pregnancy and Wilms' tumour has been found (Table 8.16). In the available studies, no association was found with paternal smoking during pregnancy (Olshan *et al.*, 1993) or before the index pregnancy (Sorahan *et al.*, 1995a).

## Maternal alcohol consumption during pregnancy

In the one available study, no association between Wilms' tumour and maternal alcohol consumption was found (Bunin *et al.*, 1987).

## Table 8.16. Summary of studies of Wilm's tumour and maternal smoking during pregnancy

| Area and period of study | Cases | | Control type[a] | Prevalence of smoking during pregnancy in mothers of controls (%) | RR[b] associated with any smoking during pregnancy | Trend[c] | Reference |
|---|---|---|---|---|---|---|---|
| | Upper age limit | Number | | | | | |
| Sweden, 1978–81[d] | 16 | 16 | HD | 29.7 | 1.8 | No | Stjernfeldt et al., 1986a |
| UK: North West, West Midlands, Yorkshire, 1980–83 | 14 | 32 | GP, H | NS | 1.0[e] | No | McKinney & Stiller, 1986 |
| USA and Canada, CCSG, 1983–86 | NS | 61 | RDD | NS | 1.0[e] | No | Buckley et al., 1986 |
| USA, Philadelphia, 1970–83 | 14 | 88 | RDD | NS | 1.0[e] | | Bunin et al., 1987 |
| Sweden, 1982–87[d] | 5 | 30 | Coh | 30.0 | 0.6 | | Pershagen et al., 1992 |
| USA and Canada, multicentre, 1984–86 | 15 | 197 | RDD | 22.4 | 0.9[f] | No | Olshan et al., 1993 |
| UK, England and Wales, 1977–81 (deaths) | 15 | 42 | B | 41.4[g] | 0.8[h] | No | Sorahan et al., 1995a |

NS, Not stated.
CCSG, Childhood Cancer Study Group.

a   HD, children hospitalized with diabetes; GP, neighbourhood controls selected through general practice; H, hospital controls; RDD, selected by random-digit dialling; Coh, cohort study; B, selected from birth records.
b   None of the relative risks was statistically significant at or below the p = 0.05 level.
c   If column is blank, no data enabling a trend to be assessed were presented. 'No', trend assessed but not found.
d   Total renal tumours.
e   No relative risk was presented. The authors stated that there was no statistically significant association.
f   Odds ratio calculated by unmatched analysis. No trend was apparent in the matched odds ratios presented.
g   Smoking before the index pregnancy.
h   Reference category comprises never smokers. RR for categories of <10 cigarettes per day (cpd), 10–19 cpd, 20–29 cpd, 30–39 cpd and 40 or more cpd, with these categories treated as a continuous variable.

## Maternal use of hair colourants during pregnancy

In the study of Wilms' tumour in the Greater Philadelphia area (USA) described above, the relative risk associated with maternal hair-dye use in pregnancy was 3.6 (95% CI 1.4–10.2, based on 32 discordant pairs) (Bunin *et al.*, 1987). The association was accounted for solely for cases diagnosed before the age of two years, for whom the relative risk associated with maternal use of hair dyes during the year preceding the birth of the index child was 15.0 (based on 16 discordant pairs, $p = 0.001$). Relative risks for ages 2–4 and 5 years and older were not statistically significant.

No overall association between maternal use of hair colourants during pregnancy and Wilms' tumour was found in a multicentre study in the USA during the period 1984–86 (Olshan *et al.* 1993). However, an elevated relative risk of 2.9 (95% CI 0.9–9.3) was apparent in a subgroup of subjects aged less than two years at the reference date.

## Hepatoblastoma

In a multicentre study of 75 cases of hepatoblastoma and 75 matched controls selected by random-digit dialling, there was no association with maternal use of vitamin or iron supplements during pregnancy, maternal or paternal smoking during pregnancy, or paternal smoking before the index pregnancy (Buckley *et al.*, 1989a). In addition, there was no statistically significant association with maternal use of 'recreational' drugs during pregnancy (4 cases, 2 controls exposed) and no association with paternal use of such drugs either during pregnancy or in the year preceding pregnancy (7 cases, 7 controls exposed). In this study, alcohol and nitrosamines were of interest in view of their potential hepatotoxicity (Buckley *et al.*, 1989a). There had been one case report of hepatoblastoma in a child with fetal alcohol syndrome (Khan *et al.*, 1979). There was no association with maternal alcohol use during pregnancy ($p$ value for trend 0.91), and the association with the mother ever having drunk alcohol (RR = 1.9) was not statistically significant. Nitrosamines induce liver tumours in experimental animals. Mothers were asked about use of face make-up, use of incense and consumption of foods likely to have contained nitroso compounds or high levels of nitrites. The only suggestion of an association was for consumption of foods containing nitroso compounds or with high nitrite levels (RR associated with daily use 3.0, 95% CI 0.9–13.5).

## Bone tumours

No association between bone tumours and maternal use of vitamins in pregnancy was apparent in the one available study (Salonen & Saxén, 1975). Holly *et al.* (1992) observed a relative risk of Ewing's sarcoma of 0.4 (95% CI 0.1–1.4) associated with consumption of vitamin and/or mixed supplements in childhood. The prevalence of use in controls was 93%. In a study of osteosarcoma in New York State, no association with reported intake of vitamin or mineral supplements was found (Gelberg *et al.*, 1997). No association between bone tumours and breast-feeding was observed in the small study of Hartley *et al.* (1988b).

Following a report of a dose–response association between osteosarcoma and exposure of male (but not female) F344/N rats to sodium fluoride, a population-based case–control study was carried out in New York State (Gelberg *et al.*, 1995). No association between osteosarcoma diagnosed at ages up to 24 years and total lifetime fluoride exposure was found. The study was based on 130 cases diagnosed during the period 1978–88 and pair-matched controls selected from live birth records. Data were obtained by interview with the parents (122 pairs) and/or the subjects themselves (64 pairs). Fluoride exposure information was obtained from questions about the use of fluoridated toothpastes and mouth rinses, and fluoride supplements. In addition, a complete residential history was obtained, which was linked with information on fluoridation of water sources. Dietary intake of fluoride was not assessed.

No association between bone tumours of all types combined and maternal smoking during pregnancy, or paternal smoking, has been identified (McKinney & Stiller, 1986; Hartley *et al.*, 1988b; Sorahan *et al.*, 1995a).

In a study of Ewing's sarcoma ($n = 208$ cases) in which two control groups were included, an association with parental smoking during pregnancy was found in comparison with sib controls ($n = 191$) but not in comparison with controls selected by random-digit dialling ($n = 204$) (Winn *et al.*, 1992). In the comparison with sib controls, the relative risk associated with maternal smoking from one month before to the end of pregnancy was 2.0 (95% CI 0.7–5.9) and that with paternal smoking was 3.7 (95% CI 1.0–13.1). A dose–response relationship was apparent for maternal smoking: compared with non-smokers, the relative risk when the mother smoked 1–19 cigarettes per day was 3.2 (95% CI 0.9–11.8) and that associated with 20+ cigarettes per day was 6.7 (95% CI 1.2–37.8). When both parents smoked compared with neither, the relative risk was 7.3 (95% CI 1.3–41.6). It is unclear whether pre-diagnostic symptoms of Ewing's sarcoma could have led to a sufficient alteration of parental smoking habits during the pregnancies leading to the birth of younger sibs to account for the inconsistency in the comparison between the two control groups.

In a smaller study (43 cases) of Ewing's sarcoma diagnosed at ages up to 31 years in the San Francisco Bay area, in which controls were selected by random-digit dialling, no association with maternal or paternal smoking during pregnancy was found (Holly *et al.*, 1992). In a study of 130 cases of osteosarcoma diagnosed at ages up to 24 years in New York State and matched controls selected from live birth certificates, no association with maternal smoking during pregnancy was found (Gelberg *et al.*, 1997).

No association between maternal alcohol consumption during pregnancy and bone tumours of all types combined (*n* = 30; Hartley *et al.*, 1988b), Ewing's sarcoma (Holly *et al.*, 1992; Winn *et al.*, 1992) or osteosarcoma (Gelberg *et al.*, 1997) has been found.

In the one available study, there was no association between Ewing's sarcoma and maternal coffee drinking during pregnancy (Winn *et al.*, 1992).

## Soft-tissue sarcoma

In small studies, no association between soft-tissue sarcoma and breast-feeding was identified (Hartley *et al.*, 1988b; Magnani *et al.*, 1989). In an exploratory study of rhabdomyosarcoma in North Carolina (USA), a positive association with eating 'organ meats' (e.g., liver, brain and tongue) was found (RR = 3.7, 95% CI 1.5–8.3; Grufferman *et al.*, 1982). Case families were reported to use less animal fat in cooking than control families (RR = 0.4, 95% CI 0.1–2.0). There were no other striking associations with dietary factors.

No association between maternal smoking during pregnancy and soft-tissue sarcoma of all types combined or rhabdomyosarcoma has been identified (Table 8.17).

In a small study in North Carolina, the relative risk of rhabdomyosarcoma associated with the father having ever smoked cigarettes was 3.9 (95% CI 1.5–9.6) (Grufferman *et al.*, 1982). The magnitude of the association was reduced (RR = 2.8, *p* = 0.07) after adjustment for family income, father's education and occupation. Subsequently, in a much larger study in which cases were ascertained from a clinical-trials group that co-ordinates treatment protocols for 80–85% of all cases of rhabdomyosarcoma in the USA, no association was found with paternal smoking in the year preceding, or any time after, the child's birth (Grufferman *et al.*, 1991b, 1993). In addition, in a hospital-based study in Padua and Turin, Italy, no association between rhabdomyosarcoma and paternal smoking before the child's birth was found (Magnani *et al.*, 1989).

In the multicentre study in the USA, no association was found with postnatal exposure to smoking by the mother or the father (Grufferman *et al.*, 1991b).

Again in the multicentre study, information was collected on use of recreational drugs and alcohol (Grufferman *et al.*, 1993). The relative risk associated with maternal use of marijuana during the year preceding the birth of the index child was 3.0 (95% CI 1.4–6.5), with maternal use of cocaine 5.1 (95% CI 1.0–25.0) and with use of any recreational drug 3.1 (95% CI 1.4–6.7). There were strong correlations between the use of marijuana and cocaine, both by the mothers and by the fathers, and therefore it was not possible to determine whether these drugs have independent effects. In addition, there were strong correlations between mothers' and fathers' use of the drugs, and therefore it was not possible to separate effects due to maternal and paternal use.

The relative risks for histological sub-types of rhabdomyosarcoma were similar to those for the total group. The mean age at diagnosis (5.4 years) of cases whose mothers used marijuana during the year before their birth was significantly lower than that of cases (7.8 years) whose mothers were non-users. A more marked difference was apparent in relation to maternal cocaine use (3.5 vs 7.7 years). This younger age at diagnosis would be consistent with a direct etiological role of these drugs.

A limitation of the study is that on average, parents were asked to recall use of the drugs eight to nine years before the interview. Therefore, recall bias was a potential problem. However in other multicentre studies in the USA, no association between mind-altering drugs and several types of childhood cancer was found (Robison *et al.*, 1989). It is difficult to see how recall bias might occur for rhabdomyosarcoma and not other forms of cancer. No evidence of recall bias was found in a study of maternal cocaine use and congenital urogenital anomalies in which the interval between exposure and interview could have been as long as 14 years (Chavez *et al.*, 1989). The reported prevalence of use in controls was similar to that in the general population surveyed by telephone in another

274

## Table 8.17. Association between soft-tissue sarcomas and smoking by either parent

| Area and period of study | Cases | | Control type[a] | Maternal smoking during pregnancy | | | Paternal smoking | | | Reference |
|---|---|---|---|---|---|---|---|---|---|---|
| | Upper age limit | N | | Prevalence in control mothers | RR[b] | Trend | Period[c] | Proportion of control fathers who smoked | RR[b] | |
| **Soft-tissue sarcoma** | | | | | | | | | | |
| UK, North West, West Midlands, Yorkshire, 1980–83 | 14 | 43 | GP, H | NS | 1.4–1.5 | No | – | – | – | McKinney & Stiller, 1986; Hartley et al., 1988b |
| Italy, Padua and Turin, 1983–84 | NS[d] | 52 | H | 34.0[e] | 0.6 | No | B- | 73.0 | 0.7 | Magnani et al., 1989 |
| USA, Colorado, Denver, 1976–83 | 14 | 26[f] | RDD | 22.4 | 1.2[g] | | B-1 | 50.0 | 0.8 | John et al., 1991 |
| **Rhabdomyosarcoma** | | | | | | | | | | |
| USA, North Carolina, 1967–76 | 14 | 33 | B | 28.0 | 1.0 | | Any | 46.0 | 3.9* | Grufferman et al., 1982 |
| Italy, Padua and Turin, 1983–84 | NS[h] | 36 | H | 34.0[e] | 0.9 | No | B- | 73.0 | 0.7 | Magnani et al., 1989 |
| USA, multicentre, 1982–88 | 20 | 322 | RDD | 36.7 | 1.0 | | B-1 | 48.4 | 1.0 | Grufferman et al., 1991b, 1993 |
| **Other soft-tissue sarcoma** | | | | | | | | | | |
| Sweden, 1982–87[i] | 5 | 15 | Coh | 30.0 | 1.2 | | – | – | – | Pershagen et al., 1992 |

NS, Not stated.
* p < 0.05.

a GP, neighbourhood controls selected through general practices; H, hospital controls; RDD, selected by random-digit dialling; B, selected from birth certificates; Coh, cohort study.
b None of the relative risks was statistically significant at or below the p = 0.05 level.
c B-7, ever exposed before the birth of the index child; B-1, during the year preceding the birth of the index child.
d Mean age at diagnosis 6.8 (±4.7).

e Smoking at any time up to child's birth.
f Number of cases whose parents were interviewed – number on whom information on smoking was available may have been somewhat lower.
g Comparison is between subjects exposed to mother's cigarette smoking during the first trimester versus subjects who were not exposed to smoking by parents and other household members before and after birth.
h Mean age at diagnosis 6.2 (±4.0).
i Tumours of connective tissue and muscle.

national study in the USA (Gfroerer & Hughes, 1991). Moreover, the absence of associations with tobacco smoking or alcohol consumption, and the similar low proportions of case and control families refusing to provide information on family income, did not suggest differential reporting of other sensitive information. Although families of cases had a lower income than families of controls, which may be attributed to control selection by random-digit dialling, the absence of an association with smoking is indirect evidence against a substantial selection bias.

With regard to biological plausibility, exposed cases were younger than unexposed cases, as already mentioned. The children, both cases and controls, of parents who reported using cocaine during the year preceding the child's birth had significantly lower birthweight than children of parents reporting no drug use. In addition, an increased prevalence of congenital anomalies of the urogenital and central nervous system has been reported in patients with rhabdomyo-sarcoma (Ruymann *et al.*, 1988). Maternal cocaine use has been associated with urogenital anomalies (Chavez *et al.*, 1989) and microcephaly (Volpe, 1992).

No association between rhabdomyosarcoma and consumption of alcohol by either parent was found, either in a large study covering the majority of cases diagnosed in the USA during the period 1982–88 (Grufferman *et al.*, 1993) or in an earlier small study in North Carolina (Grufferman *et al.*, 1982).

## Germ-cell tumours

In a multicentre study of 105 cases of malignant germ-cell tumours and 639 controls selected by random digit dialling in the USA and Canada, there was no association with maternal use of vitamin supplements during pregnancy, use of vitamin supplements by the index child or maternal coffee consumption during pregnancy (Shu *et al.*, 1995a). There was a positive association with breast-feeding for more than 12 months (RR = 3.3, 95% CI 1.2–9.2) and an inverse association with cigarette smoking by the mother during pregnancy ($p = 0.01$). These may be compatible with a role of estrogens in the etiology of these tumours. No association with maternal smoking was apparent in a small study (41 cases) of benign and malignant germ-cell tumours combined in northern England (Johnston *et al.*, 1986). No association with paternal smoking or maternal alcohol consumption was apparent in either study.

## Conclusions

So far, few studies of maternal diet during pregnancy and childhood leukaemia have been carried out. In the one available study of maternal diet and infant leukaemia, there was a statistically significant positive association between AML and dietary topoisomerase II inhibitors. Again, few investigations of the diet of the index child and leukaemia have been reported. In both studies in which information on the consumption of cured meats was provided, a raised relative risk associated with the consumption of certain types was observed. However, the validity of assessment of diet in childhood does not appear to have been evaluated. Assessment of the diet of preschool children in particular is difficult, as they eat small amounts of food at frequent intervals and often spend time under the care of several different people, so that the data, usually obtained from the mother, may be incomplete (Stein *et al.*, 1992).

No consistent association between tobacco smoking of the mother and leukaemia in the offspring is apparent. In four out of the five studies of ALL in which paternal smoking was investigated, a positive association was found. However, in some of these studies, selection bias cannot be excluded as a possible explanation for the association. No consistent association between paternal smoking and all types of leukaemia combined, or ANLL, has been observed.

Alcohol consumption has been less studied than tobacco smoking. Neither leukaemia of all types combined nor ALL has been associated consistently with maternal alcohol consumption. However, in the three available studies of AML, a positive association with maternal alcohol consumption during pregnancy was found. In two of these studies, analysis was made according to morphology, but the subgroups for which the association was strongest were not consistent between these studies.

In the one available study, a strong association between ANLL and reported use of mind-altering drugs, mainly marijuana, by the mother in the year preceding or during the index pregnancy was found. Thus, evidence appears to be emerging of a link between certain aspects of maternal lifestyle before or during pregnancy and ANLL, but not ALL.

Relatively few studies have been carried out specifically of the lymphomas. In three small studies, an inverse association between lymphomas of all types combined and breast-feeding was apparent, but in two of these selection bias may have accounted for the result. There is no consistent association between lymphomas of all types combined and smoking by either parent.

In eight out of nine studies, a positive association between brain tumours in children and maternal consumption of one or more types of cured meat during pregnancy was found. However, in some of these studies, selection bias may have occurred as a result of poor participation rates, or because families of low socioeconomic status may be under-represented when controls are selected by random-digit dialling (Greenberg, 1990), and the adequacy of others cannot be determined because they have been published only in abstract form. In addition, in most of the studies, information was sought about relatively few foods, and no evaluation of the validity of the dietary assessments appears to have been undertaken. No adjustment for total energy intake, which enables possible misclassification due to over or under-reporting of the total food intake to be taken into account (Willett, 1990), was made in any of the studies.

In five out of the six studies of brain tumours in which maternal consumption of vitamin supplements during pregnancy was investigated, an inverse association was found. A particularly intriguing finding is the inverse relationship between primitive neuroectodermal tumours of the brain and intake of dietary folate and multivitamin supplements in early pregnancy. These tumours are thought to arise from cells that also are involved in the formation of the neural tube, and folate and multivitamin supplements are known to protect against neural tube defects. So far, no other study investigating this association has been reported.

No clear relationship between brain tumours and the diet of the index child has been identified. As mentioned in relation to the studies of leukaemia, no evaluation of the validity of the assessment of childhood diet appears to have been made in these studies, and assessment of the diet of preschool children is particularly difficult.

No consistent associations between brain tumours and smoking by either parent, or with exposure of the index child to tobacco smoke after birth, are apparent. There are no consistent associations between brain tumours and maternal use of incense, consumption of alcohol, or use of hair colourants or other cosmetics.

Neuroblastoma has not been consistently associated with smoking by either parent. Concern about the possible etiological importance of maternal consumption of alcohol in pregnancy was raised by case reports of neuroblastoma in association with fetal alcohol syndrome. The results of the two available case–control studies of neuroblastoma and maternal alcohol consumption during pregnancy are inconsistent. In a single study, a positive association with use of hair colourants in pregnancy was found.

In two studies, a positive association between Wilms' tumour diagnosed before the age of two years and maternal use of hair colourants during pregnancy was reported. No association was apparent for older children. Wilms' tumour is not consistently associated with maternal smoking in pregnancy. No consistent association with consumption of tea or coffee in pregnancy is apparent.

No association between maternal smoking during pregnancy and soft-tissue sarcoma of all types combined or rhabdomyosarcoma has been found. A positive association between rhabdomyosarcoma and paternal smoking found in a small exploratory study was not confirmed in two subsequent larger studies. In one of these studies, information was obtained on use of 'recreational' drugs, and a positive association with parental use of these drugs was found.

Associations between aspects of lifestyle and retinoblastoma, bone tumours, hepatoblastoma and germ-cell tumours have been little investigated.

Overall, the absence of an association between most types of childhood cancer and tobacco smoking contrasts with the situation for cancer in adults. The lack of association does not appear to be due to poor recall. In studies in which a comparison was made between recall of smoking by the mother before or during pregnancy with that assessed by other methods, without regard to pregnancy outcome, the agreement in reported smoking behaviour was very good (Little, 1992). In most studies of childhood cancer and paternal smoking habits, the data on paternal smoking were reported by the mother. In a study in the county of Avon, England, women's reports as to their partners' smoking and drinking status agreed almost completely with the partners' own reports (Passaro *et al.*, 1997). However, women tended to report lower amounts of smoking and drinking for their partners compared to the men's self-reports. This would make a dose–response relationship more difficult to detect for paternal smoking than for maternal smoking. Another issue concerns the possibility of underlying variation in genetic susceptibility to the effects of tobacco smoke. This has been investigated in relation to some types of cancer in adults. In particular, in view of the lack of a consistent association between breast cancer and smoking, it is intriguing that an interaction between acetylator genotype and smoking in postmenopausal women was apparent in a study in which there was no overall association between breast cancer and smoking (Ambrosone *et al.*, 1996). It might be worthwhile to investigate this in relation to ALL and paternal smoking. Diet has been established to be important for a variety of cancers in adults, and it is intriguing that evidence is accumulating as regards a role in the etiology of childhood cancer.

'Recreational' drugs were associated with ANLL in one study, with rhabdomyosarcoma, again in one study, and with astrocytoma in one study but not in another. In the studies of ANLL and rhabdomyosarcoma, recall bias did not seem likely to account for the associations observed. To assess the validity of self-reported use of 'recreational' drugs during pregnancy, Hingson *et al.* (1986) randomly allocated pregnant women into a group who were told that their urine would be tested for kidney function and the presence of alcohol, marijuana, prescription and non-prescription drugs, and another group not so tested. Women told that they would be tested reported more marijuana use during pregnancy than did untested women. In addition, urine assays identified more women who used marijuana during pregnancy than were willing to admit this in the interview, even after being told that the urine would be tested. There were no differences in reported alcohol consumption or cigarette smoking during pregnancy between tested and untested women. Therefore, under-reporting of marijuana use seems likely. If this were non-differential, the relative risk associated with this exposure would be biased towards unity. It is important that replication of these findings is attempted.

# Chapter 9

# Maternal reproductive history, and maternal illness and related drug use

In this chapter, the associations between specific types of childhood cancer and maternal age, birth order and prior reproductive history are considered. The few available data on associations with other aspects of the medical history of the mother before the index pregnancy are discussed. With regard to the more extensive data on maternal illness and use of medications during the index pregnancy, this chapter deals with aspects not related to infection. Studies of possible associations with maternal infection during the index pregnancy are discussed in Chapter 7. Studies of the possible effect of diagnostic ultrasound are considered. Studies of the possible effect of intra-uterine exposure of the index child to diagnostic ionizing radiation are discussed in Chapter 4.

## Haematopoietic malignancies

### Maternal age

In most studies, no association between leukaemia and maternal age has been detected (Table 9.1). Studies of mortality due to leukaemia in the north-eastern part of the USA between the late 1940s and the early 1960s have been interpreted as showing a weak positive association with increasing maternal age, independent of an inverse association with birth order (MacMahon & Newill, 1962; Stark & Mantel, 1966, 1969). In addition, there was a positive association between maternal age and deaths due to leukaemia and lymphoma in the study of Kwa and Fine (1980), which overlapped with that of MacMahon and Newill. Because of the variation in leukaemia mortality with age of the child, and in particular because of a peak occurring in the third and fourth years of life, MacMahon and Newill examined the relationship of leukaemia mortality with maternal age according to the age at death of the child. No appreciable pattern was apparent. However, Stark and Mantel (1969) found that the maternal age effect was strongest in the fourth to eighth years of life. No maternal age effect overall, or after dividing the children by age at

death into those who died before the age of five years and those who died at older ages was apparent in a study of leukaemia deaths at ages 1–9 years between 1959 and 1965 in California (Fasal et al., 1971). Moreover, no association was found in a study based on newly incident cases in the north-eastern part of the USA during the period 1954–62, although the authors noted that their control selection method, whereby a random sample based on a stratified selection of households was selected, resulted in a larger proportion of firstborn among the controls than would have been expected on the basis of New York State vital statistics (Graham et al., 1966). In other studies, which are more recent, or based on newly incident cases, and include populations outside the USA, no association with maternal age was found.

Thus, with the exceptions of the studies of Gardner et al. (1990a) and Kaye et al. (1991), positive associations between maternal age and leukaemia have been found only in studies based on deaths. Older patients were included in the studies of Gardner et al. and Kaye et al., which might suggest that any association with maternal age was specific to cases with an older age at onset, but this is not consistent with the analysis of Stark and Mantel (1969), in which the strongest maternal age effect was associated with ages of death between the fourth and eighth years. The inconsistencies can also be interpreted as due to changes in the extent to which maternal age effects might reflect sociological rather than biological influences. With the wide availability of effective contraceptive methods since the 1960s, and the dramatic increase in induced abortions since the early 1980s in the populations in which these studies were carried out, the biological meaning of a birth at a particular age is uncertain.

### Birth order

The associations between childhood leukaemia and lymphoma and previous reproductive history are summarized in Table 9.2. In early studies of deaths due to leukaemia in childhood, a weak inverse relationship was found with

Table 9.1. Associations between haematopoietic malignancies in childhood and maternal age at the birth of the index child

| Area and period of study | Cases Dead (D), newly incident (I) or prevalent (P), upper age limit | Number | Controls Type[a] | Number | Comparison vs 20–34 years unless otherwise specified [mean age (sd) of cases, mean age (sd) of controls] | RR | Reference |
|---|---|---|---|---|---|---|---|
| **Leukaemia and lymphoma** | | | | | | | |
| USA, Massachusetts, 1947–57 and 1963–67[a] | D, 14 | 430 | P | 1384 | [28.6 (6.0), 27.6 (5.7)]* | NS | Kwa & Fine, 1980 |
| UK, North West, West Midlands and Yorkshire, 1980–83 | I, 14 | 234 | GP, H | 468 | 40+ vs ≤39 | 1.0[b] | McKinney et al., 1987 |
| **Leukaemia and non-Hodgkin lymphoma** | | | | | | | |
| UK, West Cumbria, 1950–84 | I, 24 | 74 | P[c] / P[d] | 492 / 484 | 40+ / 40+ | 5.1 / 4.0 | Gardner et al., 1990a |
| Italy, Turin, 1981–84 | I, N.S.[e] | 183 | H | 307 | [26.8 (5.8), 27.0 (5.3)] | | Magnani et al., 1990 |
| UK, West Berkshire and North Hampshire, 1972–79 | I, 4 | 54 | H / P | 216 / 108 | 30+ vs 25–29 / 30+ vs 25–29 | 0.9 / 0.7 | Roman et al., 1993 |
| **Leukaemia** | | | | | | | |
| USA, Boston, Massachusetts, 1953–56 | P, 14 | 187 | H | 44 | 36+ | 1.9 | Manning & Carroll, 1957 |
| Great Britain, 1953–55 | D, 10 | 677 | C | 739 | 40+ vs ≤39 | 2.0 | Stewart et al., 1958 |
| USA, North East Region, 1947–58[e] (white population only) | D, 14 | 2033 | P | Total population | 35+ | 1.1 | MacMahon & Newill, 1962 |
| USA, Minnesota, 1953–67 | D, 4[f] | 103 | N | 103 | 35+ | 2.4 | Ager et al., 1965 |
| USA, New York State (excl. City), Baltimore and Mineapolis-St Paul, 1959–62 | I, 14 | 309 | P | 884 | 35+ | 0.8 | Graham et al., 1966 |
| USA, Michigan, 1950–64 | D, 14 | 706 | P | Total population | 35+ | 1.1[x] | Stark & Mantel, 1966 |
| Japan, 1969–77 | I, 2 / I, 3–14 | 4607 | P | Total population | 30+ vs ≤24 | 1.0 / 0.9 | Hirayama, 1979 |
| USA, California, 1959–65 | D, 9[f,h] | 802 | P | 811 | 35+ | 1.2 | Fasal et al., 1971 |
| Finland, 1959–68 | I, 14 | 373 | P | 373 | 36+ vs ≤35 | 1.2 | Salonen & Saxen, 1975 |
| USA, California, 1975–80 | I, 14 | 255 | P | 510 | 35+ | 1.3[j] | Shaw et al., 1984 |
| USA, New York State, 1949–78 | I, 1 | 65 | P | 65 | [27.7, 25,3] | | Vianna et al., 1984 |
| China, Shanghai, 1974–86 | I, P, 14 | 309 | P | 618 | 30+ vs ≤25 | 1.1 | Shu et al., 1988 |
| Sweden, 1973–84 | I, 11 | 411 | P | 2055 | Continuous variable | 1.0 | Zack et al., 1991 |
| Mexico City, NS | I, P, 14 | 81 | H, P | 154 | NS | 1.0[l] | Fajardo-Gutiérrez et al., 1993a |
| USA and Canada, CCG, 1983–88 | I, 15 | 302 | RDD | 558 | 35+ vs 25–29 | 0.7 | Shu et al., 1996 |
| USA, Canada and Australia, NS | I, 1 | 303 | RDD | 468 | 36+ vs <20 | 0.9 | Ross et al., 1997 |

| | | | Control type | | | | Reference |
|---|---|---|---|---|---|---|---|
| **ALL** | | | | | | | |
| UK, Greater London, 1973–75 | I, 14 | 54 | E, N | [26.7, 26.6] | 54 | | Till et al., 1979 |
| The Netherlands, 1973–80 | I, 14 | 517 | P | 35+ | 509 | 0.8 | Van Steensel-Moll et al., 1985a |
| China, Shanghai, 1974–86 | I, P, 14 | 172 | P | 30+ vs ≤25 | 618 | 1.3 | Shu et al., 1988 |
| China, Shanghai, 1981–91 | I, 14 | 159 | P | [28.4, 27.8] | 159 | | Shu et al., 1995b |
| USA, Minnesota, 1969–88 | I, 17 | 337 | P | 35+ | 1336 | 2.1 | Kaye et al., 1991 |
| Sweden, 1973–84 | I, 14 | 332 | P | Continuous variable | 1660 | 1.0 | Zack et al., 1991 |
| Sweden, 1973–89 | I, 16 | 613 | P | 35+ vs 25–29 | 3065 | 1.0 | Cnattingius et al., 1995a |
| USA and Canada, CCG, 1982–91 | I, N.S.^k | 990 | C | 35+ | 1636 | 1.5* | Buckley et al., 1994 |
| | | 404 | RRD | 35+ | 440 | 1.7* | |
| *By immunophenotype:* | | | | | | | |
| Pre-B-cell | | 38 | C | 35+ | 114 | 2.0 | |
| Null-cell | | 65 | C | 35+ | 193 | 2.4 | |
| T-cell | | 158 | C | 35+ | 314 | 3.4* | |
| Common | | 286 | C | 35+ | 572 | 0.9 | |
| Unknown | | 443 | C | 35+ | 443 | 1.0 | |
| Denmark, 1968–92 | I, 14 | 704 | P | 35+ | Total population | 1.3^l | Westergaard et al., 1997 |
| **AML** | | | | | | | |
| Denmark, 1968–92 | I, 14 | 114 | P | 35+ | Total population | 1.1^l | Westergaard et al., 1997 |
| Sweden, 1973–89 | I, 14 | 84^f | P | 35+ vs 25–29 | 420 | 1.1 | Cnattingius et al., 1995b |
| **Lymphoma** | | | | | | | |
| China, Shanghai, 1981–91 | I, 14 | 82 | P | [29.6, 27.6] | 82 | | Shu et al., 1995b |
| **Non-Hodgkin lymphoma** | | | | | | | |
| Sweden, 1973–89 | I, 14 | 168 | P | N.S. | 840 | 1.0^j | Adami et al., 1996 |

NS, Not stated.
CCG, Children's Cancer Group.
* *p* < 0.05.
Control type: P, population-based, usually sampled from certificates of live birth; RDD, random-digit dialling; GP, neighbourhood, selected through general practitioner; H, hospital-based; C, children with cancer of other types.

a Studies of Kwa and Fine (1980) and MacMahon and Newill (1962) overlap.
b The authors state that the relative risk either was less than 2 or was not statistically significant at the 5% level.
c Controls matched with cases on sex and date of birth.
d In addition to sex and date of birth, controls matched with cases on parish of residence.
e Mean age of cases at diagnosis was 6.1 years.

f Cases with Down's syndrome were excluded.
g Adjusted for birth order and birth cohort; logistic regression was applied to the data in Table 1 of the original paper. The crude relative risk was 0.9.
h Singletons.
i Crude unmatched analysis of matched triplets.
j The authors stated that there were no differences between cases and controls with respect to maternal age.
k The percentages of cases aged 15 years or more were for the pre-B phenotype, 8%; the null-cell phenotype, 14%; the T-cell phenotype, 9%; the common phenotype, 7%; and ALL of unknown immunophenotype, 5%.
l Unadjusted analysis. The authors presented an analysis by five-year maternal age group adjusted for age, sex, calendar period and birth order, taking the 20–24-year age group as a reference. The risk of ALL overall and in subgroups defined by age at diagnosis tended to increase with increasing maternal age, but the trends were not statistically significant. No association was apparent for AML.

increasing birth order (Stewart *et al.*, 1958; MacMahon & Newill, 1962; Stark & Mantel, 1966).

Stewart *et al.* (1958) reported that the effect was most pronounced for deaths due to lymphatic and blast-cell leukaemias between the ages of two and four years, with a 70% higher risk for firstborn children than for other children. The authors noted that deaths in this age group were largely responsible for the striking increase in childhood deaths from leukaemia in the United Kingdom and in the USA after the Second World War. In an extension of the analysis, which included deaths in Britain during the period 1953–67 compared with healthy controls matched with cases on age, sex and area of residence, the association between reticuloen-dothelial neoplasms and birth order was independent of associations with maternal age, fetal irradiation and social class (Kneale & Stewart, 1976). Although first born children were more at risk of developing these neoplasms than other children, the risks were roughly the same for the second born children and those born later. This finding differs from the other two studies in which a trend of decreasing risk with increasing birth order was apparent after adjustment for maternal age (MacMahon & Newill, 1962, Stark & Mantel, 1966). In contrast to the finding of Stewart *et al.* (1958), MacMahon and Newill found no evidence that the birth order association for lymphatic leukaemia was different from that for other forms of leukaemia. MacMahon and Newill (1962) reported that the pattern of decreasing mortality with birth order was clearest within the group dying at ages three or four years, but was also present in the group dying at age five and over; it was not evident in the group dying before three years of age. Stark and Mantel (1969) reported that the birth order effect was strongest for leukaemia deaths in the third to tenth years of life. No association between deaths due to childhood leukaemia at age nine or under and birth order was found in California during the period 1959–65 (Fasal *et al.*, 1971).

Most studies based on newly incident or prevalent cases do not show a positive association with first birth (Table 9.2). In one of the largest of these studies, a non-significant trend of decreasing risk with increasing birth order was apparent for cases of acute lymphocytic leukaemia (ALL) diagnosed at ages 0–4 years, but not in older children (Westergaard *et al.*, 1997). This trend was more pronounced for children born during the period 1953–72 than for children born in the period 1973–92. In this study, a positive association between acute myeloid leukaemia (AML) and birth order was found (RR for birth order of two or more compared with firstborn 1.5, 95% CI 1.0–2.3, adjusted for age, sex, calendar period, and maternal age at birth of child). This was also observed in a combined analysis of data on AML diagnosed before one year of age from multicentre studies of leukaemia in the USA, Canada and Australia (Ross *et al.*, 1997).

The association between leukaemia mortality and first birth reported in early studies has been considered important in relation to hypotheses about the role of infection in childhood leukaemia (James, 1990; MacMahon, 1992b). However, this relationship has not persisted. It is interesting that a similar phenomenon was apparent for the incidence of ALL in young children in Denmark (Westergaard *et al.*, 1997). One possible explanation is that birth order is related to survival, but this is not supported by the absence of association in the mortality-based study of Fasal *et al.* (1971). MacMahon (1992b) acknowledged the possibility that the effect seen in the early studies could be due to an unidentified confounder. Another possibility is that, as with maternal age, the wide availability of effective contraceptive methods since the 1960s, and the increase in induced abortions in the early 1980s, has resulted in changes in the extent to which birth-order effects may reflect sociological rather than biological influences. Another issue which may be relevant to the interpretation of apparently conflicting results is different patterns by leukaemia sub-type, as suggested by the studies of Buckley *et al.* (1994) and Westergaard *et al.* (1997).

## Prior fetal loss

The association between childhood leukaemia and prior fetal loss has been considered in a number of studies. The relative risks of leukaemia associated with a prior history of fetal loss range between 0.3 and 1.8 (Table 9.2). There appears to be no pattern to this inconsistency in terms of study design or size. Non-differential misclassification may in part account for the inconsistency. In the interview-based studies, the proportion of controls reporting a past history of miscarriage and childbirth varied from about 10% to about 18% (Table 9.2). In a postal questionnaire-based study in the Netherlands, 23% of control mothers reported a prior history of miscarriage (Van Steensel-Moll *et al.*, 1985a). In the two studies based on information recorded in birth certificates, the proportions were 3% (Cnattingius *et al.*, 1995a) and 17% (Kaye *et al.*,

## Table 9.2. Associations between haematopoietic malignancies in childhood and previous reproductive history

| Area and period of study | Cases — Dead (D), newly incident (I) or prevalent (P), upper age limit | Number | Type of controls | Source of information | RR in firstborn vs later births | Prior miscarriage and/or stillbirth — Type of event | Prior miscarriage and/or stillbirth — Proportion of controls reporting history of this (%) | Prior miscarriage and/or stillbirth — RR | Other aspects of reproductive history | Reference |
|---|---|---|---|---|---|---|---|---|---|---|
| **Leukaemia and lymphoma** | | | | | | | | | | |
| UK, North West, West Midlands and Yorkshire, 1980–83 | I, 14 | 234 | GP, H | I | 1.0[a] | – | – | – | No association with size of sibship | McKinney et al., 1987 |
| **Leukaemia and non-Hodgkin lymphoma** | | | | | | | | | | |
| UK, West Berkshire and North Hampshire, 1972–79 | I, 4 | 54 | P | I | 3.5* | – | – | – | – | Roman et al., 1993 |
| | | | H | | 1.4 | – | – | – | – | |
| **Leukaemia** | | | | | | | | | | |
| USA, Boston, Massachusetts, 1953–56 | | 187 | H | I | 0.8 | – | – | – | – | Manning & Carroll, 1957 |
| Great Britain, 1953–55 | P, 14 | 663 | P[b] | I[b] | 1.1 | M | 13.7 | 1.5** | – | Stewart et al., 1958 |
| | D, 10 | 667 | P | I | – | SB | 3.4 | 1.1[c] | – | |
| USA, Northeast Region, 1947–58 | D, 14 | 1747 | P | B | 1.2 | SB | 4.7 | 1.1 | – | MacMahon & Newill, 1962 |
| USA, multicentre, 1958–61 | I, 15 | 459 | N | I | – | M | 9.9[d] | 1.2[e] | – | Miller, 1963 |
| | | | | | | SB | 0.8[f] | 0.5[g] | – | |
| USA, New York State (excluding city), Baltimore and Minneapolis–St Paul, 1954–62 | I, 14 | 315 | P | I | –[h] | M or SB | 16.7[i] | 1.6[i]* | – | Graham et al., 1966; Gibson et al., 1968 |
| | I, 4 | 170 | P | I | – | M or SB | 17.6 | 1.8* | – | |
| USA, Michigan, 1950–64 | D, 14 | 706 | P | B | 1.2* | – | – | – | – | Stark & Mantel, 1966 |
| USA, California, 1959–65 | D, 9 | 801 | P | B | 1.0 | – | – | – | – | Fasal et al., 1971 |
| USA, California, 1975–80 | I, 14 | 250 | P | B | 0.7* | – | – | – | – | Shaw et al., 1984 |
| USA, New York State, 1949–78 | I, 1 | 65 | P | B | –[k] | – | – | – | – | Vianna et al., 1984 |
| China, Shanghai, 1974–86 | I, P, 14 | 309 | P | I | 0.8 | M | NS | 0.5* | – | Shu et al., 1988 |
| | | | | | | SB | NS | 0.3 | – | |
| Sweden, 1973–84 | I, 11 | 411 | P | B | 1.0[l] | SB | NS | 1.0[l] | No association with number of previous live births | Zack et al., 1991 |
| Mexico City, NS | I, P, 14 | 81 | H, P | I | 1.0 | A | 24.2 | 1.3 | RR of 2.4* associated with immediately preceding pregnancy ending in abortion | Pajardo-Gutiérrez et al., 1993a |
| Greece, Attica and Crete, 1987–92 | I, 14 | 136 | H | I | 0.7 | – | – | – | – | Petridou et al., 1993 |
| UK, Oxford, Cambridge & Reading, 1962–92 | I, 30[f] | 143 | H | MR | 1.0 | – | – | – | RR of 2.1 (95% CI 0.9–4.6) associated with fertility investigations reported as ongoing at time of first antenatal clinic visit for index pregnancy | Roman et al., 1997 |
| USA, Canada and Australia, NS | I, 1 | 303 | RDD | I | 0.8[p,s] | M | NS | 1.5* | Trend of increase in risk with previous fetal deaths, p = 0.05 | Ross et al., 1997 |
| | | | | | | SB | NS | 0.9 | | |
| **ALL** | | | | | | | | | | |
| UK, Greater London, 1973–75 | I, 14 | 54 | F, N | I | – | M | 14.6[m] | 0.5[e] | – | Till et al., 1979 |
| | | | | | | SB | 1.6[j] | 1.8[g] | – | |

**Table 9.2. (contd) Associations between haematopoietic malignancies in childhood and previous reproductive history**

| Area and period of study | Cases — Dead (D), newly incident (I) or prevalent (P), upper age limit | Number | Type of controls | Source of information | RR in firstborn vs later births | Prior miscarriage and/or stillbirth — Type of event | Proportion of controls reporting history of this (%) | RR | Other aspects of reproductive history | Reference |
|---|---|---|---|---|---|---|---|---|---|---|
| The Netherlands, 1973–80 | I, 14 | 517 | P | Q | – | M / SB | 22.6 / 2.8 | 1.0 / 1.4 | – / – | Van Steensel-Moll et al., 1985a |
| France, Lyon, 1977–82 | I, NS | 158 | O | I | 1.0[r] | M | NS | 1.0[r] | – | Laval & Tuyns, 1988 |
| China, Shanghai, 1974–86 | I, P, 14 | 172 | P | I | 0.9 | – | – | – | – | Shu et al., 1988 |
| USA, Minnesota, 1969–88 | I, 17 | 337 | P | B | 0.9 | M or SB | 16.8[o] | 1.2[p] | Positive association with immediately preceding pregnancy ending in fetal loss | Kaye et al., 1991 |
| Sweden, 1973–84 | I, 11 | 332 | P | B | 1.0[i] | SB | NS | 1.0[i] | No association with number of previous live births | Zack et al., 1991 |
| Sweden, 1973–89 | I, 16 | 613 | P | B | 1.0[o] | M | 3.3 | 1.3 | No association with history of at least one year of involuntary childlessness | Cnattingius et al., 1995a |
| USA and Canada, CCG, 1982–91 | I, NS[y] | 990 / 404 | C / RDD | Q / Q | 1.0[o] / 1.0[o] | – / – | – / – | – / – | – / – | Buckley et al., 1994 |
| *By immunophenotype* | | | | | | | | | | |
| Pre-B-cell | | 38 | C | Q | 2.5[m] | – | – | – | – | |
| Null-cell | | 65 | C | Q | 1.1[p] | – | – | – | – | |
| T-cell | | 158 | C | Q | 0.8[p] | – | – | – | – | |
| Common | | 286 | C | Q | 0.9[p] | – | – | – | – | |
| Unknown | | 443 | C | Q | 0.8[p] | – | – | – | – | |
| USA, Denver, CO, 1970–83 | I, 14 | 71 | RDD | I | 0.5[p] | M | 16.8[m] | 0.9[c] | – | Savitz & Ananth, 1994 |
| Denmark, 1968–92 | I, 14 | 704 | P | B | 0.9[r] | – | – | – | Inverse association with sibship size at age 1 for 0–4-year subgroup | Westergaard et al., 1997 |
| UK, Oxford, Cambridge and Reading, 1962–92 | I, 30[t] | 113 | H | MR | 0.9 | – | – | – | – | Roman et al., 1997 |
| USA, Canada and Australia, NS | I, 1 | 181 | RDD | 0.9[o,s] | M / SB | NS / NS | 1.3 / 0.9 | – / – | Ross et al., 1997 |
| **AML** | | | | | | | | | | |
| Denmark, 1968–92 | I, 14 | 114 | P | B | 0.7 | – | – | – | Positive association with sibship size at ages 2 and 3 years | Westergaard et al., 1997 |
| Sweden, 1973–89 | I, 14 | 98 | P | I | 1.0 | M | 4.9 | 2.0 | No association with history of at least one year of involuntary childlessness | Cnattingius et al., 1995b |
| USA, Canada and Australia, NS | I, 1 | 115 | RDD | I | 0.6[o,s] | M / SB | NS / NS | 1.4 / 0.9 | Positive trend in risk with increasing birth order | Ross et al., 1997 |
| **Non-Hodgkin lymphoma** | | | | | | | | | | |
| Sweden, 1973–89 | I, 14 | 168 | P | B | 1.1 | M / SB | NS / 1.9 | 0.5 / 1.2 | No association with number of previous livebirths | Adami et al., 1996 |

NS, Not stated.

*p <0.05.

CCG, Children's Cancer Group.

Control type: P, population-based, usually sampled from certificates of live births; GP, neighbourhood, selected through general practitioner; H, hospital-based; N, neighbourhood; F, friends; O, children with severe diseases other than cancer; C, children with cancer of other types; RDD, random-digit dialling.

Source of information: B, birth certificate; I, interview, usually with mother; Q, self-completed questionnaire; MR, medical records.

Type of event: M, miscarriage; SB, stillbirth; A, abortion (type unspecified).

a The authors state that the relative risk was less than 2 or was not statistically significant at the 5% level.

b The birth rank distribution of cases was compared with national figures for the years which corresponded to the births of these children.

c Crude unmatched analysis of matched sets.

d Proportion of total pregnancies ending in miscarriage, excluding one centre in which reporting bias thought to have been severe.

e RR of miscarriage among total pregnancies in case group compared with that in the control group.

f Proportion of total births which were stillborn.

g RR of stillbirth among total births in case group compared with that in the control group.

h The authors commented that their sampling scheme resulted in a large proportion of firstborn among controls than would have been expected on the basis of vital statistics.

i Adjusted for year of birth, age of mother and birth order. When adjustment was made for pregnancy order instead of birth order, the adjusted percentage was 18.7 and the relative risk was 1.4 (p = 0.14).

j Adjusted for maternal age and birth cohort; logistic regression was applied to the data in Table 1 of the original paper. The crude relative risk was 1.1.

k Birth order was categorized into ranks 1–4 and 5+. The authors stated that there was no statistically significant difference between cases and controls matched on year of birth, sex, ethnic group and county of residence.

l Parity was treated as a continuous variable.

m Proportion of total pregnancies ending in miscarriage.

n The authors stated that there was no association.

o Calculated from proportion of cases whose mother were recorded as having prior fetal loss and the odds ratio.

p Reference category is parity of 2–3.

q The percentages of cases aged 15 years or more were for the pre-B phenotype, 8%; the null-cell phenotype, 14%; the T-cell phenotype, 9%; the common phenotype, 7%; and ALL of unknown phenotype, 5%.

r Unadjusted analysis. The authors presented analysis of birth order categorized as 1, 2, 3, 4+ and as 1, 2+ adjusted for age, sex, calender period and maternal age at birth of the index child, taking firstborn as the reference category. No overall association was apparent for ALL. For AML, the relative risk for birth order of 2 or more compared with first born was 1.5 (95% CI 1.0–2.3).

s Adjusted for maternal education.

t 92% of all leukaemia cases were aged 14 years or less at the time of diagnosis. The proportion was 96% for ALL.

1991). A positive association between leukaemia diagnosed before one year of age and number of previous fetal losses ($p = 0.05$) appeared to be due to the AML subgroup (Ross *et al.*, 1997).

## Other aspects of medical history of the mother before the index pregnancy

Few data are available on this issue. Manning and Carroll (1957) reported that a significantly higher proportion of mothers of cases with leukaemia or lymphoma had a history of hay fever, asthma or hives compared with mothers of cases with other types of cancer or mothers of controls with orthopaedic conditions excluding poliomyelitis. Till *et al.* (1979) reported that there was little difference in the frequency of atopy in parents of children with ALL and in those of controls. McKinney *et al.* (1987) observed that the medical histories of mothers of children with leukaemia or lymphoma were similar to those of mothers of controls except for skin diseases. This was more marked in medically recorded data than in the data obtained by interview. There was no striking association between history of infection in the mother before the conception of the index child and childhood leukaemia in the study of Till *et al.* (1979), but the method of control selection (nomination by parents of cases from amongst friends and neighbours to match themselves as closely as possible for age and having had a child of similar age to the index case) may have obscured any difference. In a small number of studies, maternal immune function has been assessed on the basis of blood samples taken after the diagnosis of the disease in the child (Sutton *et al.*, 1969; Chandra, 1972; Hann *et al.*, 1975; Till *et al.*, 1979; Woods *et al.*, 1987). The results of these studies have been inconsistent, perhaps because of differences in methods of control selection and perhaps due to chance, as the studies have been small, whereas a large number of tests have been performed. Alexander (1993) commented that a common factor between these studies is evidence of non-specific indicators of chronic infection in the mother.

Buckley *et al.* (1989c) reported an association between ALL and multiple sclerosis in the mother. Five mothers of 1027 cases of acute lymphoblastic cancer treated in centres participating in the Childhood Cancer Study Group in the USA and Canada reported that they had multiple sclerosis, four times (95% CI 1.3–9.3) the number expected on the basis of national rates. The excess was also apparent when comparison was made with cancers other than of the haematopoietic system, and with

children without cancer selected by random-digit dialling. No significant excess was observed for acute non-lymphoblastic leukaemia (ANLL), non-Hodgkin lymphoma or Hodgkin's disease. None of the fathers of children with any type of cancer had multiple sclerosis; the expected frequency was much lower in fathers than mothers. An important limitation of the study is that the response rate was only 50%.

## Maternal illness and use of medications during the index pregnancy

### Threatened miscarriage and hormonal treatment during pregnancy

Interest in the possible etiological importance of threatened miscarriage during pregnancy arose following the report of a positive association with childhood cancer deaths in a large study in Great Britain (Stewart *et al.*, 1958). Studies of the association with leukaemia have been inconsistent (Table 9.3). However, in the largest subsequent study, in which controls were selected randomly from the census lists, there was a significant positive association with both threatened miscarriage and "drugs to maintain the pregnancy" (Van Steensel-Moll *et al.*, 1985a). The risk of ALL was also associated with the women having had two or more previous miscarriages, use of hormones other than oral contraceptives in the year preceding conception, and hospitalization or consultation for subfertility and for miscarriages and curettage.

In a study based on obstetric records of hospitals in Oxford, Cambridge and Reading in England during the period 1962–92, in which 92% of cases were diagnosed at the age of 14 years or under (the remainder at ages up to 29 years), the relative risk associated with hormonal treatment for infertility in the periconceptional period was 2.7 (95% CI 0.6–11.9; Roman *et al.*, 1997). The relative risk associated with reported infertility investigations at the time of the first antenatal clinic visit for the index pregnancy was 2.1 (95% CI 0.9–4.6). However, in a series of childhood cancer cases in Japan in which information on ovulation induction was recorded, no instance of maternal ovulation induction was recorded among 2301 children with leukaemia (Kobayashi *et al.*, 1991).

### Oral contraceptives

McKinney *et al.* (1987) reported no association between leukaemia and lymphoma and an interval of less than three months between stopping oral contraception and conception. Van

# Table 9.3. Associations between childhood haematopoietic malignancies and cancer of all types and threatened miscarriage, and hormonal treatment during the index pregnancy

| Area and period of study | Cases Dead (D), newly incident (I) or prevalent (P), upper age limit | Cases Number | Controls Type[a] | Controls Number | Source of information[b] | Threatened miscarriage Prevalence in control mothers (%) | Threatened miscarriage RR | Hormonal treatment Prevalence of use in control mothers (%) | Hormonal treatment RR | Reference |
|---|---|---|---|---|---|---|---|---|---|---|
| **Total childhood cancer** | | | | | | | | | | |
| Great Britain, 1953–55 | D, 10 | 1299 | P | 1299 | I | 0.8 | 2.7*[e] | – | – | Stewart et al., 1958 |
| Great Britain, 1964–79 | D, 15 | 8059 | P | 8059 | I, MR | 6.9 | –[d] | 1.9 | 1.2 | Gilman et al., 1989 |
| Finland, 1959–68 | I, 14 | 972 | P | 972 | AN | – | – | 2.7 | 0.8[c] | Salonen & Saxén, 1975; Salonen, 1976 |
| Sweden, 1973–84 | I, 11 | 1230 | P | 1460 | MR | NS | 1.8 | – | – | Forsberg & Källén, 1990 |
| **Leukaemia and lymphoma** | | | | | | | | | | |
| UK, North West, West Midlands and Yorkshire, 1980–83 | I, 14 | 234 | GP, H | 468 | I MR | NS NS | 1.0[c] 1.0[c] | NS NS | 0.9 0.7 | McKinney et al., 1987 |
| **Leukaemia** | | | | | | | | | | |
| Great Britain, 1953–55 | D, 10 | 619 | P | 619 | I | 0.6 | 3.6*[e] | – | – | Stewart et al., 1958 |
| China, Shanghai, 1974–86 | I, P, 14 | 309 | P | 618 | I | NS | 1.0[f] | – | – | Shu et al., 1988 |
| **ALL** | | | | | | | | | | |
| UK, London, 1973–75 | I, 14 | 54 | F, N | 54 | Q | 3.7 | 1.5[c] | – | – | Till et al., 1979 |
| The Netherlands, 1973–80 | I, 14 | 519 | P | 507 | Q | 5.7 | 1.6* | 3.4[g] | 1.9[g] | Van Steensel-Moll et al., 1985a |
| Italy, Turin, 1981–84 | I, NS[h] | 142 | H | 307 | I | 10.4 | 1.1 | – | – | Magnani et al., 1990 |
| **ANLL** | | | | | | | | | | |
| USA and Canada, CCSG, 1980–84 | I, 17 | 204 | RDD | 204 | I | – | – | 6.4[i] | 0.8 | Robison et al., 1989 |
| The Netherlands, 1973–79 | I, 14 | 80 | P | 240 | Q | – | – | 1.7[g] | 2.5[g] | Van Duijn et al., 1994 |

NS, Not stated.
*$p < 0.05$.
CCSG, Childhood Cancer Study Group.

[a] P, population-based; GP, neighbourhood, selected through general practice; H, hospital; F, friends; N, neighbourhood; RDD, selected by random-digit dialling.
[b] I, maternal interview; MR, medical records; AN, records of antenatal clinic; Q, questionnaire
[c] Crude unmatched analysis of matched data.
[d] No relative risk was presented separately for threatened miscarriage. The relative risk for pregnancy complications other than infection, toxaemia, anaemia or Caesarean section was 1.0.
[e] The relative risk was <2 and not statistically significant.

[f] The authors state that there was no association.
[g] "Drugs to maintain the pregnancy" described as hormones, medication for threatened abortion or drugs to inhibit early labour. All of these women experienced threatened abortion. The relative risk for these drugs together, after adjustment for maternal age, number of previous miscarriages and normal medication in the year before the index pregnancy, was 2.6 (95% CI 1.2–5.5).
[h] Mean age at diagnosis of 142 cases of ALL, 22 of ANLL and 19 of non-Hodgkin lymphoma was 6.1 (S.D. 3.6).
[i] During or in year before index pregnancy.

Steensel-Moll *et al.* (1985a) observed that the reported period between discontinuation of oral contraceptive use and pregnancy was significantly longer for mothers of cases with ALL than for mothers of controls. The relative risk associated with any use of oral contraceptives before pregnancy was 1.2 (95% CI 0.9–1.6). The relative risk associated with use in the year preceding pregnancy was 1.3 (95% CI 1.0–1.8). The authors considered that the prolonged interval between cessation of use and pregnancy noted above, and the elevated risk associated with use in the year before the index pregnancy, might be evidence of an association with subfertility.

### Steroids other than gonadal hormones

No association was found between leukaemia and lymphoma and topical steroids or with hormonal pregnancy tests in a study in northern England (McKinney *et al.*, 1987). In addition, no association with steroids other than gonadal hormones was found in a large study of childhood cancer deaths in Great Britain (Gilman *et al.*, 1989).

### Anaesthesia during labour

A positive association between total childhood cancer and administration of pethidine or pethilorfan in labour was found in a small cohort study in Great Britain (Golding *et al.*, 1990; Table 9.4). The relative risk was substantially reduced and no longer statistically significant after adjustment for a number of covariates, including administration of drugs to the neonate. The main drug administered to the neonate was vitamin K; this aspect of this study has been discussed elsewhere (see section on Vitamin K in Chapter 10). In order to examine further the possible association between total childhood cancer and use of pethidine in labour and administration of vitamin K to the neonate, the authors carried out a case–control study in Bristol (Golding *et al.*, 1992a). The association with pethidine was not confirmed. In addition, no association with pethidine was found in a large study of childhood cancer deaths in Great Britain (Gilman *et al.*, 1989). The reported prevalence of exposure in mothers of controls was very much lower than in the medical record-based studies of Golding *et al.* (1990, 1992a), probably because in this study medical records were used only to confirm positive reports by the mother.

McKinney *et al.* (1987) found a positive association between haematopoietic malignancies and narcotic or opioid analgesics, mostly Distalgesic (dextropropoxyphene hydrochloride). This finding was due to the leukaemia subgroup (RR = 7.3, 95% CI 1.9–28.3). The relative risk (2.0, 95% CI 1.0–4.0) was substantially lower when analysis was restricted to reports confirmed from medical records. There was a positive association with medically recorded use of barbiturates in labour, which was due to the lymphoma subgroup (RR = 10.8, 95% CI 1.8–63.2). There was no association with maternal use of barbiturates at other times during pregnancy or maternal use of analgesics not related to anaesthetic use. No association between leukaemia or non-Hodgkin lymphoma and use of opioid analgesics, or pethidine specifically, was found in a study based on obstetric records in Oxford, Cambridge and Reading, England (Roman *et al.*, 1997).

In a study based on information recorded on the Swedish national medical birth register, Zack *et al.* (1991) found a weak but statistically significant association between leukaemia and nitrous oxide anaesthesia during labour. This association was apparent for the lymphatic leukaemia subgroup and for other types of leukaemia excluding the myeloid subgroup. However, the association with nitrous oxide was only apparent in boys and among children diagnosed with leukaemia after the age of three years, and the finding was not confirmed in a subsequent extension of the study relating specifically to lymphatic leukaemia (Cnattingius *et al.*, 1995a) or in the study in Oxford, Cambridge and Reading (Roman *et al.*, 1997).

No consistent association has been found between childhood leukaemia and Caesarean section, an indication for anaesthesia in labour (Table 9.4).

In a study using similar methods to the studies of leukaemia in Sweden (Zack *et al.*, 1991; Cnattingius *et al.*, 1995a), there was a positive association between childhood non-Hodgkin lymphoma and Caesarean section (RR = 1.6, 95% CI 1.0–2.6) and use of paracervical anaesthesia (RR = 1.8, 95% CI 1.0–3.5; Adami *et al.*, 1996). None of the other anaesthetic methods or analgesics used during delivery was associated with non-Hodgkin lymphoma.

### Other drugs

A positive association between maternal use of "cold tablets" before or during the index pregnancy and deaths due to leukaemia (Manning & Carroll, 1957) has not been confirmed in other studies. First, there was no association between maternal use of

**Table 9.4. Associations between childhood haematopoietic malignancies and cancer of all types and maternal anaesthesia during pregnancy and labour, and procedures involving this, and related drugs**

| Area and period of study | Reference | Cases: Dead (D), or newly incident (I), upper age limit | Cases: Number | Controls: Type[a] | Controls: Number | Source of information on exposure[b] | Anaesthesia or procedure including this: Type or procedure | Anaesthesia or procedure: Prevalence in control mothers (%) | Anaesthesia or procedure: RR | Drugs associated with anaesthesia: Type | Drugs: Prevalence of use in control mothers (%) | Drugs: RR |
|---|---|---|---|---|---|---|---|---|---|---|---|---|
| **Total childhood cancer** | | | | | | | | | | | | |
| Finland, 1959–68 | Salonen, 1976 | I, 14 | 972 | P | 972 | AN | – | – | – | Euphoriant analgesics / Papaverine | 0.5 / 0.6 | 2.2c / 1.2c |
| Great Britain, 1964–79 | Gilman et al., 1989 | D, 15 | 8059 | P | 8059 | I, MR | Caesarean section | NS | 1.1d | Pethidine | 0.9 | 1.4c |
| Great Britain, 1980 (1 week) | Golding et al., 1990 | I, 10 | 33c | P | 99 | N | Caesarean section | 5.1 | 0.6c | Pethidine/pethilorfan in labour | 50.0 | 4.1*f |
| UK, Bristol, 1971–91 | Golding et al., 1992a | I, 14 | 195 | H | 558 | MR | – | – | – | Pethidine in labour | 47.0g | 1.0 |
| **Leukaemia and lymphoma** | | | | | | | | | | | | |
| UK, North West, West Midlands and Yorkshire, 1980–83 | McKinney et al., 1987 | I, 14 | 234 | GP, H | 468 | I, MR / I / MR | General anaesthetic / Caesarean section | NS / NS / NS | 1.0h / 1.0h / 1.0h | Narcotic analgesics | 0.6 / NS | 8.3* / 1.4 |
| **Leukaemia and non-Hodgkin lymphoma** | | | | | | | | | | | | |
| UK, West Berkshire and North Hampshire 1972–89 | Roman et al., 1993 | I, 4 | 37 / 51 | H, P | 196 / 223 | MR / I | Caesarean section | 8.7 / 8.5 | 1.3 / 1.2 | – / – | – / – | – / – |
| **Leukaemia** | | | | | | | | | | | | |
| Sweden, 1973–84 | Zack et al., 1991 | I, 11 | 411 | P | 2055 | MR | Caesarean section | 9.8 | 1.0 | Nitrous oxide anaesthesia | 54.4 | 1.3* |
| UK, Oxford, Cambridge and Reading, 1962–92 | Roman et al., 1997 | I, 30m | 143 | H | 286 | MR | Caesarean section | 8.4 | 1.3 | Anaesthesia in labour: general / local / nitrous oxide / pethidine | 8.7 / 28.3 / 37.8 / 48.3 | 1.0 / 1.1 / 0.8 / 1.1 |
| **ALL** | | | | | | | | | | | | |
| USA, Minnesota, 1969–88 | Kaye et al., 1991 | I, 17 | 337 | B | 1336 | MR | Caesarean section | 9.4f | 1.4 | – | – | – |
| Sweden, 1973–84 | Zack et al., 1991 | I, 11 | 328j | P | 1640 | MR | Caesarean section | 9.9 | 0.9 | Nitrous oxide anaesthesia | 54.6 | 1.2* |
| Sweden, 1973–89 | Chattingius et al., 1995a | I, 16 | 613k | P | 3065 | MR | Caesarean section | NS | 1.0 | Nitrous oxide anaesthesia | NS | 1.0 |
| **AML** | | | | | | | | | | | | |
| Sweden, 1973–89 | Chattingius et al., 1995b | I, 14 | 98 | P | 490 | MR | Caesarean section | 8.8 | 2.5* | – | – | – |
| **Non-Hodgkin lymphoma** | | | | | | | | | | | | |
| Sweden, 1973–89 | Adami et al., 1996 | I, 14 | 168 | P | 840 | MR | Caesarean section | 9.5 | 1.6* | Nitrous oxide anaesthesia / Penthane / Paracervical anaesthesia | NS / NS / 4.9 | 1.0 / 1.0 / 1.8* |

NS, Not stated.   *p < 0.05.

a P, population-based; H, hospital; GP, neighbourhood, selected through general practices; B, selected from birth records.

b AN, antenatal clinic records; I, maternal interview; MR, medical records; N, data collected at home of birth of child by midwives.

c Crude unmatched analysis of matched data.

d Estimates presented in original paper differ slightly according to co-variables included in regression analysis.

e Case-control study nested in cohort.

f 1.7 when included in regression analysis with five other risk factors, all of which were inter-correlated.

g Prevalence of exposure in mothers of cases and controls.

h The authors state that the relative risk was <2 and not statistically significant.

i Estimated from proportion of cases exposed and relative risk.

j Lymphatic leukaemia: 321 of these had ALL.

k Lymphatic leukaemia: 607 of these had ALL.

l The authors state that there was no association.

m 92% of all leukaemia cases were aged 14 or less at the time of diagnosis. The proportion was 96% for ALL.

antihistamines during pregnancy and leukaemia and lymphoma in northern England (McKinney *et al.*, 1987). Second, there was no association between maternal use of "cold or cough" medications or antihistamines during or in the year before the index pregnancy and ANLL (Robison *et al.*, 1989). Third, there was no association between infant leukaemia and maternal use of cold medications around the time of pregnancy in a multicentre study in the USA (Ross *et al.*, 1996b).

In the one available study of leukaemia and maternal aspirin use during pregnancy, the association differed in comparison with the two control groups (Manning & Carroll, 1957). Gilman *et al.* (1989) reported a significant positive association between total childhood cancer deaths and analgesics and antipyretics, with a relative risk of 1.4 (*p* < 0.01). This seems to have been due largely to solid cancers (RR = 1.5, *p* < 0.01), with no marked elevation in risk for neoplasms of the reticuloendothelial system. Illnesses producing hyperthermia were associated with an increased relative risk of childhood cancer; this was mainly due to the neoplasms of the reticuloendothelial system, not solid tumours. Analgesics and antipyretics formed the majority of drugs classified as being metabolized by amino acid conjugation, the only metabolic reaction associated with childhood cancer in the analysis of Gilman *et al.* The authors note that this metabolic reaction involves the coupling of an amino acid to products of reactions such hydroxylation or oxidation, which often are toxic. The drugs in this category included aspirin, paracetamol and pethidine.

In a large study in Sweden, using data from the national medical birth registration system, there was a positive association between childhood lymphatic leukaemia and maternal hypertensive disease during pregnancy (RR = 1.4, 95% CI 1.0–1.9; Cnattingius *et al.*, 1995a). In addition, a positive association was observed with maternal renal disease (RR = 4.4, 95% CI 1.6–12.1). Mothers with hypertensive disease during pregnancy may also have underlying renal disease. A significant excess of diseases of the renal tract originating before the index pregnancy in mothers of cases with childhood cancer of all types was reported by Stewart *et al.* (1958). This finding has not been replicated. A raised relative risk of ALL associated with maternal hypertension in pregnancy was observed in the small study of Till *et al.* (1979), but not in other studies of leukaemia (Stewart *et al.*, 1958; McKinney *et al.*, 1987; Roman *et al.*,

1997). No statistically significant association has been observed with non-Hodgkin lymphoma (Adami *et al.*, 1996; Roman *et al.*, 1997). In the one available study of ANLL, there was no association with use of anti-hypertensives or diuretics (Robison *et al.*, 1989).

No association between leukaemia and lymphoma and nausea or vomiting during pregnancy (Magnani *et al.*, 1990) or use of anti-nauseants (McKinney *et al.*, 1985; Robison *et al.*, 1989) has been found. In a number of studies of childhood cancer of various types, particular attention was given to a combined preparation of doxylamine, dicyclomine and pyridoxine, marketed from 1956 in the USA under the trade name Bendectin, and in Britain from 1958 as Debendox (Orme, 1985). After the introduction of the drug, there were anecdotal reports of an association between use of the drug and genital malformation, especially in the USA, and the drug was withdrawn in 1983 on suspicion of causing birth defects, although epidemiological studies did not support any major effect (Shapiro *et al.*, 1977; MacMahon, 1981, Orme, 1985; Shiono & Klebanoff, 1989). No association between Debendox and total childhood cancer (McKinney *et al.*, 1985; Gilman *et al.*, 1989) or leukaemia and lymphoma was found (McKinney *et al.*, 1985).

In a few studies, the association between haematopoietic malignancies and maternal use of drugs having CNS effects, other than those used during labour, was investigated. In single studies, no association between leukaemia and lymphoma and benzodiazepines or pheno-thiazines (McKinney *et al.*, 1987), between leukaemia and anticonvulsants (Roman *et al.*, 1997), or between ANLL and sedatives or diet pills (Robison *et al.*, 1989) was found. In a study in the Netherlands, the relative risk of ALL associated with maternal use of sedatives or sleeping pills during pregnancy was 2.9 (95% CI 1.2–7.2; Van Steensel-Moll *et al.*, 1985a). In this study, which was based on a postal questionnaire, the prevalence of use of these drugs by control mothers was substantially lower than that reported in other studies of childhood cancer of various types (Grufferman *et al.*, 1982; Preston-Martin *et al.*, 1982; Buckley *et al.*, 1989a; Gilman *et al.*, 1989; Robison *et al.*, 1989; Birch *et al.*, 1990b; Rodvall *et al.*, 1990; Holly *et al.*, 1992; Schwartzbaum, 1992; McCredie, 1994a), so the association may be an artefact of underreporting by control mothers.

Iron can catalyse the production of oxygen radicals (Halliwell & Gutteridge, 1986). High body iron stores have been associated with an

290

increased risk of cancer of various types in adults (Stevens *et al.*, 1988; Kneckt *et al.*, 1994). There is a long history of prescribing iron supplements during pregnancy to prevent anaemia (Horn, 1988). No association between childhood leukaemia and use of iron-containing preparations during pregnancy has been found (Salonen & Saxén, 1975; Van Steensel-Moll *et al.*, 1985a; Robison *et al.*, 1989). Anaemia is an indication for giving supplemental iron. In a study based on obstetric records in Oxford, Cambridge and Reading (England) of leukaemia diagnosed up to the age of 29 years, in which 92% of 143 cases were diagnosed at ages of 14 years or less, a positive association with anaemia was found (RR = 2.4, 95% CI 1.2–5.0; Roman *et al*, 1997). Of the mothers diagnosed with anaemia, 11 cases and six controls had at least one haemoglobin measurement below 10 g/100 ml (RR = 3.8, 95% CI 1.3–11.1). In a small study in Japan, no association between anaemia and ALL of the non T-cell type was found (Nishi & Miyake, 1989).

In a multicentre study of infant leukaemia in the USA, there were suggestions of positive associations with maternal use of laxatives and anti-diarrhoeal medications around the time of the index pregnancy (Ross *et al.*, 1996b). There was no association with urinary tract infection during pregnancy or with warts for which treatment was reported. Some treatments for these conditions may inhibit topoisomerase II activity; inhibition of this activity has been postulated to cause abnormalities involving chromosomal band 11q23 (see section on maternal diet in Chapter 8 for further comment).

*Ultrasound examinations*

In three case–control studies in Great Britain, no association was found between routine ultrasound exposure in pregnancy and childhood leukaemia or childhood cancer overall (Cartwright *et al.*, 1984; Kinnier-Wilson & Waterhouse, 1984; Sorahan *et al.*, 1995b). The study of Cartwright *et al.* (1984) related to 149 cases of ALL, 77 cases of CNS tumours and 329 cases with other types of childhood malignancy, and two matched controls for each case, one selected from hospital lists, the other from general-practitioner lists. The study of Kinnier-Wilson and Waterhouse (1984) was of 665 deaths due to leukaemia and 1066 deaths due to solid tumours during the period 1972–81, and living controls matched for sex, age and locality. While no overall association was observed for leukaemia or solid tumours, a significant

increase in risk was found for the group of children who died of cancer at the age of six years or more. This may be a chance finding, as no difference in risk by age at diagnosis was found in the study of Cartwright *et al.* Another possible explanation is selective application of ultrasound to abnormal pregnancies in the early years of the study. For example, six of the 14 cases, but none of the four controls, reported in hospital records to have been exposed to prenatal ultrasound had also been exposed to prenatal X-rays. Subsequently, a study of deaths in the period 1982–84 was undertaken (Sorahan *et al.*, 1995b); cases included in the study of Cartwright *et al.* (1984) were excluded. There was no association between exposure to ultrasound in pregnancy and death of the offspring from a neoplasm of the reticuloen-dothelial system (212 cases), a solid tumour (308 cases) or from childhood cancer overall (520 cases). In addition, there was no suggestion of an increased risk for children aged six years or more. The study was limited by a poor participation rate (38%). No association between childhood leukaemia, either overall or ALL and AML specifically, diagnosed at 18 months of age or less, and intrauterine exposure to ultrasound was observed in a multicentre study in the USA and Canada (Shu *et al.*, 1994b). In addition, no association with ultrasound was observed in a population-based study of AML in the Netherlands (van Duijn *et al.*, 1994) or in a small hospital-based study of leukaemia in Mexico (Fajardo-Gutiérrez *et al.*, 1993a).

## Central nervous system tumours

### *Maternal age*

No consistent association is apparent between maternal age and CNS tumours overall (Hirayama, 1979; Johnson *et al.*, 1987; Nasca *et al.*, 1988; Birch *et al.*, 1990b), brain tumours (MacMahon & Newill, 1962; Salonen & Saxén, 1975; Gold *et al.*, 1979; Wilkins & Koutras, 1988; Wilkins & Sinks, 1990; Emerson *et al.*, 1991; Gold *et al.*, 1994; Cordier *et al.*, 1994; McCredie *et al.*, 1994b; Linet *et al.*, 1996), astrocytoma (Kuijten *et al.*, 1990; Emerson *et al.*, 1991; Bunin *et al.*, 1994b; Linet *et al.*, 1996) or other types of brain tumour (Bunin *et al.*, 1994b; Linet *et al.*, 1996).

### *Birth order and prior fetal loss*

No consistent association between tumours of the CNS and birth order or prior fetal loss has been observed (Table 9.5).

## Table 9.5. Associations between childhood tumours of the central nervous system and previous reproductive history

| Area and period of study | Cases: Dead (D), newly incident (I) or prevalent (P), upper age limit | Number | Type of controls | Source of information on exposure | RR in first born vs later births | Prior miscarriage and/or stillbirth: Type of event | Proportion of controls reporting history of this (%) | RR | Other aspects of reproductive history | Reference |
|---|---|---|---|---|---|---|---|---|---|---|
| **Central nervous system tumours** | | | | | | | | | | |
| USA, Texas, 1964–80 | D, 15 | 499 | P | B | 1.0[a] | – | – | – | – | Johnson et al., 1987 |
| UK, Northwest, West Midlands and Yorkshire, 1980–83 | I, 14 | 78 | H, GP | I | – | M / SB | NS / NS | 1.0[a] / 1.0[a] | No association with total pregnancies or live births by sex, terminations or twin pregnancies | Birch et al., 1990b |
| **Brain tumours** | | | | | | | | | | |
| USA, Northeast Region, 1947–58 | D, 14 | 777 | P | B | 1.0 | SB | 6.1 | 0.8 | – | MacMahon & Newill, 1962 |
| USA, Baltimore, 1965–75 | P, 19 | 84 | P / C | I / I | 1.7 / 1.1 | – | – | – | – | Gold et al., 1979 |
| USA, Los Angeles County, 1972–77 | I, 24 | 226 | E, N | I | 1.0[a] | A | NS | 1.0[a] | – | Preston-Martin et al., 1982 |
| USA, Ohio, 1959–79 | D, 19 | 491 | P | B | 1.0[a] | – | – | – | – | Wilkins & Koutras, 1988 |
| Canada, Southern Ontario, 1977–83 | I, 19 | 74 | P | I | 0.5* | A | 3.6 | 0.5 | – | Howe et al., 1989 |
| USA, Washington State, 1974–86 | I, 10 | 157 | P | B | 1.1 | M or SB | 32.2[b] | 1.3 | – | Emerson et al., 1991 |
| France, Ile de France, 1985–87 | I, 14 | 75 | P | I | 1.3[c] | M | 15.0 | 1.5 | – | Cordier et al., 1994 |
| Sweden, 1973–89 | I, 16 | 570 | P | B | 1.2* | M[d] | 13.3 | 0.5 | – | Linet et al., 1996 |
| Australia, New South Wales, 1985–89 | I, 14 | 82 | P | I | 1.1 | M | NS | 0.9 | – | McCredie et al., 1994a,b |
| USA, Denver, CO, 1976–83 | I, 14 | 47 | RDD | I | 1.1[e] | M | 16.8[f] | 1.2[g] | – | Savitz & Ananth, 1994 |
| **Astrocytoma** | | | | | | | | | | |
| USA, Pennsylvania, New Jersey and Delaware, 1980–86 | I, 14 | 163 | RDD | I | 1.0 | M or SB | NS | 0.5 | – | Kuijten et al., 1990 |
| USA, Washington State, 1974–86 | I, 10 | 70 | P | B | – | M or SB | 27.0[b] | 1.9[eb] | – | Emerson et al., 1991 |
| USA and Canada, CCG, 1986–89 | I, 15 | 155 | RDD | I | – | M | 23.9 | 0.8 | – | Bunin et al., 1994b |
| **Primitive neuroectodermal tumour of the brain** | | | | | | | | | | |
| USA and Canada, CCG, 1986–89 | I, 5 | 166 | RDD | I | – | M | 34.3 | 0.5* | – | Bunin et al., 1994b |

NS, Not stated.
* $p < 0.05$.
CCG, Children's Cancer Group.
Control type: P, population based, usually sampled from certificates of live birth; GP, neighbourhood, selected through general practitioner; H, hospital-based; N, neighbourhood; F, friends; C, children with cancer of other types; RDD, random digit dialling.
Source of information: B, birth certificates; I, interview, usually with mother.
Type of event: M, miscarriage; SB, stillbirth; A, abortion (type unspecified).

[a] The authors stated that there was no association.
[b] Assessed only among women reporting any prior pregnancies.
[c] Reference category is two or more previous live births.
[d] Assessed only for subset of 104 cases and 520 controls.
[e] Reference category is parity of 2–3; adjusted for per capita income.
[f] Proportion of total pregnancies ending in miscarriage.
[g] RR of miscarriage among total pregnancies in case group compared with that in control group.

## Other aspects of medical history of the mother before the index pregnancy

Little information is available. Birch *et al.* (1990b) reported an excess of diseases of the nervous system and sense organs in mothers of cases with CNS tumours. The only specific condition accounting for this excess was migraine.

## Maternal illness and use of medications during the index pregnancy

### Maternal epilepsy and use of anti-epileptic drugs and barbiturates

Interest in a possible association between childhood cancer and maternal use of anti-epileptic drugs was stimulated by the observation of an apparent excess of barbiturate use during pregnancy in mothers of cases with brain tumours compared with mothers of normal controls and with mothers of children with other types of cancer (Gold *et al.*, 1978). These observations were based on six discordant pairs. Subsequent studies of CNS tumours and childhood cancer of all types combined are summarized in Table 9.6. The association between maternal barbiturate use during pregnancy and subsequent brain tumours in children (Preston-Martin *et al.*, 1982; Howe *et al.*, 1989), or with CNS tumours in general (Goldhaber *et al.*, 1990) has not been confirmed. In addition, no case of brain tumour was observed in 177 individuals born in Rochester, Minnesota, between 1939 and 1976 who were exposed to anticonvulsants, mainly barbiturates, during the first trimester of pregnancy (Annegers *et al.*, 1979). In a study of brain tumours in New South Wales, Australia, no case or control mother reported having taken anticonvulsants or barbiturates in the month before or during the index pregnancy (McCredie *et al.*, 1994a).

Analyses of a large study of deaths due to childhood cancer in Great Britain suggested an association between total childhood cancer and epilepsy (Sanders & Draper, 1979; Gilman *et al.*, 1989). Gilman *et al.* found that the relative risk of childhood cancer associated with epilepsy when the mothers did not report having taken anticonvulsants was 1.0 (95% CI 0.5–1.8, based on 19 cases whose mothers reported epilepsy and 20 controls). The relative risk associated with reported use of anticonvulsants in the absence of reported epilepsy was 0.9 (95% CI 0.7–1.2). By contrast, a raised relative risk was found for women who reported that they had epilepsy and took anticonvulsant drugs during pregnancy (RR = 2.7, 95% CI 1.3–5.6).

In a record-linkage study of 3727 children of 3758 women hospitalized for epilepsy between 1933 and 1962 in Denmark, 49 cases of cancer were observed compared with 53.8 expected on the basis of the rate in the general population (Olsen *et al.* 1990b). The authors considered that children born after the mother's first admission for epilepsy would have been likely to have been exposed to anticonvulsant drugs during pregnancy. Among 2579 such children, 14 cancers were identified compared with 13.8 expected. There was no excess of CNS tumours among children born after the first admission of their mothers (3 cases observed, 2.2 expected).

No association between benign or malignant tumours of any type diagnosed by the age of seven years and maternal use of barbiturates or anticonvulsants, anaesthetics, muscle relaxants and stimulants combined, was found in the National Collaborative Perinatal Project, a cohort study of over 50 000 women registering for antenatal care at 12 institutions in the USA between 1959 and 1965 (Heinonen *et al.*, 1977).

### Anaesthesia during pregnancy and labour

In a study of brain tumours in Los Angeles County, six mothers of cases stated that they had undergone general anaesthesia during pregnancy, one for appendectomy and five for dental procedures; no mothers of controls reported this (Preston-Martin *et al.*, 1982; Table 9.7). Five of the women stated that sodium pentothal, a barbiturate, had been used. In a study in New South Wales, Australia, the relative risk of brain tumours associated with the mother having undergone dental surgery requiring a local anaesthetic during pregnancy was 2.0 (95% CI 0.8–6.9), and that associated with operations requiring a general anaesthetic was 4.0 (95% CI 0.4–44.1; McCredie *et al.*, 1994a). No association with general anaesthesia during pregnancy was found in a study of astrocytoma (Kuijten *et al.*, 1990).

The role of anaesthesia and pain relief in labour has also been investigated (Table 9.7). In a large study in Sweden, using information recorded in the national medical birth registration system, there was a positive association between brain tumours and maternal exposure during delivery to narcotics (RR = 1.3, 95% CI 1.0–1.6) or penthrane (RR = 1.5, 95% CI 1.1–2.0) (Linet *et al.*, 1996). The association with narcotics was apparent for high-grade astrocytoma and sub-types other than astrocytoma, medulloblastoma and ependymona. The association with penthrane was apparent for high-grade astrocytoma and medul-

## Table 9.6. Associations between childhood tumours of the central nervous system and childhood cancer of all types and maternal epilepsy and use of anti-epileptic drugs and barbiturates during pregnancy

| Area and period of study | Cases | | Controls | | Source of information on epilepsy and anti-epileptic drugs[b] | Epilepsy | | Anti-epileptics/barbiturates | | | Reference |
|---|---|---|---|---|---|---|---|---|---|---|---|
| | Dead (D), newly incident (I) or prevalent (P), upper age limit | Number | Type[a] | Number | | Prevalence in control mothers (%) | RR | Type | Prevalence of use in control mothers (%) | RR | |
| **Total childhood cancer** | | | | | | | | | | | |
| Finland, 1959–68 | I, 14 | 972 | P | 972 | AN | – | – | Barbiturates | 1.3 | 1.2[c] | Salonen, 1976 |
| Great Britain, 1953–71[d] | D, 15 | 11 169 | P | 11 169 | I, MR | 0.2 | 1.8*[c] | Phenytoin / Phenobarbitone | 0.1 / 0.1 | 1.6[c] / 1.7[c] | Sanders & Draper, 1979 |
| Great Britain, 1964–79[d] | D, 15 | 8059 | P | 8059 | I, MR | 0.4 | 1.5[c] | Anticonvulsants / Phenobarbitone | 0.1[e] / 1.7 | 2.7[f] / 0.9[c] | Gilman et al., 1989 |
| Denmark, 1943–86 | I, 65[g] | 49 | Coh | 3727[h] | MR | – | 0.9 | Inferred use of anticonvulsants[i] | – | 1.0 | Olsen et al., 1990b |
| **Central nervous system tumours** | | | | | | | | | | | |
| UK, North West, West Midlands and Yorkshire, 1980–83 | I, 14 | 78 | H, GP | 156 | I, MR | – | – | Anticonvulsants | 3.2 | 0.4 | Birch et al., 1990b |
| USA, Northern California, 1960–83 | I, 19 | 86 | Ins | 172 | MR | – | – | Barbiturates[j] | 22.7 | 1.0 | Goldhaber et al., 1990 |
| **Brain tumours** | | | | | | | | | | | |
| USA, Baltimore, MD, 1965–75 | I, P, 19 | 67 / 71 | B / OC | 67 / 71 | I / I | 3.0 / 2.8 | ∞ / ∞ | Barbiturates | 3.0 / 0.0 | 2.0 / ∞* | Gold et al., 1978, 1979 |
| USA, Los Angeles County, 1972–77 | I, 24 | 209 | E, N | 209 | I | – | – | Barbiturates[k] | 1.5 | 0.7[c] | Preston-Martin et al., 1982 |
| Canada, Toronto, 1977–83 | I, 19 | 74 | P | 138 | I | – | – | Barbiturates or dilantin | 2.9 | 0.2 | Howe et al., 1989 |
| France, Ile de France, 1985–87 | I, 14 | 75 | P | 113 | I | – | – | Barbiturates | 0.0 | ∞[l] | Cordier et al., 1994 |
| **Astrocytoma** | | | | | | | | | | | |
| USA and Canada, CCG, 1986–89 | I, 5 | 155 | RDD | 155 | I | – | – | Anti-epileptic medications | NS | 1.0[m] | Bunin et al., 1994b |
| **Primitive neuroectodermal tumour of the brain** | | | | | | | | | | | |
| USA and Canada, CCG, 1986–89 | I, 5 | 166 | RDD | 166 | I | – | – | Anti-epileptic medications | NS | 1.0[m] | Bunin et al., 1994b |

NS, Not stated.
* p < 0.05.
CCG, Children's Cancer Group.

[a] P, population-based; Coh, cohort study; H, hospital; GP, neighbourhood, selected through general practices; Ins, health insurance scheme members.
[b] I, maternal interview; MR, medical records; AN, antenatal clinic records.
[c] Crude unmatched analysis of matched pairs data.
[d] Studies overlap.
[e] Includes phenobarbitone reported to be used as an anticonvulsant.
[f] Reference group comprises subjects whose mothers did not report epilepsy or use of anticonvulsants or phenobarbitone for any reason.

[g] The average follow-up of children born before initial admission of mother to hospital for epilepsy was 37.5 years (maximum, 65). That for children born after the initial hospitalization of the mother was 22.4 years (maximum, 50).
[h] Total number of children.
[i] This part of the analysis was restricted to children born after the initial hospitalization of the mother, on the supposition that they were more likely to be exposed in utero to anticonvulsant drugs than those born before the mother's initial hospitalization.
[j] The authors state that about 50% of exposure took place only during labour and delivery.
[k] Excluding sodium pentothal used in general anaesthesia.
[l] Two cases were exposed.
[m] The authors state that there was no association.

# Table 9.7. Associations between childhood tumours of the central nervous system and maternal anaesthesia during pregnancy and labour, and procedures involving this, and related drugs

| Area and period of study | Cases Newly incident (I) or upper age limit | Controls No. | Controls Type[a] | Source of information on exposure[b] | Anaesthesia or procedure including this — Type or procedure | Prevalence in control mothers (%) | RR (95% CI) | Drugs associated with anaesthesia — Type | Prevalence of use in control mothers (%) | RR (95% CI) | Reference |
|---|---|---|---|---|---|---|---|---|---|---|---|
| **Central nervous system tumours** UK, North West, West Midlands and Yorkshire, 1980–83 | I, 14 | 78 | GP, H | I, MR | General anaesthesia | NS | 1.0[c] | – | – | – | Birch et al., 1990b |
| **Brain tumours** USA, Los Angeles County, 1972–77 | I, 24 | 209 | F, N | I | General anaesthesia | 0.0 | ∞* | Anaesthesia with sodium pentothal | 0.0 | ∞ | Preston-Martin et al., 1982 |
| Australia, New South Wales, 1985–89 | I, 14 | 82 | P | I | Operation requiring general anaesthetic | 0.6 | 4.0 | – | – | – | McCredie et al., 1994a,b |
| | | | | | Dental surgery requiring local anaesthetic | 3.0 | 2.0 | – | – | – | |
| | | | | | Anaesthesia during delivery | 72.6 | 1.9 | – | – | – | |
| | | | | | Caesarean section | 14.6 | 1.1 | – | – | – | |
| France, Ile de France, 1985–87 | I, 14 | 75 | P | I | Anaesthesia during pregnancy | NS | 1.0[c] | – | – | – | Cordier et al., 1994 |
| Sweden, 1973–89 | I, 16 | 570 | P | MR | Infiltrative anaesthesia | 15.4 | 1.2 (0.9–1.5) | Narcotics | 14.1 | 1.3 (1.0–1.6) | Linet et al., 1996 |
| | | | | | | | | Penthrane | 4.7 | 1.5 (1.1–2.0) | |
| | | | | | Caesarean section | 9.6 | 1.1 (0.8–1.5) | Sedatives and/or hypnotics | 0.7 | 1.3 (0.5–3.5) | |
| **Astrocytoma** USA, Pennsylvania, New Jersey and Delaware, 1980–86 | I, 14 | 163 | RDD | I | General anaesthesia | NS | 0.3 | – | – | – | Kuijten et al., 1990 |
| USA and Canada, CCG, 1986–89 | I, 5 | 155 | RDD | I | Dental or other surgery | 2.6 | 0.7 | – | – | – | Bunin et al., 1994b |
| | | | | | Any anaesthesia during labour | 64.5 | 0.9 | | | | |
| | | | | | Caesarean section | 21.9 | 1.8* | | | | |
| Sweden, 1973–89   low grade | I, 16 | 205 | P | MR | Infiltrative anaesthesia | 16.0 | 0.9 (0.6–1.4) | Narcotics | 14.3 | 0.9 (0.6–1.4) | Linet et al., 1996 |
| | | | | | | | | Penthrane | 6.0 | 1.0 (0.6–1.7) | |
| | | | | | Caesarean section | 9.0 | 1.3 (0.8–2.1) | Sedatives and/or hypnotics | 0.5 | 1.0 (0.1–8.6) | |
|   high grade | I, 16 | 58 | P | MR | Infiltrative anaesthesia | 15.5 | 1.3 (0.6–2.6) | Narcotics | 11.7 | 2.3 (1.1–4.7) | |
| | | | | | | | | Penthrane | 3.1 | 3.5 (1.5–8.5) | |
| | | | | | Caesarean section | 9.0 | 1.4 (0.6–3.5) | Sedatives and/or hypnotics | 1.4 | 0.0 (0.0–4.6) | |
| **Primitive neuroectodermal tumours of the brain** USA and Canada, CCG, 1986–89 | I, 5 | 166 | RD | I | Dental or other surgery | 6.0 | 0.6 | – | – | – | Bunin et al., 1994b |
| | | | | | Any anaesthetic during labour | 60.8 | 1.2 | | | | |
| | | | | | Caesarean section | 19.3 | 1.3 | | | | |

NS, Not stated.
* p < 0.05.
CCG, Children's Cancer Group.

[a] P, population-based; H, hospital; GP, neighbourhood, selected through general practices; F, friends; N, neighbourhood; RDD, selected by random-digit dialling.
[b] I, maternal interview; MR, medical records.
[c] The authors stated that there was no association.

loblastoma. No statistically significant association with anaesthesia during delivery was apparent in smaller studies (Bunin *et al.*, 1994b; McCredie *et al.*, 1994a). No consistent association with Caesarean section, an indication for anaesthetic use at the time of delivery, is apparent.

### Nitrosatable drugs

Many drugs have can undergo nitrosation *in vivo* (Carozza *et al.*, 1995). Antihistamines and diuretics are two particularly important examples.

Preston-Martin *et al.* (1982) reported a positive association between brain tumours and maternal use of antihistamines during pregnancy (RR = 3.4, *p* = 0.002). The main indication for antihistamine use was relief of the symptoms of hay fever. In other studies, no consistent association was found for brain tumours overall (Cordier *et al.*, 1994; McCredie *et al.*, 1994a), for astrocytoma (Kuijten *et al.*, 1990; Bunin *et al.*, 1994b) or for primitive neuroectodermal tumours of the brain (Bunin *et al.*, 1994b). In a large study of deaths due to childhood cancer in Great Britain, no association was found with bronchospasm relaxants (Gilman *et al.*, 1989). This category included the antihistamine diphenhydramine.

No consistent associations between brain tumours and maternal use of diuretics during pregnancy has been found (Preston-Martin *et al.*, 1982; Kuijten *et al.*, 1990; McCredie *et al.*, 1994a).

Carozza *et al.* (1995) investigated maternal gestational exposure to drugs classified as *N*-nitrosatable on the basis of published direct evaluations of nitrosatability and predictions from structure–activity relationships in 361 cases of brain tumours diagnosed at ages of 18 years or less and 1083 controls recruited by random-digit dialling. The relative risk of all types of brain tumours combined was 1.2 (95% CI 0.7–1.9). No clear association was apparent for any subgroup.

### Other maternal illnesses and medications used during pregnancy

No consistent association has been observed between brain tumours and toxaemia, pre-eclampsia or eclampsia (Birch *et al.*, 1990b; Kuijten *et al.*, 1990; Bunin *et al.*, 1994b; Linet *et al.*, 1996), antinauseants (Kuijten *et al.*, 1990; Bunin *et al.*, 1994b), hormones used during pregnancy (Gold *et al.*, 1979; Nass, 1989; Bunin *et al.*, 1994b; McCredie *et al.*, 1994a) or hormonal pregnancy tests (Birch *et al.*, 1990b). In a large study in Sweden, using information recorded in the national medical birth registration system, a positive association was found with oral contraceptive use in the three-month period preceding conception (RR = 1.6, 95% CI 1.0–2.8; Linet *et al.*, 1996). There was no association with use reported to have occurred within 30 days of the estimated date of conception. No association with preconceptional use of oral contraceptives was found in a small study in northern England (Birch *et al.*, 1990b), but the statistical power of this study was substantially lower than that of Linet *et al.* (1996).

In a few studies, the association between brain tumours and maternal use of medications having effects on the CNS other than anticonvulsants and drugs used during labour has been investigated. No association between medications such as sedatives, tranquillizers, diet pills or antidepressants and brain tumours has been found (Preston-Martin *et al.*, 1982; Birch *et al.*, 1990b; Kuijten *et al.*, 1990; Bunin *et al.*, 1994b; McCredie *et al.*, 1994a).

In three studies, data on the association between brain tumours and use of analgesics not related to anaesthetic use were presented. Bunin *et al.* (1994b) reported a relative risk associated with maternal use of prescription pain medications of 2.9 (95% CI 0.7–12.1) for astrocytoma and 2.2 (95% CI 0.7–7.5) for primitive neuroectodermal tumours of the brain. McCredie *et al.* (1994a) found a relative risk for all types of brain tumour combined and use of non-prescription drugs for pain of 2.2 (95% CI 0.7–6.6), and use of cold or cough remedies of 3.1 (95% CI 0.7–14.4). Preston-Martin *et al.* (1982) found no association between brain tumours and maternal use of aspirin during pregnancy.

No association between maternal ultrasound examination during pregnancy and brain tumours has been observed (Kinnier-Wilson & Waterhouse, 1984; Bunin *et al.*, 1994b; McCredie *et al.*, 1994a).

## Neuroblastoma

### Maternal age, birth order and prior fetal loss

There is no consistent association between maternal age and neuroblastoma (Hirayama, 1979; Greenberg, 1983; Johnson & Spitz, 1985; Carlsen, 1986; Kramer *et al.*, 1987; Neglia *et al.*, 1988; Schwartzbaum, 1992; Michaelis *et al.*, 1996; Michalek *et al.*, 1996). In addition, no consistent association with birth order or prior fetal loss has been found (Table 9.8).

## Table 9.8. Associations between childhood neuroblastoma and previous reproductive history

| Area and period of study | Cases: Dead (D), or newly incident (I), upper age limit | Number | Type of controls | Source of information on exposure | RR in first born vs later births | Prior miscarriage and/or stillbirth: Type of event | Proportion of controls reporting history of this (%) | RR | Other aspects of reproductive history | Reference |
|---|---|---|---|---|---|---|---|---|---|---|
| USA, North Carolina, 1972–81 | I, 14 | 104 | H P | MR B | 2.3*[a] 1.3[a] | SB SB | NS NS | 0.7[b] 0.9[b] | – | Greenberg, 1983 |
| USA, Texas, 1964–68 | D, 14 | 157 | P | B | 1.0[c] | M or SB | NS | 1.0[c] | – | Johnson & Spitz, 1985 |
| USA, Greater Philadelphia, 1970–83 | I, 14 | 104 | RDD | I | – | M | 13.0[d] | 1.0[e] | – | Kramer et al., 1987 |
| USA, Minnesota, 1968–NS | I, 9 | 97 | P | B | 1.2 | M or SB | 25.5 | 0.5* | No association with immediately preceding pregnancy ending in fetal loss. | Neglia et al., 1988 |
| USA, Memphis, Tennessee, 1979–68 | I, 8 | 101 | C | I | 1.0 | M or SB | 16.1 | 1.8* | RR associated with the immediately preceding pregnancy ending in fetal loss was 1.7. | Schwartzbaum, 1992 |
| USA, New York State (excl. City), 1976–87 | I, 14 | 183 | B | I | 1.3 | – | – | – | – | Michalek et al., 1996 |

NS, Not stated.
* $p < 0.05$.
Control type: H, hospital-based; P, population-based, usually sampled from certificates of live births; RDD, random-digit dialling; C, children with cancer of other types.
Source of information: MR, medical records; B, birth certificates; I, interview.
Type of event: M, miscarriage; SB, stillbirth.

[a] Reference category is birth orders of five or more.
[b] Per stillbirth.
[c] The authors state that there was no association.
[d] Proportion of total pregnancies ending in miscarriage.
[e] RR of miscarriage among total pregnancies in case group compared with that in control group.

## Other aspects of medical history of the mother before the index pregnancy

In one study of neuroblastoma, maternal medical history was examined with particular emphasis placed on a history of disorders of the CNS and on hereditary diseases (Kramer *et al.*, 1987). Of the 104 pairs of mothers in the study, 103 were negative for a history of epilepsy, seizures or other disorders of the CNS.

## Pregnancy hypertension and diuretics

Kramer *et al.* (1987) reported a positive association between neuroblastoma and both high blood pressure and toxaemia during pregnancy, based on 104 case–control pairs. However, these findings were not replicated in another study of 183 case–control pairs (Michalek *et al.*, 1996).

In the study of Kramer *et al.* (1987), positive associations with diuretic use were recorded in a comparison with controls selected by random-digit dialling (RR = 5.8, $p$ = 0.001, one-sided) and in comparison with siblings (RR = 3.0, $p$ = 0.01, one-sided). Comparison of maternal reporting of pre-eclampsia, toxaemia or high blood pressure during pregnancy after the event with medical records indicates a moderate level of agreement, (kappa between 0.4 and 0.7) (Cartwright & Smith, 1979; Martin, 1987; Little, 1992). Kramer *et al.* (1987) suggest that water retention during pregnancy, as well as toxaemia and high blood pressure, may be a consequence of increased catecholamine levels during pregnancy, which are synthesized and secreted by the majority of neuroblastomas. In the hospital-based study of Schwartzbaum (1992), the relative risk of neuroblastoma associated with use of diuretics for high blood pressure was 4.1 (95% CI 1.0–16.9, based on four exposed cases), while that associated with use of diuretics for other reasons was 1.7 (95% CI 0.4–6.5, based on three exposed cases). In the study of Michalek *et al.*, (1996), there was no association with drugs taken in pregnancy for water retention. In a study carried out in Germany in areas with high levels of caesium-137 contamination following the Chernobyl accident, no mothers of 67 cases or of 120 controls reported use of diuretics during pregnancy in response to a specific question about use of this drug (Michaelis *et al.*, 1996).

## Hormone treatment

Kramer *et al.* (1987) considered the association between maternal exposure to sex hormones before or during the index pregnancy and neuroblastoma, primarily because diethylstilbe-strol had been recognized as a transplacental human carcinogen. In a comparison of 104 cases and a similar number of controls recruited by random-digit dialling in the Greater Delaware Valley (USA), the relative risk associated with use of sex hormones in the three months before or during the index pregnancy was 2.3 ($p$ = 0.03, one-sided). Other than accidental oral contraceptive use, the main reason given for taking sex hormones was bleeding during pregnancy. In a comparison of 101 cases of neuroblastoma and 690 controls with other types of childhood cancer treated at a tertiary referral centre in Memphis (USA), no association with sex hormones was apparent (Schwartzbaum, 1992). The participation rates in this study were low, and the sociodemographic characteristics of the cases and controls whose mothers were interviewed differed from those for whom maternal interviews were not carried out. In a population-based case–control study in New York State, a positive association between neuroblastoma and use of sex hormones in pregnancy was found (RR = 3.0, 95% CI 1.3–6.9; Michalek *et al.*, 1996). 14 of 183 cases and 10 of 372 controls were exposed. The main reasons reported for hormone use were infertility, vaginal bleeding, maintaining the pregnancy and a past history of miscarriage. Information on oral contraceptive use was not sought. It would seem worthwhile to investigate the relation between neuroblastoma and intrauterine exposure to sex hormones in other studies.

Neuroectodermal tumours occurred in three of 2285 live births after conception by *in vitro* fertilization in Australia between 1979 and 1987 (White *et al.*, 1990). Two children had neuroblastoma and the other had medulloblastoma. The reported annual incidence rate of neuroblastoma in Australia is 1.0 per 100 000 children, and that of medulloblastoma is 0.4 per 100 000. The three affected children were conceived between 1985 and 1987. Two further children, one with neuroblastoma, the other with a supratentorial primitive neuroectodermal tumour were conceived during the same period after ovulation induction with clomiphene and artificial insemination. There were no data for the total number of births delivered after a similar procedure. In a series of 6236 cases of childhood cancer diagnosed during the period 1985–89 in Japan, nine cases had been born to mothers who had undergone ovulation induction (Kobayashi *et al.*, 1991). The excess was clearest for neuroblastoma, four cases of a total 187 having been conceived following ovulation induction. The other patients comprised one case of astrocytoma, one of Burkitt's lymphoma, one of malignant lymphoma not otherwise specified, one of malignant reticulosis and a suspected malignant fibrous histiocytoma.

## *Phenytoin*

A number of case reports have associated neuroblastoma with in-utero phenytoin exposure and in some cases fetal hydantoin syndrome (Pendergrass & Hanson, 1976; Sherman & Roizen, 1976; Ramilo & Harris, 1979; Seeler *et al.*, 1979; Allen *et al.*, 1980; Delgado *et al.*, 1980; Ehrenbard & Chaganti, 1981; Koren *et al.*, 1989). However, in a case series from a hospital in Toronto during 1969–86, none of the parents had had epilepsy or had been treated with phenytoin for other indications (Koren *et al.*, 1989). No association between neuroblastoma and maternal use of anti-convulsants during pregnancy was found in the one case–control study of Schwartzbaum (1992), and there was no association with maternal epilepsy in the study of Michalek *et al.* (1996).

## *Other neurally active drugs*

Case reports describing children with neuroblastoma who also had the fetal alcohol and/or fetal hydantoin syndromes stimulated interest not only in the possible role of alcohol and hydantoin in the etiology of this tumour, but also in the role of other neurally active substances (Kramer *et al.*, 1987). These authors defined 'neurally active drugs' as those which have a significant effect on the CNS, including barbiturates, amphetamines, narcotics, tranquillizers, diet pills and muscle-relaxants. In a study in the Greater Delaware Valley, these authors found a relative risk of neuroblastoma of 2.8 ($p = 0.01$, one-sided) associated with maternal use of these drugs during pregnancy. The risk associated with taking these drugs at any time before pregnancy was 1.5 (not significant). The elevated relative risk in comparison with controls selected by random-digit dialling was also apparent in comparison with siblings. A positive association with these drugs was also found in a hospital-based study in which the control group comprised children with other types of cancer (RR = 2.1, 95% CI 1.1–4.3; Schwartzbaum, 1992). However, as already discussed, the participation rate in this study was low.

## *Other maternal illnesses and medications used during pregnancy*

No consistent association has been observed with maternal use of anti-nauseants (Kramer *et al.*, 1987; Schwartzbaum, 1992). In one study, a positive association with nonprescription pain-relievers was observed, but there was no association with prescribed anti-inflammatory agents (Schwartzbaum, 1992). In another, there was a positive association with treatment for acute vaginal infections, and the infections themselves, during pregnancy (Michalek *et al.*, 1996).

## Retinoblastoma

No association between maternal age and eye tumours has been observed (Salonen & Saxén, 1975; Hirayama, 1979). One case–control study of retinoblastoma and maternal illness and medication use during pregnancy is available, a multicentre study in the USA and Canada (Bunin *et al.*, 1989a). In this study, two groups of cases without a family history were defined; (1) "non-heritable", i.e., unilateral without a constitutional 13q deletion; and (2) "sporadic heritable", i.e., bilateral, or unilateral with a constitutional 13q deletion. It was postulated that postzygotic exposures would account for cases of the former type, and prezygotic for the latter. There were 115 non-heritable and 67 sporadic heritable cases. Matched controls were selected by random-digit dialling. For both groups, there were elevated relative risks for maternal use of morning-sickness medication during pregnancy and for use of antihistamines, and there was an inverse association with anaemia. No association with other illnesses and medications, and specifically with previous fetal loss, contraceptive use at the time of conception, morning sickness or bleeding, was found.

## Wilms' tumour

### *Maternal age, birth order and prior fetal loss*

There is no consistent association between maternal age and Wilms' tumour (MacMahon & Newill, 1962; Salonen & Saxén, 1975; Hirayama, 1979; Wilkins & Sinks, 1984a,b; Bunin *et al.*, 1987; Lindblad *et al.*, 1992; Olshan *et al.*, 1993; Olson *et al.*, 1993b; Heuch *et al.*, 1996). In addition, no consistent association with birth order or prior fetal loss has been found (Table 9.9).

### *Other aspects of medical history of the mother before the index pregnancy*

In a study of Wilms' tumour, a positive association with maternal gall-bladder disorder (RR = 9.0, $p < 0.05$, based on 10 discordant pairs) was found (Bunin *et al.*, 1987).

## Table 9.9. Associations between childhood Wilms' tumour and birth order and prior fetal loss

| Area and period of study | Cases — Dead (D), or newly incident (I), upper age limit | Number | Type of controls | Source of information on exposure | RR in first born vs later births | Prior miscarriage and/or stillbirth — Type of event | Proportion of controls reporting history of this (%) | RR | Other aspects of reproductive history | Reference |
|---|---|---|---|---|---|---|---|---|---|---|
| USA, Northeast Region, 1947–58 | D, 14[a] | 311 | P | B | 1.0 | SB | 2.5 | 2.4 | – | MacMahon & Newill, 1962 |
| USA, Ohio, 1950–81 | I, NS | 105 | P | B | – | SB | NS | 1.0[b] | – | Wilkins & Sinks, 1984a,b |
| USA, Greater Philadelphia, 1970–83 | I, 14 | 88 | RDD | I | – | M | NS | 1.3 | Inverse association with history of induced abortion | Bunin et al., 1987 |
| Sweden, 1973–84 | I, 11 | 110 | P | B | 0.9[c] | SB | NS | 1.0[b] | – | Lindblad et al., 1992 |
| USA, multicentre, 1984–86 | I, 14 | 200 | RDD | Q | 1.0[b] | – | – | – | No association with "previous pregnancy history" | Olshan et al., 1993 |
| Norway, 1967–92 | I, 14 | 119 | P | B | 1.0[d] | – | – | – | No association with time since previous birth | Heuch et al., 1996 |

NS, Not stated.
Control type: P, population-based, usually sampled from certificates of live birth; RDD, selected by random-digit dialling.
Source of information: B, birth certificates; I, interview; Q, self-completed questionnaire.
Type of event: M, miscarriage; SB, stillbirth.

[a] Kidney tumours.
[b] The authors stated that there was no association.
[c] Parity was treated as a continuous variable.
[d] Incidence rate ratio for birth order ≥2 vs ≤1 1.0 (95% CI 0.7–1.5).

## Table 9.10. Associations between childhood rhabdomyosarcoma and maternal age at the birth of the index child

| Area and period of study | Cases[a] — Upper age limit | Number | Controls — Type | Number | RR associated with maternal age 30+ vs ≤29 years | Reference |
|---|---|---|---|---|---|---|
| USA, North Carolina, 1967–76 | 14 | 33 | P | 99 | 2.6* | Grufferman et al., 1982 |
| Italy, Turin and Padua, 1983–84 | NS[b] | 36 | H | 326 | 1.9* | Magnani et al., 1989 |
| USA, Connecticut, 1960–88 | 19 | 102 | P | 205 | 1.4 | Ghali et al., 1992 |

NS, Not stated.
* p < 0.05.
Control type: P, population-based; H, hospital-based.

[a] The cases were newly incident in all three studies.
[b] Mean age at diagnosis 6.2 (±4.0) years.
[c] Adjusted for social class.

## Pregnancy hypertension

Following a report of a positive association between neuroblastoma and pregnancy hypertension, this factor was investigated in a case–control study of Wilms' tumour in the Greater Philadelphia area, USA. A positive association with high blood pressure or fluid retention during pregnancy was found (RR = 5.0, 95% CI 1.2–31.2; Bunin *et al.*, 1987). This has not been confirmed in larger subsequent studies (Lindblad *et al.*, 1992; Olshan *et al.*, 1993).

## Anaesthesia during labour

In a study in Sweden, a positive association between Wilms' tumour and penthrane inhalation during labour was observed (Lindblad *et al.* 1992). This was only apparent in the subgroup of children diagnosed at four years of age or more. There was no association between Wilms' tumour and other methods of pain relief such as nitrous oxide anaesthesia. In studies in Norway and in the USA, no association with use of anaesthetics during delivery was found (Olshan *et al.*, 1993; Heuch *et al.*, 1996). No association with Caesarean section is apparent (Lindblad *et al.*, 1992; Olshan *et al.*, 1993).

## Other maternal illnesses and medications used during pregnancy

There is no consistent association with use of sex hormones during pregnancy (Bunin *et al.*, 1987; Olshan *et al.*, 1993). In the one available study, no association with maternal ultrasound examination during pregnancy was found (Olshan *et al.*, 1993).

## Hepatoblastoma

In the one available study, there was no association between hepatoblastoma and maternal age, birth order, fertility, ultrasound examination during pregnancy, or use of anti-hypertensives, diuretics, oral contraceptives and other exogenous hormones, anti-nausea medications, sedatives, tranquillizers, diet pills, cold or cough remedies or other medications during the index pregnancy or the year before it (Buckley *et al.*, 1989a).

## Bone tumours

No consistent association is apparent between maternal age and childhood bone tumours (Salonen & Saxén, 1975; Hirayama, 1979; Hartley *et al.*, 1988b).

Two studies of Ewing's sarcoma are available, both from the USA. One was of 43 cases aged up to 31 years at diagnosis and 193 controls selected by random-digit dialling (Holly *et al.*, 1992), and the other was of 208 cases diagnosed at ages up to 22 years, with a similar number of controls selected by random-digit dialling, and 191 sib controls (Winn *et al.*, 1992). There was no association with maternal age, number of previous pregnancies or with reported difficulty in becoming pregnant in the study of Winn *et al.* (1992). In the study of Holly *et al.* (1992), elevated relative risks were observed for thyroid hormone replacement taken by mothers during pregnancy and for antibiotic use, but these findings were not replicated in the study of Winn *et al.* (1992). In the study of Winn *et al.* (1992), there was a statistically significant elevated relative risk associated with maternal use of medications for nausea and vomiting in the comparison with sib controls, but this was not apparent in the comparison with controls selected by random-digit dialling or in the study of Holly *et al.* (1992). There was no association with maternal gestational spotting or cramping, severe nausea or vomiting, eclampsia, toxaemia or high blood pressure, general anaesthesia or Caesarean section, use of diuretics or other medications in either study. Thus, the limited available data on Ewing's sarcoma show no consistent association with maternal medical conditions, procedures or medications.

In two case–control studies of osteosarcoma diagnosed at ages up to 24 years, there was no association with maternal estrogen use in the year before or during the index pregnancy, (Operskalski *et al.*, 1987; Gelberg *et al.*, 1997).

## Rhabdomyosarcoma

### Maternal age and previous fetal loss

In the three available studies of rhabdomyosarcoma, relative risks of 1.4–2.6 were associated with a maternal age of 30 years or more (Table 9.10). The association was weakest in the largest study (Ghali *et al.*, 1992); no association was seen when the threshold for advanced maternal age was 35 years (RR = 0.8, 95% CI 0.3–1.8).

In a case–control study in Connecticut, a positive association with a prior history of stillbirth was observed (RR = 3.7, 95% CI 1.5–8.9; Ghali *et al.*, 1992). The finding in a small study in North Carolina of a positive association with a prior history of miscarriage (RR = 1.9, 95% CI 0.6–6.2; Grufferman *et al.*, 1982) appears to be consistent with this. However, in a study in northern England, mothers of children with soft-tissue sarcoma had a significant deficit of miscarriages compared with mothers of community or hospital controls; the deficit was largely confined to the rhabdomyosarcoma group (Hartley *et al.*, 1988b).

There was no association with birth order in the one available study (Ghali *et al.*, 1992).

## *Maternal illness and medication use during pregnancy*

Only one study specifically of rhabdomyosarcoma is available (Grufferman *et al.*, 1982). There was a positive association with maternal use of antibiotics during and in the year preceding the index pregnancy (RR = 2.7, 95% CI 1.1–6.5). There was no association with maternal use of tranquillizers, aspirin or pain or cold remedies. In a study of soft-tissue sarcoma in northern England, a positive association with pregnancy hypertension, defined to include also pre-eclampsia, oedema and albuminuria, was found (RR = 2.7, 95% CI 1.1–7.1; Hartley *et al.*, 1988b). There was no association with other maternal illnesses or medications used during pregnancy.

## Germ-cell tumours

No consistent association has been observed between maternal age and germ-cell tumours (Johnston *et al.*, 1986; Shu *et al.*, 1995a) or teratoma (Hirayama, 1979). In addition, no consistent association between germ-cell tumours and birth order or previous miscarriage is apparent (Johnston *et al.*, 1986; Shu *et al.*, 1995a).

Two case–control studies of germ-cell tumours of all types and maternal illness and medication use during pregnancy are available, one from northern England (Johnston *et al.*, 1986), the other from the USA and Canada (Shu *et al.*, 1995a). One was of 41 (25 malignant, 16 benign) cases and similar numbers of matched healthy controls selected through general practices and of hospitalized controls without neoplastic disease (Johnston *et al.*, 1986), and the other was of 105 cases with malignant germ-cell tumours and 639 controls selected by random-digit dialling (Shu *et al.*, 1995a). There was no association in either study with pregnancy hypertension, toxaemia, oedema or albuminuria, severe nausea or vomiting, threatened miscarriage or bleeding, or medication use. No association with maternal ultrasound examination during pregnancy was observed in the study of Shu *et al.* (1995a).

In a case–control study in the USA, a positive association between ovarian germ-cell tumours diagnosed before the age of 35 years and maternal use of exogenous estrogens during pregnancy was observed (RR = 3.6, 95% CI 1.2–13.1; Walker *et al.*, 1988). However, no association was found between germ-cell tumours overall, diagnosed at age 14 years or under, or specifically of ovarian germ-cell tumours, and inadvertent use of oral contraceptives during pregnancy in the study of Shu *et al.* (1995a).

## Clear-cell adenocarcinoma of the vagina and cervix and diethylstilbestrol

Diethylstilbestrol became available in 1938 and was used in the treatment and prophylaxis of threatened abortion and premature labour (Tomatis, 1989). Before 1970, clear-cell adenocarcinoma of the vagina in young women had been reported on only a few occasions (Vessey, 1989). Between 1966 and 1969, seven girls aged 15–22 years with the condition were seen at a Boston hospital (Herbst & Scully, 1970). These seven cases, together with one further case (aged 20 years at diagnosis) treated at another hospital in Boston, were included in a case–control study (Herbst *et al.*, 1971). For each case, four matched controls were selected from the records of the hospital in which the case had been born, and data on a variety of maternal exposures during pregnancy and during the lifetime of the index subjects were obtained by maternal interview. Seven of the eight mothers of cases had been treated with diethylstilbestrol, starting during the first trimester, whereas none of the control mothers reported this treatment. Six of the eight mothers of cases reported a prior pregnancy loss, compared with five of 32 mothers of controls, and three case mothers reported an episode of bleeding compared with one control mother. Similarly, in a study of five cases aged 15–19 years at diagnosis and eight controls, matched with four of the cases on hospital, data of birth, maternal age and parity, four of the mothers of cases had taken diethylstilbestrol and one dienestrol, whereas none of the control mothers had taken synthetic estrogens during pregnancy (Greenwald *et al.*, 1971). Later, clear-cell adenocarcinoma of the cervix also was shown to be related to prenatal exposure to diethylstilbestrol (Herbst *et al.*, 1972; Noller *et al.*, 1972).

The incidence of new cases of clear-cell adenocarcinoma in the available cohort studies is very low (Vessey, 1989). Giusti *et al.* (1995) estimated that the cumulative risk of clear-cell carcinoma up to the age of 34 years in women exposed to diethylstilbestrol *in utero* is between 1 in 1000 and 1 in 10 000.

## Conclusions

Diethylstilbestrol treatment of the mother during pregnancy has been causally linked with clear-cell adenocarcinoma of the vagina and cervix. The concern raised by this finding appears to have been one of the factors which stimulated investigation of the association between aspects of maternal reproductive history, including the use of exogenous sex hormones by the mother, and various types of childhood cancer.

In early studies, first-born infants had a higher risk of dying from leukaemia in childhood than later-born infants. This association is not apparent in studies based on newly incident cases, most of which are more recent. No consistent association between leukaemia and maternal age has been found. With regard to the hypothesis that maternal fertility problems are associated with ALL (Van Steensel-Moll *et al.*, 1985a), an increased risk associated with infertility investigations and hormonal treatment for infertility in the periconceptional period has been reported in a study in England, but no instance of ovulation induction was reported in a large series of childhood leukaemia cases in Japan. No consistent association is apparent with a history of fetal loss, prolonged interval between oral contraceptive discontinuation and the index pregnancy, although this has been little investigated, or threatened miscarriage during the index pregnancy.

No association between leukaemia and intrauterine exposure to ultrasound has been observed. There are inconsistent findings regarding maternal anaesthesia during labour, but no association has been found with Caesarean section, an indication for anaesthesia in labour, in any study.

No consistent association between brain or CNS tumours and maternal age, birth order or prior fetal loss has been observed. An early report of an association between brain tumours and maternal use of barbiturates during pregnancy

has not been confirmed. In some studies, an association with anaesthesia during pregnancy was found, but no consistent association with Caesarean section has been observed. In relation to the *N*-nitroso hypothesis (see Chapter 1), no consistent association between brain tumours and antihistamines or diuretics has been identified, but the statistical power of the studies to detect this was low. In a large study, a positive association with oral contraceptive use in the three-month period preceding conception was found. In smaller studies with low statistical power, no association with pre-conceptional, periconceptional or gestational use of hormones has been found.

No consistent association between neuroblastoma and maternal age, birth order or prior fetal loss has been observed. In two out of three studies, a positive association with use of sex hormones before or during the index pregnancy was found. This may be consistent with excesses of neuroblastoma reported after assisted conception. In two studies, neurally active drugs other than phenytoin have been positively associated with neuroblastoma. In two of four studies in which the association has been reported, a raised relative risk associated with maternal diuretic use during pregnancy was observed. If confirmed, the association with diuretics may be secondary to water retention consequent upon increased catecholamine levels during pregnancy caused by the presence of the tumour in the fetus.

Wilms' tumour has not consistently been associated with maternal age, birth order or prior fetal loss. No consistent association with pregnancy hypertension, anaesthesia during labour or use of sex hormones has been observed. In a single study, a positive association with maternal gall-bladder disorders was reported.

There is some evidence that the risk of rhabdomyosarcoma increases with maternal age, and in two of three studies, a positive association with a history of fetal loss was found.

The role of maternal reproductive history, maternal illness and related drug use has been little investigated for other types of childhood cancer.

# Chapter 10

# Medical history of the index child

In this chapter, the associations between childhood cancer and perinatal characteristics of the index child, namely the multiplicity of the birth, the presence of congenital anomalies, and size at birth are discussed. In addition, other aspects of perinatal health and interventions applied in the perinatal period, most notably vitamin K prophylaxis, are considered. Apart from infection, which is discussed in Chapter 7, aspects of health later in childhood have been little studied. Work on injuries, epilepsy and seizures, which have been investigated mainly in relation to brain tumours, and on growth, is reviewed.

## Perinatal and constitutional characteristics of the index child

### Multiplicity

Comparisons of concordance rates between twins of like and unlike sex have been discussed in Chapter 3.

If the intrauterine environment were important in the etiology of specific types of childhood cancer, it would be expected that if one member of a dizygotic twin pair were affected, the other would be affected more frequently than would a non-twin sib of an affected individual. The data available to test this hypothesis are very limited, but it is interesting that for leukaemia at least, in the available series (Table 3.1), no unlike-sex twin pairs were concordant, whereas there is some evidence of an increased risk to sibs of cases with childhood leukaemia.

It has been suggested that the incidence of childhood cancer in twins would differ from that in singletons because of the association between twinning and advanced maternal age, prematurity and other complications associated with twin delivery (Osborne & De George, 1964) and because of differences in prevalence of exposure to diagnostic X-rays *in utero* (Hewitt *et al.*, 1966). Studies in which the proportion of twins among series of cases of childhood cancer was compared with the proportion in the general population, and studies in which the frequency of total childhood cancer in twins was compared with that in singletons are summarized in Table 10.1. There was no excess of cancer in twins in any of the studies.

Three studies have documented an increased risk of childhood cancer associated with intrauterine exposure to X-rays of twins (Mole, 1974; Harvey *et al.*, 1985; Rodvall *et al.*, 1990). However, despite the increased frequency of prenatal X-ray exposure among twins (as high as 50–60% compared with 10% of singletons in the study of Mole (1974)), no excess of cancer has been reported. As noted by Rodvall *et al.* (1992), increased cancer risks would not be expected in the oldest cohorts studied before the time of diagnostic X-rays, for example in part of the period of study in Connecticut (Inskip *et al.*, 1991), nor in the youngest cohorts, born after improved equipment lowered exposures and ultrasonic imaging came into use. The observation by Cnattingius *et al.* (1995a) of a positive association between lymphatic leukaemia and multiplicity (RR = 2.5, 95% CI 1.0–6.0) in Swedish children aged five years or more, but not in younger children, born in the period 1973–89, may be compatible with this pattern. During the 1970s, twins were often exposed to prenatal diagnostic radiation to confirm multiple birth status or fetal position. Given the small numbers in the studies, the power of detecting any pattern of risk in twins compared with singletons in relation to cohort effects such as these is very low.

Hewitt *et al.* (1966) observed that the apparent deficit of twins among cases of childhood cancer in their series was largely of cases with co-twins of like sex. This is suggestive of a deficiency of members of monozygous pairs. Such a deficit could arise if some of the genotypes predisposing to childhood cancer also were associated with an increased risk of embryonic or fetal death. In addition, the sex ratio among cases with a co-twin of like sex was 0.86, substantially lower than in the total series, 1.26. The authors noted that in a series of leukaemia deaths in the north-eastern part of the USA, the sex ratio among

304

# Table 10.1. Associations between childhood cancer and multiple birth

*Comparison of frequency of twin births among cancer deaths with that expected in the general population*

| Area | Births in period | Ascertainment of observed cases | | | | | Calculation of expected numbers | | | O/E | Reference |
|---|---|---|---|---|---|---|---|---|---|---|---|
| | | Cancer (D, deaths; I, newly incident) | Twins[a] | Period of death or diagnosis | Upper age boundary | No. | Denominator or comparison group | Adjusted for excess infant mortality of twins | Other adjustment | | |
| USA, Northwest Region (white population only) | 1947–54 | D | B | 1947–58 | 11 | 61 | Live births in region 1947–54 | Data from New York city 1955–57 applied | – | 0.8 | MacMahon & Newill, 1962 |
| Great Britain | 1939–60 | D | MI | 1953–60 | 14 | 94 | Live births in England and Wales 1950–59 | Infant mortality of twins assumed to be five times higher than that in singletons; weighted average infant mortality, equivalent to that for England and Wales 1950–59 | For increased prevalence of exposure of twins to *in utero* X-ray and increased risk of childhood cancer associated with this exposure | 0.8 | Hewitt et al., 1966 |
| Sweden | 1973 | I | MBR | 1973–84 | 11 | 21 | Total births | No | – | 1.0[b] | Forsberg & Kallén, 1990 |

*Comparison of incidence of cancer in twins with that in singletons*

| Area | Births in period | Ascertainment of observed cases | | | | | Calculation of expected numbers | | | | O/E | Reference |
|---|---|---|---|---|---|---|---|---|---|---|---|---|
| | | Cancer (D, deaths; I, newly incident) | Twins[a] | Period of death or diagnosis | Upper age boundary | No. | Denominator or comparison group | Adjusted for excess infant mortality of twins | Data on incidence or mortality due to cancer applied | Comment | | |
| USA, California | 1940–64 | D | R | 1940–66[c] | 14 | 100 | Direct calculation of person-years | NA | Mortality data for singletons in same cohort | – | 0.9 | Jackson et al., 1969; Norris & Jackson, 1970 |
| Norway | 1967–79 | I | MBR | 1967–80 | 13 | 14 | Direct calculation of person-years by means of record linkage with death register | NA | Incidence data for births in same cohort | – | 0.9 | Windham et al., 1985 |
| USA, Connecticut | 1930–69 | I | R | 1935–80 | 14 | 31 | Indirect calculation of person-years | National data for 1950 were applied | Incidence data for Connecticut 1935–80 | National data on post-neonatal deaths were applied | 0.7 | Inskip et al., 1991 |
| Sweden | 1952–67 | D | R | 1952–83 | 15 | 41 | Direct calculation of person-years | NA | Mortality data for births in same cohort | – | 0.9 | Rodvall et al., 1992 |
| | | I | R | 1958–83 | 15 | 59 | Direct calculation of person-years by means of record linkage with death register | NA | Incidence data for births in same cohort | | 1.0 | |

NA, not applicable.

*a* B, birth certificate; MI, maternal interview; R, registry of twins; MBR, medical birth register.

*b* The authors stated that the frequency of twins among cancer cases was close to that of the total population.

*c* 1966 for leukaemia; 1967 for other cancers.

cases with a co-twin of like sex was 0.74, and that many of the deaths in twins came from a population in which the overall sex ratio for leukaemia deaths was 1.39 (MacMahon, 1962). Hewitt *et al.* considered that these observations suggest some selective elimination of males from the starting population of zygotes with a predisposition to cancer. This would be compatible with the low sex ratio defined among unaffected sibs of familial cases of childhood cancer in Great Britain (male proportion 0.71). In addition, in the British series, a history of threatened abortion followed by onset of malignant disease within six months of delivery was identified for only one boy, whereas it was identified for 13 girls. Although a deficit of like-sex pairs was identified in the series of deaths from California, this was entirely accounted for by leukaemia (Norris & Jackson, 1970). No deficit of like-sex pairs was found in Norway (Windham *et al.*, 1985) or in Connecticut (Inskip *et al.*, 1991). In the studies of Inskip *et al.* (1991) and Rodvall *et al.* (1992), substantial deficits of childhood cancer cases among twin born boys aged under five years were observed. There was a suggestion of this in the data on leukaemia from California (Jackson *et al.*, 1969), but this was not clearly apparent for deaths due to other types of childhood cancer (Norris & Jackson, 1970).

Osborne and De George (1964) suggested that the second-born member of a twin pair might be at increased risk of childhood cancer because it usually receives an extra blood transfusion from the placenta, increasing the chance of the second-born twin receiving hydatidiform, chorionic, necrotic, and other elements from the placenta compared with either the first-born twin or a singleton. In combined data on 154 twins from Great Britain (Hewitt *et al.*, 1966), California (Jackson *et al.*, 1969; Norris & Jackson, 1970) and Connecticut (Inskip *et al.*, 1991), 75 were first-born members of the pair, and 79 second-born members of the pair. In sub-group analysis, Norris and Jackson, (1970) noted that at ages 5–14 years, there were 7 first-born cancer cases and 19 second-born. By contrast, more first-born twins died of cancer at ages 0–4 years than second-born (17 as compared with 9). No significant differences in twin birth order were detectable when sex composition and birth weight were controlled. In an investigation of 1063 twins with cancer diagnosed in childhood or in early adult life in the period 1971–84 in England and Wales, and whose co-twin was born alive, the relative risk of cancer of any type in the second-born twin compared with the first-born was 0.95 (95% CI 0.84–1.08; Swerdlow *et al.*,

1996). With regard to specific types of cancer, the relative risk for leukaemia was 0.7 (95% CI 0.5–1.0). The highest relative risk was for tumours of the brain and nervous system (RR = 1.5, 95% CI 0.8–2.8). Thus, there is no evidence supporting the hypothesis proposed by Osborne and De George. Swerdlow *et al.* (1996) suggested that the excess of leukaemia in first-born twins in their study might be related to the first-born twin being at greater risk than the second-born of ascending infection or of infections acquired during the passage through the birth canal.

It has been suggested that the deficit of childhood cancer in twins observed in several series may be accounted for by the low birth weight of twins as compared to singletons (Inskip *et al.*, 1991). However, as noted by these authors, the association between birth weight and childhood cancer is unclear (see section on birth weight). In California, Jackson *et al.* (1969) observed that 69% of twins who died from leukaemia were heavier than their non-leukaemic co-twin. After adjusting for sex and birth order, there was a statistically significant intra-pair birth weight effect, with heavy leukaemic females contributing most to the test result. No such pattern was apparent for other deaths due to childhood cancer (Norris & Jackson, 1970). Inskip *et al.* (1991) noted that in slightly more than half of the incident cases of cancer in twins, the affected member of the pair was heavier than the other. These authors noted that adjustment for potential confounding was difficult in view of the close correlation between birth weight and other characteristics of pregnancy. In addition, in view of the association between low birth weight and neonatal mortality, variation in the risk of cancer associated with birth weight could be an artefact of differential survival. Inskip *et al.* (1991) suggested that if it were true that there is selective early mortality of twin fetuses or births who would otherwise have developed a cancer, a decline in the deficit of cancer in twins with time would be expected, associated with the decline in infant mortality rates. However, no such decline was apparent in the five successive decades in their study.

## Congenital anomalies

Associations between congenital anomalies and childhood cancer may provide clues as to the possible importance of prenatal exposures in the etiology of childhood cancer (Tomatis, 1989).

Studies in which the frequency of congenital anomalies in cases of childhood cancer are compared with the frequency in control series are summarized in Table 10.2. For each specific type of childhood cancer except Wilms' tumour, soft-tissue sarcomas and bone tumours, the majority of studies suggest a positive association with congenital anomalies of all types. However, the magnitude of the association varies between studies. This reflects in part the play of chance. In addition, the variation reflects differences in the groupings of congenital anomalies considered, and differences in methods of ascertainment. For example, some of the largest excesses were apparent in the study of Kobayashi *et al.* (1968) and Méhes *et al.* (1985). In the former, total anomalies recorded by paediatricians caring for the cases with cancer were compared with those in children seen at an outpatient clinic who had not been referred on grounds of malignancy or congenital anomalies. Therefore, it is possible that the cancer cases underwent a more thorough diagnostic evaluation than the control children, and it is notable that about half of the cases with cancer had minor anomalies only; no figures on this are presented for the control subjects. In the latter, the excesses were apparent only for minor abnormalities which were compared between cancer cases and control children with acute infectious diseases. While there appears to have been a specific examination protocol, it seems unlikely that the examiner would have been blind to the case–control status of the child.

In the studies in which congenital anomalies were ascertained by parental interview or questionnaire (Stewart *et al.*, 1958; Miller, 1963; Ager *et al.*, 1965; Johnston *et al.*, 1986; Bunin *et al.*, 1987; Shu *et al.*, 1988; Baptiste *et al.*, 1989; Birch *et al.*, 1990b; Magnani *et al.*, 1990; Mann *et al.*, 1993; Cordier *et al.*, 1994; Gold *et al.*, 1994; Hartley *et al.*, 1994a; McCredie *et al.*, 1994b; Shu *et al.*, 1995a), recall bias might be expected to have occurred. This would be expected to be more severe for minor than for major anomalies. However, in the study of Miller (1963), the association between leukaemia and congenital anomalies was not apparent for minor anomalies. In the studies of CNS tumours and brain tumours, the relative risks associated with congenital anomalies ascertained by parental interview are closest to unity with one exception. The exception is the study in northern England, where the relative risk obtained from parental interview data is very close to that obtained from analysis of data from medical records (Birch *et al.*, 1990b; Mann *et al.*, 1993). Therefore, recall bias may not have been a severe problem. However, substantial misclassification could have occurred. For example, in a study of the

association between parental occupation in floriculture and congenital anomalies in live births in Bogota, Colombia, Restrepo *et al.* (1990) found that physical examination of the children revealed that 53% of those reported as malformed retrospectively by the parents at interview were normal, and 8% of those reported as normal were malformed. The studies in Norway (Windham *et al.*, 1985) and Sweden (Forsberg & Källén, 1990; Zack *et al.*, 1991; Lindblad *et al.*, 1992; Adami *et al.*, 1996; Linet *et al.*, 1996) were based on medical birth registries, in which ascertainment is likely to be less complete than in registries based on multiple sources (Little, 1992). It is noteworthy that the prevalence at birth of total anomalies, and total anomalies excluding chromosomal disorders, respectively, are lower than the prevalence at birth of total major anomalies in the registries based on multiple sources in Atlanta and Iowa (Mili *et al.*, 1993a,b). It is possible that in a system based on multiple sources, detection of congenital anomalies resulting from the diagnostic work-up for childhood cancer could lead to preferential reporting of anomalies which had not required treatment. However, such a mechanism is unlikely to explain the excesses observed in the studies in Atlanta and Iowa, where only major anomalies were considered.

### Leukaemia

In some studies, the excess risk of leukaemia associated with congenital anomalies appears to be accounted for entirely by Down's syndrome (Table 10.2). The relative risk of childhood leukaemia associated with Down's syndrome is high, around 30-fold (Table 10.3). The proportion of leukaemia diagnosed by the age of 14 years attributable to Down's syndrome was estimated to be 2.7% in the study in Norway of acute leukaemia diagnosed by this age (Windham *et al.*, 1985) and 4.9% in the study in Atlanta (Mili *et al.*, 1993a), while that of leukaemia diagnosed before the age of five years in Iowa was estimated to be 1.9% (Mili *et al.*, 1993b). In record-linkage-based studies in Sweden, the relative risk of Down's syndrome associated with acute myeloid leukaemia (AML) was higher than that for lymphatic leukaemia (Zack *et al.*, 1991; Cnattingius *et al.*, 1995a,b), but the opposite was found in a record-linkage-based study in Denmark (Westergaard *et al.*, 1997).

With regard to other specific types of congenital anomaly which may be associated with childhood leukaemia, an initial report of a positive association with orofacial clefts in a study based on record-linkage in Sweden (Zack *et*

## Table 10.2. Associations between childhood cancer and congenital anomalies

| Area and period of study | Cancer cases | | | Congenital anomalies | | | Number of cancer cases with anomalies | RR | Reference |
|---|---|---|---|---|---|---|---|---|---|
| | Deaths (D), newly incident (I) or prevalent (P) | Upper age boundary | Number | Definition | Method of ascertainment | Prevalence at birth in control series (%) | | | |
| **Leukaemia** | | | | | | | | | |
| USA, multicentre, 1958–61 | I | 15 | 459 | Total major, Excluding DS[a], Minor | Parental interview | 2.0, 2.0, 7.6 | 28, 22, 36 | 3.3[b], 2.6[b], 1.0[b] | Miller, 1963 |
| USA, Minnesota, 1953–57 | D | 4 | 112 | Total, Excluding DS | Maternal interview, verified by medical records | 1.8, 0.9 | 13, 5 | 7.2*, 5.6 | Ager et al, 1965 |
| Japan, Tokyo, 1966–68 | I | NS | 175 | Total | Paediatric examination | 13.0 | 78 | 5.4* | Kobayashi et al, 1968 |
| Norway, 1967–79[c] | I | 13 | 329 | Total | Medical birth registry | 3.0[d] | 20 | 2.4* | Windham et al, 1985 |
| Switzerland, Basel and Zürich, NS | P | 22 | 51 | Minor | Paediatric examination | 38.8 | 37 | 4.9* | Méhes et al, 1985 |
| China, Shanghai, 1974–86 | I | 14 | 309 | Total, Excluding DS | Parental interview | 0.0, 0.0 | 1, 0 | ∞, 0/0 | Shu et al, 1988 |
| Sweden, 1973–84[c] | I | 11 | 411 | Total, Excluding DS | Medical birth register | 4.8, 4.7 | 31, 18 | 1.6*, 1.0[b] | Zack et al, 1991 |
| USA, Atlanta, GA, 1968–87[c] | I | 14 | 116 | Total major, Excluding DS | Registry based on multiple sources | 3.6, 3.5 | 8, 5 | 2.0, 1.2 | Mili et al, 1993a |
| USA, Iowa, 1983–88[c] | I | 4 | 102 | Total major, Excluding DS | Registry based on multiple sources | 4.5, 4.4 | 3, 1 | 1.1, 0.4 | Mili et al, 1993b |
| **ALL** | | | | | | | | | |
| Italy, Turin, 1981–84 | I | NS[e] | 142 | Total | Parental interview | 2.0 | 4 | 1.5 | Magnani et al, 1990 |
| Sweden, 1973–84[c,f] | I | 11 | 332 | Total, Excluding DS | Medical birth register | 4.8, 4.7 | 19, 16 | 1.2, 1.0 | Zack et al, 1991 |
| Germany, Mainz, NS | P | 21 | 227 | Rib abnormalities | Chest X-ray | 5.5 | 61 | 6.3* | Schumacher et al, 1992 |
| UK, North West, West Midlands, Yorkshire, 1980–83 | I | 14 | 148 | Total | Medical records | 5.4 | 11 | 1.4[b] | Mann et al, 1993 |
| USA, Denver, CO, 1976–83 | I | 14 | 71 | Major | Maternal interview | 5.2 | 6 | 2.1 | Savitz & Ananth, 1994 |
| **Lymphoma** | | | | | | | | | |
| Japan, Tokyo, 1966–8 | I | NS | 25 | Total | Paediatric examination | 13.0 | 12 | 6.2* | Kobayashi et al, 1968 |
| USA, Denver, CO, 1976–83 | I | 14 | 26 | Major | Maternal interview | 5.2 | 2 | 1.6 | Savitz & Ananth, 1994 |
| **Hodgkin's disease** | | | | | | | | | |
| Germany, Mainz, NS | P | 21 | 54 | Rib abnormalities | Chest X-ray | 5.5 | 4 | 1.4 | Schumacher et al, 1992 |

| Location, period | Type | Age | No. of cases | Defect category | Ascertainment | % | No. | Value | Reference |
|---|---|---|---|---|---|---|---|---|---|
| **Non-Hodgkin lymphoma** Germany, Mainz, NS | P | 21 | 63 | Rib abnormalities | Chest X-ray | 5.5 | 7 | 2.1 | Schumacher et al., 1992 |
| Sweden, 1973–89 | I | 14 | 168 | Total | Medical birth register | 4.4 | 5 | 0.7 | Adami et al., 1996 |
| **Nervous system tumours** Norway, 1967–79[c] | I | 13 | 215 | Total | Medical birth registry | 3.0[l] | 9 | 1.7 | Windham et al., 1985 |
| **Central nervous system tumours** USA, Texas, 1964–80 | D | 14 | 499 | Total | Birth certificate | NS | NS | 1.0[g] | Johnson et al., 1987 |
| USA, New York State, 1968–77 | I | 14 | 338 | Total | Maternal interview | 4.1 | 14 | 1.0 | Baptiste et al., 1989 |
| UK, North West, West Midlands, Yorkshire, 1980–83 | I | 14 | 78 | Total excluding small birthmarks | Paternal interview | 11.1 | 16 | 2.6 | Birch et al., 1990b; Mann et |
|  |  |  |  |  | Medical records | 5.1 | 10 | 2.7 | al., 1993 |
| Great Britain, 1971–86 | I | 14 | 4698 | Total excluding known genetic diseases | At time of registration of cancer and through postal questionnaire to family physicians | 4.2[h] | 167 | 0.9 | Narod et al., 1997 |
|  |  |  |  |  |  | 6.3[i] |  | 0.6 |  |
| **Brain tumours** Japan, Tokyo, 1966–88 | I | NS | 18 | Total | Paediatric examination | 13.0 | 8 | 2.6 | Kobayashi et al., 1968 |
| Germany, Mainz, NS | P | 21 | 234 | Rib abnormalities | Chest X-ray | 5.5 | 64 | 6.5* | Schumacher et al., 1992 |
| Sweden, 1973–89 | I | 14[j] | 570 | All types | Medical birth register | 4.5 | 25 | 1.0 | Linet et al., 1996 |
| USA, Atlanta, GA, 1968–87[c] | I | 14 | 77 | Total major | Registry based on multiple sources | 3.6 | 10 | 2.2* | Mili et al., 1993a |
| USA, Iowa, 1983–88[c] | I | 4 | 52 | Total major | Registry based on multiple sources | 4.5 | 3 | 2.1 | Mili et al., 1993b |
| USA, multicentre, 1977–81 | I | 17 | 361 | Total | Parental interview | 7.3 | 34 | 1.3 | Gold et al., 1994 |
| Australia, New South Wales, 1985–89 | I | 14 | 82 | Total | Maternal interview | 19.5 | 17 | 1.1 | McCredie et al., 1994b |
| France, Ile de France, 1985–87 | I | 14 | 75 | Total | Maternal interview | 11.0 | 5 | <1 | Cordier et al., 1994 |
| USA, Denver, CO, 1970–83 | 1 | 14 | 47 | Major | Maternal interview | 5.2 | 3 | 1.2 | Savitz & Ananth, 1994 |
| **Neuroblastoma** Japan, Tokyo, 1966–68 | I | NS | 37 | Total | Paediatric examination | 13.0 | 13 | 3.6 | Kobayashi et al., 1968 |
| USA, multicentre, 1941–64 | I | 14 | 504 | Total | Hospital records | NS | 52 | 1.0[g] | Miller et al., 1968 |
| USA, 1960–64 | D | 14 | 1535 | Total | Death certificate | NS | 9 | 1.0[g] | Miller et al., 1968 |
| UK, London, NS[k] | I | NS | 144 | Total | Paediatric examination[l] | 2.7[m] | 5 | 1.3 | Berry et al., 1970 |
| USA, North Carolina, 1972–81 | I | 14 | 104 | Total | Medical records | 10.7[n] | 121 | 1.4 | Greenberg, 1983 |
|  |  |  |  |  |  | 3.8[o] |  | 2.9 |  |
| Norway, 1967–79[c] | I | 13 | 68 | Total | Medical birth registry | 3.0[c] | 2 | 1.1 | Windham et al., 1985 |
| USA, Texas, 1964–78 | D | 14 | 157 | Total | Birth certificate | 0.6 | 3 | 3.0 | Johnson & Spitz, 1985 |
| USA, Minnesota, 1969–NS | I | 8 | 97 | Total excluding those resulting from the tumour | Birth certificate | 0.8 | 2 | 2.7 | Neglia et al., 1988 |

**Table 10.2. (contd) Associations between childhood cancer and congenital anomalies**

| Area and period of study | Cancer cases — Deaths (D), newly incident (I) or prevalent (P) | Upper age boundary | Number | Congenital anomalies — Definition | Method of ascertainment | Prevalence at birth in control series (%) | Number of cancer cases with anomalies | RR | Reference |
|---|---|---|---|---|---|---|---|---|---|
| Germany, Mainz, NS | P | 21 | 88 | Rib abnormalities | Chest X-ray | 5.5 | 29 | 8.4* | Schumacher et al., 1992 |
| UK, North West, West Midlands, Yorkshire, 1980–83 | I | 14 | 30 | Total | Hospital records | 6.7 | 3 | 1.6^c | Mann et al., 1993 |
| USA, Atlanta, GA, 1968–87^e | I | 14 | 5 | Total major | Registry based on multiple sources | 3.6 | 4 | 20.3* | Mili et al., 1993a |
| USA, Iowa, 1983–88^c | I | 4 | 34 | Total major | Registry based on multiple sources | 4.5 | 2 | 2.2 | Mili et al., 1993b |
| Great Britain, 1971–86 | I | 14 | 1208 | Total excluding known genetic diseases | At time of registration of cancer and through postal questionnaire to family physicians | 4.2^h 6.3^i | 71 | 1.4* 0.9 | Narod et al., 1997 |
| **Retinoblastoma** | | | | | | | | | |
| Japan, Tokyo, 1960–68 | | NS | 23 | Total | Paediatric examination | 13.0 | 8 | 3.6 | Kobayashi et al., 1968 |
| USA, multicentre, 1914–69 | I | 14 | 1077 | Mental retardation Other major | Hospital records | 0.4^p NS | 15 39 | 3.2* 1.0^g | Jensen & Miller, 1971 |
| Norway, 1967–79^c | I | 13 | 33 | Total | Medical birth registry | 3.0^d | 2 | 2.3 | Windham et al., 1985 |
| UK, North West, West Midlands, Yorkshire, 1980–83 | I | 14 | 6 | Total | Medical records | 16.7 | 0 | 0.0 | Mann et al., 1993 |
| USA, Atlanta, GA, 1968–87^c | I | 14 | 22 | Total major | Registry based on multiple sources | 3.6 | 4 | 4.7* | Mili et al., 1993a |
| Great Britain, 1971–86 | I | 14 | 549 | Total excluding known genetic diseases | At time of registration of cancer and through postal questionnaire to family physicians | 4.2^h 6.3^i | 36 | 1.6* 1.0 | Narod et al., 1997 |
| **Wilms' tumour** | | | | | | | | | |
| Japan, Tokyo, 1966–68 | | 14 | 19 | Total | Paediatric examination | 13.0 | 11 | 9.2* | Kobayashi et al., 1968 |
| UK, London, NS^k | I | NS | 103 | Total | Paediatric examination^l | 2.7^m | 4 | 1.4 | Berry et al., 1970 |
| USA, multicentre, 1969–81 | I | 14 | 1905 | Total | Clinical records and family questionnaire | 15.6^d | 262 | 0.9 | Breslow & Beckwith, 1982 |
| USA, Ohio, 1950–81 | I | NS | 62 | Total | Birth certificates | NS | NS | 1.0^c | Wilkins & Sinks, 1984b |
| Norway, 1967–79^c,s | I | 13 | 71 | Total | Medical birth registry | 3.0^d | 4 | 2.2 | Windham et al., 1985 |
| USA, Philadelphia, 1970–83 | I | 14 | 88 | Total excl. anomalies known to be associated with Wilms' tumour | Maternal interview | 3.4 | 13 | 4.3* | Bunin et al., 1987 |
| Sweden, 1973–84 | I | 11 | 110 | Total | Medical birth register | NS | NS | 1.0^c | Lindblad et al., 1992 |
| Germany, Mainz, NS | P | 21 | 68 | Rib abnormalities | Chest X-ray | 5.5 | 16 | 5.3* | Schumacher et al., 1992 |
| UK, North West, West Midlands, Yorkshire, 1980–83 | I | 14 | 32 | Total | Medical records | 3.1 | 5 | 5.7^b | Mann et al., 1993 |
| USA, Atlanta, GA, 1968–87^c | I | 14 | 38 | Total major | Registry based on multiple sources | 3.6 | 4 | 2.8 | Mili et al., 1993a |

| Study | | | | Category | Data source | | | | Reference |
|---|---|---|---|---|---|---|---|---|---|
| Great Britain, 1971–86 | I | 14 | 1148 | Total excluding known genetic diseases | At time of registration of cancer and through postal questionnaire to family physician | 4.2[h] 6.3[i] | 106 | 2.2* 1.5* | Narod et al., 1997 |
| **Hepatoblastoma** UK, London, NS[k] | I | NS | 40 | Total | Paediatric examination[l] | 2.7[m] | 2 | 1.9 | Berry et al., 1970 |
| UK, North West, West Midlands, Yorkshire, 1980–83 | I | 14 | 6 | Total | Medical records | 0.0 | 2 | ∞[b] | Mann et al., 1993 |
| **Sarcoma** USA, Iowa, 1983–88[c] | I | 4 | 18 | Total major | Registry based on multiple sources | 4.5 | 2 | 4.1 | Mili et al., 1993b |
| **Bone cancer** USA, multicentre, 1940–66 | I | 19 | 396 | Total excluding skeletal | Hospital records | NS | 42 | 1.0[g] | Glass & Fraumeni, 1970 |
| UK, North West, West Midlands, Yorkshire, 1980–83 | I | 14 | 35 | Total | Medical records | 11.4 | 4 | 1.0 | Hartley et al., 1988b; Mann et al., 1993 |
| **Osteosarcoma** Germany, Mainz, NS | P | 21 | 55 | Rib abnormalities | Chest X-ray | 5.5 | 3 | 1.0 | Schumacher et al., 1992 |
| Great Britain, 1971–86 | I | 14 | 549 | Total excluding known genetic diseases | At time of registration of cancer and through postal questionnaire to family physicians | 4.2[h] 6.3[i] | NS | 1.0[g] 1.0[g] | Narod et al., 1997 |
| USA, New York State, 1978–88 | I | 24 | 130 | Total | Interview with subjects and/or parents | NS | NS | 1.0[g] | Gelberg et al., 1997 |
| **Ewing's sarcoma** Germany, Mainz, NS | P | 21 | 35 | Rib abnormalities | Chest X-ray | 5.5 | 6 | 3.6* | Schumacher et al., 1992 |
| Great Britain, 1971–86 | I | 14 | 396 | Total excluding known genetic diseases | At time of registration of cancer and through postal questionnaire to family physicians | 4.2[h] 6.3[i] | 26 | 1.6 1.0 | Narod et al., 1997 |
| **Soft-tissue sarcoma** UK, North West, West Midlands, Yorkshire, 1980–83 | I | 14 | 43 | Total | Medical records | 2.3 | 6 | 6.8[b] | Hartley et al., 1988b; Mann et al., 1993 |
| Germany, Mainz, NS | P | 21 | 98 | Rib abnormalities | Chest X-ray | 5.5 | 24 | 5.6* | Schumacher et al., 1992 |
| UK, Manchester, 1954–91 | I | 14 | 181 | Serious | Parental interview, verified from medical records | – | 5 | 1.0[a] | Hartley et al., 1994a |
| USA, Denver, CO, 1970–83 | I | 14 | 26 | Major | Maternal interview | 5.2 | 3 | 2.4 | Savitz & Ananth, 1994 |
| **Rhabdomyosarcoma** USA, multicentre, 1941–67 | I | 15 | 280 | Total | Hospital records | NS | 35 | 1.0[g] | Li & Fraumeni, 1969 |
| USA, multicentre, 1982–88 | I | 20 | 249 | Total Major | Parental interview | 18.2 2.6 | 56 15 | 1.3 2.4* | Yang et al., 1995 |
| **Germ-cell tumours** UK, London, NS[k] | I | NS | 96 | Total | Paediatric examination[l] | 2.7[m] | 8 | 3.1 | Berry et al., 1970 |
| UK, North West, West Midlands, Yorkshire, 1980–83 | I | 14 | 41 | Total excluding birthmarks and naevi | Parental report, verified from medical records | 2.4 | 7 | 8.2* | Johnston et al., 1986 |

## Table 10.2. (contd) Associations between childhood cancer and congenital anomalies

| Area and period of study | Cancer cases: Deaths (D), newly incident (I) or prevalent (P) | Cancer cases: Upper age boundary | Cancer cases: Number | Congenital anomalies: Definition | Congenital anomalies: Method of ascertainment | Prevalence at birth in control series (%) | Number of cancer cases with anomalies | RR | Reference |
|---|---|---|---|---|---|---|---|---|---|
| USA and Canada, CCG, 1982–89 | I | 14 | 105 | Total | Questionnaire | NS | NS | 1.4 | Shu et al., 1995a |
| Great Britain, 1971–86 | I | 14 | 544 | Total excluding known genetic diseases | At time of registration of cancer and through postal questionnaire to family physicians | 4.2[h] / 6.3[i] | 43 | 1.9* / 1.3 | Narod et al., 1997 |
| **Total childhood cancer** Great Britain, 1953–55 | D | 10 | 1299 | NS / excluding DS[g] / excluding DS and naevi | Maternal interview | 3.5 / 3.5 / 1.9 | 75 / 57 / 23 | 1.7* / 1.3 / 0.9 | Stewart et al., 1958 |
| Japan, Tokyo, 1966–68 | I | NS | 371 | Total / Major | Paediatric examination | 13.0 / NS | 152 / 74 | 4.6* / NS | Kobayashi et al., 1968 |
| Norway, 1967–79[c] | I | 13 | 885 | Total | Medical birth registry | 3.0[d] | 42 | 1.9* | Windham et al., 1985 |
| Switzerland, Basel and Zürich, NS | P | 22 | 106 | Major / Minor | Paediatric examination | 5.7 / 34.6 | 6 / 72 | 1.0 / 4.3* | Méhes et al., 1985 |
| Sweden, 1973–84[c] | I | 11 | 1268 | Total excluding chromosomal anomalies | Medical birth registry | 3.5 | 44 | 1.0[p] | Forsberg & Källén, 1990 |
| Germany, Mainz, NS | P | 21 | 1000 | Rib abnormalities | Chest X-ray | 5.5 | 218 | 4.8* | Schumacher et al., 1992 |
| UK, North West, West Midlands, Yorkshire, 1980–83 | I | 14 | 555 | Total | Medical records | 4.9 | 60 | 2.4* | Mann et al., 1993 |
| USA, Atlanta, GA, 1968–87[c] | I | 14 | 400 | Total major | Registry based on multiple sources | 3.6 | 31 | 2.2* | Mili et al., 1993a |
| USA, Iowa, 1983–68[c] | I | 7 | 396 | Total major | Registry based on multiple sources | 4.5 | 16 | 1.5 | Mili et al., 1993b |
| USA, Denver, CO, 1976–83 | I | 14 | 242 | Major | Maternal interview | 5.2 | 21 | 2.1 | Savitz & Ananth, 1994 |

NS, Not stated.
*$p < 0.05$.

[a] DS, Down's syndrome.
[b] Crude unmatched analysis of matched data.
[c] Period of birth.
[d] Prevalence at birth in singletons (live or still born) in Norway, 1967–79 (Windham & Bjerkedal, 1984).
[e] Mean age of 142 cases of ANLL and 19 of non-Hodgkin lymphoma was 6.1 (S.D. 3.6).
[f] Lymphatic leukaemia; of 332 cases, 325 had the acute type.
[g] The authors concluded that there was no association with congenital anomalies.
[h] Controls with other types of cancer.
[i] Prevalence at birth of anomalies recorded in British Columbia Health Surveillance Registry, 1969–88.
[j] Ten children born in 1973–74 were diagnosed at ages 15–17 years.
[k] Case records of national referral centre.
[l] Anomalies discovered at autopsy or necropsy were excluded.

[m] Prevalence at birth in population-based study in Birmingham 1950–59.
[n] Hospital controls without cancer.
[o] Cases with Wilms' tumour.
[p] Based on studies of other types of childhood cancer.
[q] Prevalence at birth of anomalies detected by the age of one year in the National Collaborative Perinatal Project (Myrianthropoulos & Chung, 1974). In addition to this control series, the authors considered data from the congenital anomalies registry in Atlanta, GA, unpublished for the period 1968–78, based on multiple sources, but the comparison was made only for specific anomalies. The overall prevalence at birth of congenital anomalies in singletons in these data during the period 1969–76 was 3.3% (Layde et al., 1980).
[r] The authors stated that the frequencies of congenital anomalies among cases and controls were "remarkably similar".
[s] Renal tumours.
[t] The authors stated that reported associations with congenital anomalies were not confirmed.
[u] The authors noted that the frequency of congenital anomalies in the cases with soft-tissue sarcoma was similar to that in surveys of the general population in the UK and in the USA.

# Table 10.3. Associations between Down's syndrome and childhood leukaemia

| Study | Upper age limit | Number of cases with leukaemia | | RR (95% CI) |
|---|---|---|---|---|
| | | Total | With Down's syndrome | |
| Miller, 1963 | 15 | 459 | 6 | ∞ |
| Ager et al., 1965 | 4 | 112 | 8 | 8.5 (1.1–69.5) |
| Hirayama, 1979[a] | 14 | 4607 | 72 | 10.5 (5.1–22.5) |
| Windham et al., 1985 | 13 | 329 | 9 | 38.5 (19.8–74.7) |
| Zack et al., 1991 | 11 | 411 | 13 | 32.5 (7.3–144.0) |
| Mann et al., 1993 | 14 | 171 | 3 | ∞ |
| Mili et al., 1993a | 14 | 116 | 3 | 50.8 (10.5–148.5) |
| Mili et al., 1993b | 4 | 102 | 2 | 32.1 (3.9–116.0) |
| Cnattingius et al., 1995a | 16 | 613[b] | 8 | 20.0 (4.2–94.2) |
| Cnattingius et al., 1995b | 16 | 98[c] | 14 | ∞ (21.0–∞) |
| Westergaard et al., 1997 | 14 | 704[d] | 12 | 32 (18–57)[e] |
| | | 114[c] | 7 | 114 (53–247)[e] |

[a] Control subjects comprised children with other types of cancer.
[b] Lymphatic leukaemia; 609 of the cases had acute lymphocytic leukaemia.
[c] Acute myeloid leukaemia.
[d] Acute lymphocytic leukaemia.
[e] Adjusted for age, sex, calendar period, birth order and maternal age at birth of index child.

*al.*, 1991) was not confirmed in a continuation of that study (Cnattingius *et al.*, 1995a). Moreover, no association between childhood cancer deaths and orofacial clefts as reported at maternal interview was found in Great Britain (Blot *et al.*, 1980b). The distribution of types of childhood cancer among the cases with oral clefts was similar to that in the total series. An increased risk of renal abnormalities detected by intravenous pyelography performed as part of the standard diagnostic work-up in patients with newly diagnosed acute lymphoblastic leukaemia (ALL), compared with data from an autopsy series (Robison *et al.*, 1982), was not confirmed in a study in which renal sonography was carried out (Méhes *et al.*, 1985). An excess of rib abnormalities ascertained from chart X-rays was observed in 227 cases of ALL compared with 200 control children, 30 of whom were healthy and the remainder of whom had bronchitis, pneumonia, trauma, tuberculosis or gastro-enteritis (Schumacher *et al.*, 1992). Excesses were also observed for other tumour types (Table 10.2).

In a study of 20 029 children with cancer in Great Britain during the period 1971–86, excluding those with cancers which could be attributed to known genetic diseases, the frequency of anomalies was significantly lower in children with leukaemia or lymphoma (2.6%) than in those with solid tumours (4.8%) (Narod *et al.*, 1997). This would be compatible with leukaemias and lymphomas being more likely than solid tumours to be due to mutation occurring at later stages of tissue development, in cells committed to form blood and lymphatic elements.

*Lymphoma*

Except in the study of Kobayashi *et al.* (1968), no noteworthy associations between lymphoma and congenital anomalies have been observed (Table 10.2).

*Central nervous system tumours*

The largest study of tumours of the CNS and congenital anomalies was carried out in Great Britain (Narod *et al.*, 1997). In this study, cases with known genetic disease were excluded. The overall frequency of anomalies was lower than that for most other solid tumours. There was an excess of hydrocephalus both in comparison with children with other types of cancer and in comparison with the number expected on the basis of data from the British Columbia Health Surveillance Registry. This may be due to obstruction secondary to the tumour. Spina

bifida and other anomalies of the spine were more common in cases than in the British Columbia series. However, the excess of spina bifida may reflect the higher prevalence at birth in the United Kingdom than in western Canada (Little & Elwood, 1992b). Two children with medulloblastoma were reported to have Rubinstein–Taybi syndrome. This syndrome was not reported for any other children with cancer. In a series of 724 cases of Rubinstein–Taybi syndrome, 4 of 13 cases diagnosed with childhood cancer had brain tumours (Miller & Rubinstein, 1995). In other studies, the highest relative risks of CNS or brain tumours associated with congenital anomalies of all types are of the order of 2.5 (Table 10.2). A statistically significant excess has been found only in one study (Mili *et al.*, 1993a). However, in this study, five of the ten cases of CNS tumour associated with congenital anomaly were associated with hydrocephalus, and in some of these, the hydrocephalus may have been secondary to the tumour. By contrast, in the study of Mann *et al.* (1993), in which the relative risk associated with congenital anomalies of all types recorded in medical records was 2.7, none of the cases with CNS tumours was documented as having had hydrocephalus. In the studies of Mili *et al.* (1993a,b), neurofibromatosis was included among the congenital anomalies. In the study of Baptiste *et al.* (1989) neurofibromatosis was reported by the mothers of 13 cases verified from medical reports, whereas none of 676 mothers of controls reported this disease in their child. There was no association with other types of congenital anomaly. In one study, an excess of rib abnormalities ascertained from chest X-rays was observed (Schumacher *et al.*, 1992).

*Neuroblastoma*

In all but two studies of neuroblastoma, the relative risk associated with congenital anomalies of all types is in the range of unity to under 4, and was not statistically significant (Table 10.2). Any apparent excess might have been an artefact, as a neuroblastoma which undergoes spontaneous regression may be more likely to be diagnosed in children with congenital anomalies than in unaffected children (Mili *et al.*, 1993a).

With regard to specific types of congenital anomaly which may be associated with neuroblastoma, there are case reports of neuroblastoma associated with congenital heart disease (Bolande, 1977; Rosti *et al.*, 1996). Publication bias makes this possible association difficult to interpret, but it is interesting that an apparent predominance of conotruncal heart malformations has been reported (Rosti *et al.*, 1996). While it has been suggested that abnormal neural crest cell migration and development might be a unifying factor which would account for the coexistence of conotruncal malformations and neuroblastoma, there appear to be no reports of an excess of other anomalies of structures considered to arise from cranial neural crest cells, such as orofacial clefts (Werler *et al.*, 1990). In one study, an excess of rib abnormalities ascertained from chest X-rays was observed (Schumacher *et al.*, 1992). The occurrence of neuroblastoma in patients with the fetal hydantoin syndrome has been documented in several case reports (Pendergrass & Hanson, 1976; Sherman & Roizen, 1976; Allen *et al.*, 1980; Ehrenbard & Chaganti, 1981). In a study of 6484 cases of neuroblastoma recorded in cancer registries in seven European countries, there were no cases of Down's syndrome (Satgé *et al.*, 1997). This may be linked with the hypoplasia of the sympathetic nervous system observed in those with Down's syndrome.

## Retinoblastoma

In small studies, retinoblastoma has been positively associated with congenital anomalies (Table 10.2), but there has been no specificity with regard to the type of anomaly. In the large multicentre study in the USA based on hospital records, Jensen and Miller (1971) observed a significant excess of mental retardation among cases of retinoblastoma compared with the frequency among cases of other types of childhood cancer—neuroblastoma, bone cancer, rhabdomyosarcoma and childhood Hodgkin's disease—studied by similar methods. No excess was apparent for other major anomalies. In the large study in Great Britain, an excess of ventricular septal defects was observed in comparison with cases with other types of cancer and the prevalence at birth in British Columbia (Narod *et al.*, 1997).

## Wilms' tumour

The results of studies of the association between Wilms' tumour and total congenital anomalies are inconsistent (Table 10.2). For example, in the largest study (1905 cases of Wilms' tumour), there was no association with congenital anomalies overall (Breslow & Beckwith, 1982), whereas a positive association was apparent in another large (1148 cases) study (Narod *et al.*, 1997). In the study of Breslow and Beckwith (1982), comparison was made only with external data. First, comparison was made

with data from the National Collaborative Perinatal Project, in which the infants were given several thorough paediatric examinations before they were discharged from the hospital after birth, a paediatric examination at four months of age, and a paediatric–neurologic examination at one year of age (Myrianthopoulos & Chung, 1974). The prevalence at birth of anomalies detected up to one year of age in these data was 15.6%, whereas in the series of Wilms' tumour patients, the frequency of anomalies detected up to the age of 15 years was 13.8%. Second, comparison was made with data from Atlanta from a congenital anomalies registry based on multiple sources of ascertainment. The prevalence at birth of congenital anomalies among the cases with Wilms' tumour was substantially lower than in births in Atlanta. As acknowledged by the authors, the periods of study, source populations and methods of ascertainment differed between the Wilms' tumour series and the comparison series. The authors noted that the Wilms' tumour patients were examined intensively at diagnosis and had surgical exploration of the kidney and other abdominal organs which would have tended to elevate the prevalence at birth for some conditions. In the comparison with both external series, Wilms' tumour patients had a high frequency of aniridia, cryptorchidism, hypospadias, and hemihypertrophy. There was also an excess of fused kidney, double collecting system and other anomalies of the urinary system, but this almost certainly reflects differences in diagnostic opportunity conferred by surgical exploration of the kidney and abdomen in cases of Wilms' tumour. The aniridia–Wilms' tumour syndrome accounts for the excess of aniridia, and some of the excess of cryptorchidism. The mean age at diagnosis of boys with cryptorchidism or hypospadias was younger than the mean age for all boys with Wilms' tumour. The mean age of diagnosis for patients with hemihypertrophy was very similar to that of the total series. The frequency of total congenital anomalies in bilateral cases was more than twice that among unilateral cases. The difference was particularly strong for hemihypertrophy and hypospadias and other anomalies of the male genitalia. There was no difference in the frequency of congenital anomalies between unilateral multicentric cases and unicentric cases.

In the study of Narod *et al.* (1997), comparison was made both with cases with other types of cancer and with an external comparison series, the British Columbia Health Surveillance

Registry. The prevalence of anomalies was higher for Wilms' tumour (8.1%) than for any other type of childhood cancer in these data. As observed in other studies, there was an apparent excess of anomalies of the urogenital system. An association with ventricular septal defect, apparent in an earlier analysis of these data (Stiller *et al.*, 1987), was confirmed.

In a multicentre study in Europe (Italy, France, Germany and The Netherlands), the findings of a younger age of diagnosis for patients with aniridia, cryptorchidism and hypospadias were confirmed, as well as the lack of a younger age at diagnosis for patients with hemihypertrophy (Pastore *et al.*, 1988). However, in a small study (176 patients) in Brazil, the mean age at diagnosis of patients with congenital anomalies was higher than that of the remaining patients (Franco *et al.*, 1991).

Bunin *et al.* (1987) reported a relative risk for a Wilms' tumour associated congenital anomaly in the index child of 1.5 (95% CI 0.3–8.3). Although ten of the 88 cases were known to have one of these anomalies, mothers of only five of them reported the anomaly during the interview. Two other mothers of cases reported anomalies that could not be validated in medical or tumour registry records. Thirteen cases were reported to have a congenital anomaly other than one known to be associated with Wilms' tumour (RR = 4.3, 95% CI 1.0–27.6). The anomaly was validated for ten cases. The authors stated that no anomaly or group of anomalies predominated.

Recent molecular genetic studies have identified a candidate gene for anomalies of the genitourinary tract and Wilms' tumour (Francke, 1990; Gessler *et al.*, 1990; Pritchard-Jones & Hastie, 1990).

In one study, an excess of rib abnormalities ascertained from chest X-rays has been observed (Schumacher *et al.*, 1992).

### Bone tumours

In a multicentre study in the USA based on hospital records, bone cancer appeared to be related to a variety of antecedent skeletal defects, but not to non-skeletal anomalies (Glass & Fraumeni, 1970; Table 10.2). The authors considered that some of the excess of skeletal defects in the same bone as the primary cancer may have represented misdiagnosis, and the reporting of skeletal defects of distant bones may have reflected increased awareness among the orthopaedic surgeons who cared for most of the patients. No clear association between osteosarcoma and congenital anomalies has been observed (Operskalski *et al.* 1987; Gelberg *et al.*,

1997). In one study, an excess of rib abnormalities ascertained by chest X-ray was found for Ewing's sarcoma but not for osteosarcoma (Schumacher *et al.*, 1992). Other studies do not show a consistent association between Ewing's sarcoma and skeletal anomalies (Nakissa *et al.*, 1985; Winn *et al.*, 1992; Narod *et al.*, 1997).

In a multicentre case–control study of Ewing's sarcoma in the USA, an excess of hernias and heart conditions was observed in cases compared with one of the two control groups, but not both (Winn *et al.*, 1992). The majority of hernias were umbilical or inguinal, occurred early in life and were surgically treated. The cardiac problems were mainly functional heart murmurs not involving hospitalization or surgery. Neither hernias nor heart defects were associated with Ewing's sarcoma in a case–control study in California (Holly *et al.*, 1992) or in the large study in Great Britain involving internal comparison with other types of cancer and external comparison with data from British Columbia (Narod *et al.*, 1997).

### Soft-tissue sarcoma

No clear association between soft-tissue sarcoma and congenital anomalies of all types has been found (Table 10.2). In one study, an excess of rib abnormalities ascertained by chest X-ray was found (Schumacher *et al.*, 1992).

In a study of children and adolescents autopsied with rhabdomyosarcoma in the USA and in Great Britain (Ruymann *et al.*, 1988), the frequency of anomalies of the genitourinary system was similar to that found in the large study of Wilms' tumour in the USA (Breslow & Beckwith, 1982), while the frequency of anomalies of the musculoskeletal system, of aniridia, and of hemihypertrophy was lower than in that study. In comparison with both the study of Wilms' tumour and with data from the National Collaborative Perinatal Project (Myrianthopoulos & Chung, 1974), there was an excess of anomalies of the CNS, of the upper alimentary tract and digestive system, of the cardiopulmonary system, and of accessory spleens. The authors stated that about half of the anomalies of the CNS would probably not have been discovered except by autopsy, but the frequency of these anomalies was still substantially increased as compared with the other two series.

In a multicentre case–control study in the USA, in which data on congenital anomalies in the index child were obtained by parental interview, the relative risk of rhabdomyosarcoma associated with major congenital malformations was 2.4 (95% CI 0.9–6.2; Yang *et al.*, 1995). Six of the 15 cases with these malformations had developed the rhabdomyosarcoma of the same or at an adjacent site; two had both in the extremities, two were in the genitourinary system, and two were in the head and neck. A further two cases had clubfoot at birth and later developed rhabdomyosarcoma in their arms.

## Germ-cell tumours

In three out of the four available studies, an excess of congenital anomalies has been found in patients with germ-cell tumours compared with control subjects (Table 10.2). There was insufficient information in these studies to evaluate the role of cryptorchidism, a well established risk factor for testicular cancer in adults. High frequencies of anomalies have also been reported in case series (Carney *et al.*, 1972; Fraumeni *et al.*, 1973; Birch *et al.*, 1982). In particular, sacrococcygeal teratoma has been associated with pelvic anomalies such as meningocoele, spina bifida, sacral defects, imperforate anus and hypospadias (Fraumeni *et al.*, 1973), and these anomalies have usually been ascribed to the effects of tumour growth during embryonic development (Berry *et al.*, 1970). This may, at least in part, be a result of particularly careful investigation of the pelvic area. Of the 134 children with germ-cell tumours described by Birch *et al.* (1982), one had encephalocoele, five spina bifida aperta and two spina bifida occulta. Neural tube defects were also present in six of the stillborn siblings of these children (Birch, 1980). However, in another study of germ-cell tumours, the frequency of neural tube defects in relatives was similar to that in the relatives of controls (Johnston *et al.*, 1986). In some series, an association between sacrococcygeal teratoma and duplication anomalies of the hindgut has been reported (Fraumeni *et al.*, 1973; Lemire & Beckwith, 1982). This has given rise to the postulate that sacrococcygeal teratoma is a form of incomplete monozygotic twinning (Schinzel *et al.*, 1979). It has been suggested that sacrococcygeal teratoma is at one extreme of a spectrum of consequences resulting from abnormal segregation of the blastomere, ranging from sacrococcygeal teratoma through fetus-in-fetu, conjoined twins to uncomplicated monozygotic twinning (Gross & Clatworthy, 1951; Potter, 1962).

## Total childhood cancer

The association between childhood cancer of all types and congenital anomalies of all types (Table 10.2) is in part accounted for by chromosomal anomalies. Exclusion of children with Down's syndrome reduces the relative risk from 1.7 to 1.3 in the study of Stewart *et al.* (1958) and from 1.9 to 1.4 in the study of Windham *et al.* (1985). In addition, it is noteworthy that no association was apparent in the study of Forsberg and Källén (1990), in which children with chromosomal abnormalities were excluded. In a study in northern England, a marked excess of congenital anomalies in cases persisted after excluding cases with chromosomal anomalies and disorders of known genetic etiology (Mann *et al.*, 1993). Powell *et al.* (1995) observed that, in Asian children with cancer in the West Midlands (England), congenital malformations, as recorded in hospital notes, were three times as frequent in Muslims (21 of 101) as in non-Muslims (7%: 6 of 86). This excess was associated for by autosomal recessive and dominant disorders.

Except for Down's syndrome and leukaemia, and aniridia and hemihypertrophy and Wilms' tumour, there is little support for specific associations between specific types of congenital anomaly and specific types of childhood cancer. However, most types of childhood cancer are weakly associated with congenital anomalies of all types. If there were associations between childhood cancer and specific congenital anomalies, this would provide a more specific clue as to the nature and timing of the prenatal influence. In the study in Atlanta (Mili *et al.*, 1993a), four children with pyloric stenosis developed cancer (standardized incidence ratio 7.5, 95% CI 2.0–19.3). Narod *et al.* (1997) observed that in six studies combined, including the study of Mili *et al.* (1993a), the types of cancer described in children with pyloric stenosis included leukaemia (8 cases), brain tumours (8 cases), Wilms' tumour (8 cases), neuroblastoma (7 cases), lymphoma (4 cases), germ-cell tumours (2 cases) and retinoblastoma (1 case).

Congenital hemihypertrophy has been associated not only with Wilms' tumour but also with hepatoblastoma (Fraumeni *et al.*, 1968) and adrenocortical neoplasia (Fraumeni & Miller, 1967). The majority of tumours develop on the hypertrophied side of the body (Bolande, 1977). Hemihypertrophy is associated with the visceral cytomegaly syndrome and with hamartomas, and hamartomas have been reported to occur excessively with Wilms' tumour and adrenocortical neoplasia (Miller, 1968).

## Birth weight

Birth weight has been considered to be a marker of potential unspecified intrauterine environmental exposures of the fetus. Gold *et al.* (1979) suggested that the association between higher birth weight and childhood cancer might be related to a greater number of cells in heavier infants. A greater number of cells would result from more cell divisions, which would increase the vulnerability to carcinogenic exposure. The associations between low birth weight and childhood cancer have been less studied than those with high birth weight. Low birth weight in itself may represent either prematurity or intrauterine growth retardation. In developed countries, which are the only ones in which associations between birth weight and childhood cancer have been considered, the most important single factor in the etiology of low birth weight is maternal cigarette smoking, followed by poor gestational nutrition and low pre-pregnancy weight (Kramer, 1987). For gestational duration, only pre-pregnancy weight, prior history of prematurity or spontaneous abortion, in-utero exposure to diethylstilbestrol and cigarette smoking have well established causal effects, and the majority of prematurity occurring in both developing and developed countries remains unexplained (Kramer, 1987).

## Leukaemia

The results of studies of the association between childhood leukaemia and high birth weight are inconsistent (Table 10.4). There is no clear pattern in the inconsistency with respect to study period or geographical area. In subgroup analyses by age, the strongest associations have been observed in young children (Hirayama, 1979; Daling *et al.*, 1984; Robison *et al.*, 1987; Shu *et al.*, 1988; Kaye *et al.*, 1991; Cnattingius *et al.*, 1995a; Ross *et al.*, 1997). However, the boundaries of the age groups differed between these studies. In an analysis stratified by immunophenotype, cases with ALL in all subgroups tended to be heavier at birth than their controls (Buckley *et al.*, 1994). In a recent study in Denmark, there was no association between ALL and birth weight in children aged under two years at diagnosis, but the relative risk of AML associated with increasing birth weight for children aged 0–1 years at diagnosis was higher than for older children (Westergaard *et al.*, 1997). In a combined analysis of leukaemia diagnosed before the age of one year in which data were obtained by maternal interview from three multicentre case–control studies in the USA, Canada and Australia, there was a significant trend of increase in risk with increasing birth weight; this was apparent for ALL (Ross *et al.*, 1997). For AML, the risk was fairly constant over all the weight categories examined.

Doll (1989) suggested that a possible explanation for boys being at a higher risk of childhood leukaemia than girls was that their slightly higher birth weight resulted in their having a relatively large number of cells at risk in the tissues from which the leukaemias arose. If this were true, any association with high birth weight would be expected to be stronger in populations in which the sex ratio in leukaemia cases was high. In the studies in which information on both characteristics was presented, sex ratios ranging from 1.1 to 1.5 were observed in populations in which no association with high birth weight was apparent (Shaw *et al.*, 1984; Eisenberg & Sorahan, 1987; Zack *et al.*, 1991), while the sex ratios in the two studies in which there was an association with high birth weight were 1.2 in Shanghai (Shu *et al.*, 1988) and 1.3 in California (Fasal *et al.*, 1971). Thus, the available evidence does not support this explanation. Ross *et al.* (1996a) postulated that high levels of insulin-like growth factor-1 (IGF-1) might produce both a larger baby and contribute to leukaemogenesis. In many studies, a positive correlation between IGF-1 levels in umbilical cord blood and birth weight has been observed. IGF-1 appears to be important in blood formation.

## Tumours of the central nervous system

There is no clear association between birth weight and tumours of the CNS or brain of all types combined (Table 10.4). However, the relative risks of astrocytoma associated with birth weight greater than 4000 g are consistently greater than unity.

## Wilms' tumour

In the largest studies, a positive association between high birth weight and Wilms' tumours has been observed (Table 10.4). In a large national study in the USA, in which birth weights were available for 46% of patients, birth weights were particularly elevated for patients in whom Wilms' tumour occurred in conjunction with Beckwith–Wiedemann syndrome (*n* = 20), hemihypertrophy (*n* = 45), or perilobar nephrogenic rests (*n* = 304; Leisenring *et al.*, 1994). The birthweights of patients with intralobar nephrogenic rests only (*n* = 266), and of those without associated anomalies or precursor lesions (*n* = 792), were slightly but significantly higher than those of the general population, adjusted for gender, ethnic group and year of birth. This suggests that the growth factor excess postulated to contribute to the etiology of Wilms' tumour (Miller *et al.*, 1964;

## Table 10.4. Associations between childhood cancer and birth weight

| Area and period of study | Deaths (D), newly incident (I), or prevalent (P) cases, upper age boundary | Source of information on birth weight | Total number of cases | Difference between means (cases minus controls) | Association with High birth weight — Threshold> | RR | Low birth weight (<2500 g) — RR | Reference |
|---|---|---|---|---|---|---|---|---|
| **Leukaemia and lymphoma** UK, North West, West Midlands and Yorkshire, 1980–83 | I, 14 | I, GP, H | 234 | Not significant | – | – | – | McKinney et al., 1987 |
| **Leukaemia and non-Hodgkin lymphoma** UK, West Berkshire and North Hampshire, 1972–89 | I, 4 | H, I | 54 | – | 3500 g | 0.6–1.0 | – | Roman et al., 1993 |
| **Leukaemia** USA, Los Angeles, 1936–59 | P, 15 | H | 275 | – | 50th %ile | 1.1 | – | Stowens et al., 1961 |
| USA, North East Region, 1947–58 (white children only) | D, 11 | B | 1323 | 23 g | 3859 g | 1.2 | 0.8 | MacMahon & Newill, 1962 |
| USA, California, 1959–65[d] | D, 9 | B | 800 | 45 g | 3859 g for girls; 4086 g for boys | 1.6[e] | 1.0[f] | Fasal et al., 1971 |
| Japan, 1969–77 | I, 2 / I, 14[f] | CR / CR | 1040 / 2120 | – / – | 4000 g / 4000 g | 1.7*[c] / 1.2[g] | – / – | Hirayama, 1979 |
| USA, California, 1975–80 | I, 14 | B | 255 | 30 g | – | – | – | Shaw et al., 1984 |
| USA, Washington State, 1974–82 | I, 2 | B | NS | – | 4000 g | 2.2* | – | Daling et al., 1984 |
| Norway, 1967–79[a,b] | I, 13 | B | 329 | – | – | – | 0.9 | Windham et al., 1985 |
| Great Britain, 1965–70  girls: / boys: | D, 14 | B, GP, I | 517 / 690 | –34 g / –3 g | 3972 g | 1.0[h] / 1.2[h] | 1.0[h] / 1.3[h] | Eisenberg & Sorahan, 1987 |
| China, Shanghai, 1974–86 | I, 14 | I | 309 | – | 3500 g | 1.7*[i] | – | Shu et al., 1988 |
| Sweden, 1973–84[a] | I, 11 | B | 411 | – | No association | – | – | Zack et al., 1991 |
| Mexico City, NS | I, P, 14 | I | 81 | – | 3500 g | 2.2* | – | Fajardo-Gutiérrez et al., 1993a |
| USA, Canada and Australia, NS | I, 1 | I | 303 | – | 4001 g | 2.3*[m] | – | Ross et al., 1997 |
| UK, Oxford, Cambridge and Reading, 1962–92 | I, 30[d] | H | 143 | – | 3501 g | 1.2 | 1.1 | Roman et al., 1987 |
| **ALL** USA, Bethesda, MD, 1969–70  boys: / girls: | P, 14 | I | 41 / 31 | 57 g / 199 g | – / – | – / – | – / – | Wertelecki & Mantel, 1973 |
| China, Shanghai, 1974–86 | I, 14 | I | 191 | – | 3500 g | 1.5[l] | – | Shu et al., 1988 |
| Italy, Turin, 1981–84 | I, NS[j] | I | 142 | – | – | – | 1.3 | Magnani et al., 1990 |
| USA, Minnesota, 1969–NS[z] | I, NS | B | 219 | Not significant | 3500 g / 4000 g | 1.0, 1.0[zj] / 0.7, 1.0[zj] | – / – | Robison et al., 1987 |
| USA, Minnesota, 1969–88[z] | I, 18 | B | 337 | – | 3500 g / 4000 g | 1.1 / 1.2 | – / – | Kaye et al., 1991 |
| Sweden, 1973–84[u] | I, 11 | B | 325 | No association | No association | – | – | Zack et al., 1991 |

# Table 10.4. (contd) Associations between childhood cancer and birth weight

| Area and period of study | Deaths (D), newly incident (I), or prevalent (P) cases, upper age boundary | Source of information on birth weight | Total number of cases | Difference between means (cases minus controls) | Association with High birth weight Threshold> | Association with High birth weight RR | Low birth weight (<2500 g) RR | Reference |
|---|---|---|---|---|---|---|---|---|
| Sweden, 1973–89[u] | I, 16 | B | 613 | – | 4500 g | 1.7* | 1.0[x] | Cnattingius et al., 1995a |
| USA and Canada, CCG, 1982–91 | I, NS[y] | Q | 990[aa] 404[zb] | – – | 3632 g 3632 g | 1.6[az] 1.4[z] | – – | Buckley et al., 1994 |
| USA, Denver, CO, 1976–83 | I, 14 | I | 71 | – | 4001 g | 0.7[ik] | 0.8[ik] | Savitz & Ananth, 1994 |
| UK, Oxford, Cambridge and Reading, 1962–92 | I, 30[ad] | H | 113 | – | 3501 g | 1.3 | 0.9 | Roman et al., 1987 |
| USA, Canada and Australia, NS | I, 1 | I | 181 | – | 4001 g | 2.5*[zm] | – | Ross et al., 1997 |
| Denmark, 1973–92 | I, 14 | B | 413 | – | 4510 g | 1.5[d,x] | 0.7[d,x] | Westergaard et al., 1997 |
| **AML** USA, Canada and Australia, NS | I, 1 | I | 115 | – | 4001 g | 2.2[zn] | – | Ross et al., 1997 |
| Denmark, 1973–92 | I, 14 | B | 65 | – | 4010 g | 1.7[d,x] | – | Westergaard et al., 1997 |
| **Other reticuloendothelial neoplasms** Great Britain, 1965–70 | D, 14 | B, GP, I | girls: 79 boys: 185 | 20 g –31 g | 3972 g | 1.7[h] 1.0[h] | 1.4[h] 0.8[h] | Eisenberg & Sorahan, 1987 |
| **Lymphoma** USA, North East Region, 1947–58 (white children only) | D, 11 | B | 182 | 45 g | 3859 g | 1.4 | 0.8 | MacMahon & Newill, 1962 |
| Japan, 1969–77 | I, 2 I, 14[k] | CR | 750 | – | 4000 g | 0.3[s] 1.3[s] | – | Hirayama, 1979 |
| UK, North West, West Midlands and Yorkshire, 1980–83 | I, 14 | I, GP, H | 63 | –173 g* | – | – | – | McKinney et al., 1987 |
| USA, Denver, CO, 1976–83 | I, 14 | I | 26 | – | 4001 g | 3.3[jk,zl] | 0.4[zk] | Savitz & Ananth, 1994 |
| **Non-Hodgkin lymphoma** Sweden, 1973–89 | I, 14 | B | 168 | –·–·–·– | No association | –·–·–·– | –·–·–·– | Adami et al., 1996 |
| **Solid tumours** Great Britain, 1965–70 | D, 14 | B, GP, I | girls: 652 boys: 772 | 43 g 11 g | 3972 g | 1.3[h] 1.0[h] | 1.1[h] 1.0[h] | Eisenberg & Sorahan, 1987 |
| **Nervous system tumours** Norway, 1967–79[b] | I, 13 | B | 215 | – | – | – | 0.8 | Windham et al., 1985 |
| **Central nervous system tumours** Japan, 1969–77 | I, 2 I, 14[k] | CR | 1027 | – | 4000 g | 1.1[s] 2.0[s] | – | Hirayama, 1979 |
| USA, Texas, 1964–80 | D, 14 | B | 499 | "None" | – | – | – | Johnson et al., 1987 |
| UK, North West, West Midlands, Yorkshire, 1980–83 | I, 14 | I, GP, H | 78 | –25 g[l] | – | – | – | Birch et al., 1990b |
| **Brain tumours** USA, North East Region, 1947–58 (white children only) | D, 11 | B | 603 | 41 g | 3859 g | 0.9 | 0.8 | MacMahon & Newill, 1962 |
| USA, Baltimore, 1965–75 | I, 19 | I | 84 | 181 g[m] | 3629 g | 0.9, 2.6[n] | – | Gold et al., 1979 |

| Location, period | Code 1 | Code 2 | n | | Birth weight | OR | OR | Reference |
|---|---|---|---|---|---|---|---|---|
| USA, Los Angeles County, 1972–77 | I, 24 | I | 209 | 51 g | — | — | — | Preston-Martin et al., 1982 |
| USA, Texas, 1964–80 | D, 14 | B | 499 | "None" | — | — | — | Johnson et al., 1987 |
| USA, Ohio, 1959–78 | D, 19 | B | 491 | "None" | — | — | — | Wilkins & Koutras, 1988 |
| Canada, Southern Ontario, 1977–83 | I, 19 | I | 74 | — | 3630 g | 1.1 | — | Howe et al., 1989 |
| USA, Washington State, 1974–86 | I, 10 | B | 157 | — | 4000 g | 1.4* | — | Emerson et al., 1991 |
| USA, Ohio, 1975–82 | I, 19 | I | 110 | "None" | — | — | — | Wilkins & Sinks, 1990 |
| Australia, New South Wales, 1985–89 | I, 14 | I | 82 | — | 3636 g | 0.9 | — | McCredie et al., 1994b |
| France, Ile de France, 1985–87 | I, 14 | I | 75 | — | No association | — — — | — | Cordier et al., 1994 |
| Sweden, 1973–89 | I, 14[zd] | B | 570 | — | 4500 g | 1.3[zz] | 0.9[zx] | Linet et al., 1996 |
| USA, Denver, CO, 1976–83 | I, 14 | I | 47 | — | 4001 g | 2.3[zk] | 1.6[zk] | Savitz & Ananth, 1994 |
| **Astrocytoma** |  |  |  |  |  |  |  |  |
| US, Greater Delaware Valley, 1980–86 | I, 9 | I | 96 | — | 4000 g | 1.4[u] | 0.3[p] | Nass, 1989 (subset of data of Kuijten et al. (1990)) |
| USA, Pennsylvania, New Jersey and Delaware, 1980–86 | I, 14 | I | 163 | — | 4000 g | 2.9[p] | — | Kuijten et al., 1990 |
| USA, Washington State, 1974–86 | I, 10 | B | 70 | — | 4000 g | 1.9* | — | Emerson et al., 1991 |
| USA and Canada, CCG, 1986–89 | I, 5 | I | 155 | — | 4000 g | 1.2 | — | Bunin et al., 1994b |
| Sweden, 1973–89 | I, 14[zd] | B | 263 | — | 4000 g | 2.3[f,zx] | 0.8[zx] | Linet et al., 1996 |
| **Primitive neuroectodermal tumour of the brain** |  |  |  |  |  |  |  |  |
| USA and Canada, CCG, 1986–89 | I, 5 | I | 166 | — | 4000 g | 1.3 | — | Bunin et al., 1994b |
| **Neuroblastoma** |  |  |  |  |  |  |  |  |
| Japan, 1969–77 | I, 2 / I, 14[k] | CR | 1041 | — | 4000 g | 1.4[g] / 0.7[x] | — | Hirayama, 1979 |
| USA, North Carolina, 1972–81 | I, 14 | H / B | 104 | — | 4500 g | 6.1[x,u] / 1.8[x,s] | — | Greenberg, 1983 |
| USA, Washington State, 1974–82 | I, 2 | B | NS | — | 4000 g | 2.2* | — | Daling et al., 1984 |
| USA, Texas, 1964–78 | D, 14 | B | 157 | — | — | — | 3.2* | Johnson & Spitz, 1985 |
| Norway, 1967–79[a,b] | I, 13 | B | 68 | — | — | — | 0.5 | Windham et al., 1985 |
| USA, Minnesota, 1969–NS | I, 8 | B | 97 | — | 4000 g | 1.0 | — | Neglia et al., 1988 |
| USA, Memphis, Tennessee, 1979–86 | I, 8 | I | 99 | — | 3805 g | 0.9[u] | — | Schwartzbaum, 1992 |
| **Retinoblastoma** |  |  |  |  |  |  |  |  |
| Japan, 1969–77 | I, 2 / I, 14[k] | CR | 918 | — | 4000 g | 0.8[s] / 0.5[s] | — | Hirayama, 1979 |
| Norway, 1967–79[a,b] | I, 13 | B | 33 | — | — | — | 0.5 | Windham et al., 1985 |
| USA and Canada, CCSG, 1982–85 sporadic heritable non heritable | I, NS | I | 67 / 115 | "None" / "None" | — / — | — / — | — / — | Bunin et al., 1989a |

## Table 10.4. (contd) Associations between childhood cancer and birth weight

| Area and period of study | Deaths (D), newly incident (I), or prevalent (P) cases, upper age boundary | Source of information on birth weight | Total number of cases | Difference between means (cases minus controls) | Association with High birth weight Threshold | RR | Low birth weight (<2500 g) RR | Reference |
|---|---|---|---|---|---|---|---|---|
| **Wilms' tumour** | | | | | | | | |
| USA, North East Region, 1947–58[v] (white children only) | D, 11 | B | 233 | 68 g | 3859 g | 1.5 | 1.4 | MacMahon & Newill, 1962 |
| Japan, 1969–77 | I, 2 / I, 14[k] | CR | 507 | – | 4000 g | 2.0[g] / 2.7[x] | – / – | Hirayama, 1979 |
| USA, Connecticut, 1935–73 | I, 19 | B | 149 | "None" | – | – | – | Kantor et al., 1979 |
| USA, Washington State, 1974–82 | I, 2 | B | NS | – | 4000 g | 3.3* | – | Daling et al., 1984 |
| USA, Ohio, 1950–81 | I, NS | B | 62 | "None" | – | – | – | Wilkins & Sinks, 1984b |
| Norway, 1967–79[a,b,v] | I, 13 | B | 71 | – | – | – | 0.0 | Windham et al., 1985 |
| USA, Philadelphia, 1970–83 | I, 14 | I | 88 | "None" | – | – | – | Bunin et al., 1987 |
| Sweden, 1973–84 | I, 11 | B | 110 | – | 4000 g | 1.2 | – | Lindblad et al., 1992 |
| USA, multicentre, 1984–86 | I, 14 | Q | 200 | – | 4500 g | 0.6 | 0.4 | Olshan et al., 1993 |
| USA, multicentre, 1979–93 | I, 15 | H | 1852 | 120 g | – | – | – | Leisenring et al., 1994 |
| Norway, 1967–93 | I, 14 | B | 119 | – | 4000 g | 1.2 | – | Heuch et al., 1996 |
| **Bone tumours** | | | | | | | | |
| Japan, 1969–77 | I, 2 / I, 14[k] | CR | 139 | – | 4000 g | 0.0[t] / 0.0[t] | – | Hirayama, 1979 |
| USA, Washington State, 1974–82 | I, 2 | B | NS | – | 4000 g | 0.0 | – | Daling et al., 1984 |
| UK, North West, West Midlands and Yorkshire, 1980–83 | I, 14 | I, GP, H | 30 | –284 g* | – | – | – | Hartley et al., 1988a |
| **Ewing's sarcoma** | | | | | | | | |
| USA, San Francisco Bay Area, 1978–86 | I, 31 | I | 43 | "None" | – | – | – | Holly et al., 1992 |
| USA, multicentre, 1983–85 | I, 22 | I | 208 | 28 g | – | – | – | Winn et al., 1992 |
| **Osteosarcoma** | | | | | | | | |
| USA, New York State, 1978–88 | I, 24 | B | 130 | – | 3665 g | 0.9[gh] | 1.9 | Gelberg et al., 1997 |
| **Soft-tissue sarcoma** | | | | | | | | |
| Japan, 1969–77 | I, 2 / I, 14[k] | CR | 219 | – | 4000 g | 1.3[g] / 0.7[x] | – / – | Hirayama, 1979 |
| USA, Washington State, 1974–82 | I, 2 | B | NS | – | 4000 g | 2.7 | – | Daling et al., 1984 |
| UK, North West, West Midlands and Yorkshire, 1980–83 | I, 14 | I, GP, H | 43 | 65 g | – | – | – | Hartley et al., 1988b |
| USA, Denver, CO, 1976–83 | I, 14 | I | 26 | – | 4001 g | 1.7[gk] | 1.4[gk] | Savitz & Ananth, 1994 |
| **Rhabdomyosarcoma** | | | | | | | | |
| USA, North Carolina, 1967–76 | I, 14 | I | 33 | – | 3401 g | 0.9 | – | Grufferman et al., 1982 |

| Study (country, period) | Source | BW source | No. | Difference | Mean birthweight | RR | RR | Reference |
|---|---|---|---|---|---|---|---|---|
| USA, Connecticut, 1960–88 | I, 19 | B | 79 | – | 3349 g | 1.6 | 0.6 | Ghali et al., 1992 |
| **Germ-cell tumours** | | | | | | | | |
| UK, North West, West Midlands and Yorkshire, 1980–83 | I, 14 | L, GP, H | 41 | 229 g* | – | – | – | Hartley et al., 1988a |
| USA and Canada, CCG, 1982–89 | I, 14 | Q | 105 | – | 4000 g | 2.4[v,x] | – | Shu et al., 1995a |
| **Teratoma (benign or of unspecified nature)** | | | | | | | | |
| Japan, 1969–77 | I, 2 / I, 14[k] | CR | 47 | – | 4000 g | 1.7* / 1.5[g] | – | Hirayama, 1979 |
| **Total childhood cancer** | | | | | | | | |
| USA, North East Region, 1947–58 | D, 11 | B | 2802 | 41 g | 3859 g | 1.1 | 0.9 | MacMahon & Newill, 1962 |
| Finland, 1959–68[u] | I, 14 | A | 939 | 30 g | – | – | – | Salonen & Saxén, 1975 |
| USA, Washington State, 1974–82 | I, 15 | B | 681 | – | 4000 g | 1.4[c] | 1.0[c] | Daling et al., 1984 |
| Norway, 1967–79[a,b] | I, 13 | B | 885 | – | – | – | 0.6 | Windham et al., 1985 |
| UK, North West, West Midlands and Yorkshire, 1980–83 | I, 14 | L, GP, H | 555 | Not significant | – | – | – | Hartley et al., 1988a |
| Sweden, 1973–84[zi] | I, 11 | B | 1268 | – | – | – | 1.2 | Forsberg & Källén, 1990 |
| UK, Bristol, 1971–81 | I, 14 | H | 195 | – | 3500 g | 1.1 | 1.0 | Golding et al., 1992a |
| USA, Denver, CO, 1976–83 | I, 14 | I | 242 | – | 4001 g | 1.1[zm] | 1.0 | Savitz & Ananth, 1994 |

NS, Not stated.

\* $p < 0.05$

CCG, Children's Cancer Group.

Source of information on birthweight: B, birth certificates or medical birth registry; I, interview with parent (usually mother); GP, general practitioner; H, hospital records; CR, cancer register; Q, questionnaire.

[a] Period of birth.
[b] Singleton births only; births with congenital anomalies excluded.
[c] Adjusted for sex and year of birth.
[d] Singleton births known to have survived the first year of life and excluding those with Down's syndrome.
[e] Adjusted for maternal age, social class and sex.
[f] Crude odds ratio.
[g] Reference category was <3500 g.
[h] Reference category was 2866–3235 g (101–114 oz).
[i] Reference category birth weight <3000 g; adjusted for age, sex, birth order, rural residence, prenatal and paternal preconceptional X-ray exposure, chloramphenicol and syntomycin use, mother's age at menarche and maternal occupational exposure during pregnancy.
[j] Mean age of diagnosis of 142 cases of ALL, 22 of ANLL and 19 of non-Hodgkin lymphoma was 6.1 (S.D. 3.6).
[k] Age range 3–14 years.
[l] Based on information from medical records. There was no difference between the groups in median birth weight reported at parental interview.
[m] With normal controls. Compared with controls with other types of childhood cancer, the difference was –91 g.
[n] Compared with matched controls with (1) malignancies of other types; and (2) non known malignant disease respectively.
[o] Unmatched analysis of matched pairs.
[p] Category comprises subjects weighing less than 2501g at birth.
[q] Reference category was <1500 g.

[r] Control group was children hospitalized for reasons other than cancer; relative risk in comparison with children hospitalized for Wilms' tumour was 0.6.
[s] Group was population-based.
[t] Term births only. There was no association with birth weight in preterm births.
[u] Controls comprised children with other types of childhood cancer.
[v] Renal tumours.
[w] "Malignant neoplasm of soft part".
[x] Category 3000–3499 g.
[y] The percentages of cases aged 15 years or more were for the pre-B phenotype, 8%; the null-cell phenotype, 14%; the T-cell phenotype, 9%; the common phenotype, 7%; and ALL of unknown immunophenotype, 5%.
[z] Reference category <2724 g.
[za] Comparison with controls with other types of cancer.
[zb] Comparison with controls selected by random-digit dialling.
[zc] Reference category ≤3000 g.
[zd] Ten children born in 1973–74 were diagnosed at ages 15–17 years.
[ze] Reference category 3500–3999 g.
[zf] Reference category 3010–3509 g.
[zg] Adjusted for age, sex, calendar period, maternal age at birth of index child, and birth order.
[zh] Reference category 1984–2977 g.
[zi] Studies overlap.
[zj] One control group was matched on date and county of birth, the other on year of birth.
[zk] Reference category 2500–4000 g.
[zl] After adjustment for maternal smoking, year of diagnosis and wire code; unadjusted RR = 1.1 (95% CI 0.7–6.3).
[zm] After adjustment for year of diagnosis.
[zn] Reference category ≤3000 g.
[zo] 92% diagnosed before age 15 years. The proportion for ALL was 94%.

Olshan, 1986) may not be limited to those with specific overgrowth syndromes. The birthweights of patients with aniridia (*n* = 10) were significantly lower than those of the general population.

## Other types of childhood cancer

No consistent pattern of association between birth weight and neuroblastoma or retinoblastoma is apparent (Table 10.4). Associations between birth weight and other types of childhood cancer have been little studied. In the three available studies, an inverse association between birth weight and bone tumours was observed. However, no association was apparent in the few available studies relating specifically to Ewing's sarcoma or to osteosarcoma. Significant positive associations between birth weight and germ-cell tumours have been reported (Table 10.4). As increased birth weight has been associated with an elevated endogenous estrogen level, this finding may be compatible with an etiological role for estrogen exposure (Shu *et al.*, 1995a). However, in studies of testicular cancer in adults, an inverse association has been found with high birth weight (Depue *et al.*, 1983; Brown *et al.*, 1986).

In summary, the five available studies of astrocytoma, two of which overlap, suggest a positive association with high birth weight. In the largest studies, a positive association between Wilms' tumour and high birth weight was observed. There appears to be a consistent positive association between germ-cell tumours and high birth weight. Some, but not all studies, suggest a positive association between leukaemia and high birth weight, and this may be restricted to young children. The relationship between birth weight and other types of childhood cancer either is inconsistent or has been little studied.

# Other perinatal characteristics and related interventions

## Length at birth

No consistent association has been observed between length of the child at birth and total childhood cancer (Salonen & Saxén, 1975), leukaemia and lymphoma (McKinney *et al.*, 1987; Zack *et al.*, 1991; Adami *et al.*, 1996), Wilms' tumour (Lindblad *et al.*, 1992; Heuch *et al.*, 1996), Ewing's sarcoma (Holly *et al.*, 1992), osteosarcoma (Operskalski *et al.*, 1987; Gelberg *et al.*, 1997) or rhabdomyosarcoma (Grufferman *et al.*, 1982).

## Apgar score

A Swedish record-linkage based study has shown an elevated risk of brain tumours (RR = 1.6, 95% CI 1.1–2.5) among children with one-minute Apgar scores of six or less (Linet *et al.*, 1996). In a Norwegian record-linkage-based study, the relative risk of Wilms' tumour associated with a one-minute Apgar score of eight or less was 2.2 (95% CI 1.2–3.9; Heuch *et al.*, 1996). No clear association between Apgar score and total childhood cancer has been found in the three studies in which this has been assessed (Salonen & Saxén, 1975; Hartley *et al.*, 1988a; Forsberg & Källén, 1990). In an analysis of a subset of the data of Hartley *et al.* (1988a), no association was found between Apgar score and leukaemia and lymphoma (McKinney *et al.*, 1987). In the one available study carried out using methods similar to those of Linet *et al.* (1996), no association was found between Apgar score and non-Hodgkin lymphoma in children (Adami *et al.*, 1996).

## Jaundice

In a study based on linkage of the medical birth register with the cancer register in Sweden for cases born and diagnosed in the period 1973–84, a positive association was found between "physiologic icterus" and total childhood cancer (RR = 1.4, 95% CI 1.1–1.9; Forsberg & Källén, 1990). Relative risks of 1.5 or more were observed for leukaemia, other haematopoietic neoplasms, kidney tumours, and tumours of the connective tissue or muscle. Further analyses have been published in relation to leukaemia (Zack *et al.*, 1991), lymphatic leukaemia (Cnattingius *et al.*, 1995a), non-Hodgkin lymphoma (Adami *et al.*, 1996), brain tumours (Linet *et al.*, 1996) and Wilms' tumour (Lindblad *et al.*, 1992), based at least in part on the same cases, but with five controls per case instead of two.

Zack *et al.* (1991) found a positive association between physiological jaundice and myeloid leukaemia (RR = 6.7, 95% CI 1.9–23.7) but not lymphatic leukaemia (RR = 1.4, 95% CI 0.9–2.4). The lack of association with lymphatic leukaemia was confirmed in an extension of this study (Cnattingius *et al.*, 1995a) and in studies of ALL (Magnani *et al.*, 1990; Buckley *et al.*, 1994; Roman *et al.*, 1997). The positive association with AML reported by Zack *et al.* (1991) remained apparent in an extension of the study (RR = 2.5; 95% CI 1.2–5.0; Cnattingius *et al.*, 1995b). However, when cases with Down's syndrome were excluded, the relative risk was reduced and no longer statistically significant (RR = 1.7, 95% CI 0.8–4.0).

In a hospital-based study in Turin, Italy, during the period 1981–84, two of 19 children with non-Hodgkin lymphoma were reported to have had neonatal jaundice, compared with five of 307 controls (RR = 7.1, 95% CI 4.0–12.6; Magnani *et al.*, 1990). By contrast, in a study in Sweden, no association between phototherapy and non-Hodgkin lymphoma was found (Adami *et al.*, 1996).

In the initial report of Forsberg and Källén (1990), the relative risk of brain tumours associated with "physiologic icterus" was 1.2 (95% CI 0.6–2.1). No association was found in an extension of this study and there was no association between brain tumours and treatment with phototherapy (Linet *et al.*, 1996).

In the one available study on Wilms' tumour and physiological jaundice, the relative risk was 2.3 (95% CI 1.1–5.0; Lindblad *et al.*, 1992).

In small studies, there was no association between neonatal jaundice and rhabdomyosarcoma (Grufferman *et al.*, 1982), hepatoblastoma (Buckley *et al.*, 1989a) or germ-cell tumours (Shu *et al.*, 1995a).

## Photosensitizing lighting and leukaemia

Ben-Sasson and Davis (1992) postulated that exposure to photosensitizing lighting immediately after birth may cause ALL in childhood. The authors noted that there have been persistent unexplained increases in the incidence of this disease in the USA in the past 20 years, while the intensity of lighting in newborn nurseries in that country has increased five- to ten-fold during this period. Strong illumination from fluorescent lamps and other light sources, around a wavelength of 400 nanometres, can activate protoporphyrin. This may lead to production of superoxides and free radicals that can induce breaks in DNA. They noted that the results of the study of Zack *et al.* (1991), in which increases in the risk of leukaemia were independently associated with neonatal physiological jaundice and exposure to supplemental oxygen, being stronger for children born later in the study period than for those born around the mid-point of the study, may be compatible with this hypothesis. In particular, the association with supplemental oxygen may be relevant as the mechanism proposed involves the transformation of oxygen into harmful metabolites. However, it is difficult to reconcile the particularly high relative risk (8.4, 95% CI 2.1–34.1) with this exposure for children born in the earliest part of the study (1973 and 1974) with this hypothesis. Moreover,

in an extension of the study of Zack *et al.* (1991), no association between lymphatic leukaemia and phototherapy, physiological jaundice or exchange transfusion was found (Cnattingius *et al.*, 1995a). In addition, there was no association between total leukaemia or ALL specifically and phototherapy, as recorded on obstetric notes in a study in Oxford, Cambridge and Reading (England) (Roman *et al.*, 1997). There was no association between phototherapy or exchange transfusion and total childhood cancer in a study carried out in the north of England in the early 1980s, in which the children would have been born from 1965 onwards (Hartley *et al.*, 1988a).

If the hypothesis that exposure to photosensitizing lighting has a causal role in childhood ALL were true, it might be expected that children born in hospital would be at higher risk of the disease than those born at home. There was no association between total childhood cancer and home or hospital confinement in the study of Hartley *et al.* (1988a), or in analyses relating to leukaemia and lymphoma based on the same data-set (McKinney *et al.*, 1987). In response to the hypothesis of Ben-Sasson and Davis (1992), Van Steensel-Moll *et al.* (1992) reanalysed data from a case–control study of childhood leukaemia carried out in The Netherlands in 1981–82 (Van Steensel-Moll *et al.*, 1985a,b). As phototherapy was not widely used in neonatal care until the late 1960s, only children born in 1970 or later were included in the analysis. There was a weak association between ALL and birth in hospital as compared to home (RR = 1.3, 95% CI 1.0–1.7, adjusted for social class, birth order and maternal age). When the comparison was made between children born in hospital without medical indication and children born at home, to control for possible confounding due to medical reasons for delivery in hospital which may have been related to the risk of ALL, the relative risk was unchanged. Seven cases of ALL and one control were reported to have been hospitalized for neonatal hyperbilirubinaemia (RR = 3.6, 95% CI 0.9–57.4). These children were treated with phototherapy. There was no association between neonatal hyperbilirubinaemia and ALL for children born before 1970, suggesting that the neonatal jaundice itself was not associated with ALL. There was no association between ANLL and hospital or home confinement. The authors noted that the investigation on which their analysis was based was not designed to study the association between fluorescent light and childhood leukaemia, and no detailed information concerning intensity and duration of potential exposure was available, and other explanations could be provided for the association with hospital delivery.

Olsen *et al.* (1996) carried out a cohort study of 55 120 newborn children treated with phototherapy for hyperbilirubinaemia identified from the Danish national hospital discharge register for 1979–89. Neonates recorded as immature (*n* = 10 384) or as having haemolytic disease of the newborn (*n* = 926) were excluded. Twenty-eight cases of ALL were ascertained by means of linkage with the national cancer register, compared with 24.6 expected (standardized incidence ratio 1.1, 95% CI 0.8–1.7). The standardized incidence ratio for other types of leukaemia was 1.6 (95% CI 0.6–3.3: 6 cases observed, 3.8 expected). No association was apparent for other types of childhood cancer. On the basis of a random sample of neonates notified in the hospital discharge register as having hyperbilirubinaemia diagnosed in the period 1980–81 in one of three different hospital departments, it was estimated that 85 to 90% of children in Denmark were treated with prolonged (average 71 hours, range 24–188 hours) irradiation with light at wavelengths of 420–470 nm. As no effect was apparent at these intense levels of therapeutic exposure, it seems unlikely that the much lower levels found in nurseries would be hazardous.

Miller (1992) observed that the apparent increase in incidence of childhood ALL in the USA, one of the observations on which the hypothesis of Ben-Sasson and Davis is based, is likely to be an artefact of change in diagnostic accuracy, with leukaemias formerly classified as of uncertain cell type becoming classified as ALL as a result of use of cell surface markers and the identification of the common ALL antigen. In other populations, no unequivocal evidence of a trend in the incidence of childhood ALL has been found (see Chapter 2).

In a study of myeloid leukaemia in Sweden during the period 1973–89, there was a positive association with phototherapy (RR = 7.5, 95% CI 1.8–31.9; Cnattingius *et al.*, 1995b). This association was attenuated when cases with Down's syndrome were excluded (RR = 4.3, 95% CI 0.9–21.9).

### Supplemental oxygen use

In a record-linkage-based study in Sweden, an association of borderline statistical significance was found between total childhood cancer and neonatal hypoxia (odds ratio 1.3, 95% CI 0.99–1.78; Forsberg & Källén, 1990). The association was mainly due to the group "other or unspecified tumours". A weak non-significant association with leukaemia was apparent (RR = 1.5), and in an extension of the study, a positive association between leukaemia and supplemental oxygen use was found (RR = 2.6, 95% CI 1.3–4.9; Zack *et al.*, 1991). Only 1.5% of controls and 4% of cases received this therapy. No specific diagnosis or procedure was associated with its use. The occurrence of Down's syndrome, in which a high prevalence at birth of congenital heart defects may increase exposure to supplemental oxygen, did not account for the increased use of the therapy in cases. In a further extension of the study, the relative risk of lymphatic leukaemia associated with supplemental oxygen use was 1.9 (95% CI 1.2–3.2), adjusted for postpartum asphyxia (Cnattingius *et al.*, 1995a). The relative risk of AML associated with supplemental oxygen use, excluding cases with Down's syndrome, was 1.7 (95% CI 0.4–6.5; Cnattingius *et al.*, 1995b).

In other studies of the effect of supplemental oxygen in Sweden using similar methods, no association with non-Hodgkin lymphoma was found (Adami *et al.*, 1996), and only a weak association with brain tumours (RR = 1.5, 95% CI 0.9–2.5; Linet *et al.*, 1996). In subgroup analysis, a higher relative risk was observed for astrocytoma, but this did not differ significantly from that for all subtypes combined. In a study of germ-cell tumours in which data were obtained by means of a postal questionnaire to parents, no association with the child having supplemental oxygen within six months of birth was found (Shu *et al.*, 1995a).

### Vitamin K

Studies of the association between childhood cancer and vitamin K administered in the perinatal period are summarized in Table 10.5.

In a cohort study based on 16 193 infants delivered in Great Britain in one week of April 1970, in whom 33 cases of cancer occurred, an unexpected statistically significant association was found between childhood cancer and drug administration in the first week of life (Golding *et al.*, 1990). Sixteen of the 18 cases who had received drugs in the first weeks of life had received vitamin K. Within the cohort, a comparison was made between the 33 cases and 99 controls matched with the cases for the age of the mother at the birth of the child, parity, social class, marital status at delivery, and whether the birth was single or multiple. Statistically significant associations were identified not only with drug administration during the first week of

## Table 10.5. Associations between childhood cancer and vitamin K administered in the perinatal period

| Area and period of birth of children | Age group | Type of preparation containing vitamin K | Method of determining route of administration | Route of administration | Prevalence of exposure in controls (%) | Group or subgroup | Cases | Controls | RR (95% CI) | Adjusted for | Reference |
|---|---|---|---|---|---|---|---|---|---|---|---|
| Great Britain, 1970 | 0–9 years | NA | NA | Any | 31.2[a] | All cancer | 33 | 99 | 2.6 (1.3–5.2)[a] | Social class, smoking during pregnancy, X-ray in pregnancy, term delivery and pethidine in labour | Golding et al., 1990 |
| UK, Bristol, 1965–87 | 0–14 years | Konakion[k] | Recorded in medical records or imputed on the basis of year of birth, type of delivery, and whether or not infant admitted to special care | Intra-muscular[b] Oral | 40.6[c] | All cancer | 180 | 544 | 2.2 (1.1–4.4)[d] 1.2 (0.5–2.7)[d] | Hospital and year of delivery | Golding et al., 1992a |
|  |  |  |  | Intra-muscular[b] | 35.1[c] | Leukaemia Cancer other than leukaemia | –[e] –[g] | 544 544 | 2.7 (1.3–5.2)[f] 1.7 (1.0–2.8)[f] |  |  |
|  |  |  | Recorded in medical records | Intra-muscular[b] | NS | All cancer | NS | NS | 2.0 (1.2–3.3)[f] |  |  |
| Sweden, full-term non-instrumental deliveries, 1973–89 | 30 days–17 years | Konakion[k] | Imputed on the basis of hospital policy | Intra-muscular | 78.4 | All cancer Leukaemia | 2287 708 | 1 357 734[h] 1 357 734[h] | 1.0 (0.9–1.2)[j] 0.9 (0.7–1.2)[j] | Year of birth | Eklund et al., 1993 |
| 1982–89 | 30 days–9 years |  |  |  | 66.2 | All cancer Leukaemia | 722 250 | 655 454[h] 655 454[h] | 1.1 (0.9–1.4)[j] 1.2 (0.7–2.1)[j] |  |  |
| USA, multicentre, 1959–66 | 0–8 years | All brands[l] | Review of records prospectively completed by labour and delivery room observers | Intra-muscular[l] | 71.2 | All cancer Leukaemia Cancer other than leukaemia | 44 15 29 | 226 NS NS | 0.8 (0.4–1.7)[d] 0.5 (0.1–1.6)[d] 1.1 (0.5–2.6)[d] | – | Klebanoff et al., 1993 |
| Denmark, 1945–54, 1975–84 | 1–12 years | Konakion[k] | Imputed from recommended practice as no vitamin K for births 1945–54; intramuscular administration 1975–84 | NA | NA | All cancer Leukaemia | NS NS | 1 421 808 1 421 808 | 1.3 (1.2–1.4) 1.0 (0.9–1.1) | – | Olsen et al., 1994 |
| UK, Cambridge, Oxford and Reading, 1951–NS | 0–14 years | Konakion[k] | Determined from medical records, with route derived from hospital practice when the route was not recorded | Intra-muscular | 95.3 | Leukaemia | 91 | 171 | 1.2 (0.7–2.3) | Admission for special care and mode of delivery | Ansell et al., 1996 |
|  |  |  | Imputed from hospital policy | Intra-muscular | 74.2 | Leukaemia | 132 | 264 | 1.1 (0.5–2.6) | Type of region (urban or rural), social class and prematurity | von Kries et al., 1996 |
| Germany, Lower Saxony, 1975–93 | 30 days–14 years | Konakion[k] | Determined from medical records | Intra-muscular or subcutaneous | 61.0 | Leukaemia, brain tumours, nephroblastoma, neuroblastoma and rhabdomyosarcoma Leukaemia Brain tumours, neuroblastoma, neuroblastoma and rhabdomyosarcoma | 272 136 136 | 334 334 334 | 1.0 (0.7–1.5)[f] 1.0 (0.6–1.5)[f] 1.2 (0.8–1.8)[f] | Age, sex, type of region, social class and prematurity |  |

NS, Not stated.   NA, Not applicable.

[a] Drugs given to neonate. 16 of 18 cases and 27 of 30 controls who received drugs were given vitamin K.

[b] The authors state that a few instances of intravenous administration were combined with those who received vitamin K intramuscularly.

[c] Calculated for 507 controls with information also on type of delivery and admission to special care. The frequency of intramuscularly administered vitamin K in one hospital was 59.4%, in the other 23.9%. That for oral administration was 13.8% and 54.1% respectively.

[d] Reference category is no vitamin K exposure.

[e] 74 cases of leukaemia were ascertained; it is not stated how many were included in the analysis.

[f] Reference category is either no vitamin K exposure or vitamin K administered by the oral route only.

[g] 143 cases of childhood cancer other than leukaemia were ascertained; it is not stated how many were included in the analysis.

[h] Total number of births imputed as having vitamin K administered intramuscularly or orally.

[i] Reference category is vitamin K administered orally.

[j] One child in the sample received vitamin K orally.

[k] Konakion contained phenol, Cremophor EL and propylene glycol (Rennie & Kelsall, 1994).

[l] When Konakion was used, the preparation contained phenol, polysorbate-80 (rather than Cremophor EL) and propylene glycol (Rennie & Kelsall, 1994).

life, but also with antenatal X-rays, antenatal smoking, non-term delivery and use of pethidine or pethilorfan in labour. Only two of the 33 cases had fewer than two of these risk factors, whereas 47% of the controls had either no or only one risk factor. All but four of the mothers of the 16 cases who had received vitamin K had received pethidine or pethilorfan in labour. In logistic regression analysis carried out on the whole cohort, in which social class was included with the other variables already mentioned, the relative risk associated with drug administration in the first week of life was 2.6 (95% CI 1.3–5.2). This relationship was found in the absence of an association with neonatal abnormalities in the child.

This unexpected association with neonatal administration of vitamin K was examined in a subsequent study of 195 children with cancer diagnosed in the period 1971–91 and who had been born in two major maternity hospitals in Bristol in the period 1965–87, compared with 558 controls identified from the delivery books (Golding *et al.*, 1992a). The cases were ascertained from the oncology register of the regional paediatric oncology unit and from the national registry of children's tumours. The basic method of control selection was to select every 300th birth in each year in each hospital. In view of the observation that the immediate effects of oral and intramuscular doses of vitamin K have been shown to be different, even though the dose was identical, the investigators sought to distinguish the effects of administration intramuscularly and by the oral route. However, the route of vitamin K administration was often not recorded in the neonatal notes. When this was not clearly described, a probable route was identified on the basis of year of birth, the type of delivery and whether or not the infant was admitted to special care; the probable route was identified blind to case–control status.

Based on 180 cases (92.3% of those whose notes were available) and 544 controls (97.5% of those whose notes were available), the relative risk of childhood cancer associated with intramuscular vitamin K was 2.0 (95% CI 1.3–3.0) when compared with oral vitamin K or no vitamin K. The relative risk of leukaemia associated with intramuscular vitamin K was 2.7 (95% CI 1.3–5.2), and that of other types of childhood cancer was 1.7 (95% CI 1.0–2.8). Thus, there was no clear difference in the association by type of childhood cancer. When the analysis was confined to records where the route was clearly stated, the odds ratio for total childhood cancer was 2.0 (95% CI 1.2–3.3). The odds ratio

for oral vitamin K compared to no vitamin K was 1.2 (95% CI 0.5–2.7). These results could not be accounted for by other factors associated with the administration of intramuscular vitamin K, such as type of delivery or admission to a special care baby unit. These risks were adjusted for hospital and year of delivery.

Data were collected on 319 variables in all controls and 111 cases of cancer ascertained from the oncology register of the regional paediatric oncology unit. These data were not obtained for the remaining 84 cancer cases. Of these variables, presence of rubella antibody, resuscitation using intermittent positive pressure, and paediatric estimation of gestation, were statistically significant at the 1% level, which is what would be expected by chance. Adjustment for these or other variables reported to be associated with childhood cancer or known to be indicators for administering intramuscular vitamin K had little effect on the odds ratio of childhood cancer associated with vitamin K.

As acknowledged by the authors, there was a large number of instances in which the information on potentially confounding variables was not available, for example 20% for smoking in pregnancy. Medical records may not necessarily be reliable sources of information about pregnancy and childbirth (Hewson & Bennett, 1987; Oakley *et al.*, 1990), and this, together with the fact that potential confounding was assessed only for a subset of cases, constitutes a major limitation of the study. In the study of Golding *et al.* (1992a), the relationship between the type of delivery and intramuscular administration of vitamin K differed markedly between the two hospitals (Carstensen, 1992; Draper & Stiller, 1992). The association with childhood cancer is largely accounted for by data from one of the hospitals only in which virtually all of the control infants who received intramuscular vitamin K had been born following an assisted delivery. This raises the issue as to whether bias arose in control selection in that hospital; it would be relevant to know the distribution by hospital of study subjects, either whose notes were not available or from whose notes receipt of vitamin K could not be established.

Nineteen of the cases were diagnosed in the first year of life. The possibility was considered that these cancers might have been present before the child was born and therefore could not have been initiated by an injection of vitamin K. The association persisted after excluding these nineteen cases from analysis. When the analysis was restricted to subjects who would have been followed for at least ten years, by considering only those born in the period 1971–80, the relative risk of total childhood cancer associated with intramuscular vitamin K was 1.9 (95% CI 1.1–3.4), similar to that assessed for all subjects.

Golding *et al.* (1992a) noted that in England and Wales, an increase in the incidence of leukaemia was observed in children born between 1962 and 1974 (Stiller & Draper, 1982). The authors considered that this increase was compatible with an increase in the use of intramuscular vitamin K of the order of 2% per year, on the basis of national birth surveys in Great Britain in 1958 and 1970.

Draper and Stiller (1992) considered time trends in the incidence of childhood leukaemia in relation to (1) data on the use of intramuscular vitamin K use from the British national birth surveys in 1958 and 1970, and from a national survey of special care baby units in 1982; and (2) sales figures for the period 1958–83 of ampoules of a type (Konakion 1 mg) which has been almost the sole source of intramuscular vitamin K in the UK since 1958. As noted by Golding *et al.* (1992a), the increase in the incidence of leukaemia between 1962 and 1974 is compatible with a relative risk of around 2.0 associated with intramuscular vitamin K and the increase in the rate of its administration between 1958 and 1972. However, the data on vitamin K use suggest that, if causal, the trend of increase in the incidence of leukaemia should have continued up to 1982, whereas no increase since the early 1970s has been observed (Draper & Stiller, 1992). This analysis is limited by the usual problems of ecological studies and, in particular, there is some debate as to the extent to which the increase in vitamin K use is by oral or intramuscular administration (Draper & Stiller, 1992; Golding *et al.*, 1992b).

Ekelund *et al.* (1993) investigated the association between childhood cancer and intramuscular administration of vitamin K in a study in Sweden based on linkage of the medical birth registry and the national cancer registry. The study was restricted to full-term infants (gestation 37–42 weeks) who survived and who were born in 1973–89 after a delivery without use of forceps or vacuum extraction. This restriction was imposed because intramuscular administration of vitamin K is often preferred for pre-term and complicated deliveries. The infants were followed up to 1 January 1992. Cancers diagnosed within 30 days of birth were regarded as congenital and were excluded from analysis. Routines for administration of vitamin K were

obtained from all 95 maternity hospitals. In order to determine the validity of this information, 102 infants with cancer and 100 control infants were randomly selected from among those who, according to the routine exposure information, received intramuscular vitamin K, and 94 infants with cancer and 100 control infants from those who should have received oral vitamin K. Copies of the original medical charts were reviewed for these 396 infants. The individual information could not be found for a substantial proportion of the infants (55% of those who would have been expected to receive the vitamin intramuscularly and 25% of those who would have been expected to have received it orally). The difference in the proportion is because the infants' individual medical charts usually indicated the dose of vitamin K given but not how it was administered, but the route of administration was often obvious from the information about the dose. When the method of administration of vitamin K was recorded, it agreed with the stated routine method of administration in 92% of cases. The authors considered that the proportion of misclassification (8%) was probably overestimated, because incomplete information was probably given more often when the method of administration was the same as the routine method. If this were true, the proportion of misclassification could have been low as 4% for routine intramuscular administration and 7% for routine oral administration.

The relative risk of total childhood cancer associated with intramuscular administration of vitamin K as compared with oral administration was 1.0 (95% CI 0.9–1.2, after stratification for year of birth) (Ekelund *et al.*, 1993). The relative risk for leukaemia was 0.9 (95% CI 0.7–1.2). When the analysis was subdivided to include births delivered during the period 1973–81, and thereby including cancers diagnosed at ages up to 18 years, the relative risk for total childhood cancer was 0.96 and for leukaemia 0.83. For births delivered during the period 1982–89, that is including only cancers diagnosed at ages up to ten years, the relative risks were 1.1 and 1.2 respectively. There was no difference in the cumulative prevalence of cancer among those infants born in hospitals where routine neonatal administration of vitamin K was intramuscular and among those where routine administration was oral. During the period 1973–89, vitamin K was given intramuscularly to a total of 78.4% of approximately 1.4 million births; the vitamin was given orally to 19.7% of the infants. Both methods of treatment were used in parallel for 0.4% of the infants, and the vitamin was given before delivery to the mothers of 1.3% of the infants. The authors note that the doses of vitamin K given in Sweden were similar to those given in the United Kingdom, and the same preparation was used (Phytomenadione (vitamin K1), Konakion).

There was no association between childhood cancer and prenatal exposure to vitamin K in a cohort study in the USA (Klebanoff *et al.*, 1993). The study was based on follow-up to the age of seven or eight years of 54 795 liveborn children of pregnant women enrolled between 1959 and 1966 in 12 centres. Stillborn infants with cancer and neonates whose cancer was diagnosed or strongly suspected during the first day of life were excluded because vitamin K could not have been a factor in these cases. Vitamin K was administered in the delivery room or the nursery, and information about administration was recorded along with other events during and after delivery by labour and delivery observers who were not involved in the clinical care of the mother or the child. Among 54 795 liveborn children, 48 developed cancer after the first day of life. The prevalence of administration of vitamin K increased from 56% to 86% from 1959 to 1966. Exposure status was unknown for four case children. The relative risk of total childhood cancer associated with vitamin K exposure was 0.8 (95% CI 0.4–1.7). That of leukaemia was 0.5 (95% CI 0.1–1.6, based on 15 cases). The relative risk of total childhood cancer associated with the use of Aquamephyton and Konakion, the only brands currently approved for use in the USA, was 0.6; that for children who received brands of vitamin K containing phenol was 0.7. In this study, only one child received vitamin K orally. A particular strength of this study is that the records on neonatal events were part of a research study and so were more complete than routinely collected medical data. None of the brands used in the centres in this study contained the vehicle used in the United Kingdom.

Von Kries *et al.* (1996) carried out a case–control study of children born in 162 obstetric hospitals in Lower Saxony (Germany) during the period 1975–93, when only one vitamin K preparation, the same as the one used in the United Kingdom, was licensed for neonatal vitamin K prophylaxis. Of a total of 218 children with leukaemia identified as eligible, information regarding vitamin K prophylaxis was obtained for 136 (62%). For each leukaemia case, one control was selected from the municipality where the patient lived at the time of diagnosis (local control), and a second one from a municipality selected at random in Lower Saxony by means of a population-weighted sampling scheme (state control). These controls were matched with cases by sex and date of birth. Case and control families were contacted initially by being sent a questionnaire. If a control family refused to collaborate in the study, or did not return the questionnaire within three months, another control family was invited. A number of control families returned the questionnaire after more than three months, by which time another family had been invited. Thus, in total, 305 local and 308 state controls were invited to participate.

Information regarding vitamin K prophylaxis was obtained for 174 (57%) of the local controls and 160 (52%) of the state controls. As the study was performed as part of a population-based case–control study to explore possible causes of childhood leukaemia in Lower Saxony, a third control group for the leukaemia study was identified. This comprised cases with brain tumours, nephroblastoma, neuroblastoma and rhabdomyosarcoma. No population-based controls were selected for these cases, but they were used as additional cases in the vitamin K study. Of a total of 246 potentially eligible cases of this type, information on vitamin prophylaxis was obtained for 136 (55%). Data on vitamin K prophylaxis were abstracted from the birth report blind to the case–control status of each child. Information on the dose and route of vitamin K prophylaxis was obtained from the birth record or the delivery book for 196 (72%) of the 272 cases of leukaemia and other tumours, and 211 (63%) of the 334 controls. When this information was not available, the index child was assumed to have the same vitamin K exposure as the child nearest to the index baby in the delivery book with the same route of delivery and same perinatal morbidity (9 cases and 6 controls). When this could not be established, staff who worked in the delivery unit at the time when the index child was born were asked what kind of vitamin K prophylaxis the index baby would have received, giving the birth weight and route of delivery (63 cases and 109 controls). Finally, similar information was sought from medical staff who did not work in the delivery unit at the time the index child was born (4 cases and 4 controls).

In the comparison with local controls, the relative risk of leukaemia associated with intramuscular or subcutaneous administration of vitamin K compared with oral or no vitamin K prophylaxis was 1.24 (95% CI 0.68–2.25). In the comparison with state controls, the relative risk was 0.82 (95% CI 0.50–1.36). When the control groups were pooled, the relative risk was close to unity. The relative risk for brain tumours, nephroblastoma, neuroblastoma and rhab-domyosarcoma combined was 1.19 (95% CI 0.77–1.83). When the analysis was repeated for subjects for whom vitamin K prophylaxis had been documented in birth records or delivery books, the results were almost unchanged, except the comparison of leukaemia cases versus local controls, for whom the relative risk increased to 2.03 (95% CI 0.69–5.97). When the analyses were repeated for parenteral prophylaxis versus no prophylaxis, most of the relative risks were slightly decreased.

Analysis of the subgroup of cases of leukaemia in children aged one to six years was made, as this was considered to be a relatively homogenous sub-group, most of the cases having common ALL. It is not clear whether the decision to make this subgroup analysis was specified in the original study protocol, or was *post hoc*. The relative risk versus both control groups combined was 1.22 (95% CI 0.69–2.15), in the comparison with state controls 0.99 (95% CI 0.52–1.90) and in comparison with local controls 2.28 (95% CI 0.94–5.54). There was no difference regarding the source of information on the vitamin K prophylaxis between cases and controls. The increased relative risk in the comparison with local controls could not be explained by any of the potential confounders. It would be expected that the policy of administration of vitamin K would be more likely to be similar for cases and local controls than for cases and state controls. Therefore, the relative risk would be expected to be closer to unity in the comparison between cases and local controls than in the other comparison, whereas the opposite was observed. The elevated relative risk in the comparison with local controls may be a chance result in subgroup analysis with multiple testing, as acknowledged by the authors.

In a case–control study of childhood leukaemia based on births in three hospitals in different parts of England (Cambridge, Oxford and Reading), no association with intramuscular vitamin K, either as determined from hospital records or as imputed from hospital policy, was found (Ansell *et al.*, 1996). In addition, no association was found specifically for ALL. Subsequently, Roman *et al.* (1997) reported a more detailed analysis of data relating to leukaemia and non-Hodgkin lymphoma

diagnosed before the age of 30 years in subjects whose obstetric records were stored in the same three hospitals. 92% of the cases of leukaemia were diagnosed at age 14 years or less; these cases, and their controls, were included in the report of Ansell *et al.* (1996). There was no association between leukaemia and intramuscular vitamin K administration either recorded in the notes (RR = 1.2, 95% CI 0.7–2.1) or imputed from information about hospital policy (RR = 1.2, 95% CI 0.5–2.4). In view of the finding of von Kries *et al.* (1996), ALL diagnosed between the ages of one and six years was considered; the relative risk associated with recorded administration was 0.6 (95% CI 0.7–2.2), and that with imputed administration was again 0.6 (95% CI 0.2–1.7).

Olsen *et al.* (1994) compared the cumulative risk of childhood cancer among children born during the period 1945–54 (*n* = 835 430), in which no vitamin K was administered, those born during the period 1960–69 (*n* = 797 472), in which pregnant women received oral vitamin K, and those born during the period 1975–84 (*n* = 586 378), in which virtually all newborns received vitamin K intramuscularly. There was a small increase in risk for all tumour types combined, due mainly to lymphoma in boys and neuroblastoma in both sexes. There was no trend for childhood leukaemia. The preparation used was the same as that employed in the United Kingdom (Draper & McNinch, 1994).

In the USA, where the American Academy of Pediatrics advocated universal neonatal vitamin K prophylaxis in 1961 (Vitamin K Ad Hoc Task Force, 1993), no increase in the incidence of leukaemia occurred in 1969–84 compared with 1947–50 (Miller, 1992). However, vitamin K prophlylaxis was mandatory in only five states until 1987 (Tulchinsky *et al.*, 1993) and together with data from the study of Klebanoff *et al.* (1993), this raises questions about the universality of prophylaxis with vitamin K in the USA, which Miller (1992) assumed when commenting on this trend (Passmore *et al.*, 1993). In countries such as the USA (Vitamin K Ad Hoc Task Force, 1993) and Australia (NHMRC, 1994), where intramuscular vitamin K has been recommended as routine after delivery, the incidence of leukaemia is no higher than in the United Kingdom (see Chapter 2).

In New Zealand, there was a statistically significant increase in the incidence of leukaemia in children aged 0–4 years between 1953–57 and 1988–90; this was due to ALL from 1973–77 onwards (Dockerty *et al.* 1996). Intramuscular vitamin K was available for use in neonates in New Zealand from the late 1960s, although it was reported to have been given routinely in at least one hospital as early as 1962. Therefore, time trends in New Zealand might be consistent with the vitamin K hypothesis.

Golding *et al.* (1992a) discussed the biological plausibility of the possible relationship between childhood cancer and vitamin K. Concentrations of the level observed in the plasma of infants 12–24 hours after injection have been shown to increase sister chromatid exchanges in human placental lymphocytes *in vitro* and sheep fetal lymphocytes *in vitro* (Israels *et al.*, 1987). However, in a small series of human neonates, no increase in sister chromatid exchanges in peripheral blood lymphocytes was observed (Cornelissen *et al.*, 1991). In addition to vitamin K, Konakion used in the countries in which the studies in Europe were carried out contains phenol, cremophor EL and propylene glycol (Rennie & Kelsall, 1994). Therefore, if a positive association had been confirmed, the components of the preparation other than vitamin K might have been responsible for the effect. While phenol has been suspected to be carcinogenic (Chayen, 1992), the available evidence is inadequate to evaluate its potential carcinogenicity (IARC, 1989b). The majority of adverse effects of phenol have been observed at high exposures, whereas those received after an injection of Konakion are very low. In the study of Klebanoff *et al.* (1993), the relative risk of cancer among children who received brands of vitamin K containing phenol was lower than that for all brands.

As indicated by Golding *et al.* (1992a), the possible association with intramuscular vitamin K has stimulated a reappraisal of the risks and benefits of neonatal prophylaxis with this vitamin (Hull, 1992). The most important benefit, prevention of late onset haemorrhagic disease, is not as substantial when the vitamin is administered orally (von Kries, 1992). The finding in two studies (Golding *et al.*, 1990, 1992a) of an increased risk of total childhood cancer associated with intramuscular vitamin K administration to neonates in the United Kingdom has not been confirmed by analytical studies in Germany, Sweden or the USA. A study of time trends in Denmark, although limited by changes in ascertainment, does not suggest any relationship with the introduction of the prophylaxis. The positive association between leukaemia of all types and vitamin K reported by Golding *et al.* (1992a) has not been confirmed by analytical studies in England, Germany, Sweden and the USA. However, the possibility of a small increase in the risk of ALL occurring at ages around those of the peak incidence in childhood cannot yet be excluded, in view of the increased risk at ages 1–6 years found in comparison with one of two control groups in Germany (von Kries *et al.*, 1996) and the time trend data from New Zealand (Dockerty *et al.*, 1996), although such an increase was not apparent in a study in Cambridge, Oxford and Reading (Roman *et al.*, 1997). Further case–control and ecological studies in progress (Draper & McNinch, 1994) should help resolve this issue.

## Allergies

In view of the postulated importance of immunological factors in the development of certain tumours, there have been a number of investigations of the association between cancer and a history of asthma, hay fever, hives and other allergy-related diseases in adults (Vena *et al.*, 1985). The available data on the relation between allergies and cancer in children are summarized in Table 10.6. The limited data, mainly based on maternal interview, do not suggest any consistent relationship for haematopoietic malignancies, and there was no noteworthy association with other specific types of childhood cancer in single studies.

## Injuries

Any association with an injury may be the result of incidental diagnosis of a tumour during the investigations leading to its management, although it also has been suggested that diagnostic X-ray exposure associated with such investigation may play a direct causal role (see Chapter 4). Most of the studies in which this issue has been assessed have been of brain tumours and head injuries.

### Brain tumours and head injuries

Among subjects with brain tumours diagnosed under the age of 20 years in the Minneapolis–St Paul Metropolitan Area, Minnesota, in 1963, eight of 20 cases as compared with two of 20 matched controls had either been delivered following prolonged labour or by forceps associated with breech delivery (Choi *et al.*, 1970). The authors suggested that these events might have inflicted mechanical trauma to the heads of the subjects. Subsequently, Preston-Martin *et al.* (1982) observed that four of 209 cases of brain tumour were described by their mothers as severely bruised about the face and head at birth, whereas no controls were so described. Howe *et al.* (1989) reported a relative risk associated with reported birth injury or

# Table 10.6. Associations between childhood cancer and allergy

| Area and period of study | Cases | | Controls | | Method of determining allergy in child[b] | Type of allergy | Frequency in controls (%) | RR | Reference |
|---|---|---|---|---|---|---|---|---|---|
| | Dead (D), newly incident (I) or prevalent (P), upper age limit | Number | Type[a] | Number | | | | | |
| **Leukaemia and lymphoma** USA, Boston MA, 1953–56 | P, 14 | 210 | H OC | 50 93 | I | Any | 12.0 10.8 | 2.4 2.7* | Manning & Caroll, 1957 |
| **Leukaemia and non-Hodgkin lymphoma** Italy, Turin, 1981–84 | I, P, NS[c] | 183 | H | 307 | I | Any Asthma | NS 12.1 | 0.4* 0.5 | Magnani *et al.*, 1990 |
| **Leukaemia** USA, Minnesota, 1953–57 | D, 4 | 112 | N | 112 | MR | Eczema Asthma Hives | 1.8 2.8 1.8 | 1.0 0.7 1.0 | Ager *et al.*, 1965 |
| **ALL** UK, London, 1973–75 | I, 14 | 54 | F, N | 121 | I | Any atopic | 10.0 | 1.6 | Till *et al.*, 1979 |
| Japan, Hokkaido, 1981–87 | I, P, 14[d] | 63 | H | 126 | I | Asthma or atopic dermatitis | NS | 0.3* | Nishi & Miyake, 1989 |
| **Neuroblastoma** USA, North Carolina, 1972–81 | I, 14 | 104 | H | 208 | MR | Any Asthma | 11.2 1.5 | 0.2* 1.7 | Greenberg, 1983 |
| **Soft-tissue sarcoma** Italy, Padua and Turin, 1983 | I, P, NS[e] | 52 | H | 326 | I | Any | NS | 0.7 | Magnani *et al.*, 1989 |
| **Rhabdomyosarcoma** USA, North Carolina, 1967–76 | I, 14 | 33 | P | 99 | I | Asthma | 4.0 | 2.3 | Grufferman *et al.*, 1982 |
| **Germ-cell tumours** USA and Canada, CCG, 1982–89 | I, 14 | 105 | RDD | 639 | Q | Allergy medicine | 12.1 | 1.1 | Shu *et al.*, 1995a |
| **Total childhood cancer** Great Britain, 1953–55 | D, 9 | 1299 | P | 1299 | I | Any | 1.9 | 1.1 | Stewart *et al.*, 1958 |
| UK, North West, West Midlands and Yorkshire, 1980–83 | I, 14 | 555 | GP, H | 1110 | I, MR | Contact dermatitis and other eczema | NS | <1.0[f] | Hartley *et al.*, 1988a |

NS, Not stated.
* p < 0.05

[a] P, population-based; H, hospital; OC, other types of cancer; N, neighbourhood; F, friends; GP, neighbourhood, selected through general practitioner.

[b] I, maternal interview; MR, medical records; Q, questionnaire.
[c] Mean age at diagnosis 6.1 (S.D. 3.6) years.
[d] Non-T-cell type.
[e] Mean age at diagnosis 6.8 (±4.7) years.
[f] The authors stated that there was an inverse association.

trauma of 2.2 (95% CI 0.9–5.6), but no association with delivery complications was reported. No association with head trauma at birth (RR = 0.6, 95% CI 0.3–1.2) was found by McCredie *et al.* (1994b), although these authors noted that the increased relative risk (1.9, 95% CI 0.9–3.7) associated with use of anaesthetics during delivery could be an indicator of trauma to the child, as an anaesthetic is more likely to be given for a difficult birth. In a large record-linkage-based study in Sweden, there was no association between brain tumours (*n* = 570) and birth injury at any specific anatomical site (Linet *et al.*, 1996). The relative risk associated with birth injuries of any type was 1.0 (95% CI 0.7–1.7).

Regarding head injuries later in life, Preston-Martin *et al.* (1982) reported a positive association with head injury requiring hospital-ization (RR = 3.0, *p* = 0.07, based on 12 discordant pairs), but there was no association with head injury for which any kind of medical treatment was received (RR = 1.0, based on 92 discordant pairs). Howe *et al.* (1989) found a significant positive association between head and neck injuries requiring medical attention (RR = 3.2, 95% CI 1.4–7.1); a weaker association was found when all reported head and neck injuries were considered (RR = 1.9, 95% CI 0.9–4.3). These workers found that there was only a weak association (correlation coefficient = 0.2) between head and neck injuries and history of skull X-rays, and that positive associations with head injuries and with skull X-rays taken at least five years before the diagnosis were unchanged when both were included in the logistic regression model simultaneously. It therefore seems unlikely that the occurrence of a head injury would have precipitated the diagnosis of a brain tumour. No association with head injury for which the child was reported to have been seen by a doctor or nurse was found in the study of McCredie *et al.* (1994b) and Cordier *et al.* (1994) found no association with reported head trauma in childhood.

No association between astrocytoma and head injury with loss of consciousness was found in the study of Kuijten *et al.* (1990). By contrast, Bunin *et al.* (1994b) found that astrocytoma cases were somewhat more likely than controls to have had a head injury that required medical attention (RR = 2.2, 95% CI 0.9–5.2, adjusted for income level). In the same study, the relative risk of primitive neuroectodermal tumours of the brain associated with head injuries was 0.9 (95% CI 0.4–2.2).

In summary, there are no consistent associations with head injury in the perinatal period or later life, either with brain tumours overall or specifically with astrocytoma.

*Other types of childhood cancer*

In a study of deaths due to childhood cancer in Great Britain during the period 1953–55, a moderate excess of fractures and burns or scalds within two years of the date of diagnosis of leukaemia was reported (Stewart *et al.*, 1958).

Neglia *et al.* (1988) found that the relative risk of neuroblastoma associated with "birth injuries/other significant conditions" was 4.1 (95% CI 0.8–42.0). The proportion of controls for whom this was reported was 0.8%. Operskalski *et al.* (1987) found that osteosarcoma was associated with prior injury to the tumour site. Fewer than 10% of cases had such injuries, and none of them was a fracture. There was no association with prior injury overall, that is, irrespective of site.

## Epilepsy, seizures, barbiturates and tumours of the central nervous system

Following experiments in animals suggesting that barbiturates might be carcinogenic, and a report of an increased incidence of tumours of the CNS in adult patients treated for epilepsy with phenobarbitone, phenytoin or primidone (Clemmesen *et al.*, 1974), the relationship between barbiturate use in the index child and brain tumours in childhood, and the underlying condition, has been investigated (Table 10.7).

Gold *et al.* (1979) found that seven of 84 children with brain tumours had epilepsy many years before their tumour was diagnosed; only one child in each of the control groups (73 normal controls and 78 cancer controls) was so affected. These authors also found a non-significant positive association with postnatal exposure to barbiturates (Gold *et al.*, 1978). This was not statistically significant; three of the five exposed cases took barbiturates for seizures beginning 8–14 years before the diagnosis of the tumour. McCredie *et al.* (1994b) found that three of 82 cases of brain tumour and one of 164 controls had epilepsy—the association was not statistically significant after exclusion of symptoms that occurred within six months of the diagnosis of the brain tumour, and there was no association with reported use of anticonvulsant medication by the child. Preston-Martin *et al.* (1982) found that a total of 19 cases but no controls had taken drugs for seizures. The interval between occurrence of first seizure and diagnosis was 2–4 years for nine

# Table 10.7. Associations between epilepsy, seizures, barbiturate use and tumours of the central nervous system in children

| Area and period of study | Number of cases | Controls Type[a] | Number | Method of assessing exposure[b] | Epilepsy Prevalence in controls (%) | RR | Seizures Prevalence in controls (%) | RR | Barbiturates Indication | Prevalence of use in controls (%) | RR | Reference |
|---|---|---|---|---|---|---|---|---|---|---|---|---|
| USA, Baltimore, MD, 1965–75 | 84 | B | 73 | I | 1.4 | 6.6[e] | – | – | NS[d] | 2.9 | 2.5 | Gold et al., 1978, 1979 |
| | | OC | 78 | | 1.3 | 7.0[e] | – | – | | 2.8 | 2.5 | |
| USA, Los Angeles County, 1972–77 | 209 | F, N | 209 | I | 0.0 | ∞ | 0.0 | ∞ | Seizures | 0.0 | ∞ | Preston-Martin et al., 1982 |
| | | | | | | | | | Other than seizures | 4.2[e] | 0.9[e] | |
| Canada, Toronto, 1977–83 | 74 | P | 138 | I | – | – | – | – | Any | 1.4[f] | 4.4 | Howe et al., 1989 |
| USA, Northern California, 1960–83 | 237 | Ins | 474 | MR | 1.1 | 5.1* | – | – | Any | 15.2 | 1.4[g] | Goldhaber et al., 1990 |
| | | | | | | | | | Other than epilepsy | 14.6 | 1.3 | |
| Australia, New South Wales, 1985–89 | 82 | P | 164 | I | 0.6 | 5.6[h] | 4.3[h,i] | 0.8[h,i] | – | – | – | McCredie et al., 1994b |
| France, Ile de France, 1985–87 | 75 | P | 113 | I | 5.3[j] | 1.0[j] | – | 1.0[j] | Any | 2.7 | 2.1 | Cordier et al., 1994 |

NS, Not stated.
* P < 0.05.

[a] B, selected from file of birth certificates; OC, other types of cancer; F, friends; N, neighbourhood; Ins, members of a health insurance plan; P, population-based.
[b] I, maternal interview; MR, medical records.
[c] Crude unmatched analysis of matched data.
[d] Of the five cases who took barbiturates, three took these for seizures beginning 8–14 years before the diagnosis of the tumour, one took them for emotional problems two years before diagnosis, and one took them for two concussions 13 years before diagnosis.
[e] Based on 190 pairs, after exclusion of 19 pairs in which the patients had epilepsy.
[f] Phenobarbital, dilantin, meberal and tryptizol.
[g] After control for history of epilepsy.
[h] Up to six months before diagnosis.
[i] Fits due to high fever.
[j] Up to one year before diagnosis.

cases (47%); 5–8 years for five cases (26%) and more than 9 years for a further five cases. There was no association with postnatal use of barbiturates for conditions other than seizures. An elevated relative risk of brain tumours in association with anticonvulsant use was reported by Howe *et al.* (1989), and in association with use of barbiturates by Cordier *et al.* (1994). These associations were not statistically significant. No information was given on the timing of use.

Using medical records for subjects who were members of a health insurance plan, Goldhaber *et al.* (1990) found a positive association between tumours of the CNS diagnosed at ages up to 19 years and history of epilepsy (RR = 5.1, 95% CI 0.9–2.2), mainly due to gliomas. Relative to never-use of barbiturates, the risk associated with use for less than one week was 1.4 (95% CI 0.9–2.3), with use for periods between one week and one year 2.7 (95% CI 0.7–10.0) and with use for periods of longer than one year 4.4 (95% CI 1.5–12.8). The great majority of subjects with epilepsy had been exposed to barbiturates, all for greater than a week, whereas only 9% of those exposed to barbiturates for indications other than epilepsy had taken the drugs for more than a week. Therefore, the association with duration was no longer apparent after adjustment for a history of epilepsy. No association with barbiturate use was apparent in subjects without such a history (RR = 1.3, 95% CI 0.8–2.1). The indications other than epilepsy included gastrointestinal disorders (51% of non-epileptic case users, 30% of non-epileptic control users), febrile seizures (7% and 28% respectively), sleep or emotional disorders (20% in each group) and asthma (20% and 17% respectively). There was no association with barbiturate use when the interval between first use and tumour diagnosis was two years or less, or ten years or more. In the interval between three and nine years, the relative risk was 1.8 (95% CI 1.0–3.0)—the rationale for selecting intervals of these lengths was not specified. Other subgroup analyses suggested that the association was restricted to boys. The lack of a pattern to the variations in the association by subgroups suggests that the association was due to chance. Seizures may be an early manifestation of tumour development; cohort studies of adults treated with phenobarbital for epilepsy have shown an excess risk of brain cancer, particularly gliomas, in the early stages of follow-up, which declined with increasing duration of use, a pattern which would be consistent with inclusion of patients with undiagnosed brain tumours that led to seizures and exposure to phenobarbital for their control (Goldhaber *et al.*, 1990). Slow-growing tumours have been reported to give rise to seizures which may predate tumour diagnosis by 20 years or more (Mathieson, 1975). The prevalence of exposure to barbiturates (15% in controls) in the study of Goldhaber *et al.* (1990), which was based on medical records, was substantially higher than those recorded in the other studies, in which this information was determined by interview.

In a study in Rochester, Minnesota, reported only in a letter, no cases of brain tumour were observed in 8291 person-years of follow-up contributed by 666 children who had experienced febrile convulsions and 91 children placed on long-term regimens of anticonvulsants, usually phenobarbital (Annegers *et al.*, 1979).

In summary, there is a consistent positive association between brain tumours and a history of epilepsy and/or use of barbiturates in the index child. However, the possibility that this association is secondary to the presence of the tumour before its diagnosis cannot be excluded.

## Other illnesses in the index child

In a record-linkage-based study in Sweden, the relative risk of brain tumours associated with neonatal distress, related treatments or both was in the range 1.4–1.6 (Linet *et al.*, 1996). The risk remained elevated after exclusion of subjects aged under two years. The effects of specific neonatal conditions and the related treatments could not be disentangled. In an interview-based study in New South Wales, Australia, the relative risk associated with "breathing problems immediately after birth" was 1.7 (95% CI 0.7–4.0), while that associated with "health problems in first 2 weeks" was 1.2 (95% CI 0.7–2.4; McCredie *et al.*, 1994b). These findings, although as yet unconfirmed, are interesting in view of the possible role of oxygen deprivation and excess in brain cell damage during a period of rapid cell division, and in view of the fact that DNA damage is less efficiently repaired in brain cells than in other cells (Linet *et al.*, 1996).

In a study of all types of childhood cancer in northern England, there was a positive association with increasing numbers of illnesses reported over the age of six months (Hartley *et al.*, 1988a). This was largely attributable to an excess of "symptoms, signs and ill-defined conditions" (ICD9 780–799) reported in cases. The authors noted that this was particularly striking for brain tumours. The association was apparent in comparison both with controls selected through general practices and in comparison with hospital controls. No association between brain tumours and serious illnesses in childhood other than fits due to high fever, epilepsy and meningitis was observed by McCredie *et al.* (1994b).

In multicentre studies in north America, no association between aspects of the medical history of the index child and Wilms' tumour (Olshan *et al.*, 1993) or hepatoblastoma (Buckley *et al.*, 1989a) has been found. In the latter study, no patients were reported to have had a prior liver disease.

Holly *et al.* (1992) reported a positive association between Ewing's sarcoma and the index child having taken an overdose of medication or poisons (RR = 4.4, 95% CI 1.4–13.5). The association persisted when the analysis was restricted to subjects who were reported to have seen a physician as a result of the episode (RR = 9.3, 95% CI 1.9–46.5). The authors noted that there was no specificity in the type of agent reported to be involved in the episodes. The intervals between episode and diagnosis in cases, and episode and interview in controls, were similar. In addition, the mean age when the episode occurred was similar between cases and controls. For these reasons, and in view of the absence of other reports of such an association, the possibility cannot be excluded that the association reflects the operation of an unidentified confounder.

Goodman *et al.* (1978) found that 80% of adolescent cases of osteosarcoma had abnormal growth hormone responses to glucose stimulation. However, Operskalski *et al.* (1987) reported that there was no association between osteosarcoma and metabolic and other growth-related disorders, including diabetes and other abnormalities of carbohydrate metabolism. While acromegaly, a syndrome caused by excessive secretion of growth hormone usually due to a pituitary adenoma, has been associated with an increased risk of neoplasia, osteosarcoma has not been one of the tumours observed (Bengtsson, 1993).

## Height

Adult stature has been investigated in studies of cancers typically occurring in middle or old age because it is considered to be a marker of the effects of nutrition in childhood or adolescence (Albanes *et al.*, 1988). Adult stature is also under genetic control. Height has been investigated in a number of studies of cancer in children, in part in order to assess the long-term effects of therapy.

There have been conflicting observations about the associations of height at diagnosis and childhood cancer (Table 10.8). It is difficult to resolve the inconsistencies for at least three reasons. First, in several studies, the cases have included those admitted to clinical trials or protocol treatment programmes, and it is unknown to what extent cases with a particularly poor prognosis, which might be related to height, have been included. Where a participation rate is specified, this has often been less than 70%. Second, in many studies, the height of cases has been compared with national standards, and does not take account of regional variations which may be related to social class. In relation to ALL, it might be expected that cases would be taller than expected because of the relationship with social class (see Chapter 2; McWhirter *et al.*, 1983), but this has been observed only in one study (Broomhall *et al.*, 1983). Third, it is possible that a prediagnostic sign of childhood cancer is alteration of growth velocity. For example, it has been suggested that the association between brain tumours in children and low height and weight for age (Howe *et al.*, 1989) may be due to a prediagnostic effect of the tumour on growth hormone levels (Kuijten & Bunin, 1993). Information on height before diagnosis was reported only in two studies, both of osteosarcoma (Broström *et al.*, 1979; Gelberg *et al.*, 1997).

Interest in the possible association between height and osteosarcoma and Ewing's sarcoma was stimulated by the observation of a resemblance between the curves for growth in stature by age and sex and mortality due to bone cancer according to the same parameters (Ederer *et al.*, 1965) and by the observation of an excess risk of canine bone cancer among larger breeds of dog (Tjalma, 1966). In three of the four available studies, no association between Ewing's sarcoma and height at diagnosis was observed (Table 10.8). In one of the two available studies of height recorded before diagnosis and osteosarcoma, a positive association was found (Gelberg *et al.*, 1997). Due to a substantial amount of missing data, the possibility that selection bias influenced the results cannot be excluded. No consistent association between osteosarcoma and height at diagnosis was observed (Table 10.8). In childhood, osteosarcomas of the long bones predominate, whereas later there is a more equal division between long and flat bones (Weinfeld & Dudley, 1962; Parkin *et al.*, 1993b). In addition, osteosarcomas of the long bones of the arm tend to occur earlier than those in the leg, which may

# Table 10.8. Associations between childhood cancer and height

| Area and period of study | Cases — Upper age limit | Cases — Eligibility | N (participation rate, %) | Comparison standard | Timing of assessment | Result | Reference |
|---|---|---|---|---|---|---|---|
| **ALL** | | | | | | | |
| USA, Charleston, SC, NS | NS | Admitted to protocol treatment programmes | 50 | NS | Diagnosis | Cases were shorter than normal. | Westphal et al., 1979 |
| UK, multicentre, 1972–73 | Boys, 12 Girls, 10 | Admitted to clinical trial | 140 96 | National data for UK | Diagnosis | Cases were taller than normal. | Broomhall et al., 1983 |
| USA, multicentre, 1979–81 | 20 | Admitted to clinical trial | 127 | National data for USA | Diagnosis | Boys aged <4 years at diagnosis were shorter than normal. There were no other differences. | Berry et al., 1983 |
| Australia, Queensland, 1975–81 | Boys, 12 Girls, 10 | Recorded in cancer registry | 59 | National data for Australia | Presentation | No association | McWhirter et al., 1983 |
| USA and Canada, multicentre, 1972–75 | 17 | Disease-free and not receiving maintenance chemotherapy.[a] | 140 (75) | National data for USA | Diagnosis | No association | Robison et al., 1985 |
| Japan, Tokyo, 1977–NS | NS | | 44 | Controls matched for age, sex and period selected from among patients admitted because of acute illness. | Pre-treatment | Mean height of cases was slightly less than that of controls. | Bessho, 1986 |
| USA, Memphis, TN, 1962–85 | 17 | | 1591 | National data for USA | Diagnosis | No association | Pui et al., 1987 |
| **Brain tumours** | | | | | | | |
| Canada, Toronto, 1977–83 | 19 | All cases | 74 (60) | Age- and sex-matched population controls | Diagnosis | There was a significant association with low height for age. | Howe et al., 1989 |
| **Osteosarcoma** | | | | | | | |
| USA, Boston, 1945–65 | 18 | | 85 (65) | Children with primary cancer other than of the bones. | Diagnosis | Cases were taller than controls. | Fraumeni, 1967 |
| USA, Pittsburgh, 1951–71 | 17 | Patients with paraosteal tumours, tumours of the mandible or maxilla, thought to be secondary, or associated with Paget's disease, were excluded. | 35 (65) | National data for USA | Diagnosis | Cases were taller than normal. | Scranton et al., 1975 |
| Sweden, 1972–74 | 25 | Patients with paraosteal tumours or with clinical evidence of metastases upon admission to hospital were excluded. | 19 (43) | Data from an urban community in Sweden | 8.0 years Diagnosis | No association No association | Broström et al., 1979 |
| USA, Los Angeles County, 1972–82 | 24 | | 60 (66) | Sex, ethnic group and birth year matched controls, selected from among friends and neighbours. | Diagnosis | No association. Growth rates of cases and controls just before diagnosis were similar. | Operskalski et al., 1987 |

| Location & period | No. of cases | Comments (cases) | No. of controls | Controls | Age at measurement | Result | Reference |
|---|---|---|---|---|---|---|---|
| USA, Memphis, TN, 1962–85 | 17 | | 150 | National data for USA. | Diagnosis | No association | Pui *et al.*, 1987 |
| USA, New York State, 1978–88 | 24 | Cases with previous cancers and children under the age of 3 years were excluded. | 91[b] | Controls randomly selected from live birth records. | One year before diagnosis | Significant trend of increasing risk with increasing height one year before diagnosis ($p = 0.01$)[c] | Gelberg *et al.*, 1997 |
| **Ewing's sarcoma** USA, Boston, 1945–65 | 18 | | 82 (65) | Children with primary cancer other than of the bones. | Diagnosis | Cases were taller than controls. | Fraumeni, 1967 |
| USA, multicentre, 1972–78 | 18 | Admitted to clinical trial. | 291 (94) | National data for USA. | Diagnosis | Girls were smaller than normal. There was no association for boys. | Pendergrass *et al.*, 1984 |
| USA, Memphis, TN, 1962–85 | 17 | | 113 | National data for USA. | Diagnosis | No association | Pui *et al.*, 1987 |
| USA, San Francisco Bay Area, 1978–86 | 31 | Recorded in cancer registry. | 43 (86) | Age- and sex-matched controls selected by random-digit dialling. | Diagnosis | No association | Holly *et al.*, 1992 |

NS, Not stated.

[a] The study was designed primarily to assess the effects of therapy on growth.
[b] Interviews were completed for 130 (76%) of osteosarcoma cases ascertained. 85% of cases (or their parents) gave consent to having height and weight information abstracted from medical and school records. Information was returned by 52% of the doctors and 82% of the schools.
[c] In addition to an unmatched analysis of 91 cases compared with 96 controls, a matched analysis based on 67 pairs was carried out. The *p* value for trend was 0.02.

be due to more rapid growth of the humerus early in life (Price, 1958; Parkin *et al.*, 1993b). In a study of cancer registrations in England and Wales during the period 1962–84, sex differences in bone cancer risk at puberty, especially for osteosarcoma and Ewing's sarcoma, paralleled known sex differences in skeletal growth (dos Santos Silva & Swerdlow, 1993).

Dos Santos Silva and Swerdlow (1993) found an analogous pattern for rhabdomyosarcoma. They observed that sex differences in the adolescent peak of rhabdomyosarcoma paralleled sex variations in muscle growth velocity at these ages, and that muscle development is subject to the same hormonal stimuli as bone. No association between rhabdomyosarcoma and height at diagnosis was found in a hospital-based study in Memphis, Tennessee (Pui *et al.*, 1987).

Only in one study have associations between height at diagnosis and Hodgkin's disease, non-Hodgkin lymphoma, ANLL, retinoblastoma, neuroblastoma, and Wilms' tumour in children been assessed (Pui *et al.*, 1987). Compared with published national standards, no significant deviations from population norms were found for any of these categories after adjustment for multiple significance testing. In a national study in the USA of more than 3000 patients with Wilms' tumour, heights and weights at diagnosis were significantly higher for the subgroups of patients with Beckwith–Wiedemann syndrome or hemihypertrophy, and height was lower for those with aniridia, cryptorchidism or hypospadias, when compared to other patients with Wilms' tumour (Leisenring *et al.*, 1994).

## Conclusions

The risk of childhood leukaemia is elevated in children with Down's syndrome. In some studies, this association appears to account for the excess risk of leukaemia associated with congenital anomalies of any type. The results of studies of the association between childhood leukaemia diagnosed at all ages and high birth weight are inconsistent. In subgroup analysis by age, the strongest associations are apparent in young children. An initial report of an association between leukaemia and jaundice was subsequently shown to be confined to the acute myeloid type. This relationship may have been secondary to a strong association between acute myeloid leukaemia and Down's syndrome. No association between ALL and jaundice has been found. The hypothesis that exposure to photo-sensitizing lighting immediately after birth may

be a cause of ALL was not supported by a cohort study of newborns treated with phototherapy for hyperbilirubinaemia, by a record-linkage-based case–control study in which information on phototherapy had been collected prospectively, by two studies of the effects of hospital versus home confinement, or by data on time trends. An initial report of an association between leukaemia and intramuscular vitamin K prophylaxis has not been confirmed by other studies in England, Germany, Sweden and the USA. However, the possibility of a small increase in the risk of ALL occurring at ages around those of the peak incidence in childhood cannot be excluded entirely in view of the results of the German case–control study and time trend data from New Zealand.

No consistent association between brain tumours and congenital anomalies of all types combined has been observed. Associations with congenital anomalies of the CNS may be artefactual. While there is no clear association between birth weight and brain tumours of all types combined, there is a consistent positive association between astrocytoma and high birth weight. Other aspects of perinatal characteristics have been less investigated for brain tumours than for leukaemia. However, in two studies in which such investigation was made, raised risks in association with neonatal distress or related treatments were observed. No consistent association between brain tumours and head injury in the perinatal period or later in life is apparent. There is a consistent positive association between brain tumours and a history of epilepsy in the index child and/or use of barbiturates by the child, but this may be secondary to the presence of the tumour before its diagnosis.

Neuroblastoma does not appear to develop in children with Down's syndrome. This may be attributable to the hypoplasia of the sympathetic nervous system observed in those with Down's syndrome. No clear association between neuroblastoma and birth weight has been observed.

Wilms' tumour is associated with aniridia, hemihypertrophy, cryptorchidism and hypospadias. While some of the excess risk for cryptochidism and hypospadias may be attributable to the fact that cases with Wilms' tumour are likely to undergo particularly thorough examination of the urogenital system, recent molecular genetic studies have identified a candidate gene for anomalies of the genitourinary tract and Wilms' tumour. In the largest studies, a consistent positive association between Wilms' tumour and high birth weight has been observed. This does not appear to be due entirely to the association with specific overgrowth syndromes.

There appears to be an excess of congenital anomalies of all types combined in cases with germ-cell tumours. It is unclear whether this is attributable to anomalies of specific types, and bias of ascertainment may have influenced the findings. There is a consistent positive association between germ-cell tumours and high birth weight. This may be compatible with a role of estrogen exposure in the etiology of germ-cell tumours.

With regard to other types of childhood cancer, no clear associations between congenital anomalies and lymphoma, retinoblastoma, bone tumours or soft-tissue sarcoma have been observed. No consistent association between retinoblastoma and birth weight is apparent. Associations between birth weight and other types of childhood cancer have been little studied.

# Chapter 11

# Conclusions

In relation to specific types of childhood cancer, the factors that have been investigated are classified in this chapter according to whether (1) they are generally accepted as being of etiological importance; (2) they have been identified as associated with the disease with some degree of consistency; (3) they have not been consistently associated with the disease; (4) they were identified as associated with the disease in one or two studies but this has not been investigated further; (5) they have not been associated with the disease in most of the available studies. This information has been tabulated for the leukaemias (Table 11.1), the lymphomas (Table 11.2), central nervous system tumours (Table 11.3), neuroblastoma (Table 11.4) and Wilms' tumour (Table 11.5). Within each category in each table, the factors have been listed in the order in which they have been discussed in the text; there is no ranking of the strength of evidence other than into the five categories defined.

## The leukaemias

Evidence on possible etiological factors investigated in relation to leukaemia is summarized in Table 11.1. In many of the studies, the disease was not considered by subtype. Acute lymphatic leukaemia (ALL) generally accounts for 75–80% of total childhood leukaemia (Parkin *et al.*, 1989). Leukaemia is associated with high socioeconomic status in many studies. Spatial clustering has been identified in studies in Great Britain, Greece and Hong Kong, but not in Sweden or in metropolitan areas of the USA. The units of space considered in the study in the USA were larger than those used in the analyses in other countries, and therefore the effects of small-scale geographical clustering may have been diluted. In studies in Great Britain, there have been consistent positive associations with measures of population mixing. In some of these studies, estimates of the population at risk may have been inaccurate, although in certain analyses, the results were shown to be similar when

different estimates of the denominator population were applied. Population mixing also has been associated with excesses of childhood leukaemia in Hong Kong. High rates of mortality due to childhood leukaemia in Greece and Italy between the late 1950s and early 1970s may be attributable to mass migration from rural areas, and high rates in Israel during the late 1950s to mass immigration. However, excesses of mortality due to childhood leukaemia have not been associated with rapid population influx in France or with the growth of tourism in Greece. Data from other populations are needed on these issues.

These findings have been interpreted as supporting an infectious etiology for the disease (Alexander, 1993; Greaves & Alexander, 1993). According to Greaves' (1988) hypothesis, ALL of the common B-cell precursor type is postulated to arise from two spontaneous mutations, one *in utero* at a stage of multiplication of B-cell precursors and the other postnatally following the infant's first contact with a diverse range of antigens. Mathematical modelling, analogy with other paediatric tumours, experimental studies with avian oncogenes *in vitro* and studies on leukaemias in transgenic mice suggest that a minimum of two mutations is required for the development of acute leukaemia (Greaves, 1993). In the absence of a virus containing two (or more) oncogenes, these mutations will occur sequentially and independently. A leading candidate for the cause of the postulated first mutation has been paternal occupational exposure to ionizing radiation resulting in germ-cell mutation, suggested by the study in West Cumbria (Gardner *et al.*, 1990a), but in view of a lack of corroborative evidence from studies in Canada (McLaughlin *et al.*, 1992, 1993b), France (Pobel & Viel, 1997), Germany (Michaelis *et al.*, 1994) and Scotland (Kinlen *et al.*, 1993b), it seems likely that the effect of paternal occupational exposure in West Cumbria is due to other factors. The association with paternal occupational exposure to solvents (Table 11.1) might reflect germ-cell mutation, but might also be compatible with an effect of postnatal

## Table 11.1. Summary of factors investigated in relation to leukaemia in children

*Factors generally accepted as associated with leukaemia*
  Ataxia telangiectasia, Fanconi's anaemia in the index child
  Neurofibromatosis type 1 in the index child
  Certain types of hereditary immunodeficiency in the index child
  Tumour of the central nervous system as main type of second primary tumour
  Intrauterine exposure to diagnostic X-rays (early studies)
  Down's syndrome in the index child

*Factors which have been associated with leukaemia with some degree of consistency*
  High socioeconomic status
  Spatial clustering
  HLA-haplotype sharing in sibs
  Postnatal exposure to pesticides
  Maternal occupational exposure to metals (ANLL)
  Paternal occupational exposure to solvents
  Population mixing
  Paternal smoking (ALL)
  Maternal alcohol consumption during pregnancy (ANLL)
  Neonatal jaundice (AML, possibly secondary to Down's syndrome)

*Factors for which the evidence is inconsistent*
  Familial aggregation of acute leukaemia
  Excesses in the vicinity of nuclear reprocessing plants
  Paternal preconceptional occupational exposure to ionizing radiation
  Preconceptional X-ray exposure of the mother or father
  Postnatal exposure to diagnostic and therapeutic ionizing radiation
  Residential exposure to electromagnetic fields
  Maternal and paternal occupational exposure to pesticides
  Maternal immune function
  Infection during the first six months of life
  Infection at any time during the child's lifetime
  B.C.G. vaccination of the index child
  Contact of the index child with pets
  Maternal smoking during pregnancy
  Paternal smoking (all types combined, ANLL)
  Maternal alcohol consumption during pregnancy (all types combined, ALL)
  Birth order
  Elevated maternal age
  Previous fetal loss
  Interval between discontinuation of oral contraceptive use and the conception of the index child
  Threatened miscarriage of index pregnancy
  Intrauterine exposure to ultrasound
  Maternal anaesthesia during labour
  High birth weight
  Neonatal exposure to photosensitizing lighting (ALL)
  Intramuscular vitamin K prophylaxis
  Allergy in the index child
  Height of the index child

*Factors for which associations indicated in one or two studies do not appear to have been investigated further*
  Maternal dietary topoisomerase II inhibitors (AML)
  Consumption of cured meats by the index child
  Incense burning during the index pregnancy
  Multiple sclerosis in the mother
  Skin diseases in the mother or in the father
  Maternal consumption of milk during pregnancy (inverse association for ALL of the non-T-cell type)
  Use of chloramphenicol or syntomycin by the index child
  Attendance of the index child at a crèche during the first two years of life (inverse association)
  Use of cod liver oil by the index child
  Use of mind-altering drugs by the mother in the year preceding or during the index pregnancy (ANLL)
  Maternal use of anti-nauseants during pregnancy (ANLL)

*Factors not associated with leukaemia in most of the available studies*
  Paternal age
  Paternal occupational exposure to hydrocarbons
  Maternal use of antibiotics during pregnancy
  Caesarean section
  Neonatal jaundice (ALL)

---

ALL, Acute lymphocytic leukaemia
AML, Acute myeloid leukaemia
ANLL, Acute non-lymphocytic leukaemia

exposure of the index child, as chlorinated solvents have been detected in the exhaled air of workers for several hours after exposure. Similarly, it is difficult to determine whether the association between paternal smoking and ALL is due to preconceptional, gestational or postnatal effects. In view of the absence of an association with maternal smoking, a preconceptional effect seems to be most likely. Cigarette smoke has been shown to be mutagenic in prokaryotes, fungi/green plants and insects, and cigarette smoke condensate in these organisms and also in mammalian cells *in vitro* (IARC, 1986a). The initial mutation could be a somatic mutation *in utero*, and the increased risk associated with exposure to diagnostic X-rays in pregnancy suggests that a mutation *in utero* is possible (Greaves, 1993).

Other intrauterine exposures have not clearly been linked with the disease (Table 11.1), although it is interesting that in a few studies, acute non-lymphocytic leukaemia (ANLL) has been associated with maternal alcohol consumption during pregnancy and with maternal occupational exposure to metals.

A study of immunoglobulin heavy chain gene rearrangements in 61 cases of B-cell precursor ALL in children showed that 87.5% of cases aged three years or less lacked N regions, compared with only 11% of cases above this age (Wassermann *et al.*, 1992). Recent data on monozygotic twins concordant for ALL show that these leukaemias are clonally initiated *in utero* in one twin but spread to the co-twin via placental anastomoses that occur in monochorionic placentae (Ford *et al.*, 1993; Greaves, 1993). Low concordance rates for leukaemia in twins indicate that an *in utero* event itself is insufficient for the development of clinical leukaemia, and support the concept of a second postnatal event.

Exposure to infection during the lifetime of the index child is the leading suspect in initiating the postulated postnatal event. However, direct evidence is lacking. No consistent association has been identified with infections during the child's lifetime (Table 11.1). In addition, there is a report of a positive association with use of chloramphenicol or syntomycin by the index child. In two studies, an inverse association with attendance of the index child at a crèche during the first two years of life was found. It would be relevant to examine this association in other countries such as France, where attendance at a crèche or 'halte-garderie' is common from the age of two months. In some studies, there appears to be an association between ALL and

HLA-Cw3 and Cw4 antigens, and there is a preliminary report of associations between common ALL and HLA-DP1 genotypes. Thus, the possible relationship with postnatal infection may be mediated by genetic susceptibility. As yet, little information is available specifically for leukaemia in relation to vaccination and breast-feeding. These issues are being pursued in studies currently in progress in Canada, New Zealand, Great Britain and the USA (Coleman *et al.*, 1992). In the case–control design typically employed in analytical epidemiological studies of childhood cancer, obtaining information on prior infection is extremely difficult. Serological studies give no information on the timing of infection, and the possibility cannot be excluded that cases will be especially prone to infection during the pre-clinical period. Certain infections may be clinically silent, and parents may not recollect the particular type of infection diagnosed. Greaves and Alexander (1993) suggested that candidate viruses could be evaluated by a combination of laboratory, sero-epidemiological and case–control studies. Subsequently, precise hypotheses could be tested using biological samples from large prospective cohorts of high-risk individuals.

Another exposure which might induce the postulated postnatal event is to pesticides (Table 11.1). The available data are inadequate to assess whether the association is apparent only for certain specific agents. In addition, use of pesticides may be a marker of rural isolation, so the possibility that the association is secondary to confounding by patterns of exposure to infection which may be due to population mixing cannot be excluded. Much of the data considered by IARC working groups (IARC, 1983, 1986b) was inadequate to determine the mutagenicity of pesticides in short-term tests. Evidence of the mutagenicity in cellular systems was classified as sufficient for the insecticides methyl parathion and trichlorfon, the herbicides diallate and sulfallate, and the fungicide captan, but the available evidence was insufficient as to the possible mutagenic effects on mammalian cells.

At the time of writing, it seems unlikely that exposure to electromagnetic fields is a major cause of childhood leukaemia. While in four out of five studies, there was a positive association between childhood leukaemia and calculated historical exposure to magnetic fields, no association with measured magnetic fields was found in a large study in which measurements were obtained for most of the reference period for more than 80% of the study subjects. This suggests that the lack of a consistent association in other studies based on measured magnetic fields may not entirely be the result of these being a poor indicator of past exposure.

In regard to the hypothesis that maternal fertility problems are associated with ALL (van Steensel-Moll *et al.*, 1985a), an increased risk associated with infertility investigations and hormonal treatment for infertility in the peri-conceptional period has been reported in a study in England, but no instance of ovulation induction was reported in a large series of childhood leukaemia cases in Japan. No consistent association is apparent with a history of previous fetal loss, prolonged interval between oral contraceptive discontinuation and the index conception (although this has been little investigated), or threatened abortion during the index pregnancy.

## The lymphomas

Studies in endemic areas have indicated that Burkitt's lymphoma is associated with Epstein–Barr virus (Table 11.2). However, this association does not explain the geographical distribution of Burkitt's lymphoma, its relationship with age, or the observation that in general predominantly boys are affected. The factor most discussed in relation to these features is persistent and heavy infection with malaria, as the geographical distributions of holoendemic malaria and Burkitt's lymphoma are similar. If true, this may depend on the vectorial capacity, rather than the simple occurrence of falciparum malaria. The proportion of cases of Burkitt's lymphoma associated with Epstein–Barr virus is lower in areas of low and intermediate incidence of the lymphoma than in endemic areas, and the

sub-types of the virus involved may differ.

Other than the investigations of Burkitt's lymphoma, little work has been done specifically on lymphomas in children. Outside Africa, South America, parts of Asia, and the Mediterranean area, Burkitt's lymphoma accounts only for a minority of cases of non-Hodgkin lymphoma in children. Non-Hodgkin lymphoma was included with leukaemia in several studies with case ascertainment starting in the 1950s because of possible confusion in diagnosis. Work specifically on non-Hodgkin disease in children would now be of interest in view of the rise in incidence reported in children and adults combined (Coleman *et al.*, 1993). Non-Hodgkin lymphoma has been reported in children infected with HIV. HIV may become an important cause of childhood cancer. Epstein–Barr virus has been detected in high proportions of tumour samples from paediatric cases of Hodgkin's disease.

## Central nervous system tumours

Evidence on factors of possible importance in the etiology of tumours of the central nervous system is summarized in Table 11.3. There is an increased risk of cancer in sibs, but the evidence regarding the occurrence of cancer in other relatives is inconsistent. In the available studies, a positive association between astrocytoma and high birth weight has been observed.

The *N*-nitroso hypothesis does not appear to be well supported. No consistent association between brain tumours and smoking of either parent, or with exposure of the index child to tobacco smoke after birth, is apparent. The associations with maternal use of incense, consumption of beer, or use of hair colourants or

---

**Table 11.2. Summary of factors investigated in relation to lymphomas in children**

*Factors generally accepted as associated with lymphoma*
  Certain types of hereditary immunodeficiency in the index child
  Ataxia telangiectasia in the index child
  Neurofibromatosis type 1 in the index child
  Epstein–Barr virus infection (endemic Burkitt's lymphoma)

*Factors for which the evidence is inconsistent*
  Residential exposure to electromagnetic fields
  Persistent and heavy infection with malaria (endemic Burkitt's lymphoma)

*Factors for which associations indicated in one or two studies do not appear to have been investigated further*
  Excess risk of brain tumours in relatives of children with non-Hodgkin lymphoma
  Presence of *Euphorbia tirucalli* plant in the home (endemic Burkitt's lymphoma)
  Epstein–Barr virus infection (Hodgkin's disease)
  HIV infection (non-Hodgkin lymphoma)
  Asian ethnic group (mainly Indian sub-continent) within the UK (Hodgkin's disease)

HIV, Human immunodeficiency virus

**Table 11.3. Summary of factors investigated in relation to tumours of the central nervous system (CNS) in children**

*Factors generally accepted to be associated with CNS tumours*
 Neurofibromatosis (mainly type 1) in the index child
 Tuberous sclerosis in the index child
 Gorlin syndrome in the index child
 Turcot's syndrome in the index child
 Increased risk of cancer in sibs
 Leukaemia as main type of second primary tumour
 Intrauterine exposure to diagnostic X-rays (early studies)

*Factors which have been associated with CNS tumours with some degree of consistency*
 Maternal consumption of cured meats during the index pregnancy
 Maternal use of vitamin supplements during early pregnancy
 High birth weight (astrocytoma)

*Factors for which the evidence is inconsistent*
 Ethnic group
 Socioeconomic status
 Risk of cancer in relatives other than sibs
 Index child's exposure to diagnostic X-rays
 Residential exposure to electromagnetic fields
 Paternal occupational exposure to electromagnetic fields
 Pesticide exposure during the index pregnancy or during the lifetime of the index child
 Paternal occupational exposure to hydrocarbons
 Paternal employment in the aircraft industry
 Contact of the index child with animals
 Tonsillectomy in the index child
 Diet, including vitamin supplement use, of the index child
 Maternal smoking during pregnancy
 Smoking by the father
 Postnatal exposure of the index child to tobacco smoke
 Maternal beer consumption during the index pregnancy
 Maternal use of face make-up during pregnancy
 Incense burning during the index pregnancy
 Maternal age
 Birth order
 Previous fetal loss
 Maternal use of barbiturates during pregnancy
 General anaesthesia during pregnancy
 Caesarean section
 Maternal use of antihistamines during pregnancy
 Maternal use of diuretics during pregnancy
 Maternal use of exogenous hormones
 Congenital anomalies in the index child
 Birthweight (all types combined)
 Head injury in the index child

*Factors for which associations indicated in one or two studies do not appear to have been investigated further*
 Maternal intake of folate during pregnancy (PNET)
 Maternal use of marijuana during pregnancy or in the month preceding pregnancy (astrocytoma)
 Maternal use of anti-nauseants during pregnancy (astrocytoma)
 Neonatal distress and related treatments

*Factors not associated with brain tumours in most of the available studies*
 Paternal age
 Maternal use of hair colourants during pregnancy

*Factors thought to be secondary to the presence of the tumour*
 Hydrocephalus
 Epilepsy and related use of anticonvulsants

PNET, Primitive neuroectodermal tumours

other cosmetics, have been less studied than those with tobacco smoking, but are not consistent in the available studies. No consistent association with maternal use of antihistamines or diuretics in pregnancy has been found. In seven out of eight studies, a positive association between brain tumours in children and maternal consumption of one or more types of cured meat during pregnancy was found. However, in some of these studies, the association may be accounted for by selection bias, and the adequacy of others cannot be determined as they have been published only as abstracts. In addition, in most of the studies, information was sought about relatively few foods, and no evaluation of the validity of the dietary assessments appears to have been undertaken. No clear relationship between brain tumours and the diet of the index child has been identified. As yet, no analysis according to estimated total burden of *N*-nitroso compounds (Choi, 1985) has been published.

In five out of six studies of brain tumours in which maternal consumption of vitamin supplements during pregnancy was investigated, an inverse association was observed. One of these studies related specifically to the category of primitive neuroectodermal tumours, defined to include medulloblastomas, neuroblastomas in the brain, ependymoblastomas and pineoblastoma (Bunin *et al.*, 1993). There is considerable dispute as to the categorization of embryonal tumours of the central nervous system, which has arisen from the unresolved histogenesis of cerebellar medulloblastoma (Kleihues *et al.*, 1993). There is general agreement that this tumour is derived from an immature precursor cell, but this has not been identified. Nevertheless, a most exciting finding is that 'primitive neuroectodermal tumours', 90% of which were medulloblastomas, have been associated with estimated maternal folate intake during pregnancy, and with use of multivitamin supplements during the first six weeks of pregnancy. If these associations are real, it might be expected that there would be an association between these tumours and neural tube defects, for which a protective effect of folate supplementation has been described (MRC Vitamin Study Research Group, 1991; Little, 1995). Such an association has been reported in a study of childhood brain tumours (Narod *et al.*, 1997), but was not specific to medulloblastoma, and may have been an artefact of comparison with an inappropriate control group. It would be interesting to explore this issue in areas of high prevalence at birth of neural tube defects, namely the north-west parts of the British Isles, north-east China and perhaps parts of India and the Middle East (Little & Elwood, 1992b). A direct approach would be to study red cell folate levels in samples of blood taken early in pregnancy. It would be prohibitively expensive to undertake this in a prospective cohort study, but it may be possible to identify stored samples from cohort studies already undertaken and to match these to cancer registries. Another approach would be to examine folate levels in mothers of cases and controls, on the assumption that a deficiency in folate absorption or metabolism is relevant, as has been postulated

for neural tube defects (Yates *et al.*, 1987; Bower and Stanley, 1989; Wild *et al.*, 1993), and to determine the 5,10-methylenetetrahydrofolate reductase genotype, which also has been associated with spina bifida (van der Put *et al.*, 1995; Whitehead *et al.*, 1995).

Early reports suggesting an association between brain tumours and residential exposure to magnetic fields have not been confirmed. No consistent association between central nervous system tumours and inferred paternal occupational exposure to electromagnetic fields has been observed.

## Neuroblastoma

Fewer investigations have been made on neuroblastoma than on the leukaemias or tumours of the central nervous system. There are consistent reports of an increase in the incidence of neuroblastoma. In most areas in which this has been observed, no systematic screening for neuroblastoma has been in operation. In two out of three studies, a positive association with use of sex hormones before or during the index pregnancy was found. This may be consistent with excesses of neuroblastoma reported after assisted conception. Earlier reports of associations with maternal consumption of alcohol, use of neurally active drugs, and use of hair colourants during pregnancy (Table 11.4) do not appear to have been investigated further. Recent reports suggest an association with parental occupational exposure to pesticides.

There is considerable diversity in the clinical behaviour of neuroblastoma, which has been interpreted as evidence of biological diversity, and confirmed by molecular genetic studies (Tonini, 1993). It would be relevant to pool data from several centres and attempt to analyse potential risk factors by biological sub-type.

## Wilms' tumour

In earlier work, Wilms' tumour was considered as an 'index tumour' for the purposes of evaluating completeness of ascertainment but more recently, considerable geographical variation in incidence has been documented. While a subset of cases of Wilms' tumour is known to be of genetic etiology, the importance of genetic factors in etiology is less substantial than suggested in early studies. A consistent association between high birth weight and Wilms' tumour is apparent in the largest studies. This does not appear to be due

## Table 11.4. Summary of factors investigated in relation to neuroblastoma in children

*Factors which have been associated with neuroblastoma with some degree of consistency*
Maternal use of sex hormones before or during the index pregnancy

*Factors for which the evidence is inconsistent*
Thyroid cancer as main type of second primary tumour
Paternal occupational exposure to electromagnetic fields
Maternal smoking during pregnancy
Paternal smoking
Maternal use of anticonvulsants during pregnancy
Maternal age
Birth order
Previous fetal loss
Maternal use of diuretics during pregnancy (may be secondary to pre-symptomatic disease in the fetus)
Birth weight

*Factors for which associations indicated in one or two studies do not appear to have been investigated further*
Low socioeconomic status
Congenital anomalies in relatives of cases
Parental occupational exposure to pesticides
Maternal alcohol consumption during pregnancy (the two available studies are inconsistent)
Maternal use of hair colourants during pregnancy
Maternal use of neurally active drugs other than phenytoin during pregnancy

*Factors consistently not associated with neuroblastoma in the available studies*
Specific genetic syndromes

## Table 11.5. Summary of factors investigated in relation to Wilms' tumour

*Factors generally accepted as associated with Wilms' tumour*
Aniridia
Hemihypertrophy
Denys–Drash syndrome
Beckwith–Wiedemann syndrome
Anomalies of the genitourinary tract

*Factors which have been associated with Wilms' tumour with some degree of consistency*
Ethnic group (blacks in the USA)
Paternal employment in occupations potentially involving exposure to metals
Exposure to pesticides
High birth weight

*Factors for which the evidence is inconsistent*
Risk of cancer in relatives of patients with Wilms' tumour
Elevated paternal age
Paternal occupational exposure to hydrocarbons
Paternal occupational exposure to lead
Maternal consumption of tea and coffee during pregnancy
Maternal smoking during pregnancy
High birth weight
Maternal age
Birth order
Previous fetal loss
Pregnancy hypertension
Maternal anaesthesia during labour
Maternal use of sex hormones

*Factors for which associations indicated in one or two studies do not appear to have been investigated further*
Ethnic origin (decreased risk in Asians, mainly originating from the Indian subcontinent, in the UK)
Maternal vaginal infection during pregnancy
Maternal antibiotic use during pregnancy
Maternal use of hair colourants during pregnancy (Wilms' tumour diagnosed before the age of two years)
Mother diagnosed with a gall-bladder disorder or gallstones during pregnancy
Neonatal jaundice

entirely to the association with specific overgrowth syndromes. The only other factor to have been associated with Wilms' tumour with some consistency is paternal employment in occupations potentially involving exposure to metals or to pesticides (Table 11.5). In future studies, there is a need to consider sub-types of the disease.

# Other specific types of cancer

The two-mutation hypothesis proposed to account for the occurrence of retinoblastoma in both hereditary and sporadic forms has become the paradigm for considering the role of genetic factors in the etiology of cancer. There is a paternal predominance of *de novo* mutation, but no strong paternal age effect has been observed. In studies with a short follow-up, most second primary tumours are osteosarcomas and soft-tissue sarcomas. Melanoma has been observed in studies with longer follow-up, and has been reported in excess in the families of patients with retinoblastoma. In two studies, an association with paternal employment involving welding has been observed. Only one study has been made of sporadic heritable and non-heritable forms of the disease (Bunin *et al.*, 1989a, 1990a). With regard to the sporadic heritable type, positive associations were found with paternal preconceptional employment in the armed forces and in the metal industry, and with X-ray examination of the lower abdomen or back and smoking of the father before conception. A number of maternal exposures during pregnancy were found to be associated with the non-heritable form of the disease (X-ray, morning sickness medication), while there were inverse associations with anaemia and multivitamin use.

Hepatoblastoma is associated with familial adenomatous polyposis. Only one analytical epidemiological study of hepatoblastoma is available (Buckley *et al.*, 1989a). The only significantly associated paternal exposure was to metals. There was also a significant association with maternal occupational exposure to metals; in addition, significant associations were found with maternal occupational exposure to petroleum products, paints and pigments. No evidence was found to support the primary study hypotheses relating to hepatitis infection, maternal estrogen exposure, alcohol consumption, smoking or potential sources of nitrosamines.

No consistent association between height and osteosarcoma or Ewing's sarcoma has been found, contrary to early studies. In the two available case–control studies of osteosarcoma, there was no association with maternal estrogen use during pregnancy, no consistent association with maternal occupation, and no clear association with birth weight, length at birth or presence of congenital anomalies in the index child. In the earlier study, a weak association was apparent with intrauterine exposure to diagnostic radiation, whereas this was not observed in the more recent study. This pattern is consistent with observations for other types of childhood cancer. The two available studies of Ewing's sarcoma show positive associations with paternal employment in agriculture. In one of these, this appears to have been due to pesticides, but there was no association with use of pesticides in the home.

In several areas, the incidence of soft-tissue sarcoma appears to be increasing. Soft-tissue sarcoma has been observed to aggregate with other tumours in families with an autosomal dominant pattern, recognized as the Li–Fraumeni syndrome. However, this accounts for only a small proportion of cases. Soft-tissue sarcoma also is associated with neurofibromatosis type 1, but again this association accounts only for a very small proportion of cases. A weak association between maternal age over 30 years and rhabdomyosarcoma has been observed in the three available studies, although in the largest study, this was not apparent when maternal age over 35 years was considered (Ghali *et al.*, 1992). The two available studies indicate a positive association with prior fetal loss. A positive association between rhabdomyosarcoma and smoking by the father found in an early exploratory study was not confirmed in subsequent studies. One of these was specifically designed to test the hypothesis that paternal smoking was causal (Grufferman *et al.*, 1993) and questions about other aspects of lifestyle were asked of parents in order to minimize the possibility of biased reporting of smoking habits. Unexpected positive associations with use of recreational drugs were found in this large study, but it was not possible to clarify whether maternal or paternal exposure was relevant.

In several locations, the incidence of germ-cell tumours appears to be rising. There appears to be an excess of congenital anomalies of all types combined in cases with germ-cell tumours. It is unclear whether this is attributable to anomalies of specific types, and bias of ascertainment may have influenced the findings. There is a consistent positive association between germ-cell tumours and high birth weight. This may be compatible with a role of estrogen exposure in the etiology of germ-cell tumours, as was postulated by Shu *et al.* (1995a).

Diethylstilbestrol treatment of the mother during pregnancy has been causally linked with clear-cell adenocarcinoma of the vagina and cervix.

# Final comments

The problem of childhood cancer has stimulated a new area of epidemiological inquiry, namely the health effects of exposure to electromagnetic fields, and a great deal of methodological development in the analysis of clustering and clusters, following the observation of excesses of haematopoietic malignancies in young people in the vicinity of some nuclear plants. Although the weight of evidence now available does not support a major role for electromagnetic fields or ionizing radiation other than that received in diagnostic X-ray examinations *in utero*, these are important areas of public concern and further studies are in progress (Coleman *et al.*, 1992). The studies of electromagnetic fields have highlighted the more general problems of exposure assessment and selection bias of controls. Aspects relevant to clinical practice include the associations with vitamin K suggested in studies in Great Britain, but subsequently not confirmed in studies in Sweden and the USA.

A recurrent issue in the concluding points relating to specific types of cancer has been the need for assessment of associations for sub-types. In view of the rarity of childhood cancer, multicentre studies are needed in order to have adequate numbers by sub-type for analysis. This poses the challenge of standardization of classification, but this is not insurmountable in view of the experience of cooperative clinical trials in Europe and in North America. As emphasized in much recent epidemiological literature, improvement in methods of assessing exposure is needed (Armstrong *et al.*, 1992). In the context of the case–control study, which is the design used in almost all analytical epidemiological studies of childhood cancer, recall bias is a major concern, but no severe unidirectional bias has been detected in studies where differences in information collected retrospectively and that obtained before pregnancy outcome was known were compared between mothers who experienced adverse reproductive outcome and other mothers (Little, 1992). This issue has not, however, been explored in relation to childhood cancer, and certain exposures have received a great deal of publicity in this context. With regard to illnesses affecting, and drugs used by, the index child, the parents of the child and perhaps other family members, use of medical records is valuable but should be used in parallel with, rather than supplanting, information collected by interview. With regard to measurements in the human body or its products, the main tissue considered in studies of childhood cancer has been blood. Studies which seek to use biomarkers in blood are likely to face difficulties in meeting ethical guidelines (Garralda, 1993) and possibly poor participation rates, especially in relation to control subjects. These problems may in part be solved by the development of techniques suitable for the analysis of very small blood volumes (Elliott *et al.*, 1991a) and of saliva (Malamud, 1992).

Most of the available studies of childhood cancer have been carried out in North America or in Europe. It is important that studies are carried out in other countries.

# References

Adami, H-O., Glimelius, B., Sparén, P., Holmberg, L., Krusemo, U.B. & Pontén, J. (1992) Trends in childhood and adolescent cancer survival in Sweden 1960 through 1984. *Acta Oncol.*, **31**, 1–10

Adami, J., Glimelius, B., Cnattingius, S., Ekbom, A., Hoar Zahm, S., Linet, M. & Zack, M. (1996) Maternal and perinatal factors associated with non-Hodgkin's lymphoma among children. *Int. J. Cancer*, **65**, 774–777

Ager, E. A., Schuman, L.M., Wallace, H.M., Rosenfield, A.B. & Gullen, W.H. (1965) An epidemiological study of childhood leukaemia. *J. Chron. Dis.*, **18**, 113–132

Ahlbom, A., Feychting, M., Koskenvuo, M., Olsen, J.H., Pukkala, E., Schulgen, G. & Verkasalo, P. (1993) Electromagnetic fields and childhood cancer. *Lancet*, **342**, 1295–1296

Aickin, M., Chapin, C.A., Flood, T.J., Englender, S. J. & Caldwell, G.G. (1992) Assessment of the spatial occurrence of childhood leukaemia mortality using standardized rate ratios with a simple linear Poisson model. *Int. J. Epidemiol.*, **21**, 649–655

Aikhionbare, H.A., Yakuba, A.M. & Apolayan, A.E. (1988) Neuroblastoma, an under-diagnosed tumour: a 7-year experience in Zaria. *Ann. Trop. Paediatr.*, **8**, 149–152

Ajiki, W., Hanai, A., Tsukuma, H., Hiyama, T. & Fujimoto, I. (1994) Incidence of childhood cancer in Osaka, Japan, 1971–1988: Reclassification of registered cases by Birch's scheme using information on clinical diagnosis, histology and primary site. *Jpn. J. Cancer Res.*, **85**, 139–146

Ajiki, W., Hanai, A., Tzukuma, H., Hiyama, T. & Fujimoto, I. (1995) Survival rates of childhood cancer patients in Osaka, Japan, 1975–1984. *Jpn. J. Cancer Res.*, **86**, 13–20

al-Sheyyab, M., Muir, K.R., Cameron, A.H., Raafat, F., Pincott, J.R., Parkes, S.E. & Mann, J.R. (1993) Malignant epithelial tumours in children: incidence and aetiology. *Med. Pediat. Oncol.*, **21**, 421–428

Alaoui, F.M. (1988) Rabat: Hospital for Children, 1983–85. In: Parkin D.M., Stiller C.A., Draper, G.J., Bieber, C.A., Terracini, B. & Young, J.L., eds, *International Incidence of Childhood Cancer* (IARC Scientific Publication No. 87), Lyon, IARC, pp. 33–35

Albanes, D., Jones, D.Y., Schatzkin, A., Micozzi, M. S. & Taylor, P.R. (1988) Adult stature and risk of cancer. *Cancer Res.*, **48**, 1658–1662

Alderson, M.R. & Nayak, R. (1971) A study of space-time clustering in Hodgkin's disease in the Manchester region. *Br. J. Prev. Soc. Med.*, **25**, 168–173

Alderson, M.R. & Nayak, R. (1972) Epidemiology of Hodgkin's disease. *J. Chron. Dis.*, **25**, 253–259

Alexander, F., Ricketts, T.J., McKinney, P.A. & Cartwright, R.A. (1989a) Cancer registration of leukaemias and lymphomas: results of a comparison with a specialist registry. *Commun. Med.*, **11**, 81–89

Alexander, F.E., Williams, J., McKinney, P.A., Ricketts, T.J. & Cartwright, R.A. (1989b) A specialist leukaemia/lymphoma registry in the UK. Part 2: Clustering of Hodgkin's disease. *Br. J. Cancer*, **60**, 948–952

Alexander, F., Cartwright, R., McKinney, P.A. & Ricketts, T.J. (1990a) Investigation of spatial clustering of rare diseases: childhood malignancies in North Humberside. *J. Epidemiol. Commun. Health*, **44**, 39–46

Alexander, F.E., Cartwright, R.A., McKinney, P.A. & Ricketts, T.J. (1990b) Leukaemia incidence, social class and estuaries: an ecological analysis. *J. Public Health Med.*, **12**, 109–117

Alexander, F.E., McKinney, P.A. & Cartwright, R.A. (1990c) Radon and leukaemia. *Lancet*, **335**, 1336–1337

Alexander, F.E., Ricketts, T.J., McKinney, P.A. & Cartwright, R.A. (1990d) Community lifestyle characteristics and risk of acute lymphoblastic leukaemia in children. *Lancet*, **336**, 1461–1465

Alexander, F.E. (1991) Investigations of localised spatial clustering, and extra-Poisson variation. In: Draper G.J., ... ukaemia ... 1966–83 ... No. 53), ... ght, R.A. ... g small ... raphical ... twright, ... ics and ... K. Eur. J. ... twright, ... cs and ... . Int. J. ... ldhood ... e for a ... K.C. & ... ity of ... phoma ... er, 65, 583–588

Alexander, F.E., Cartwright, R.A. & McKinney, P.A. (1992b) Paternal occupations of children with leukaemia. *Br. Med. J.*, **305**, 715–716

Alexander, F. E. (1993) Viruses, clusters and clustering of childhood leukaemia: a new perspective? *Eur. J. Cancer*, **29A**, 1424–1443

Alexander, F.E., McKinney, P.M. & Cartwright, R.A. (1993) Migration patterns of children with leukaemia and non-Hodgkin's lymphoma in three areas of northern England. *J. Pub. Health Med.* **15**, 9–15

Alexander, F.E. & Boyle, P., eds (1996) *Methods for Investigating Localised Clustering of Disease* (IARC Scientific Publication No. 135), Lyon, IARC

Alexander, F.E., Leon, D.A. & Cartwright, R.A. (1996) Isolation, car ownership, and small area variation in incidence of acute lymphoblastic leukaemia in children. *Paediat. Perinatal Epidemiol.*, **10**, 411–417

Alexander, F.E., Chan, L.C., Lam, T.H., Yuen, P., Leung, N.K., Ha, S.Y., Yuen, H.L., Li, C.K., Li, C.K., Lau, Y.L. & Greaves, M.F. (1997) Clustering of childhood leukaemia in Hong Kong: association with the childhood peak and common acute lymphoblastic leukaemia and with population mixing. *Br. J. Cancer*, **75**, 457–463

Allen, R.W., Jr, Ogden, B., Bentley, F.L. & Jung, A.L. (1980) Fetal hydantoin syndrome, neuroblastoma and hemorrhagic disease in a neonate. *J. Am. Med. Assoc.*, **244**, 1464–1465

Ambach, W. & Rehwald, W. (1994) Studies may have had inadequate statistical power. *Br. Med. J.*, **309**, 1300

Ambrosch, F., Wiedermann, G. & Krepler, P. (1986) Studies on the influence of BCG vaccination on infantile leukaemia. International Symposium of BCG Vaccines and Tuberculins, Budapest, Hungary, 1983. *Develop. Biol. Standard*, **58**, 419–424

Ambrosone, C.B., Freudenheim, J.L., Graham, S., Marshall, J.R., Vena, J.E., Brasure, J.R., Michalek, A.M., Laughlin, R., Nemoto, T., Gillenwater, K.A., Harrington, A.M. & Shields, P.G. (1996) Cigarette smoking, N-acetyltransferase 2 genetic polymorphisms, and breast cancer risk. *J. Am. Med. Assoc.*, **276**, 1494–1501

Andersson, M., Juel, K., Ishikawa, Y. & Storm, H.H. (1994) Effects of preconceptional irradiation on mortality and cancer incidence in the offspring of patients given injections of Thorotrast. *J. Natl. Cancer Inst.*, **86**, 1866–1870

Annegers, J.F., Kurland, L.T. & Hauser, W.A. (1979) Brain tumors in children exposed to barbiturates. *J. Natl. Cancer Inst.*, **63**, 3

Ansell, P., Bull, D. & Roman, E. (1996) Childhood leukaemia and intramuscular vitamin K: findings from a case-control study. *Br. Med. J.*, **313**, 204–205

Anwar, N., Kingma, D.W., Bloch, A.R., Mourad, M., Raffeld, M., Franklin, J., Magrath, I., el Bolkainy, N. & Jaffe, E.S. (1995) The investigation of Epstein-Barr viral sequences in 41 cases of Burkitt's lymphoma from Egypt: epidemiologic correlations. *Cancer*, **76**, 1245–1252

Archer, V.E. (1987) Association of nuclear fallout with leukaemia in the United States. *Arch. Environ. Health*, **42**, 263–271

Aricò, M., Caselli, D., D'Argenio, P., Del Mistro, A.R., DeMartino, M., Livadiotti, S., Santoro, N. & Terragna, A. (1991) Malignancies in children with human immunodeficiency virus type 1 infection. *Cancer*, **68**, 2473–2477

Armstrong, B.K., White, E. & Saracci, R. (1992) *Principles of Exposure Assessment in Epidemiology*, Oxford, Oxford University Press

Armstrong, A.A., Alexander, F.E., Pinto Paes, R., Morad, N.A., Gallagher, A., Krajewski, A.S., Jones, D.B., Angus, B., Adams, J., Cartwright, R.A., Onions, D.E. & Jarrett, R.F. (1993) Association of Epstein-Barr virus with pediatric Hodgkin's disease. *Am. J. Pathol.*, **142**, 1683–1688

Artzt, K. & Bennett, D. (1972) A genetically caused embryonal ectodermal tumor in the mouse. *J. Natl. Cancer Inst.*, **48**, 141–158

Austin, D.F., Karp, S., Dworsky, R. & Henderson, B.E. (1975) Excess leukemia in cohorts of children born following influenza epidemics. *Am. J. Epidemiol.*, **101**, 77–83

Australian Paediatric Cancer Registry (1994) *Childhood Cancer Incidence in Australia 1977–86*, Brisbane, Australian Paediatric Cancer Registry

Auvinen, A., Hakama, M., Arvela, H., Hakulinen, T., Rahola, T., Suomela, M., Söderman, B. & Rytömaa, T. (1994) Fallout from Chernobyl and incidence of childhood leukaemia in Finland, 1976–92. *Br. Med. J.*, **309**, 151–154

Aya, T., Kinoshita, T., Imai, S., Koizumi, S., Mizuno, F., Osato, T., Satoh, C., Oikawa, T., Kuzumaki, N., Ohigashi, H. & Koshimizu, K. (1991) Chromosome translocation and c-MYC activation by Epstein-Barr virus and *Euphorbia tirucalli* in B lymphocytes. *Lancet*, **337**, 1190

Bacchi, M.M., Bacchi, C.E., Alvarenga, M., Miranda, R., Chen, Y.Y. & Weiss, L.M. (1996) Burkitt's lymphoma in Brazil: strong association with Epstein-Barr virus. *Modern Pathology*, **9**, 63–67

Bader, J.L. & Miller, R.W. (1978) Neurofibromatosis and childhood leukemia. *J. Pediatr.*, **92**, 925–929

Bailar, J.C., Eisenberg, H. & Mantel, M. (1970) Time between pairs of leukemia cases. *Cancer*, **25**, 1301–1303

Banks, P.M. (1992) Changes in diagnosis of non-Hodgkin's lymphomas over time. *Cancer Res.*, **52**, 5453S–5455S

Baptiste, M., Nasca, P., Metzger, B., Field, N., MacCubbin, P., Greenwald, P., Armbrustmacher, V., Waldman, J. & Carlton, K. (1989) Neurofibromatosis and other disorders among children with CNS tumors and their families. *Neurology*, **39**, 487–492

Barber, R. & Spiers, P. (1964) Oxford survey of childhood cancer: progress report II. *Monthly Bull. Min. Health*, **23**, 46–52

Barlow, D.P. (1995) Gametic imprinting in mammals. *Science*, **270**, 1610–1613

Barnes, N., Cartwright, R.A., O'Brien, C., Roberts, B., Richards, I.D.G. & Bird, C.C. (1987) Spatial patterns in electoral wards with high lymphoma incidence in Yorkshire health region. *Br. J. Cancer*, **56**, 169–172

Barona, P., Sierrasesúmaga, L., Antillón, F. & Villa-Elízaga, I. (1993) Study of HLA-antigens in patients with osteosarcoma. *Hum. Hered.*, **43**, 311–314

Barton, D.E., David, F.N. & Merrington, M. (1965) A criteria for testing contagion in time and space. *Ann. Hum. Genet. (Lond.)*, **29**, 97–102

Bartsch, H. (1991) N-Nitroso compounds and human cancer: where do we stand? In: O'Neill I.K., Chen J. & Bartsch H., eds, *Relevance to Human Cancer of N-Nitroso Compounds, Tobacco Smoke and Mycotoxins* (IARC Scientific Publications No. 105), Lyon, IARC, pp. 1–10

Bartsch, H., Ohshima, H. & Pignatelli, B. (1988) Inhibitors of endogenous nitrosation. Mechanism and implications in human cancer prevention. *Mutat. Res.*, **202**, 307–324

Baverstock, K., Egloff, B., Pinchera, A., Ruchti, C. & Williams, D. (1992) Thyroid cancer after Chernobyl. *Nature*, **359**, 21–22

Ben-Sasson, S.A. & Davis, D.L. (1992) Neonatal exposure to protoporphyrin-activating lighting as a contributing cause of childhood acute lymphocytic leukemia. *Cancer Causes Control*, **3**, 385–387

Bender, A.P., Robison, L.L., Kashmiri, S.V.S., McClain, K.L., Woods, W.G., Smithson, W.A., Heyn, R., Finlay, J., Schuman, L.M., Renier, C. & Gibson, R. (1988) No involvement of bovine leukemia virus in childhood acute lymphoblastic leukemia and non-Hodgkin's lymphoma. *Cancer Res.*, **48**, 2919–2922

Bengtsson, B.-A. (1993) Acromegaly and neoplasia. *J. Pediat. Endocrinol.*, **6**, 73–78

Beral, V. & Reeves, G. (1992) Childhood thyroid cancer in Belarus. *Nature*, **359**, 680–681

Bernard, J.L., Bernard-Couteret, E., Coste, D., Thyss, A., Scheiner, C., Perrimond, H., Mariani, R., Deville, A., Michel, G., Gentet, J.C. & Raybaud, C. (1993a) Childhood cancer incidence in the south-east of France. *Eur. J. Cancer*, **29A**, 2284–2291

Bernard, J.L., Bernard-Couteret, E. & Coste, D. (1993b) Neuroblastoma incidence in south-east France. *Int. J. Cancer*, **54**, 702

Berry, C.L., Keeling, J. & Hilton, C. (1970) Coincidence of congenital malformation and embryonic tumours of childhood. *Arch. Dis. Child.*, **45**, 229–231

Berry, D.H., Elders, M.J., Crist, W., Land, V., Lui, V., Sexauer, A.C. & Dickinson, L. (1983) Growth in children with acute lymphocytic leukemia: a Pediatric Oncology Group study. *Med. Pediatr. Oncol.*, **11**, 39–45

Bertazzi, P.-A. (1989) Industrial disasters and epidemiology. *Scand. J. Work Environ. Health*, **15**, 85–100

Bertin, M. & Lallemand, J. (1992) Augmentation des cancers de la thyroïde de l'enfant en Bélarus. *Ann. Endocrinol.*, **53**, 173–177

Besag, J. & Newell, J. (1991) The detection of clusters in rare diseases. *J. R. Statist. Soc.*, **154A**, 143–155

Besag, J., Newall, J. & Craft, A. (1991) The detection of small-area anomalies in the database. In: Draper G.J., ed., *The Geographical Epidemiology of Childhood Leukaemia and Non-Hodgkin Lymphomas in Great Britain, 1966–83* (Studies on Medical and Population Subjects No. 53), London, HMSO, pp. 101–107

Bessho, F. (1986) Height at diagnosis in acute lymphocytic leukaemia. *Arch. Dis. Child.*, **61**, 296–299

Bessho, F. (1989) Acute non-lymphocytic leukemia is not a major type of childhood leukemia in Japan. *Eur. J. Cancer Clin. Oncol.*, **25**, 729–732

Bessho, F., Hashizume, K., Nakajo, T. & Kamoshita, S. (1991) Mass screening in Japan increased the detection of infants with neuroblastoma without a decrease in cases in older children. *J. Pediatrics*, **119**, 237–241

Betuel, H., Freidel, A. C., Gebuhrer, L. & ARTMO Cooperative Group (1981) HLA antigens and haplotypes in families of leukaemic patients, eventual recipients of a bone marrow graft. In: Touraine, J.L., Gluckman, E. & Griscelli, C., eds, *Bone Marrow Transplantation in Europe. Volume II: Proceedings of the Fifth European Symposium on Bone Marrow Transplantation, Courchevel, Savoie, France; March 16–18, 1981.* Amsterdam, Excerpta Medica, Vol. II, pp. 255–263

Biggar, R.J. & Nkrumah, F.K. (1979) Burkitt's lymphoma in Ghana: urban–rural distribution, time–space clustering and seasonality. *Int. J. Cancer,* **232**, 330–336

Biggar, R.J., Gardiner, C., Lennette, E.T., Collins, W.E., Nkrumah, F.K. & Henle, W. (1981) Malaria, sex, and place of residence as factors in antibody response to Epstein-Barr virus in Ghana, West Africa. *Lancet,* **ii**, 115–118

Birch, J.M. (1980) Anencephaly in stillborn sibs of children with germ cell tumours. *Lancet,* **i**, 1257

Birch, J.M. (1988) Manchester Children's Tumour Registry 1954–1970 and 1971–1983. In: Parkin, D.M., Stiller, C.A., Draper, G.J., Bieber, C.A., Terracini, B., Young, J.L., eds, *International Incidence of Childhood Cancer* (IARC Scientific Publications No. 87), Lyon, IARC, pp. 299–304

Birch, J.M. (1994) Li–Fraumeni syndrome. *Eur. J. Cancer,* **30A**, 1935–1941

Birch, J.M. & Blair, V. (1988) Increase in childhood carcinomas in north-west England. *Lancet,* **i**, 833

Birch, J.M. & Marsden, H.B. (1987) A classification scheme for childhood cancer. *Int. J. Cancer,* **40**, 620–624

Birch, J.M., Swindell, R., Marsden, H.B. & Morris Jones, P.H. (1981) Childhood leukaemia in north west England 1954–1977: epidemiology, incidence and survival. *Br. J. Cancer,* **43**, 324–329

Birch, J.M., Marsden, H.B. & Swindell, R. (1982) Pre-natal factors in the origin of germ cell tumors of childhood. *Carcinogenesis,* **3**, 75–80

Birch, J.M., Mann, J.R., Cartwright, R.A., Draper, G.J., Waterhouse, J.A., Hartley, A.L., Johnston, H.E., McKinney, P.A., Stiller, C.A. & Hopton, P.A. (1985) The Inter-Regional Epidemiological Study of Childhood Cancer (IRESCC). Study design, control selection and data collection. *Br. J. Cancer,* **52**, 915–922

Birch, J.M., Hartley, A.L., Blair, V., Kelsey, A.M., Harris, M., Teare, M.D. & Jones, P.H. (1990a) Cancer in the families of children with soft tissue sarcoma. *Cancer,* **66**, 2239–2248

Birch, J.M., Hartley, A.L., Teare, M.D., Blair, V., McKinney, P.A., Mann, J.R., Stiller, C.A., Draper, G.J., Johnston, H.E., Cartwright, R.A. & Waterhouse, J.A.H. (1990b) The Inter-Regional Epidemiological Study of Childhood Cancer (IRESCC): case-control study of children with central nervous system tumours. *Br. J. Neurosurg.,* **4**, 17–26

Bishop, D.T. & Hall, N.R. (1994) The genetics of colorectal cancer. *Eur. J. Cancer,* **30A**, 1946–1956

Bithell, J.F. & Draper, G.J. (1995) Apparent association between benzene and childhood leukaemia: methodological doubts concerning a report by Knox. *J. Epidemiol. Commun. Health,* **49**, 437–439

Bithell, J.F. & Stewart, A.M. (1975) Pre-natal irradiation and childhood malignancy: a review of British data from the Oxford survey. *Br. J. Cancer,* **31**, 271–287

Bithell, J.F. & Stiller, C.A. (1988) A new calculation of the carcinogenic risk of obstetric X-raying. *Stat. Med.,* **7**, 857–864

Bithell, J.F., Draper, G.J. & Gorbach, P.D. (1973) Association between malignant disease in children and maternal virus infections. *Br. Med. J.,* **1**, 706–708

Bithell, J.F., Dutton, S.J., Draper, G.J. & Neary, N.M. (1994) Distribution of childhood leukaemias and non-Hodgkin's lymphomas near nuclear installations in England and Wales. *Br. Med. J.,* **309**, 501–505

Black, R.J., Sharp, L. & Urquhart, J.D. (1991) An analysis of the geographical distribution of childhood leukaemia and non-Hodgkin lymphomas in Great Britain using areas of approximately equal population size. In: Draper, G.J., ed., *The geographical epidemiology of childhood leukaemia and non-Hodgkin lymphomas in Great Britain, 1966–83* (Studies on Medical and Population Subjects No. 53), London, HMSO, pp. 61–67

Black, R.J., Urquhart, J.D., Kendrick, S.W., Bunch, K.J., Warner, J. & Adams Jones, D. (1992) Incidence of leukaemia and other cancers in birth and schools cohorts in the Dounreay area. *Br. Med. J.,* **304**, 1401–1405

Black, R.J., Sharp, L., Harkness, E.F. & McKinney, P.A. (1994) Leukaemia and non-Hodgkin's lymphoma: incidence in children and young adults resident in the Dounreay area of Caithness, Scotland in 1968–91. *J. Epidemiol. Commun. Health,* **48**, 232–236

Black, R.J., Sharp, L. & Urquhart, J.D. (1996) Analysing the spatial distribution of disease using a method of constructing geographical areas of approximately equal population size. In: Alexander, F.E. & Boyle, P., eds, *Methods for Investigating Localized Clustering of Disease* (IARC Scientific Publications No. 135), Lyon, IARC, pp. 28–39

Blair, V. & Birch, J.M. (1994a) Patterns and temporal trends in the incidence of malignant disease in children: I. Leukaemia and lymphoma. *Eur. J. Cancer,* **30A**, 1490–1498

Blair, V. & Birch, J.M. (1994b) Patterns and temporal trends in the incidence of malignant disease in children: II. Solid tumours of childhood. *Eur. J. Cancer,* **30A**, 1498–1511

Blot, W.J., Draper, G., Kinlen, L. & Kinnier-Wilson, M. (1980a) Childhood cancer in relation to prenatal exposure to chickenpox. *Br. J. Cancer,* **42**, 342–344

Blot, W.J., Stiller, C.A. & Kinnier-Wilson, L.M. (1980b) Oral clefts and childhood cancer. *Lancet,* **i**, 722

Boice, J.D., Jr (1990) Studies of atomic bomb survivors. Understanding radiation effects. *J. Am. Med. Assoc.,* **264**, 622–623

Boice, J. & Linet, M. (1994) Fallout from Chernobyl – Editorial authors' response. *Br. Med. J.,* **309**, 1300

Bolande, R.P. (1977) Childhood tumors and their relationship to birth defects. In: Mulvihill, J.J., Miller, R.W. & Fraumeni, J.F., Jr, eds, *Genetics of Human Cancer,* New York, Raven Press, pp. 43–75

Bonaïti-Pellié, C. & Briard-Guillemot, M.L. (1980) Excess of cancer deaths in grandparents of patients with retinoblastoma. *J. Med. Genet.,* **17**, 95–101

Bonaïti-Pellié, C., Chompret, A., Tournade, M.F., Hochez, J., Moutou, C., Zucker, J.M., Steschenko, D., Brunat-Mentigny, M., Roche, H., Tron, P., Frappaz, D., Munzer, M., Bachelot, C., Dusol, F., Sommelet-Olive, D. & Lemerle, J. (1992) Genetics and epidemiology of Wilms' tumor: the French Wilms' tumor study. *Med. Pediat. Oncol.,* **20**, 284–291

Bonde, J.P.E., Olsen, J.H. & Hansen, K.S. (1992) Adverse pregnancy outcome and childhood malignancy with reference to paternal welding exposure. *Scand. J. Work Environ. Health,* **18**, 169–177

Bondy, M., Lustbader, E.D., Buffler, P.A., Schull, W.J., Hardy, R.J. & Strong, L.C. (1991) Genetic epidemiology of childhood brain tumors. *Genet. Epidemiol.,* **8**, 253–267

Bondy, M.L., Strom, S.S., Colopy, M.W., Brown, B.W. & Strong, L.C. (1994) Accuracy of family history of cancer obtained through interviews with relatives of patients with childhood sarcoma. *J. Clin. Epidemiol.,* **47**, 89–96

Bone Tumor Committee of Japanese Orthopedic Association. (1982) *Bone Tumor Registry in Japan: The Incidence of Bone Tumors in Japan,* Tokyo. National Cancer Centre, pp. 122–123

Booth, K., Burkitt, D.P., Bassett, D.J., Cooke, R.A. & Biddulph, J. (1967) Burkitt lymphoma in Papua, New Guinea. *Br. J. Cancer,* **21**, 657–664

Bower, C. & Stanley, F.J. (1989) Dietary folate as a risk factor for neural-tube defects: evidence from a case-control study in Western Australia. *Med. J. Aust.,* **150**, 613–619

Bowie, C. (1987) The validity of a cancer register in leukaemia epidemiology. *Commun. Med.,* **9**, 152–159

Boyle, P. (1989) Relative value of incidence and mortality data in cancer research. *Recent Results in Cancer Research,* **114**, 41–63

Bradley, D. (1992) An orange a day helps to keep sperm OK. *New Scientist,* **133**, 20

Breslow, N.E. (1984) Extra-Poisson variation in log-linear models. *Appl. Stat.,* **33**, 38–44

Breslow, N.E. & Beckwith, J.B. (1982) Epidemiological features of Wilms' tumor: results of the National Wilms' Tumor Study. *J. Natl. Cancer Inst.,* **68**, 429–436

Breslow, N.E. & Langholz, B. (1983) Childhood cancer incidence: Geographical and temporal variations. *Int. J. Cancer,* **32**, 703–716

Breslow, N., Olshan, A., Beckwith, J.B. & Green, D.M. (1993) Epidemiology of Wilms tumor. *Med. Pediat. Oncol.,* **21**, 172–181

Breslow, N., Olshan, A., Beckwith, J.B., Moksness, J., Feigl, P. & Green, D. (1994) Ethnic variation in the incidence, diagnosis, prognosis and follow-up of children with Wilms' tumor. *J. Natl. Cancer Inst.,* **86**, 49–51

Breslow, N.E., Olson, J., Moksness, J., Beckwith, J.B. & Grundy, P. (1996) Familial Wilms' tumor: a descriptive study. *Med. Pediat. Oncol.*, **27**, 398–403

Brodeur, P. (1989a) Annals of Radiation. The hazards of electromagnetic fields. I – Power lines. *New Yorker* (12 June), 51–88

Brodeur, P. (1989b) Annals of Radiation. The hazards of electromagnetic fields. II – Something is happening. *New Yorker* (19 June), 47–73

Brodeur, P. (1989c) Annals of Radiation. The hazards of electromagnetic fields. III – Video display terminals. *New Yorker* (26 June), 39–68

Broomhall, J., May, R., Lilleyman, J.S. & Milner, R.D.G. (1983) Height and lymphoblastic leukaemia. *Arch. Dis. Child.*, **58**, 300–301

Bross, I.D.J. & Gibson, R. (1970) Cats and childhood leukemia. *J. Med.*, **1**, 180–187

Bross, I.D.J. & Natarajan, N. (1972) Leukemia from low-level radiation. Identification of susceptible children. *New Engl. J. Med.*, **287**, 107–110

Bross, I.D., Bertell, R. & Gibson, R. (1972) Pets and adult leukemia. *Am. J. Pub. Health*, **62**, 1520–1531

Broström, L.A., Adamson, U., Filipsson, R. & Hall, K. (1979) Longitudinal growth and dental development in osteosarcoma patients. *Acta Orthop. Scand.*, **51**, 755–759

Brown, L.M., Pottern, L.M. & Hoover, R.N. (1986) Prenatal and perinatal risk factors for testicular cancer. *Cancer Res.*, **46**, 4812–4816

Brown, L.M., Blair, A., Gibson, R., Everett, G.D., Cantor, K.P., Schuman, L.M., Burmeister, L.F., Van Lier, S.F. & Dick, F. (1990) Pesticide exposures and other agricultural risk factors for leukaemia among men in Iowa and Minnesota. *Cancer Res.*, **50**, 6585–6591

Browning, D. & Gross, S. (1968) Epidemiological studies of acute childhood leukemia. *Am. J. Dis. Child.*, **116**, 576–585

Brownson, R.C., Reif, J.S., Chang, J.C. & Davis, J.R. (1990) An analysis of occupational risks for brain cancer. *Am. J. Pub. Health*, **80**, 169–172

Brubaker, G., Geser, A. & Pike, M.C. (1973) Burkitt's lymphoma in the North Mara district of Tanzania 1964–70: failure to find evidence of time–space clustering in a high risk isolated rural area. *Br. J. Cancer*, **28**, 469–472

Buckley, J.D., Hobbie, W.L., Ruccione, K., Sather, H.N., Woods, W.G. & Hammond, G.D. (1986) Maternal smoking during pregnancy and the risk of childhood cancer (letter). *Lancet*, **ii**, 519–520

Buckley, J.D., Sather, H., Ruccione, K., Rogers, P.C., Haas, J.E., Henderson, B.E. & Hammond, G.D. (1989a) A case-control study of risk factors for hepatoblastoma. *Cancer*, **64**, 1169–1176

Buckley, J.D., Robison, L.L., Swotinsky, R., Garabrant, D.H., LeBeau, M., Manchester, P., Nesbit, M.E., Odom, L., Peters, J.M., Woods, W.G. & Hammond, D.G. (1989b) Occupational exposures of parents of children with acute nonlymphocytic leukemia: a report from the Children's Cancer Study Group. *Cancer Res.*, **49**, 4030–4037

Buckley, J.D., Gilchrist, G.S., Ruccione, K., Sather, H.N., Woods, W.G. & Hammond, G.D. (1989c) Multiple sclerosis in mothers of children with acute lymphoblastic leukemia. *Leukemia*, **3**, 736–739

Buckley, J.D., Buckley, C.M., Ruccione, K., Sather, H.N., Waskerwitz, M.J., Woods, W.G. & Robison, L.L. (1994) Epidemiological characteristics of childhood acute lymphocytic leukaemia. Analysis by immunophenotype. *Leukemia*, **8**, 856–864

Buckley, J.D., Buckley, C.M., Breslow, N.E., Draper, G.J., Roberson, P.K. & Mack, T.M. (1996) Concordance for childhood cancer in twins. *Med. Pediat. Oncol.*, **26**, 223–229

Budowle, B., Acton, R., Barger, B., Blackstock, R., Crist, W., Go, R.C., Humphrey, G.B., Ragab, A., Roper, M., Vietti, T. & Dearth, J. (1982) Properdin factor B and acute lymphocytic leukemia (ALL). *Cancer*, **50**, 2369–2371

Budowle, B., Dearth, J., Bowman, P., Melvin, S., Crist, W., Go, R., Kim, T., Iyer, R., Roseman, J., Barger, B. & Acton, R. (1985) Genetic predisposition to acute lymphocytic leukemia in American blacks. *Cancer*, **55**, 2880–2882

Bunin, G.R., Kramer, S., Marrero, O. & Meadows, A.T. (1987) Gestational risk factors for Wilms' tumor: results of a case–control study. *Cancer Res.*, **47**, 2972–2977

Bunin, G.R., Meadows, A.T., Emanuel, B.S., Buckley, J.D., Woods, W.G. & Hammond, G.D. (1989a) Pre- and postconception factors associated with sporadic heritable and nonheritable retinoblastoma. *Cancer Res.*, **49**, 5730–5735

Bunin, G.R., Nass, C.C., Kramer, S. & Meadows, A.T. (1989b) Parental occupation and Wilms' tumor: results of a case–control study. *Cancer Res.*, **49**, 725–729

Bunin, G.R., Petrakova, A., Meadows, A.T., Emanuel, B.S., Buckley, J.D., Woods, W.G. & Hammond, G.D. (1990a) Occupation of parents of children with retinoblastoma: a report from the Children's Cancer Study Group. *Cancer Res.*, **50**, 7129–7133

Bunin, G.R., Ward, E., Kramer, S., Rhee, C.A. & Meadows, A.T. (1990b) Neuroblastoma and parental occupation. *Am. J. Epidemiol.*, **131**, 776–780

Bunin, G.R., Kuijten, R.R., Buckley, J.D., Rorke, L.B. & Meadows, A.T. (1993) Relation between maternal diet and subsequent primitive neuroectodermal brain tumors in young children. *New Engl. J. Med.*, **329**, 536–541

Bunin, G.R., Kuijten, R.R., Boesel, C.P., Buckley, J.D. & Meadows, A.T. (1994a) Maternal diet and risk of astrocytic glioma in children: a report from the Children's Cancer Group. *Cancer Causes Control*, **5**, 177–187

Bunin, G.R., Buckley, J.D., Boesel, C.P., Rorke, L.B. & Meadows, A.T. (1994b) Risk factors for astrocytic glioma and primitive neuroectodermal tumor of the brain in young children: a report from the Children's Cancer Group. *Cancer Epidemiol. Biomarkers Prev.*, **3**, 197–204

Bunin, G.R., Feuer, E.J., Witman, P.A. & Meadows, A.T. (1996) Increasing incidence of childhood cancer: report of 20 years experience from the Greater Delaware Valley Pediatric Tumor Registry. *Paediat. Perinatal Epidemiol.*, **10**, 319–338

Burch, P.R.J. (1970) Prenatal radiation exposure and childhood cancer. *Lancet*, **ii**, 1189

Burch, P.R.J. (1971) Prenatal radiation exposure and childhood cancer. *Lancet*, **i**, 43

Burke, E., Li, F.P., Janov, A.J., Batter, S., Grier, H. & Goorin, A. (1991) Cancer in relatives of survivors of childhood sarcoma. *Cancer*, **67**, 1467–1469

Burkitt, D.P. (1969) Etiology of Burkitt's lymphoma – an alternative hypothesis to a vectored virus. *J. Natl. Cancer Inst.*, **42**, 19–28

Butland, B.K., Muirhead, C.R. & Draper, G.J. (1990) Radon and leukaemia. *Lancet*, **335**, 1338–1339

Byrne, J., Mulvihill, J.J., Connelly, R.R., Austin, D.A., Holmes, G.E., Holmes, F.F., Latourette, H.B., Meigs, J.W., Strong, L.C. & Myers, M.H. (1988) Reproductive problems and birth defects in survivors of Wilms' tumor and their relatives. *Med. Pediat. Oncol.*, **16**, 233–240

Carlsen, N.L.T. (1986) Epidemiological investigations on neuroblastomas in Denmark 1943–1980. *Br. J. Cancer*, **54**, 977–988

Carlsen, N.L.T. (1996) Neuroblastomas presenting in the first year of life: Epidemiological differences from those presenting at older ages. *Cancer Detect. Prev.*, **20**, 251–261

Carney, J.A., Thompson, D.P., Johnson, C. & Lynn, H.B. (1972) Teratomas in children: clinical and pathologic aspects. *J. Pediatr. Surg.*, **7**, 271–282

Carozza, S.E., Olshan, A.F., Faustman, E.M., Gula, M.J., Kolonel, L.N., Austin, D.F., West, E.D., Weiss, N.S., Swanson, G.M., Lyon, J.L., Hedley-Whyte, T., Gilles, F.H., Aschenbrener, C. & Leviton, A. (1995) Maternal exposure to *N*-nitrosatable drugs as a risk factor for childhood brain tumours. *Int. J. Epidemiol.*, **24**, 308–312

Carstensen, J. (1992) Intramuscular vitamin K and childhood cancer. *Br. Med. J.*, **305**, 710

Cartwright, A. & Smith, C. (1979) Some comparisons of data from medical records and from interviews with women who had recently had a live birth or stillbirth. *J. Biosoc. Sci.*, **11**, 49–64

Cartwright, R.A., McKinney, P.A., Hopton, P.A., Birch, J.M., Hartley, A.L., Mann, J.R., Waterhouse, J.A., Johnston, H.E., Draper, G.J. & Stiller, C. (1984) Ultrasound examinations in pregnancy and childhood cancer. *Lancet*, **ii**, 999–1000

Cartwright, R.A., McKinney, P.A., Alexander, F.E. & Ricketts, J. (1988) Leukaemia in young children. *Lancet*, **ii**, 960

Cartwright, R.A., Alexander, F.E., McKinney, P.A. & Ricketts, T.J. (1990) *Leukaemia and Lymphoma: an Atlas of Distribution within Areas of England and Wales. 1984–1988*, London, Leukaemia Research Fund

Cassimos, C., Sklavunu-Zurukzoglu, S., Catriu, D. & Panajiotidu, C. (1973) The frequency of tonsillectomy and appendectomy in cancer patients. *Cancer, 32*, 1374–1379

Cavalli-Sforza, L.L. & Bodmer, W.F. (1971) *The Genetics of Human Populations*, San Francisco, W. H. Freeman, p. 98

Cavdar, A.O., Yavuz, G., Babacan, E., Gozdasoglu, S., Unal, E., Ertem, U., Pamir, A., Yucesan, S., Gokcora, H., Uluoglu, O. & Ikinciogullari, A. (1994) Burkitt's lymphoma in Turkish children: clinical, viral (EBV) and molecular studies. *Leukemia Lymphoma, 14*, 323–330

Centres for Disease Control Vietnam Experience Study. (1988) Health status of Vietnam veterans. III. Reproductive outcomes and child health. *J. Am. Med. Assoc., 259*, 2715–2719

Cerhan, J.R., Wallace, R.B., Folsom, A.R., Potter, J.D., Munger, R.G. & Prineas, R.J. (1993) Transfusion history and cancer risk in older women. *Annals Internal Med., 119*, 8–15

Chaganti, R.S.K., Miller, D.R., Meyers, P.A. & German, J. (1979) Cytogenetic evidence of the intrauterine origin of acute leukemia in monozygotic twins. *New Engl. J. Med., 18*, 1032–1034

Chamberlain, J. (1996) Screening for cancers of other sites: lung, stomach, oral and neuroblastoma. In: Chamberlain, J. & Moss, S., eds, *Evaluation of Cancer Screening*, London, Springer, pp. 137–157

Chan, K.W., Pollack, M.S., Braun, D., O'Reilly, R.J. & Dupont, B. (1982) Distribution of HLA genotypes in families of patients with acute leukemia. *Transplantation, 33*, 613–615

Chandley, A.C. (1991) On the paternal origin of de novo mutation in man. *J. Med. Genet., 28*, 217–223

Chandra, R.K. (1972) Serum immunoglobulin levels in children with acute lymphoblastic leukaemia and their mothers and sibs. *Arch. Dis. Child., 47*, 618–620

Chavez, G.F., Mulinare, J. & Cordero, J.F. (1989) Maternal cocaine use during early pregnancy as a risk factor for congenital urogenital anomalies. *J. Am. Med. Assoc., 262*, 795–798

Chayen, J. (1992) Intramuscular vitamin K and childhood cancer. *Br. Med. J., 305*, 710

Chen, R., Mantel, N. & Klingberg, M.A. (1984) A study of three techniques for time-space clustering in Hodgkin's disease. *Stat. Med., 3*, 173–184

Chen, W.G., Chen, Y.Y., Bacchi, M.M., Bacchi, C.E., Alvarenga, M. & Weiss, L.M. (1996) Genotyping of Epstein-Barr virus in Brazilian Burkitt's lymphoma and reactive lymphoid tissue. *Am. J. Pathol., 148*, 17–23

Chintu, C., Athale, U.H. & Patil, P.S. (1995) Childhood cancers in Zambia before and after the HIV epidemic. *Arch. Dis. Child., 73*, 100–105

Choi, B.C.K. (1985) N-Nitroso compounds and human cancer. *Am. J. Epidemiol., 121*, 737–743

Choi, N.W., Schuman, L.M. & Gullen, W.H. (1970) Epidemiology of primary central nervous system neoplasms. II: Case-control study. *Am. J. Epidemiol., 91*, 467–485

Clarke, E.A., McLaughlin, J. & Anderson, T.W. (1991) *Childhood Leukaemia around Canadian Nuclear Facilities – Phase II. Final Report*. A report prepared for the Atomic Energy Control Board, Ottawa, Canada

Clarkson, B.D. & Boyse, E.A. (1971) Possible explanation of the high concordance for acute leukaemia in monozygotic twins. *Lancet, i*, 699–701

Clavel, J. & Hémon, D. (1997) Leukaemia near La Hague nuclear plant. Bias could have been introduced into study. *Br. Med. J., 314*, 1553

Clemmesen, J., Fuglsang-Frederiksen, V. & Plum, C. M. (1974) Are anticonvulsants oncogenic? *Lancet, ii*, 705–707

Cliff, A.D. & Ord, J.K. (1981) *Spatial Processes: Models and Applications*, London, Pion

Cnattingius, S., Zack, M.M., Ekbom, A., Gunnarskog, J., Kreuger, A., Linet, M. & Adami, H.O. (1995a) Prenatal and neonatal risk factors for childhood lymphatic leukemia. *J. Natl. Cancer Inst., 87*, 908–914

Cnattingius, S., Zack, M., Ekbom, A., Gunnarskog, J., Linet, M. & Adami, H.O. (1995b) Prenatal and neonatal risk factors for childhood myeloid leukemia. *Cancer Epidemiol. Biomarkers Prev., 4*, 441–445

Cocco, P., Bernardinelli, L. & Biddau, P. (1993) Childhood leukemia in south west Sardinia (Italy). *Tumori, 79*, 244–245

Cocco, P., Rapallo, M., Targhetta, R., Biddau, P.F. & Fadda, D. (1996) Analysis of risk factors in a cluster of childhood acute lymphoblastic leukemia. *Arch. Environ. Health, 51*, 242–244

Coebergh, J.W.W., van der Does-van den Berg, A., van Wering, E.R., van Steensel-Moll, H.A., Valkenburg, H.A., van't Veer, M.B., Schmitz, P.I.M. & van Zanen, G.E. (1989) Childhood leukaemia in The Netherlands, 1973–1986: temporary variation of the incidence of acute lymphocytic leukaemia in young children. *Br. J. Cancer, 59*, 100–105

Coebergh, J.W.W., van der Does-van den Berg, A., Kamps, W.A., Rammeloo, J.A., Valkenburg, H.A. & van Wering, E.R. (1991) Malignant lymphomas in children in the Netherlands in the period 1973–1985: Incidence in relation to leukemia: A report from the Dutch Childhood Leukemia Study Group. *Med. Pediat. Oncol., 19*, 169–174

Coebergh, J.W.W., van der Heijden, L.H. & Janssen-Heijnen, M.L.G. (1995) *Cancer Incidence and Survival in the Southeast of the Netherlands 1955–1994* (A report from the Eindhoven Cancer Registry) Eindhoven, IKZ Comprehensive Cancer Centre South

Coghill, R.W., Steward, J. & Philips, A. (1996) Extra low frequency electric and magnetic fields in the bedplace of children diagnosed with leukaemia: a case-control study. *Eur. J. Cancer Prev., 5*, 153–158

Cole, P., MacMahon, B. & Aisenberg, A. (1968) Mortality from Hodgkin's disease in the United States. *Lancet, ii*, 1371–1376

Coleman, M.P., Bell, C.M.J., Taylor, H.L. & Primic-Zakelj, M. (1989) Leukaemia and residence near electricity transmission equipment: a case-control study. *Br. J. Cancer, 60*, 793–798

Coleman, M., Wahrendorf, J. & Demaret, E. (1992) *Directory of On-Going Research in Cancer Epidemiology* (IARC Scientific Publications No. 117), Lyon, IARC

Coleman, M.P., Estève, J., Damiecki, P., Arslan, A. & Renard, H. (1993) *Trends in Cancer Incidence and Mortality* (IARC Scientific Publications No. 121). Lyon, IARC

Collman, G.W., Loomis, D.P. & Sandler, D.P. (1991) Childhood cancer mortality and radon concentration in drinking water in North Carolina. *Br. J. Cancer, 63*, 626–629

COMARE (Committee on Medical Aspects of Radiation in the Environment) (1988) *Investigation of the Possible Increased Incidence of Leukaemia in Young People near Dounreay Nuclear Establishment, Caithness, Scotland*, London, HMSO

COMARE (Committee on Medical Aspects of Radiation in the Environment) (1996) *Fourth Report. The Incidence of Cancer and Leukaemia in Young People in the Vicinity of the Sellafield Site, West Cumbria: Further Studies and an Update of the Situation since the Publication of the Report of the Black Advisory Group in 1984*, London, Department of Health

Commission of the European Communities (1990) *Radiation Protection: Feasibility of Studies on Health Effects in Western Europe due to the Reactor Accidents at Chernobyl and Recommendations for Research*. D.G. Science, Research and Development, EVR 12551

Comstock, G.W., Livesay, V.T. & Webster, R.G. (1971) Leukaemia and B.C.G. – a controlled trial. *Lancet, ii*, 1062–1063

Comstock, G.W., Martinez, I. & Livesay, V.T. (1975) Efficacy of BCG vaccination in prevention of cancer. *J. Natl. Cancer Inst., 54*, 835–839

Conard, R.A. (1984) Late radiation effects in Marshall Islanders exposed to fallout twenty-eight years ago. In: Boice, J.D., Jr & Fraumeni, F., Jr, eds, *Radiation Carcinogenesis: Epidemiology and Biological Significance*, New York, Raven Press, pp. 57–71

Cook-Mozaffari, P.J., Ashwood, F.L., Vincent, T., Forman, D. & Alderson, M. (1987) *Cancer Incidence and Mortality in the Vicinity of Nuclear Installations, England and Wales 1959–80* (Studies on Medical and Population Subjects No. 51), London, HMSO

Cook-Mozaffari, P.J., Darby, S.C., Doll, R., Forman, D., Hermon, C., Pike, M.C. & Vincent, T. (1989a) Geographical variation in mortality from leukaemia and other cancers in England and Wales in relation to proximity to nuclear installations, 1969–78. *Br. J. Cancer*, 59, 476–485

Cook-Mozaffari, P., Darby, S. & Doll, R. (1989b) Cancer near potential sites of nuclear installations. *Lancet*, ii, 1145–1147

Cook-Mozaffari, P., Darby, S. & Doll, R. (1990) Bracken spores and leukaemia. *Lancet*, i, 736

Cordier, S., Iglesias, M.J., Le Gosater, C., Guyot, M. M., Mandereau, L. & Hemon, D. (1994) Incidence and risk factors for childhood brain tumors in the Ile de France. *Int. J. Cancer*, 59, 776–782

Cornelissen, M., Smeets, D., Merkx, G., De Abreu, R., Kollee, L. & Monnens, L. (1991) Analysis of chromosome aberrations and sister chromatid exchanges in peripheral blood lymphocytes of newborns after vitamin K prophylaxis at birth. *Pediat. Res.*, 30, 550–553

Correa, P. & O'Conor, G.T. (1971) Epidemiologic patterns of Hodgkin's disease. *Int. J. Cancer*, 8, 192–201

Courot, M., Hochereau-de Reviers, M.T. & Ortavant, R. (1970) Spermatogenesis. In: Johnson, A.D., Gomes, W.R. & Vandemark, N.L., eds, *The Testis*, New York, Academic Press, p. 390

Court-Brown, W.M., Doll, R. & Bradford Hill, A. (1960) Incidence of leukaemia after exposure to diagnostic radiation *in utero*. *Br. Med. J.*, ii, 1539–1544

Court-Brown, W.M. & Doll, R. (1961) Leukaemia in childhood and young adult life. Trends in mortality in relation to aetiology. *Br. Med. J.*, 1, 981–988

Craft, A.W., Openshaw, S. & Birch, J.M. (1985) Childhood cancer in the Northern Region, 1968–82: incidence in small geographical areas. *J. Epidemiol. Commun. Health*, 39, 53–57

Craft, A.W., Parker, L., Openshaw, S., Charlton, M., Newell, J., Birch, J.M. & Blair, V. (1993) Cancer in young people in the north of England, 1968–85; analysis by census wards. *J. Epidemiol. Commun. Health*, 47, 109–115

Crispen, R.G. & Rosenthal, S.R. (1976) BCG vaccination and cancer mortality. *Cancer Immunol. Immunother.*, 1, 139–142

Cuzick, J. & Edwards, R. (1990) Spatial clustering for inhomogeneous populations. *J. R. Statist. Soc.*, 52B, 73–104

Daigle, A.E. (1987) Epidemiologic study of etiologic factors in Ewing's sarcoma (abstract). *Dissertation Abstracts International*, 47, 2861-B

Daling, J.R., Starzyk, P., Olshan, A.F. & Weiss, N.S. (1984) Birth weight and the incidence of childhood cancer. *J. Natl. Cancer Inst.*, 72, 1039–1041

Danis, R.P. & Keith, L.G. (1982) Some observations concerning leukaemia in twins. *Acta Genet. Med. Gemmellol.*, 31, 173–177

Darby, S.C. & Doll, R. (1987) Fallout, radiation doses near Dounreay, and childhood leukaemia. *Br. Med. J.*, 294, 603–607

Darby, S.C. & Reeves, G.K. (1991) Lessons of Chernobyl. *Br. Med. J.*, 303, 1347–1348

Darby, S.C., Olsen, J.H., Doll, R., Thakrar, B., Brown, P.D., Storm, H.H., Barlow, L., Langmark, F., Teppo, L. & Tulinius, H. (1992) Trends in childhood leukaemia in the Nordic counties in relation to fallout from atmospheric nuclear weapons testing. *Br. Med. J.*, 304, 1005–1009

Daugaard, S., Hørding, U. & Schiødt, T. (1991) Ewing's sarcoma and Epstein-Barr virus. *Eur. J. Cancer*, 27, 1334

Dausset, J., Gluckman, E., Lemarchand, F., Nunez-Roland, A., Contu, L. & Hors, J. (1977) Excès de HLA-A2 parmi les malades atteints d'aplaisie médullaire et de maladie de Fanconi. *Nouv. Rev. Fr. Hématol.*, 18, 315–324

Dausset, J., Colombani, J. & Hors, J. (1982) Major histocompatibility complex and cancer, with special reference to human familial tumours (Hodgkin's disease and other malignancies). *Cancer Surveys*, 1, 119–147

Davignon, L., Lemonde, P., Robillard, P. & Frappier, A. (1970) BCG vaccination and leukaemia mortality. *Lancet*, ii, 638

Davignon, L., Lemonde, P., St-Pierre, J. & Frappier, A. (1971) BCG vaccination and leukaemia mortality. *Lancet*, i, 799

Davis, S., Rogers, M.A.M. & Pendergrass, T.W. (1987) The incidence and epidemiologic characteristics of neuroblastoma in the United States. *Am. J. Epidemiol.*, 126, 1063–1074

Davis, M.K., Savitz, D. & Graubard, B.I. (1988) Infant feeding and childhood cancer. *Lancet*, ii, 365–368

Davis, J.R., Brownson, R.C., Garcia, R., Bentz, B.J. & Turner, A. (1993) Family pesticide use and childhood brain cancer. *Arch. Environ. Contam. Toxicol.*, 24, 87–92

de-Thé, G., Geser, A., Day, N.E., Tukei, P.M., Williams, E.H., Beri, D.P., Smith, P.G., Dean, A.G., Bornkamm, G.W., Feorino, P. & Henle, W. (1978) Epidemiological evidence for a causal relationship between Epstein-Barr virus and Burkitt's lymphoma: results of the Ugandan prospective study. *Nature*, 274, 756–761

de-Thé, G. (1985) Epstein-Barr virus and Burkitt's lymphoma worldwide: The causal relationship revisited. In: Lenoir, G., O'Conor, G. & Olweny, C.L.M., eds, *Burkitt's Lymphoma: A Human Cancer Model* (IARC Scientific Publications No. 60), Lyon, IARC, pp. 165–176

De Moor, P. & Louwagie, A. (1985) Distribution of HLA genotypes in sibs of patients with acute leukaemia. *Scand. J. Haematol.*, 34, 68–70

de Nully Brown, P., Hertz, H., Olsen, J.H., Yssing, M., Scheibel, E. & Jensen, O.M. (1989) Incidence of childhood cancer in Denmark 1943–1984. *Int. J. Epidemiol.*, 18, 546–555

de Nully Brown, P., Olsen, J.H., Hertz, H., Carstensen, B. & Bautz, A. (1995) Trends in survival after childhood cancer in Denmark, 1943–87: a population-based study. *Acta Paediat.*, 84, 316–324

de Vathaire, F., François, P., Schlumberger, M., Schweisguth, O., Hardiman, C., Grimaud, E., Oberlin, O., Hill, C., Lemerle, J. & Flamant, R. (1992) Epidemiological evidence for a common mechanism for neuroblastoma and differentiated thyroid tumour. *Br. J. Cancer*, 65, 425–428

Deapen, D.M. & Henderson, B.E. (1986) A case-control study of amyotrophic lateral sclerosis. *Am. J. Epidemiol.*, 123, 790–799

DeCaprio, J.A., Ludlow, J.W., Figge, J., Shew, J.Y., Huang, C.M., Lee, W.H., Marsilio, E., Paucha, E. & Livingston, D.M. (1988) SV40 large tumor antigen forms a specific complex with the product of retinoblastoma susceptibility gene. *Cell*, 54, 275–283

Delgado, A., Molina, J., Muñoz, M., Egues, J. & Martinez Penuela, J.M. (1980) Neuroblastoma en niño con síndrome fetal hidantoínico. *An. Esp. Pediat.*, 13, 433–436

Department of Health and Social Services. (1989) *Investigation into Patterns of Disease with Possible Association with Radiation in Northern Ireland. Final Report of the Independent Committee* (Chairman: Professor Sidney Lowry) Belfast, HMSO

Depue, R.H., Pike, M.C. & Henderson, B.E. (1983) Estrogen exposure during gestation and risk of testicular cancer. *J. Natl. Cancer Inst.*, 71, 1151–55

der Kinderen, D.J., Koten, J.W., Nagelkerke, N.J.D., Tan, K.E.W.P., Beemer, F.A. & Den Otter, W. (1988) Non-ocular cancer in patients with hereditary retinoblastoma and their relatives. *Int. J. Cancer*, 41, 499–504

Desmeules, M., Mikkelsen, T. & Mao, Y. (1992) Increasing incidence of primary malignant brain tumors: influence of diagnostic methods. *J. Natl. Cancer Inst.*, 84, 442–445

Devesa, S.S. & Fears, T. (1992) Non-Hodgkin's lymphoma time trends: United States and international data. *Cancer Res.*, 52, 5432S–5440S

Diamond, E.L., Schmerler, H. & Lilienfeld, A.M. (1973) The relationship of intra-uterine radiation to subsequent mortality and development of leukemia in children. A prospective study. *Am. J. Epidemiol.*, 97, 283–313

Dickman, S. (1991) Chernobyl effects not as bad as feared. *Nature*, 351, 335

Dockerty, J.D., Cox, B. & Cockburn, M.G. (1996) Childhood leukaemias in New Zealand: time trends and ethnic differences. *Br. J. Cancer*, 73, 1141–1147

Dolk, H., Shaddick, G., Walls, P., Grundy, C., Thakrar, B., Kleinschmidt, I. & Elliott, P. (1997a) Cancer incidence near radio and television transmitters in Great Britain. I. Sutton Coldfield transmitter. *Am. J. Epidemiol.*, 145, 1–9

Dolk, H., Elliott, P., Shaddick, G., Walls, P. & Thakrar, B. (1997b) Cancer incidence near radio and television transmitters in Great Britain. II. All high power transmitters. *Am. J. Epidemiol.*, 145, 10–17

Doll, R. (1989) The epidemiology of childhood leukaemia. *J. R. Statist. Soc.*, 152, 341–351

Doll, R. & Wakeford, R. (1997) Risk of childhood cancer from fetal irradiation. *Br. J. Radiol.*, 70, 130–139

Donovan, J.W., MacLennan, R. & Adena, M. (1984) Vietnam service and the risk of congenital anomalies. A case-control study. *Med. J. Aust.*, 140, 394–397

Dorak, M.T. & Burnett, A.K. (1992) Major histocompatibility complex, t-complex, and leukemia. *Cancer Causes Control*, 3, 273–282

Dorak, M.T. & Chalmers, E.A. (1992) HLA and leukemia: is it a simple allelic association? *Turk. J. Pediatr.*, 34, 55–59

dos Santos Silva, I. & Swerdlow, A.J. (1991) Ovarian germ cell malignancies in England: epidemiological parallels with testicular cancer. *Br. J. Cancer*, 63, 814–818

dos Santos Silva, I. & Swerdlow, A. J. (1993) Sex differences in the risks of hormone dependent cancers. *Am. J. Epidemiol.*, 138, 10–28

Dousset, M. (1989) Cancer mortality around La Hague nuclear facilities. *Health Phys.*, 56, 875–884

Dovan, T., Kaune, W.T. & Savitz, D. (1993) Repeatability of measurements of residential magnetic fields and wire codes. *Bioelectromagnetics*, 14, 145–159

Draper, G.J. (1989) General overview of multigeneration carcinogenesis in man, particularly in relation to exposure to chemicals. In: Napalkov, N.P., Rice, J.M., Tomatis, L. & Yamasaki, H., eds, *Perinatal and Multigeneration Carcinogenesis* (IARC Scientific Publications No. 96), Lyon, IARC, pp. 275–278

Draper, G.J. & Elliott, P. (1991) Variations in incidence rates and factors affecting them – summary. In: Draper, G.J., ed., *The Geographical Epidemiology of Childhood Leukaemia and Non-Hodgkin Lymphomas in Great Britain, 1966–83* (Studies on Medical and Population Subjects No. 53), London, HMSO, pp. 57–59

Draper, G. & McNinch, A. (1994) Vitamin K for neonates: the controversy. *Br. Med. J.*, 308, 867–868

Draper, G.J. & Stiller, C.A. (1992) Intramuscular vitamin K and childhood cancer. *Br. Med. J.*, 305, 709

Draper, G.J., Heaf, M.M. & Kinnier-Wilson, L.M. (1977) Occurrence of childhood cancers among sibs and estimation of familial risks. *J. Med. Genet.*, 14, 81–90

Draper, G.J., Sanders, B.M. & Kingston, J.E. (1986) Second primary neoplasms in patients with retinoblastoma. *Br. J. Cancer*, 53, 661–671

Draper, G.J., Vincent, T.J., O'Connor, C.M. & Stiller, C.A. (1991a) Socio-economic factors and variations in incidence rates between County Districts. In: Draper, G., ed., *The Geographical Epidemiology of Childhood Leukaemia and Non-Hodgkin Lymphomas in Great Britain, 1966–83* (Studies on Medical and Population Subjects No. 53), London, HMSO, pp. 37–45

Draper, G.J., Stiller, C.A., O'Connor, C.M. & Vincent, T.J. (1991b) Introduction and objectives. In: Draper, G., ed., *The Geographical Epidemiology of Childhood Leukaemia and Non-Hodgkin Lymphomas in Great Britain, 1966–83* (Studies on Medical and Population Subjects No. 53), London, HMSO, pp. 1–6

Draper, G.J., Sanders, B.M., Brownbill, P.A. & Hawkins, M.M. (1992) Patterns of risk of hereditary retinoblastoma and applications to genetic counselling. *Br. J. Cancer*, 66, 211–219

Draper, G.J., Stiller, C.A., Cartwright, R.A., Craft, A.W. & Vincent, T.J. (1993) Cancer in Cumbria and in the vicinity of the Sellafield nuclear installation, 1963–90. *Br. Med. J.*, 306, 89–91

Draper, G.J., Kroll, M.E. & Stiller, C.A. (1994) Childhood cancer. *Cancer Surveys*, 19/20, 493–517

Draper, G.J., Sanders, B.M., Lennox, E.L. & Brownbill, P.A. (1996) Patterns of childhood cancer among siblings. *Br. J. Cancer*, 74, 152–158

Drews, C.D. & Greenland, S. (1990) The impact of differential recall on the results of case-control studies. *Int. J. Epidemiol.*, 19, 1107–1112

Drews, C.D., Kraus, J.F. & Greenland, S. (1990) Recall bias in a case-control study of sudden infant death syndrome. *Int. J. Epidemiol.*, 19, 405–411

Drews, C., Greenland, S. & Flanders, W.D. (1993) The use of restricted controls to prevent recall bias in case-control studies of reproductive outcomes. *Ann. Epidemiol.*, 3, 86–92

Druckrey, H., Preussmann, R. & Ivankovic, S. (1969) N-Nitroso compounds in organotropic and transplacental carcinogenesis. *Ann. N. Y. Acad. Sci.*, 163, 676–696

Drut, R., Hernández, A. & Pollono, D. (1990) Incidence of childhood cancer in La Plata, Argentina, 1977–1987. *Int. J. Cancer*, 45, 1045–1047

Drut, R.M., Day, S., Drut, R. & Meisner, L. (1994) Demonstration of Epstein-Barr viral DNA in paraffin-embedded tissues of Burkitt's lymphoma from Argentina using the polymerase chain reaction and in situ hybridization. *Pediat. Pathol.*, 14, 101–109

Duncan, M.H., Wiggins, C.L., Samet, J.M. & Key, C.R. (1986) Childhood cancer epidemiology in New Mexico's American Indians, Hispanic whites and non-hispanic whites, 1970–82. *J. Natl. Cancer Inst.*, 76, 1013–1018

Dyson, N., Howley, P. M., Munger, K. & Harlow, E. (1989) The human papilloma virus-16 E7 oncoprotein is able to bind to the retinoblastoma gene product. *Science*, 243, 934–940

Ederer, F., Myers, M.H. & Mantel, N. (1964) A statistical problem in space and time: do leukemia cases come in clusters? *Biometrics*, 20, 626–638

Ederer, F., Miller, R.W. & Scotto, J. (1965) US childhood cancer mortality patterns, 1950–1959. *J. Am. Med. Assoc.*, 192, 593–596

Ehrenbard, L.T. & Chaganti, R.S.K. (1981) Cancer in the fetal hydantoin syndrome. *Lancet*, ii, 97

Eisenberg, D.E. & Sorahan, T. (1987) Birth weight and childhood cancer deaths. *J. Natl. Cancer Inst.*, 78, 1095–1100

Ekelund, H., Finnström, O., Gunnarskog, J., Källen, B. & Larsson, Y. (1993) Administration of vitamin K to newborn infants and childhood cancer. *Br. Med. J.*, 307, 89–91

Elliott, J., Coulter-Mackie, M.B., Jung, J.H., Rodenhiser, D.I. & Singh, S.M. (1991a) A method for transforming lymphocytes from very small blood volumes suitable for paediatric samples. *Hum. Genet.*, 86, 615–616

Elliott, P., McGale, P. & Vincent, T.J. (1991b) Description of population data and definitions of areas. In: Draper, G., ed., *The Geographical Epidemiology of Childhood Leukaemia and Non-Hodgkin Lymphomas in Great Britain, 1966–83* (Studies on Medical and Population Subjects No. 53), London, HMSO, pp. 17–23

Elwood, J.M., Elwood, J.H. & Little, J. (1992) Diet. In: Elwood, J.M., Little, J. & Elwood, J.H., eds, *Epidemiology and Control of Neural Tube Defects*, Oxford, Oxford University Press, pp. 521–603

Emerson, J.C., Malone, K.E., Daling, J.R. & Starzyk, P. (1991) Childhood brain tumor risk in relation to birth characteristics. *J. Clin. Epidemiol.*, 44, 1159–1166

Eng, C., Li, F.P., Abramson, D.H., Ellsworth, R.M., Wong, F. L., Goldman, M.B., Seddon, J., Tarbell, N. & Boice, J.D., Jr (1993) Mortality from second tumors among long-term survivors of retinoblastoma. *J. Natl. Cancer Inst.*, 85, 1121–1128

Erickson, J.D., Mulinare, J., McClain, P.W., Fitch, T. G., James, L.M., McClearn, A.B. & Adams, M.J., Jr (1984) Vietnam veterans' risks for fathering babies with birth defects. *J. Am. Med. Assoc.*, 252, 903–912

Ericsson, J.L., Karnström, L. & Mattsson, B. (1978) Childhood cancer in Sweden, 1958–1974. *Acta Paediatr. Scand.*, 67, 425–432

European Network of Cancer Registries (1995) *European Cancer Incidence and Mortality Database (EUROCIM) User Manual*, 2nd edition, Lyon, IARC

Evans, I.A. & Galpin, O.P. (1990) Bracken and leukaemia. *Lancet*, 335, 231

Evans, D.G., Farndón, P.A., Burnell, L.D., Gattamaneni, H.R. & Birch, J.M. (1991) The incidence of Gorlin syndrome in 173 consecutive cases of medulloblastoma. *Br. J. Cancer*, 64, 959–961

Evans, G., Burnell, L., Campbell, R., Gattamaneni, H. R. & Birch, J. (1993) Congenital anomalies and genetic syndromes in 173 cases of medulloblastoma. *Med. Pediat. Oncol.*, 21, 433–434

Evatt, B.L., Chase, G.A. & Heath, C.W. (1973) Time-space clustering among cases of acute leukemia in two Georgia counties. *Blood,* **41,** 265–272

Fabia, J. & Thuy, T.D. (1974) Occupation of father at time of birth of children dying of malignant diseases. *Br. J. Prev. Soc. Med.,* **28,** 98–100

Fajardo-Gutiérrez, A., Garduno-Espinosa, J., Yamamoto-Kimura, L., Hernandez-Hernandez, D.M., Mejia-Arangure, M., Gomez-Delgado, A., Farfan-Canto, J.M., Ortiz-Fernandez, A. & Martinez-Garcia, M.C. (1993a) Factores de riesgo asociados al desarrollo de leucemia en ninos. *Bol. Med. Hosp. Infant. Mex.,* **50,** 248–257

Fajardo-Gutiérrez, A., Garduño-Espinosa, J., Yamamoto-Kimura, L., Hernández-Hernández, D.M., Gómez-Delgado, A., Mejía-Aranguré, M., Cartagena-Sandoval, A. & del Carmen Martínez-García, M. (1993b) Residencia cercana a fuentes eléctricas de alta tensión y su asociación con leucemia en niños. *Bol. Med. Hosp. Infant. Mex.,* **50,** 32–37

Farwell, J. & Flannery, J.T. (1984a) Cancer in relatives of children with central-nervous system neoplasms. *New Engl. J. Med.,* **311,** 749–753

Farwell, J. & Flannery, J.T. (1984b) Second primaries in children with central nervous system tumors. *J. Neurooncol.,* **2,** 371–375

Farwell, J.R., Dohrmann, G.J., Marrett, L.D. & Meigs, J.W. (1979) Effect of SV40 virus-contaminated polio vaccine on the incidence and type of CNS neoplasms in children: a population-based study. *Trans. Am. Neurol. Assoc.,* **104,** 261–264

Fasal, E., Jackson, E.W. & Klauber, M.R. (1971) Birth characteristics and leukemia in childhood. *J. Natl. Cancer Inst.,* **47,** 501–509

Fedrick, J. & Alberman, E.D. (1972) Reported influenza in pregnancy and subsequent cancer in the child. *Br. Med. J.,* **2,** 485–488

Feingold, L., Savitz, D.A. & John, E.M. (1992) Use of job-exposure matrix to evaluate parental occupation and childhood cancer. *Cancer Causes Control,* **3,** 161–169

Feldman, J.G., Lee, S.L. & Seligman, B. (1976) Occurrence of acute leukemia in females in a genetically isolated population. *Cancer,* **38,** 2548–2550

Feychting, M. & Ahlbom, A. (1992) *Magnetic Fields and Cancer in People Residing near Swedish High Voltage Power Lines* (IMM-rapport 6/92), Stockholm, Karolinska Institute

Feychting, M. & Ahlbom, A. (1993) Magnetic fields and cancer in children residing near Swedish high-voltage power lines. *Am. J. Epidemiol.,* **138,** 467–481

Feychting, M. & Ahlbom, A. (1995) Electromagnetic fields and childhood cancer: meta-analysis. *Cancer Causes Control,* **6,** 275–279

Feychting, M., Schulgen, G., Olsen, J.H. & Ahlbom, A. (1995) Magnetic fields and childhood cancer – a pooled analysis of two Scandinavian studies. *Eur. J. Cancer,* **31A,** 2035–2039

Filippini, G., Farinotti, M., Lovicu, G., Maisonneuve, P. & Boyle, P. (1994) Mothers' active and passive smoking during pregnancy and risk of brain tumours in children. *Int. J. Cancer,* **57,** 769–774

Fine, P.E.M., Adelstein, A.M., Snowman, J., Clarkson, J.A. & Evans, S.M. (1985) Long term effects of exposure to viral infections *in utero. Br. Med. J.,* **290,** 509–511

Ford, D.D., Paterson, J.C.S. & Treuting, W.L. (1959) Fetal exposure to diagnostic X-rays, and leukemia and other malignant diseases in childhood. *J. Natl. Cancer Inst.,* **22,** 1093–1104

Ford, A.M., Ridge, S.A., Cabrera, M.E., Mahmoud, H., Steel, C.M., Chan, L.C. & Greaves, M. (1993) *In utero* rearrangements in the trithorax-related oncogene in infant leukaemias. *Nature,* **363,** 358–360

Foreman, N.K. & Pearson, A.D. (1993) Maternal diet and primitive neuroectodermal brain tumors in children. *New Engl. J. Med.,* **329,** 1963

Forman, D., Cook-Mozaffari, P., Darby, S., Davey, G., Stratton, I., Doll, R. & Pike, M. (1987) Cancer near nuclear installations. *Nature,* **329,** 499–505

Forsberg, J.G. & Källén, B. (1990) Pregnancy and delivery characteristics of women whose infants develop child cancer. *APMIS,* **98,** 37–42

Franceschi, S., Serraino, D., Carbone, A., Talamini, R. & La Vecchia, C. (1989) Dietary factors and non-Hodgkin's lymphoma: a case-control study in the northeastern part of Italy. *Nutr. Cancer,* **12,** 333–341

Francke, U. (1990) A gene for Wilms tumour? *Nature,* **343,** 692–694

Franco, E.L., de Camargo, B., Saba, L. & Marques, L.A. (1991) Epidemiological and clinical correlations with genetic characteristics of Wilms' tumor: results of the Brazilian Wilms' Tumor Study Group. *Int. J. Cancer,* **48,** 641–646

Franssila, K.O. & Harach, J.R. (1986) Occult papillary carcinoma of the thyroid in children and young adults. A systemic autopsy study in Finland. *Cancer,* **58,** 715–719

Fraumeni, J.F., Jr (1967) Stature and malignant tumors of bone in childhood and adolescence. *Cancer,* **20,** 967–973

Fraumeni, J.F., Jr & Glass, A.G. (1970) Rarity of Ewing's sarcoma among US Negro children. *Lancet,* **i,** 366–367

Fraumeni, J.F., Jr & Li, F.P. (1969) Hodgkin's disease in childhood: an epidemiologic study. *J. Natl. Cancer Inst.,* **42,** 681–691

Fraumeni, J.F., Jr & Miller, R.W. (1967) Adrenocortical neoplasms with hemihypertrophy, brain tumors and others. *J. Pediat.,* **70,** 129–138

Fraumeni, J.F., Jr, Ederer, F. & Handy, V.H. (1966) Temporal–spatial distribution of childhood leukemia in New York State. *Cancer,* **19,** 996–1000

Fraumeni, J.F., Miller, R.W. & Hill, J.A. (1968) Primary carcinoma of the liver in childhood: an epidemiologic study. *J. Natl. Cancer Inst.,* **40,** 1087–1099

Fraumeni, J.F., Jr., Manning, M.D. & Mitus, W.J. (1971) Acute childhood leukemia: epidemiologic study by cell type of 1,263 cases at the Children's Cancer Research Foundation in Boston, 1947–65. *J. Natl. Cancer Inst.,* **46,** 461–470

Fraumeni, J.F., Li, F.P. & Dalager, N. (1973) Teratomas in children: epidemiologic features. *J. Natl. Cancer Inst.,* **51,** 1425–1430

Freeman, A.I., Lieberman, N., Tidings, J., Bross, I. & Glidewell, O. (1971) Previous tonsillectomy and the incidence of acute leukaemia of childhood. *Lancet,* **i,** 1128

Fulton, J.P., Cobb, S., Preble, L., Leone, L. & Forman, E. (1980) Electrical wiring configurations and childhood leukemia in Rhode Island. *Am. J. Epidemiol.,* **111,** 292–296

Furmanchuk, A.W., Averkin, J.I., Egloff, B., Ruchti, C., Abelin, T., Schappi, W. & Korotkevich, E.A. (1992) Pathomorphological findings in thyroid cancers of children from the Republic of Belarus: a study of 86 cases occurring between 1986 ('post-Chernobyl') and 1991. *Histopathology,* **21,** 401–408

Gahrton, G., Wahren, B., Killander, D. & Foley, G.E. (1971) Epstein-Barr and other herpes virus antibodies in children with acute leukemia. *Int. J. Cancer,* **8,** 242–249

Gale, R.P. (1987) Immediate medical consequences of nuclear accidents: lessons from Chernobyl. *J. Am. Med. Assoc.,* **258,** 625–628

Gale, R.P. & Butturini, A. (1991) Perspective: Chernobyl and leukemia. *Leukemia,* **5,** 441–442

Garber, J.E., Goldstein, A.M., Kantor, A.F., Dreyfus, M.G., Fraumeni, J.F., Jr & Li, F.P. (1991) Follow-up study of twenty-four families with Li-Fraumeni syndrome. *Cancer Res.,* **51,** 6094–6097

Gardner, M.J. (1989) Review of reported increases of childhood cancer rates in the vicinity of nuclear installations in the UK. *J. R. Statist. Soc.,* **152A,** 307–325

Gardner, M.J. (1991) Father's occupational exposure to radiation and the raised level of childhood leukemia near the Sellafield nuclear plant. *Environ. Health Perspect.,* **94,** 5–7

Gardner, M.J. (1992) Paternal occupations of children with leukaemia. *Br. Med. J.,* **305,** 715

Gardner, M.J. & Snee, M.P. (1990) Leukaemia and lymphoma among young people near Sellafield. *Br. Med. J.,* **300,** 678

Gardner, M.J., Hall, A.J., Downes, S. & Terrell, J.D. (1987a) Follow-up study of children born to mothers resident in Seascale, West Cumbria (birth cohort). *Br. Med. J.,* **295,** 822–827

Gardner, M.J., Hall, A.J., Downes, S. & Terrell, J.D. (1987b) Follow-up study of children born elsewhere but attending schools in Seascale, West Cumbria (schools cohort). *Br. Med. J.,* **295,** 819–822

Gardner, M.J., Snee, M.P., Hall, A.J., Powell, C.A., Downes, S. & Terrell, J.D. (1990a) Results of case–control study of leukaemia and lymphoma among young people near Sellafield nuclear plant in West Cumbria. *Br. Med. J.*, **300**, 423–429

Gardner, M.J., Hall, A.J., Snee, M.P., Downes, S., Powell, C.A. & Terrell, J.D. (1990b) Methods and basic data of case–control study of leukaemia and lymphoma among young people near Sellafield nuclear plant in West Cumbria. *Br. Med. J.*, **300**, 429–434

Garralda, E. (1993) Venepuncture distress and research in childhood. *Lancet*, **341**, 832

Gelberg, K.H., Fitzgerald, E.F., Hwang, S. & Dubrow, R. (1995) Fluoride exposure and childhood osteosarcoma: A case-control study. *Am. J. Pub. Health*, **85**, 1678–1683

Gelberg, K.H., Fitzgerald, E.F., Hwang, S. & Dubrow, R. (1997) Growth and development and other risk factors for osteosarcoma in children and young adults. *Int. J. Epidemiol.*, **26**, 272–278

Geser, A., de Thé, G., Lenoir, G., Day, N.E. & Williams, E.H. (1982) Final case reporting from the Ugandan prospective study of the relationship between EBV and Burkitt's lymphoma. *Int. J. Cancer*, **29**, 397–400

Geser, A., Brubaker, G. & Draper, C.C. (1989) Effect of a malaria suppression program on the incidence of African Burkitt's lymphoma. *Am. J. Epidemiol.*, **129**, 740–752

Gessler, M., Poustka, A., Cavenee, W., Neve, R.L., Orkin, S.H. & Bruns, G.A.P. (1990) Homozygous deletion in Wilms tumours of a zinc-finger gene identified by chromosome jumping. *Nature*, **343**, 774–778

Gfroerer, J.C. & Hughes, A.L. (1991) The feasibility of collecting drug abuse data by telephone. *Public Health Rep.*, **106**, 384–393

Ghali, M.H., Yoo, K.Y., Flannery, J.T. & Dubrow, R. (1992) Associations between childhood rhabdomyosarcoma and maternal history of stillbirths. *Int. J. Cancer*, **50**, 365–368

Gibson, R.W., Bross, I.D.J., Graham, S., Lilienfeld, A.M., Schuman, L.M., Levin, M.L. & Dowd, J.E. (1968) Leukemia in children exposed to multiple risk factors. *New Engl. J. Med.* **279**, 906–909

Gibson, B.E.S., Eden, O.B., Barrett, A., Stiller, C.A. & Draper, G.J. (1988) Leukaemia in young children in Scotland. *Lancet*, **ii**, 630

Giles, G., Waters, K., Thursfield, V. & Farrugia, H. (1995) Childhood cancer in Victoria, Australia, 1970–1989. *Int. J. Cancer*, **63**, 794–797

Gilliam, A.G. & Walter, W.A. (1958) Trends of mortality from leukemia in the United States 1921–55. *Public Health Reports (Washington)*, **73**, 773–784

Gillis, C.R. & Hole, D.J. (1984) Childhood leukaemia in coastal areas of West Scotland 1969–83. *Lancet*, **ii**, 872

Gilman, E.A. & Knox, E.G. (1991) Temporal-spatial distribution of childhood leukaemias and non-Hodgkin lymphomas in Great Britain. In: Draper, G.J., ed., *The Geographical Epidemiology of Childhood Leukaemia and Non-Hodgkin Lymphomas in Great Britain, 1966–83* (Studies on Medical and Population Subjects No. 53), London, HMSO, pp. 77–99

Gilman, E.A. & Knox, E.G. (1995) Childhood cancers: space-time distribution in Britain. *J. Epidemiol. Commun. Health*, **49**, 158–163

Gilman, E.A., Kneale, G.W., Knox, E.G. & Stewart, A.M. (1988) Pregnancy X-rays and childhood cancers: effects of exposure age and radiation dose. *J. Radiol. Prot.*, **8**, 3–8

Gilman, E.A., Kinnier-Wilson, L.M., Kneale, G.W. & Waterhouse, J.A.H. (1989) Childhood cancers and their association with pregnancy drugs and illnesses. *Paediat. Perinatal Epidemiol.*, **3**, 66–94

Githens, J.H., Elliot, F.E. & Saunders, L.H. (1965) The relation of socioeconomic factors to incidence of childhood leukemia. *Public Health Reports*, **80**, 573–578

Giusti, R.M., Iwamoto, K. & Hatch, E.E. (1995) Diethylstilbestrol revisited: A review of the long-term health effects. *Annals Internal Med.*, **122**, 778–788

Glaser, S.L. & Swartz, W.G. (1990) Time trends in Hodgkin's disease incidence. The role of diagnostic accuracy. *Cancer*, **66**, 2196–2204

Glass, A.G. & Fraumeni, J.F., Jr. (1970) Epidemiology of bone cancer in children. *J. Natl. Cancer Inst.*, **44**, 187–199

Glass, A.G. & Mantel, N. (1969) Lack of time-space clustering of childhood leukemia in Los Angeles County, 1960–64. *Cancer Res.*, **29**, 1995–2001

Glass, A.G., Hill, J.A. & Miller, R.W. (1968) Significance of leukemia clusters. *J. Pediatr.*, **73**, 101–107

Glass, A.G., Mantel, N., Gunz, F.W. & Spears, G.F.S. (1971) Time-space clustering of childhood leukemia in New Zealand. *J. Natl. Cancer Inst.*, **47**, 329–336

Glass, S., Gray, M., Eden, O.B. & Hann, I. (1987) Scottish validation study of cancer registration data childhood leukaemia 1968–1981 – I. *Leukemia Res.*, **11**, 881–885

Gold, E., Gordis, L., Tonascia, J. & Szklo, M. (1978) Increased risk of brain tumors in children exposed to barbiturates. *J. Natl. Cancer Inst.*, **61**, 1031–1034

Gold, E., Gordis, L., Tonascia, J. & Szklo, M. (1979) Risk factors for brain tumors in children. *Am. J. Epidemiol.*, **109**, 309–319

Gold, E.B., Diener, M.D. & Szklo, M. (1982) Parental occupations and cancer in children. A case-control study and review of the methodological issues. *J. Occup. Med.*, **24**, 578–584

Gold, E.B., Leviton, A., Lopez, R., Gilles, F.H., Hedley-Whyte, E.T., Kolonel, L.N., Lyon, J.L., Swanson, G.M., Weiss, N.S., West, D., Aschenbrener, C. & Austin, D.F. (1993) Parental smoking and risk of childhood brain tumors. *Am. J. Epidemiol.*, **137**, 620–628

Gold, E.B., Leviton, A., Lopez, R., Austin, D.F., Gilles, F.H., Hedley-Whyte, E.T., Kolonel, L.N., Lyon, J.L., Swanson, G.M., Weiss, N.S., West, D.W. & Aschenbrener, C. (1994) The role of family history in risk of childhood brain tumors. *Cancer*, **73**, 1302–1311

Goldhaber, M.K., Selby, J.V., Hiatt, R.A. & Quesenberry, C.P. (1990) Exposure to barbiturates *in utero* and during childhood and risk of intracranial and spinal cord tumors. *Cancer Res.*, **50**, 4600–4603

Golding, J., Paterson, M. & Kinlen, L.J. (1990) Factors associated with childhood cancer in a national cohort study. *Br. J. Cancer*, **62**, 304–308

Golding, J., Greenwood, R., Birmingham, K. & Mott, M. (1992a) Childhood cancer, intramuscular vitamin K and pethidine given during labour. *Br. Med. J.*, **305**, 341–346

Golding, J., Greenwood, R. & Mott, M. (1992b) Intramuscular vitamin K and childhood cancer. *Br. Med. J.*, **305**, 711

Goodman, M.A., McMaster, J.H., Drash, A.L., Diamond, P.E., Kappakas, G.S. & Scranton, P.E., Jr (1978) Metabolic and endocrine alterations in osteosarcoma patients. *Cancer*, **42**, 603–610

Goodman, M.T., Yoshizawa, C.N. & Kolonel, L.N. (1989) Ethnic patterns of childhood cancer in Hawaii between 1960 and 1984. *Cancer*, **64**, 1758–1763

Goodrich, D.W. & Lee, W.H. (1990) The molecular genetics of retinoblastoma. *Cancer Surv.*, **9**, 529–554

Gordis, L., Szklo, M., Thompson, B., Kaplan, E. & Tonascia, J.A. (1981) An apparent increase in the incidence of acute nonlymphocytic leukemia in black children. *Cancer*, **47**, 2763–2768

Graham, S., Levin, M.L., Lilienfeld, M., Schuman, L.M., Gibson, R., Dowd, J.E. & Hempelmann, L. (1966) Preconception, intrauterine, and postnatal irradiation as related to leukemia. *Natl. Cancer Inst. Monogr.*, **19**, 347–371

Gray, J.I. (1981) Formation of *N*-nitroso compounds in foods. In: Scanlan, R.A. & Tannenbaum, S.R., eds, *N-Nitroso Compounds*, Washington, DC, American Chemical Society, pp. 165–180

Gray, M., Glass, S., Eden, O.B., Hann, I.M. & Gibson, B. (1987) Scottish validation study of cancer registration data childhood leukaemia 1968–1981, bone marrow review – II. *Leukaemia Res.*, **11**, 887–889

Greaves, M.F. (1988) Speculations on the cause of childhood acute lymphoblastic leukaemia. *Leukemia*, **2**, 120–125

Greaves, M. (1993) A natural history for pediatric acute leukaemia. *Blood*, **82**, 1043–1051

Greaves, M.F. & Alexander, F.E. (1993) An infectious etiology for common acute lymphoblastic leukemia in childhood? *Leukemia*, **3**, 349–360

Greaves, M.F., Pegram, S.M. & Chan, L.C. (1985) Collaborative group study of the epidemiology of acute lymphoblastic leukaemia subtypes: Background and first report. *Leukemia Res.*, **9**, 715–733

Greaves, M.F., Colman, S.M., Beard, M.E.J., Bradstock, K., Cabrera, M.E., Chen, P.M., Jacobs, P., Lam-Po-Tang, P.R., MacDougall, L.G., Williams, C.K. & Alexander, F.E. (1993) Geographical distribution of acute lymphoblastic leukemia subtypes: Second Report of the Collaborative Group Study. *Leukemia*, 7, 27–34

Green, D.M., Fine, W.E. & Li, F.P. (1982) Offspring of patients treated for unilateral Wilms' tumor in childhood. *Cancer*, 49, 2285–2288

Green, D.M., Tarbell, N.J. & Schamberger, R.C. (1997) Solid tumors of chidhood. In: DeVita, V.T., Jr, Hellman, S. & Rosenberg, S.A., eds, *Cancer: Principles and Practice of Oncology*, fifth edition, New York, Lippincott-Raven, pp. 2091–2130

Greenberg, R.S. (1983) *The Population Distribution and Possible Determinants of Neuroblastoma in Children*, Chapel Hill, NC, University of North Carolina

Greenberg, R.S. & Shuster, J.L., Jr (1985) Epidemiology of cancer in children. *Epidemiol. Rev.*, 7, 22–48

Greenberg, E.R. (1990) Random digit dialing for control selection. A review and a caution on its use in studies of childhood cancer. *Am. J. Epidemiol.*, 131, 1–5

Greenberg, R.S., Grufferman, S. & Cole, P. (1983) An evaluation of space-time clustering in Hodgkin's disease. *J. Chron. Dis.*, 36, 257–262

Greene, M.H., Fraumeni, J.F. & Hoover, R. (1977) Nasopharyngeal cancer among young people in the United States: racial variations by cell type. *J. Natl. Cancer Inst.*, 58, 1267–1270

Greenwald, P., Barlow, J.J., Nasca, P.C. & Burnett, W.S. (1971) Vaginal cancer after maternal treatment with synthetic estrogens. *New Engl. J. Med.*, 285, 390–392

Grimson, R.C., Aldrich, T.E. & Drane, J.W. (1992) Clustering in sparse data and an analysis of rhabdomyosarcoma incidence. *Stat. Med.*, 11, 761–768

Gross, R.E. & Clatworthy, H.W. (1951) Twin fetuses in fetu. *J. Pediat.*, 38, 502–508

Grufferman, S. & Delzell, E. (1984) Epidemiology of Hodgkin's disease. *Epidemiol. Rev.*, 6, 76–106

Grufferman, S., Cole, P., Smith, P.G. & Lukes, R.J. (1977) Hodgkin's disease in siblings. *New Engl. J. Med.*, 296, 248–250

Grufferman, S., Wang, H.H., DeLong, E.R., Kimm, S.Y.S., Delzell, E.S. & Falletta, J.M. (1982) Environmental factors in the etiology of rhabdomyosarcoma in childhood. *J. Natl. Cancer Inst.*, 68, 107–113

Grufferman, S., Gula, M.J., Olshan, A.F., Falletta, J.M., Pendergrass, T.W., Buckley, J. & Maurer, H.M. (1991a) *In utero* X-ray and risk of childhood rhabdomyosarcoma. *Paediatr. Perinat. Epidemiol.*, 5, A6–A7

Grufferman, S., Gula, M.J., Olshan, A.F., Falletta, J.M., Buckley, J., Pendergrass, T.W. & Maurer, H.M. (1991b) Absence of an association between parents' cigarette smoking and risk of rhabdomyosarcoma in their children. *Paediatr. Perinat. Epidemiol.*, 5, A17

Grufferman, S., Schwartz, A.G., Ruymann, F.B. & Maurer, H.M. (1993) Parents' use of cocaine and marijuana and increased risk of rhabdomyosarcoma in their children. *Cancer Causes Control*, 4, 217–224

Grundy, G.W., Creagan, E.T. & Fraumeni, J.F., Jr (1973) Non-Hodgkin's lymphoma in childhood: epidemiologic features. *J. Natl. Cancer Inst.*, 51, 767–776

Grundy, P., Koufos, A., Morgan, K., Li, F.P., Meadows, A.T. & Cavenee, W.K. (1988) Familial predisposition to Wilms' tumour does not map to the short arm of chromosome 11. *Nature*, 336, 374–376

Gunz, F.W. (1964) Leukaemia in New Zealand and Australia. *Pathol. Microbiol.*, 27, 697–704

Gunz, F.W. & Spears, G.F.S. (1968) Distribution of acute leukaemia in time and space. Studies in New Zealand. *Br. Med. J.*, 4, 604–608

Gunz, F.W. & Veale, A.M.O. (1969) Leukemia in close relatives – accident or predisposition? *J. Natl. Cancer Inst.*, 42, 517–524

Gunz, F.W., Gunz, J.P., Veale, A.M.O., Chapman, C.J. & Houston, I.B. (1975) Familial leukaemia: a study of 909 families. *Scand. J. Haematol.*, 15, 117–131

Gurney, J.G., Davis, S., Schwartz, S.M., Mueller, B.A., Kaune, W.T. & Stevens, R.G. (1995) Childhood cancer occurrence in relation to power line configurations: A study of potential selection bias in case-control studies. *Epidemiology*, 6, 31–35

Gurney, J.G., Davis, S., Severson, R.K., Fang, J.Y., Ross, J.A. & Robison, L.L. (1996a) Trends in cancer incidence among children in the U.S. *Cancer*, 78, 532–541

Gurney, J.G., Mueller, B.A., Davis, S., Schwartz, S.M., Stevens, R.G. & Kopecky, K.J. (1996b) Childhood brain tumor occurrence in relation to residential power line configurations, electric heating sources, and electric appliance use. *Am. J. Epidemiol.*, 143, 120–128

Gurney, J.G., Pogoda, J.M., Holly, E.A., Hecht, S.S. & Preston-Martin, S. (1997) Aspartame consumption in relation to childhood brain tumor risk: results from a case–control study. *J. Natl. Cancer Inst.*, 89, 1072–1074

Gutensohn, N. & Cole, P. (1977) Epidemiology of Hodgkin's disease in the young. *Int. J. Cancer*, 19, 595–604

Gutensohn, N.M. & Shapiro, D.S. (1982) Social class risk factors among children with Hodgkin's disease. *Int. J. Cancer*, 30, 433–435

Gutiérrez, M.I., Bhatia, K., Barriga, F., Diez, B., Muriel, F.S., de Andreas, M.L., Epelman, S., Risueño, C. & Magrath, I.T. (1992) Molecular epidemiology of Burkitt's lymphoma from South America: differences in breakpoint location and Epstein-Barr virus association from tumors in other world regions. *Blood*, 79, 3261–3266

Gwinn, M., Pappaioanou, M., George, J.R., Hannon, W.H., Wasser, S.C., Redus, M.A., Hoff, R., Grady, G.F., Willoughby, A., Novello, A.C., Petersen, L.R., Dondero, T.J. & Curran, J.W. (1991) Prevalence of HIV infection in childbearing women in the United States. Surveillance using newborn blood samples. *J. Am. Med. Assoc.*, 265, 1704–1708

Hafez, M., El-Tahan, H., El-Morsi, Z., Al-Tonbary, Y., El-Ziny, M., Sirag, S. & El-Serafi, M. (1985) Genetic–environmental interaction in acute lymphatic leukemia. In: Müller, H. & Weber, W., eds, *Familial Cancer* (1st Int. Res. Conf.), Basel, Karger, pp. 161–166

Hakulinen, T., Hovi, L., Karkinen-Jääskeläinen, M., Penttinen, K. & Saxén, L. (1973) Association between influenza during pregnancy and childhood leukaemia. *Br. Med. J.*, 4, 265–267

Hakulinen, T., Salonen, T. & Teppo, L. (1976) Cancer in the offspring of fathers in hydrocarbon-related occupations. *Br. J. Prev. Soc. Med.*, 30, 138–140

Hakulinen, T., Andersen, A.A., Malker, B., Pukkala, E., Schou, G. & Tulinius, H. (1986) Trends in cancer incidence in the Nordic Countries. *Acta Pathol. Microbiol. Immunol. Scand.*, Supple. 288, 1–151

Halliwell, B. & Gutteridge, J.M. (1986) Oxygen free radicals and iron in relation to biology and medicine: some problems and concepts. *Arch. Biochem. Biophys.*, 246, 501–514

Hann, H.W.L., London, W.T., Sutnick, A.I., Blumberg, B.S., Lustbader, E., Carim, H.M., Evans, A.E., Kay, H.E. & MacLennan, I.C. (1975) Studies of parents of children with acute leukemia. *J. Natl. Cancer Inst.*, 54, 1299–1305

Harach, H.R. & Williams, E.D. (1995) Childhood thyroid cancer in England and Wales. *Br. J. Cancer*, 72, 777–783

Harnden, D.G. (1985) Inherited factors in leukaemia and lymphoma. *Leukemia Res.*, 9, 705–707

Hartley, S.E. & Sainsbury, S.E. (1981) Acute leukaemia and the same chromosome abnormality in monozygotic twins. *Hum. Genet.*, 58, 408–410

Hartley, A.L., Birch, J.M., Marsden, H.B. & Harris, M. (1986) Breast cancer risk in mothers of children with osteosarcoma and chondrosarcoma. *Br. J. Cancer*, 54, 819–823

Hartley, A.L., Birch, J.M., McKinney, P.A., Blair, V., Teare, M.D., Carrette, J., Mann, J.R., Stiller, C.A., Draper, G.J., Johnston, H.E., Cartwright, R.A. & Waterhouse, J.A.H. (1988a) The Inter-Regional Epidemiological Study of Childhood Cancer (IRESCC): past medical history in children with cancer. *J. Epidemiol. Commun. Health*, 42, 235–242

Hartley, A.L., Birch, J.M., McKinney, P.A., Teare, M.D., Blair, V., Carrette, J., Mann, J.R., Draper, G.J., Stiller, C.A., Johnston, H.E., Cartwright, R.A. & Waterhouse, J.A.H. (1988b) The Inter-Regional Epidemiological Study of Childhood Cancer (IRESCC): case-control study of children with bone and soft tissue sarcomas. *Br. J. Cancer*, **58**, 838–842

Hartley, A.L., Birch, J.M., Blair, V., Teare, M.D., Marsden, H.B. & Harris, M. (1991a) Cancer incidence in the families of children with Ewing's tumor. *J. Natl. Cancer Inst.*, **83**, 955–956

Hartley, A.L., Birch, J.M. & Blair, V. (1991b) Malignant disease in the mothers of a population-based series of young adults with bone and soft tissue sarcomas. *Br. J. Cancer*, **63**, 416–419

Hartley, A.L., Birch, J.M., Blair, V. & Kelsey, A.M. (1994a) Malformations in children with soft tissue sarcoma and in their parents and siblings. *Paediat. Perinatal Epidemiol.*, **8**, 423–432

Hartley, A.L., Birch, J.M., Blair, V., Kelsey, A.M. & Morris Jones, P.H. (1994b) Foetal loss and infant deaths in families of children with soft-tissue sarcoma. *Int. J. Cancer*, **56**, 646–649

Harvey, E.B., Boice, J.D., Honeyman, M. & Flannery, J.T. (1985) Prenatal X-ray exposure and childhood cancer in twins. *New Engl. J. Med.*, **312**, 541–545

Hatch, M. & Susser, M. (1990) Background gamma radiation and childhood cancers within ten miles of a US nuclear plant. *Int. J. Epidemiol.*, **19**, 546–552

Hatch, M.C., Beyea, J., Nieves, J.W. & Susser, M. (1990) Cancer near the Three Mile Island nuclear plant: radiation emissions. *Am. J. Epidemiol.*, **132**, 397–412

Havery, D.C. & Fazio, T. (1983) Survey of baby bottle rubber nipples for volatile N-nitrosamines. *J. Assoc. Offic. Analyt. Chem.*, **66**, 1500–1503

Hawkins, M.M., Draper, G.J. & Kingston, J.E. (1987) Incidence of second primary tumours among childhood cancer survivors. *Br. J. Cancer*, **56**, 339–347

Hawkins, M.M., Draper, G.J. & Winter, D.L. (1995a) Cancer in the offspring of survivors of childhood leukaemia and non-Hodgkin lymphomas. *Br. J. Cancer*, **71**, 1335–1339

Hawkins, M.M., Winter, D.L., Burton, H.S. & Potok, M.H. (1995b) Heritability of Wilms' tumor. *J. Natl. Cancer Inst.*, **87**, 1323–1324

Hayes, F.A. & Green, A.A. (1983) Neuroblastoma. *Pediatr. Ann.*, **12**, 366–373

Health and Safety Executive (1993) *HSE Investigation of Leukaemia and Other Cancers in the Children of Male Workers at Sellafield*. London, HSE

Heasman, M.A., Kemp, I.W., MacLaren, A.M., Trotter, P., Gillis, C.R. & Hole, D.J. (1984) Incidence of leukaemia in young persons in west of Scotland. *Lancet*, **i**, 1188–1189

Heasman, M.A., Kemp, I.W., Urquhart, J.D. & Black, R. (1986a) Childhood leukaemia in northern Scotland. *Lancet, **i**, 266

Heasman, M.A., Kemp, I.W., Urquhart, J.D. & Black, R. (1986b) Leukaemia and lymphatic cancer in young people near nuclear installations (correction to Heasman et al. 1986a). *Lancet*, **i**, 385

Heasman, M.A., Urquhart, J.D., Black, R.J. & Kemp, I.W. (1987) Leukaemia in young persons in Scotland: a study of its geographical distribution and relationship to nuclear installations. *Health Bull.*, **45**, 147–151

Heath, C.W., Jr (1988) Investigation of cancer case clusters: possibilities and limitations. In: Miller R.W., Watanabe, S., Fraumeni, J.F., Jr, Sugimura, T., Takayama, S. & Sugano, H., eds., *Unusual Occurrences as Clues to Cancer Etiology*, Tokyo, Japan Scientific Societies Press; London, Taylor & Francis, pp. 27–35

Heath, C.W. & Hasterlik, R.J. (1963) Leukemia among children in a suburban community. *Am. J. Med.*, **34**, 796–812

Hecht, S.S. & Hoffmann, D. (1991) N-Nitroso compounds and tobacco-induced cancer in man. In: O'Neill, I.K., Chen, J. & Bartsch, H., eds, *Relevance to Human Cancer of N-Nitroso Compounds, Tobacco Smoke and Mycotoxins* (IARC Scientific Publications No. 105), Lyon, IARC, pp. 54–61

Heidemann, R.L., Freeman, C.R., Packer, R.J., Rorke, L.B. & Albright, L.A. (1993) Tumors of the central nervous system. In: Pizzo, P.A. & Poplack, D.G., eds, *Principles and Practice of Pediatric Oncology*, 2nd ed., Philadelphia, Lippincott, pp. 633–681

Heinonen, O.P., Slone, D. & Shapiro, S. (1977) *Birth Defects and Drugs in Pregnancy*, Littleton, MA, Publishing Sciences Group

Hemminki, K., Saloniemi, I., Salonen, T., Partanen, T. & Vainio, H. (1981) Childhood cancer and parental occupation in Finland. *J. Epidemiol. Commun. Health*, **35**, 11–15

Hems, G. & Stuart, A. (1971) BCG and leukaemia. *Lancet*, **i**, 183

Henshaw, D.L., Eatough, J.P. & Richardson, R.B. (1990) Radon as a causative factor in induction of myeloid leukaemia and other cancers. *Lancet*, **335**, 1008–1012

Herbst, A.L. & Scully, R.E. (1970) Adenocarcinoma of the vagina in adolescence: a report of 7 cases including 6 clear-cell carcinomas (so called Mesonephromas). *Cancer*, **25**, 745–757

Herbst, A.I., Ulfelder, H. & Poskanzer, D.C. (1971) Adenocarcinoma of the vagina. *New Engl. J. Med.*, **284**, 878–881

Herbst, A.L., Kurman, R.J., Scully, R.E. & Poskanzer, D.C. (1972) Clear-cell adenocarcinoma of the genital tract in young females. *New Engl. J. Med.*, **287**, 1259–1264

Heuch, J.M., Heuch, I. & Kvåle, G. (1996) Birth characteristics and risk of Wilms' tumours: a nationwide prospective study in Norway. *Br. J. Cancer*, **74**, 1148–1151

Hewitt, D. (1955) Some features of leukaemia mortality. *Br. J. Prev. Soc. Med.*, **9**, 81–88

Hewitt, D., Lashof, J.C. & Stewart, A.M. (1966) Childhood cancer in twins. *Cancer*, **19**, 157–161

Hewson, D. & Bennett, A. (1987) Childbirth research data: medical records or women's reports? *Am. J. Epidemiol.*, **125**, 484–491

Heyn, R., Haeberlen, V., Newton, W.A., Ragab, A.H., Raney, R.B., Tefft, M., Wharam, M., Ensign, L.G. & Maurer, H.M. (1993) Second malignant neoplasms in children treated for rhabdomyosarcoma. *J. Clin. Oncol.*, **11**, 262–270

Hicks, N., Zack, M., Caldwell, G.G., Fernbach, D.J. & Falletta, J.M. (1984) Childhood cancer and occupational radiation exposure in parents. *Cancer*, **53**, 1637–1643

Higginson, J., Muir, C.S. & Muñoz, N. (1992) *Human Cancer: Epidemiology and Environmental Causes* (Cambridge Monographs on Cancer Research), Cambridge, Cambridge University Press

Hill, A.B. (1965) The environment and disease: association or causation? *Proc. R. Soc. Med.*, **58**, 295–300

Hill, C. & Laplanche, A. (1990) Overall mortality and cancer mortality around French nuclear sites. *Nature*, **347**, 755–757

Hingson, R., Zuckerman, B., Amaro, H., Frank, D.A., Kayne, H., Sorenson, J.R., Mitchell, J., Parker, S., Morelock, S. & Timperi, R. (1986) Maternal marijuana use and neonatal outcome: uncertainty posed by self-reports. *Am. J. Pub. Health*, **76**, 667–669

Hirayama, T. (1979) Descriptive and analytical epidemiology of childhood malignancy in Japan. In: *Recent Advances in Managements of Children with Cancer*, Tokyo, The Children's Cancer Association of Japan, pp. 27–43

Hjalmars, U., Kulldorff, M. & Gustafsson, G. (1994) Risk of acute childhood leukaemia in Sweden after the Chernobyl reactor accident. *Br. Med. J.*, **309**, 154–157

Hjalmars, U., Kulldorff, M., Gustafsson, G. & Nagarwalla, N. (1996) Childhood leukaemia in Sweden: Using GIS and a spatial scan statistic for cluster detection. *Stat. Med.*, **15**, 707–715

Hoar, S.K., Morrison, A.S., Cole, P. & Silverman, D.T. (1980) An occupation and exposure linkage system for the study of occupational carcinogenesis. *J. Occup. Med.*, **11**, 722–726

Hocking, B., Gordon, I.R., Grain, H.L. & Hatfield, G.E. (1996) Cancer incidence and mortality and proximity to TV towers. *Med. J. Aust.*, **165**, 601–605

Hoffmann, W., Kranefeld, A. & Schmitz-Feuerhake, I. (1993) Radium-226-contaminated drinking water: hypothesis on an exposure pathway in a population with elevated childhood leukaemia. *Environ. Health Perspect.*, Supple. **101**, 113–115

Holland, W.W., Doll, R. & Carter, C.O. (1962) Mortality from leukaemia and other cancers among patients with Down's syndrome (mongols) and among their parents. *Br. J. Cancer,* **16**, 177–186

Holly, E.A., Aston, D.A., Ahn, D.K. & Kristiansen, J.J. (1992) Ewing's bone sarcoma, paternal occupational exposure, and other factors. *Am. J. Epidemiol.,* **135**, 122–129

Hoover, R.N. (1976) Bacillus Calmette-Guérin vaccination and cancer prevention: a critical review of the human experience. *Cancer Res.,* **36**, 652–654

Hopton, P.A., McKinney, P.A., Cartwright, R.A., Mann, J.R., Birch, J.M., Hartley, A.L., Waterhouse, J.A., Johnston, H.E., Draper, G.J. & Stiller, C.A. (1985) X-rays in pregnancy and the risk of childhood cancer. *Lancet,* **ii**, 773

Horn, E. (1988) Iron and folate supplements during pregnancy: supplementing everyone treats those at risk and is cost effective. *Br. Med. J.,* **297**, 1325–1327

Hornstein, L. (1977) Adrenal carcinoma in a child with a history of fetal-alcohol syndrome. *Lancet,* **ii**, 1292

Howe, G.R., Burch, J.D., Chiarelli, A.M., Risch, H.A. & Choi, B.C.K. (1989) An exploratory case–control study of brain tumors in children. *Cancer Res.,* **49**, 4349–4352

Hsieh, C.C., Walker, A.M. & Hoar, S.K. (1983) Grouping occupations according to carcinogenic potential: occupation clusters from an exposure linkage system. *Am. J. Epidemiol.,* **117**, 575–589

Huff, V., Compton, D.A., Chao, L.Y., Strong, L.C., Geiser, C.F. & Saunders, G.F. (1988) Lack of linkage of familial Wilms' tumour to chromosomal band 11p13. *Nature,* **336**, 377–378

Huff, V., Meadows, A., Riccardi, V.M., Strong, L.C. & Saunders, G.F. (1990) Parental origin of de novo constitutional deletions of chromosomal band 11p13. *Am. J. Human Genet.,* **47**, 155–160

Hull, D. (1992) Vitamin K and childhood cancer. *Br. Med. J.,* **305**, 326–327

Hummel, M., Anagnostopoulos, I., Korbjuhn, P. & Stein, H. (1995) Epstein-Barr virus in B-cell non-Hodgkin's lymphomas: unexpected infection patterns and different infection incidence in low- and high-grade types. *J. Pathol.,* **175**, 263–271

IARC (1983) *IARC Monographs on the Evaluation of the Carcinogenic Risk of Chemicals to Humans. Volume 30. Miscellaneous Pesticides,* Lyon, IARC

IARC (1986a) *IARC Monographs on the Evaluation of the Carcinogenic Risk of Chemicals to Humans. Volume 38. Tobacco Smoking,* Lyon, IARC

IARC (1986b) *IARC Monographs on the Evaluation of the Carcinogenic Risk of Chemicals to Humans. Volume 41. Some Halogenated Hydrocarbons and Pesticide Exposures,* Lyon, IARC

IARC (1987) *IARC Monographs on the Evaluation of Carcinogenic Risks to Humans. Supplement 7. Overall Evaluations of Carcinogenicity: An Updating of IARC Monographs Volumes 1 to 42,* Lyon, IARC

IARC (1989a) *IARC Monographs on the Evaluation of Carcinogenic Risks to Humans. Volume 46. Diesel and Gasoline Engine Exhausts and Some Nitroarenes,* Lyon, IARC, pp. 147–148

IARC (1989b) *IARC Monographs on the Evaluation of the Carcinogenic Risk of Chemicals to Humans. Volume 47. Some Organic Solvents, Resin Monomers and Related Compounds, Pigments and Occupational Exposures in Paint Manufacture and Painting,* Lyon, IARC, pp. 43–77

IARC (1991) *IARC Monographs on the Evaluation of Carcinogenic Risks to Humans. Volume 53. Occupational Exposures in Insecticide Application, and Some Pesticides,* Lyon, IARC

IARC (1993) *IARC Monographs on the Evaluation of Carcinogenic Risks to Humans. Volume 57. Occupational Exposures of Hairdressers and Barbers and Personal Use of Hair Colourants; Some Hair Dyes, Cosmetic Colourants, Industrial Dyestuffs and Aromatic Amines,* Lyon, IARC, pp. 43–118

Imaizumi, Y., Shinozaki, N. & Aoki, H. (1975) Inbreeding in Japan: results of a nation-wide study. *Jap. J. Hum. Genet.,* **20**, 91–107

Independent Advisory Group (1984) *Investigation of the Possible Increased Incidence of Cancer in West Cumbria* (Chairman Sir Douglas Black), London, HMSO

Infante-Rivard, C., Mur, P., Armstrong, B., Alverez-Dardet, C. & Bolumar, F. (1991) Acute lymphoblastic leukaemia among Spanish children and mothers' occupation: a case-control study. *J. Epidemiol. Commun. Health,* **45**, 11–15

Infante-Rivard, C. (1995) Electromagnetic field exposure during pregnancy and childhood leukaemia. *Lancet,* **346**, 177

Innis, M.D. (1965) Immunisation and childhood leukaemia. *Lancet,* **i**, 605

Innis, M.D. (1972) Nephroblastoma: possible index cancer of childhood. *Med. J. Aust.,* **1**, 18–20

Inskip, P.D., Harvey, E.B., Boice, J.D., Jr, Stone, B.J., Matanoski, G., Flannery, J.T. & Fraumeni, J.F., Jr (1991) Incidence of childhood cancer in twins. *Cancer Causes Control,* **2**, 315–324

Inskip, P.D., Linet, M.S. & Heineman, E.F. (1995) Etiology of brain tumors in adults. *Epidemiol. Rev.,* **17**, 382–414

Ishimura, T., Ichimaru, M. & Mihami, M. (1981) *Leukaemia Incidence among Individuals Exposed In utero, Children of Atomic Bomb Survivors and their Controls, Hiroshima and Nagasaki, 1945–1979* (RERF Tech Rep 11–81), Hiroshima, Radiation Effects Research Foundation

Israels, L.G., Friesen, E., Jansen, A.H. & Israels, E.D. (1987) Vitamin $K_1$ increases sister chromatid exchange *in vitro* in human leukocytes and *in vivo* in fetal sheep cells: A possible role for "vitamin K deficiency" in the fetus. *Pediat. Res.,* **22**, 405–408

Issa, J.P.J. & Baylin, S.B. (1996) Epigenetics and human disease. *Nature Med.,* **2**, 281–282

Ito, Y. (1985) Vegetable activators of the viral genome and the causation of Burkitt's lymphoma and naso-phayrngeal carcinoma. In: Epstein, M.A. & Achong, B.C., eds, *The Epstein–Barr Virus – Recent Advances,* London, Heinemann Medical, pp. 209–234

Ivankovic, S. & Druckrey, H. (1968) Transplacental induction of malignant tumors of the nervous system. I. Ethyl-nitroso-urea (ENU) in BD IX rats. *Z. Krebsforsch.,* **71**, 320–360

Ivanov, E.P., Tolochko, G., Lazarev, V.S. & Shuvaeva, L. (1993) Child leukaemia after Chernobyl. *Nature,* **365**, 702

Iversen, T. (1966) Leukaemia in infancy and childhood – a material of 570 Danish cases. *Acta Paediat. Scand., Supple.* **167**, 9–219

Jablon, S. & Kato, H. (1970) Childhood cancer in relation to prenatal exposure to atomic bomb radiation. *Lancet,* **ii**, 1000–1003

Jablon, S., Belsky, J.L., Tachikawa, K. & Steer, A. (1971) Cancer in Japanese exposed as children to atomic bombs. *Lancet,* **i**, 927–932

Jablon, S., Hrubec, Z., Boice, J.D., Jr & Stone, B.J. (1990) *Cancer in Populations Living near Nuclear Facilities* (NIH Publication 90–874), Bethesda, MD, Public Health Service, Dept. of Health and Human Services

Jablon, S., Hrubec, Z. & Boice, J.D. (1991) Cancer in populations living near nuclear facilities. *J. Am. Med. Assoc.,* **265**, 1403–1408

Jackson, E.W., Norris, F.D. & Klauber, M.R. (1969) Childhood leukemia in California-born twins. *Cancer,* **23**, 913–919

Jackson, J.D. (1992) Are the stray 60-Hz electromagnetic fields associated with the distribution and use of electric power a significant cause of cancer? *Proc. Natl. Acad. Sci.,* **89**, 3508–3510

Jadayel, D., Fain, P. & Upadhyaya, M. (1990) Paternal origin of new mutations in Von Recklinghausen neurofibromatosis. *Nature,* **343**, 558–559

Jaffe, E.S., Raffeld, M., Medeiros, L.J. & Stetler-Stevenson, M. (1992) An overview of the classification of non-Hodgkin's lymphomas: An integration of morphological and phenotypical concepts. *Cancer Res.,* **52**, 5447S–5452S

James, W.H. (1990) Further evidence for the hypothesis that one cause of childhood leukaemia is infection. *Paediat. Perinatal Epidemiol.,* **4**, 113–117

Jamrozik, K., White, R. & Misch, K. (1988) Cancer Registry of Papua New Guinea, 1979–83. In: Parkin, D.M., Stiller, C.A., Draper, G.J., Bieber, C.A., Terracini, B. & Young, J.L., eds, *International Incidence of Childhood Cancer.* (IARC Scientific Publications No 87), Lyon, IARC, pp. 335–337

Janerich, D.T. & Polednak, A.P. (1983) Epidemiology of birth defects. *Epidemiol. Rev.*, **5**, 16–37

Jensen, R.D. & Miller, R.W. (1971) Retinoblastoma: epidemiologic characteristics. *New Engl. J. Med.* **285**, 307–311

Ji, B.T., Shu, X.O., Linet, M.S., Zheng, W., Wacholder, S., Gao, Y.T., Ying, D.M. & Jin, F. (1997) Paternal cigarette smoking and the risk of childhood cancer among offspring of nonsmoking mothers. *J. Natl. Cancer Inst.*, **89**, 238–244

Joffe, M. (1992) Validity of exposure data derived from a structured questionnaire. *Am. J. Epidemiol.*, **135**, 564–570

John, E.M., Savitz, D.A. & Sandler, D.P. (1991) Prenatal exposure to parents' smoking and childhood cancer. *Am. J. Epidemiol.*, **133**, 123–132

Johnson, C.C. & Spitz, M.R. (1985) Neuroblastoma: case-control analysis of birth characteristics. *J. Natl. Cancer Inst.*, **74**, 789–792

Johnson, C.C., Annegers, J.F., Frankowski, R.F., Spitz, M.R. & Buffler, P.A. (1987) Childhood nervous system tumors – an evaluation of the association with paternal occupational exposure to hydrocarbons. *Am. J. Epidemiol.*, **126**, 605–613

Johnson, C.C. & Spitz, M.R. (1989) Childhood nervous system tumours: an assessment of risk associated with paternal occupations involving use, repair or manufacture of electrical and electronic equipment. *Int. J. Epidemiol.*, **18**, 756–762

Johnston, H.E., Mann, J.R., Williams, J., Waterhouse, J.A., Birch, J.M., Cartwright, R.A., Draper, G.J., Hartley, A.L., McKinney, P.A., Hopton, P.A. & Stiller, C.A. (1986) The Inter-Regional Epidemiological Study of Childhood Cancer (IRESCC): case–control study in children with germ cell tumors. *Carcinogenesis*, **7**, 717–722

Jones, T.L., Shih, C.H., Thurston, D.H., Ware, B.J. & Cole, P. (1993) Selection bias from differential residential mobility as an explanation for associations of wire codes with childhood cancer. *J. Clin. Epidemiol.*, **46**, 545–548

Jones, S.M., Phillips, P.C., Molloy, P.T., Lange, B.J., Needle, M.N. & Biegel, J.A. (1995) Congenital anomalies and genetic disorders in families of children with central nervous system tumours. *J. Med. Genet.*, **32**, 627–632

Junaid, T.A. & Babalola (1988) Ibadan Cancer Registry, 1960–1984. In: Parkin, D.M., Stiller, C.A., Draper, G.J., Bieber, C.A., Terracini, B. & Young, J.L., eds, *International Incidence of Childhood Cancer* (IARC Scientific Publications No. 87), Lyon, IARC, pp. 37–41

Kaatsch, P., Haaf, G. & Michaelis, J. (1995) Childhood malignancies in Germany – methods and results of a nationwide registry. *Eur. J. Cancer*, **31A**, 993–999

Kafuko, G.W. & Burkitt, D.P. (1970) Burkitt's lymphoma and malaria. *Int. J. Cancer*, **6**, 1–9

Kahn, P. (1993) A grisly archive of key cancer data. *Science*, **259**, 448–451

Kantor, A.F., Curnen, M.G.M., Meigs, J.W. & Flannery, J.T. (1979) Occupations of fathers of patients with Wilms's tumour. *J. Epidemiol. Commun. Health*, **33**, 253–256

Kato, M.V., Ishizaki, K., Shimizu, T., Ejima, Y., Tanooka, H., Takayama, J., Kaneko, A., Toguchida, J. & Sasaki, M.S. (1994) Parental origin of germ-line and somatic mutations in the retinoblastoma gene. *Human Genet.*, **94**, 31–38

Katz, L. & Steinitz, R. (1988) Israel Cancer Registry, 1970–1979. In: Parkin, D.M., Stiller, C.A., Draper, G.J., Bieber, C.A., Terracini, B. & Young, J.L., eds, *International Incidence of Childhood Cancer*. (IARC Scientific Publications No. 87), Lyon, IARC, pp. 175–180

Kaune, W.T., Stevens, R.G., Callahan, N.J., Severson, R.K. & Thomas, D.B. (1987) Residential magnetic and electric fields. *Bioelectromagnetics*, **8**, 315–335

Kaune, W.T. & Savitz, D.A. (1994) Simplification of the Wertheimer–Leeper wire code. *Bioelectromagnetics*, **15**, 275–282

Kaye, S.A., Robison, L.L., Smithson, W.A., Gunderson, P., King, F.L. & Neglia, J.P. (1991) Maternal reproductive history and birth characteristics in childhood acute lymphoblastic leukemia. *Cancer*, **68**, 1351–1355

Kazakov, V.S., Demidchik, E.P. & Astakhova, L.N. (1992) Thyroid cancer after Chernobyl. *Nature*, **359**, 21

Keith, L., Brown, E.R., Fields, C. & Stepto, R. (1973) Age group differences of twins with leukemia. In: Dutcher, R.M. & Chieco-Bianchi, L., eds, *Unifying Concepts of Leukaemia*, Bibl Haematol., no. 39, Basel, Karger, pp. 1125–1135

Kemeny, J.G.C. (1979) *Report of the President's Commission on the Accident at Three Mile Island, the Need for Change: The Legacy of Three Mile Island*. Washington, DC, US Government Printing Office

Kenney, L.B., Nicholson, H.S., Brasseux, C., Mills, J.L., Robison, L.L., Zeltzer, L.K., Meadows, A.T., Reaman, G.H. & Byrne, J. (1996) Birth defects in offspring of adult survivors of childhood acute lymphoblastic leukemia. *Cancer*, **78**, 169–176

Khan, A., Bader, J.L., Hoy, G.R. & Sinks, L.F. (1979) Hepatoblastoma in child with fetal alcohol syndrome. *Lancet*, **i**, 1403–1404

Khoury, M.J., James, L.M. & Erickson, J.D. (1994) On the use of affected controls to address recall bias in case–control studies of birth defects. *Teratology*, **49**, 273–281

Kingston, J.E., Hawkins, M.M., Draper, G.J., Marsden, H.B. & Kinnier-Wilson, L.M. (1987) Patterns of multiple primary tumours in patients treated for cancer during childhood. *Br. J. Cancer*, **56**, 331–338

Kinlen, L. (1988) Evidence for an infective cause of childhood leukaemia: comparison of a Scottish new town with nuclear reprocessing sites in Britain. *Lancet*, **ii**, 1323–1327

Kinlen, L. (1992) Childhood leukaemia on Greek islands. *Lancet*, **i**, 252–253

Kinlen, L.J. (1993) Can paternal preconceptional radiation account for the increase of leukaemia and non-Hodgkin's lymphoma in Seascale? *Br. Med. J.*, **306**, 1718–1721

Kinlen, L.J. (1994) Leukaemia. In: Doll, R., Fraumeni, J.F. & Muir, C.S., eds, *Trends in Cancer Incidence and Mortality. Cancer Surveys*, **19/20**, 475–491

Kinlen, L.J. (1995) Epidemiological evidence for an infective basis in childhood leukaemia. *Br. J. Cancer*, **71**, 1–5

Kinlen, L.J. & John, S.M. (1994) Wartime evacuation and mortality from childhood leukaemia in England and Wales in 1945–9. *Br. Med. J.*, **309**, 1197–1202

Kinlen, L.J. & Petridou, E. (1995) Childhood leukemia and rural population movements: Greece, Italy, and other countries. *Cancer Causes Control*, **6**, 445–450

Kinlen, L.J. & Pike, M.C. (1971) BCG vaccination and leukaemia. *Lancet*, **ii**, 398–402

Kinlen, L.J., Clarke, K. & Hudson, C. (1990) Evidence from population mixing in British new towns 1946–85 of an infective basis for childhood leukaemia. *Lancet*, **336**, 577–582

Kinlen, L.J. & Hudson, C. (1991) Childhood leukaemia and poliomyelitis in relation to military encampments in England and Wales in the period of national military service, 1950–63. *Br. Med. J.*, **303**, 1357–1362

Kinlen, L.J., Hudson, C.M. & Stiller, C.A. (1991) Contacts between adults as evidence for an infective origin of childhood leukaemia: an explanation for the excess near nuclear establishments in West Berkshire? *Br. J. Cancer*, **64**, 549–554

Kinlen, L.J., O'Brien, F., Clarke, K., Balkwill, A. & Matthews, F. (1993a) Rural population mixing and childhood leukaemia: effects of the North Sea oil industry in Scotland, including the area near Dounreay nuclear site. *Br. Med. J.*, **306**, 743–748

Kinlen, L.J., Clarke, K. & Balkwill, A. (1993b) Paternal preconceptional radiation exposure in the nuclear industry and leukaemia and non-Hodgkin's lymphoma in young people in Scotland. *Br. Med. J.*, **306**, 1153–1158

Kinlen, L.J., Dickson, M. & Stiller, C.A. (1995) Childhood leukaemia and non-Hodgkin's lymphoma near large rural construction sites, with a comparison with Sellafield nuclear site. *Br. Med. J.*, **310**, 763–768

Kinnier-Wilson, L.M. & Draper, G.J. (1974) Neuroblastoma, its natural history and prognosis: A study of 487 cases. *Br. Med. J.*, **3**, 301–307

Kinnier-Wilson, L.M. & Waterhouse, J.A.H. (1984) Obstetric ultrasound and childhood malignancies. *Lancet*, **ii**, 997–999

Klauber, M.R. (1968) A study of clustering of childhood leukemia by hospital of birth. *Cancer Res.*, **28**, 1710–1712

Klauber, M.R. & Mustacchi, P. (1970) Space-time clustering of childhood leukemia in San Francisco. *Cancer Res.*, **30**, 1969–1973

Klebanoff, M.A., Read, J.S., Mills, J.L. & Shiono, P.H. (1993) The risk of childhood cancer after neonatal exposure to vitamin K. *New Engl. J. Med.*, **329**, 905–908

Klebanoff, M.A., Clemens, J.D. & Read, J.S. (1996) Maternal smoking during pregnancy and childhood cancer. *Am. J. Epidemiol.*, **144**, 1028–1033

Kleihues, P., Burger, P.C. & Scheithauer, B.W. (1993) The new WHO classification of brain tumours. *Brain Pathol.*, **3**, 255–268

Kneale, G.W. & Stewart, A.M. (1976) Mantel-Haenszel analysis of Oxford data. I. Independent effects of several birth factors including fetal irradiation. *J. Natl. Cancer Inst.*, **56**, 879–883

Kneale, G.W. & Stewart, A.M. (1978) Pre-cancers and liability to other diseases. *Br. J. Cancer*, **37**, 448–457

Kneale, G.W. & Stewart, A.M. (1980) Pre-conception X-rays and childhood cancers. *Br. J. Cancer*, **41**, 222–226

Kneale, G.W. & Stewart, A.M. (1987) Childhood cancers in the UK and their relation to background radiation. *Radiation and Health, The Biological Effects of Low-level Exposure to Ionizing Radiation*, Chichester, Wiley, pp. 203–220

Kneale, G.W., Stewart, A.M. & Kinnier-Wilson, L.M. (1986) Immunizations against infectious diseases and childhood cancers. *Cancer Immunol. Immunother.*, **21**, 129–132

Knekt, P., Reunanen, A., Takkunen, H., Aromaa, A., Heliövaara, M. & Hakulinen, T. (1994) Body iron stores and risk of cancer. *Int. J. Cancer*, **56**, 379–382

Knishkowy, B. & Baker, E.L. (1986) Transmission of occupational disease to family contacts. *Am. J. Ind. Med.*, **9**, 543–550

Knox, G. (1964) Epidemiology of childhood leukaemia in Northumberland and Durham. *Br. J. Prev. Soc. Med.*, **18**, 17–24

Knox, E.G. (1994) Leukaemia clusters in childhood: geographical analysis in Britain. *J. Epidemiol. Commun. Health*, **48**, 369–376

Knox, E.G. & Gilman, E. (1992a) Leukaemia clusters in Great Britain. I. Space-time interactions. *J. Epidemiol. Commun. Health*, **46**, 566–572

Knox, E.G. & Gilman, E. (1992b) Leukaemia clusters in Great Britain. 2. Geographical concentrations. *J. Epidemiol. Commun. Health*, **46**, 573–576

Knox, E.G. & Gilman, E.A. (1997) Hazard proximities of childhood cancers in Great Britain from 1953–80. *J. Epidemiol. Commun. Health*, **51**, 151–159

Knox, E.G., Stewart, A. & Kneale, G. (1980) Childhood leukaemia and mother-foetus infection. *Br. J. Cancer*, **42**, 158–161

Knox, E.G., Stewart, A.M. & Kneale, G.W. (1983) Foetal infection, childhood leukaemia and cancer. *Br. J. Cancer*, **48**, 849–852

Knox, E.G., Marshall, T. & Barling, R. (1984) Leukaemia and childhood cancer in twins. *J. Epidemiol. Commun. Health*, **38**, 12–16

Knox, E.G., Stewart, A.M., Kneale, G.W. & Gilman, E.A. (1987) Prenatal irradiation and childhood cancer. *J. Soc. Radiol. Protect.*, **7**, 177–189

Knox, E.G., Stewart, A.M., Gilman, E.A. & Kneale, G.W. (1988) Background radiation and childhood cancers. *J. Radiol. Prot.*, **8**, 9–18

Knudson, A.G. (1971) Mutation and cancer: statistical study of retinoblastoma. *Proc. Natl. Acad. Sci. USA*, **68**, 820–823

Knudson, A.G. & Strong, L.C. (1972) Mutation and cancer: a model for Wilms' tumor of the kidney. *J. Natl. Cancer Inst.*, **48**, 313–324

Kobayashi, N., Furukawa, T. & Takatsu, T. (1968) Congenital anomalies in children with malignancy. *Paediatr. Univ. Tokyo*, **16**, 31–37

Kobayashi, N., Matsui, I., Tanimura, M., Nagahara, N., Akatsuka, J., Hirayama, T. & Sato, K. (1991) Childhood neuroectodermal tumours and malignant lymphoma after maternal ovulation induction. *Lancet*, **338**, 955

Koide, O., Watanabe, Y. & Sato, K. (1980) A pathological survey of intracranial germinoma and pinealoma in Japan. *Cancer*, **45**, 2119–2130

Koren, G., Demitrakoudis, D., Weksberg, R., Rieder, M., Shear, N.H., Sonely, M., Shandling, B. & Spielberg, S.P. (1989) Neuroblastoma after prenatal exposure to phenytoin: cause and effect? *Teratology*, **40**, 157–162

Koufos, A., Grundy, P., Morgan, K., Aleck, K.A., Hadro, T., Lampkin, B.C., Kalbakji, A. & Cavenee, W.K. (1989) Familial Wiedemann–Beckwith syndrome and a second Wilms' tumor locus both map to 11p15.5. *Am. J. Hum. Genet.*, **44**, 711–719

Kramárová, E., Stiller, C.A., Ferlay, J., Parkin, D.M., Draper, G.J., Michaelis, J., Neglia, J. & Qureshi, S. (1996) *International Classification of Childhood Cancer 1996* (IARC Technical Reports No. 29), Lyon, IARC

Kramer, M.S. (1987) Determinants of low birth weight: methodological assessment and meta-analysis. *Bull. WHO*, **65**, 663–737

Kramer, S., Ward, E., Meadows, A.T. & Malone, K.E. (1987) Medical and drug risk factors associated with neuroblastoma: a case-control study. *J. Natl. Cancer Inst.*, **78**, 797–804

Kraut, A., Tate, R. & Tran, N. (1994) Residential electric consumption and childhood cancer in Canada (1971–1986). *Arch. Environ. Health*, **49**, 156–159

Krishnamurthy, S. & Dhar, M. (1991) Cancer and other causes of childhood mortality in Bombay, India. *Cancer*, **68**, 1848–1853

Kristensen, P. & Andersen, A. (1992) A cohort study on cancer incidence in offspring of male printing workers. *Epidemiology*, **3**, 6–10

Kristensen, P., Andersen, A., Irgens, L.M., Bye, A.S. & Sundheim, L. (1996) Cancer in offspring of parents engaged in agricultural activities in Norway: incidence and risk factors in the farm environment. *Int. J. Cancer*, **65**, 39–50

Kryscio, R.G., Myers, M.H., Prusiner, S.T., Heise, H.W. & Christine, B.W. (1973) The space-time distribution of Hodgkin's disease in Connecticut, 1940–1969. *J. Natl. Cancer Inst.*, **50**, 1107–1110

Kuijten, R.R. & Bunin, G.R. (1993) Risk factors for childhood brain tumors. *Cancer Epidemiol. Biomarkers Prev.*, **2**, 277–288

Kuijten, R.R., Bunin, G.R., Nass, C.C. & Meadows, A.T. (1990) Gestational and familial risk factors for childhood astrocytoma: results of a case-control study. *Cancer Res.*, **50**, 2608–2612

Kuijten, R.R., Bunin, G.R., Nass, C.C. & Meadows, A.T. (1992) Parental occupation and childhood astrocytoma: results of a case-control study. *Cancer Res.*, **52**, 782–786

Kuijten, R.R., Strom, S.S., Rorke, L.B., Boesel, C.P., Buckley, J.D., Meadows, A.T. & Bunin, G.R. (1993) Family history of cancer and seizures in young children with brain tumors: a report from the Childrens Cancer Group (United States and Canada). *Cancer Causes Control*, **4**, 455–464

Kurita, S., Kamei, Y. & Ota, K. (1974) Genetic studies on familial leukemia. *Cancer*, **34**, 1098–1101

Kushner, B.H. & Helson, L. (1985) Monozygotic siblings discordant for neuroblastoma: etiologic implications. *J. Pediatr.*, **107**, 405–409

Kushner, B.H., Gilbert, F. & Helson, L. (1986) Familial neuroblastoma. Case reports, literature review, and etiologic considerations. *Cancer*, **57**, 1887–1893

Kuzmack, A.M. (1987) Comment on Lagakos, Wessen and Zelen. *J. Am. Stat. Assoc.*, **82**, 703

Kwa, S.L. & Fine, L.J. (1980) The association between parental occupation and childhood malignancy. *J. Occup. Med.*, **22**, 792–794

Lagakos, S.W., Wessen, B.J. & Zelen, M. (1986) An analysis of contaminated well water and health effects in Woburn, Massachusetts. *J. Am. Stat. Assoc.*, **81**, 583–596

Lamy, M.E., Favart, A.M., Cornu, C., Mendez, M., Segas, M. & Burtonboy, G. (1982) Study of Epstein Barr virus (EBV) antibodies: IgG and IgM anti-VCA, IgG anti-EA and Ig anti-EBNA obtained with an original microtiter technique: serological criterions of primary and recurrent EBV infections and follow-up of infectious mononucleosis, sero-epidemiology of EBV in Belgium based on 5178 sera from patients. *Acta Clin. Belgica*, **37**, 281–298

Lancaster, H.O. & Clements, F.W. (1965) Immunisation and childhood leukaemia. *Lancet*, **i**, 654–655

*Lancet* (1990) Childhood leukaemia: an infectious disease? (Editorial). *Lancet*, **336**, 1477

Land, C.E., McKay, F.W. & Machado, S.G. (1984) Childhood leukemia and fallout from the Nevada nuclear tests. *Science*, **223**, 139–144

Langford, I. (1991) Childhood leukaemia mortality and population change in England and Wales 1969–73. *Soc. Sci. Med.*, **33**, 435–440

Langford, I. & Bentham, G. (1990) Infectious aetiology of childhood leukaemia. *Lancet*, **336**, 945

Laplanche, A. & de Vathaire, F. (1994a) Leukaemia mortality in French communes (administrative units) with a large and rapid population increase. *Br. J. Cancer*, **69**, 110–113

Laplanche, A. & de Vathaire, F. (1994b) Reply to letter from Dr Kinlen. *Br. J. Cancer*, **70**, 181

Larsen, R.J., Holmes, C.L. & Heath, C.W. (1973) A statistical test for measuring unimodal clustering: a description of the test and of its application to cases of acute leukemia in metropolitan Atlanta, Georgia. *Biometrics*, **29**, 301–309

Lathrop, G.D., Wolfe, W.H., Albanese, R.A. & Moynahan, P.M. (1984) Air Force Health Study (Project Ranch Hand II). In: *An Epidemiologic Investigation of Health Effects in Air Force Personnel Following Exposure to Herbicides. Baseline Morbidity Study Results*, San Antonio, TX, United States Air Force School of Aerospace Medicine, Brooks Air Force Base

Laval, G. & Tuyns, A.J. (1988) Environmental factors in childhood leukaemia. *Br. J. Ind. Med.*, **45**, 843–844

Law, G. & Roman, E. (1997) Leukaemia near La Hague nuclear plant. Study design is questionable. *Br. Med. J.*, **314**, 1553

Layde, P.M., Erickson, J.D., Falek, A. & McCarthy, B.J. (1980) Congenital malformation in twins. *Am. J. Hum. Genet.*, **32**, 69–78

Leck, I. & Steward, J.K. (1972) Incidence of neoplasms in children born after influenza epidemics. *Br. Med. J.*, **4**, 631–634

Leisenring, W.M., Breslow, N.E., Evans, I.E., Beckwith, J.B., Coppes, M.J. & Grundy, P. (1994) Increased birth weights of national Wilms' tumor study patients suggest a growth factor excess. *Cancer Res.*, **54**, 4680–4683

Leiss, J.K. & Savitz, D.A. (1995) Home pesticide use and childhood cancer: A case–control study. *Am. J. Pub. Health*, **85**, 249–252

LeMasters, S.K. & Bove, K.E. (1980) Genetic/environmental significance of multifocal nodular renal blastema. *Am. J. Pediatr. Hematol. Oncol.*, **2**, 81–87

Lemire, R.J. & Beckwith, J.B. (1982) Pathogenesis of congenital tumors and malformations of the sacrococcygeal region. *Teratology*, **25**, 201–213

Leogrande, G. & Jirillo, E. (1993) Studies on the epidemiology of child infections in the Bari area (south Italy). VII. Epidemiology of Epstein-Barr virus infections. *Eur. J. Epidemiol.*, **9**, 368–372

Levi, F., La Vecchia, C., Lucchini, F., Negri, E. & Boyle, P. (1995) Patterns of childhood cancer mortality: America, Asia and Oceania. *Eur. J. Cancer*, **31A**, 771–782

Li, F.P. & Fraumeni, J.F. (1969) Rhabdomyosarcoma in children: epidemiologic study and identification of a familial cancer syndrome. *J. Natl. Cancer Inst.*, **43**, 1365–1373

Li, F.P., Tu, J., Liu, F. & Shiang, E.L. (1980) Rarity of Ewing's sarcoma in China. *Lancet*, **i**, 1255

Li, F.P., Williams, W.R., Gimbrere, K., Flamant, F., Green, D.M. & Meadows, A.T. (1988) Heritable fraction of unilateral Wilms tumor. *Pediatrics*, **81**, 147–149

Lilly, F., Boyse, E.A. & Old, L.J. (1964) Genetic basis of susceptibility to viral leukaemogenesis. *Lancet*, **ii**, 1207–1209

Lin, R.S. & Lu, P.Y. (1989) *An Epidemiologic Study of Childhood Cancer in Relation to Residential Exposure to Electromagnetic Fields*. Paper presented at DOE/EPRI Annual Review of Research on Biological Effects of 50/60 Hz Electrical and Magnetic Fields (cited by Gordon, I., *et al.*, 1990, Epidemiological studies of cancer and powerline frequency electromagnetic fields: a meta-analysis. University of Melbourne Statistical Consulting Centre Report No. 242)

Lin, R.S., Dischinger, P.C., Conde, J. & Farrell, K.P. (1985) Occupational exposure to electromagnetic fields and the occurrence of brain tumors. An analysis of possible associations. *J. Occup. Med.*, **6**, 413–419

Lindblad, P., Zack, M., Adami, H.O. & Ericson, A. (1992) Maternal and perinatal risk factors for Wilms' tumor: a nationwide nested case–control study in Sweden. *Int. J. Cancer*, **51**, 38–41

Linet, M.S. (1985) *The Leukemias: Epidemiologic Aspects*, New York, Oxford University Press

Linet, M.S. & Devesa, S.S. (1991) Descriptive epidemiology of childhood leukaemia. *Br. J. Cancer*, **63**, 424–429

Linet, M.S., Stewart, W.F., Van Natta, M.L., McCaffrey, L.D. & Szklo, M. (1987) Comparison of methods for determining occupational exposure in a case–control interview study of chronic lymphocytic leukemia. *J. Occup. Med.*, **29**, 136–141

Linet, M.S., Gridley, G., Cnattingius, S., Nicholson, H.S., Martinsson, U., Glimelius, B., Adami, H.O. & Zack, M. (1996) Maternal and perinatal risk factors for childhood brain tumors (Sweden). *Cancer Causes Control*, **7**, 437–448

Linet, M.S., Hatch, E.E., Kleinerman, R.A., Robison, L.L., Kaune, W.T., Friedman, D.R., Severson, R.K., Haines, C.M., Hartsock, C.T., Niwa, S., Wacholder, S. & Tarone, R.E. (1997) Residential exposure to magnetic fields and acute lymphoblastic leukemia in children. *New Engl. J. Med.*, **337**, 1–7

Little, J. (1992) Ascertainment, registration and assessment of exposure. In: Elwood, J.M., Little, J. & Elwood, J.H., eds, *Epidemiology and Control of Neural Tube Defects*, Oxford, Oxford University Press, pp. 37–95

Little, M.P. (1993) A comparison of the risks of leukaemia in the offspring of the Japanese bomb survivors and those of the Sellafield workforce with those in the offspring of the Ontario and Scottish workforces. *J. Radiol. Prot.*, **13**, 161–175

Little, J. (1995) Is folic acid pluripotent? A review of the associations with congenital anomalies, cancer and other diseases. In: Ioannides, C., ed., *Drugs, Diet and Disease*, Volume 1. *Mechanistic Approaches to Cancer*, New York, Ellis Horwood, pp. 262–308

Little, J. & Elwood, J.M. (1992a) Clustering in time and space. In: Elwood, J.M., Little, J. & Elwood, J.H., eds, *Epidemiology and Control of Neural Tube Defects*, Oxford, Oxford University Press, pp. 247–305

Little, J. & Elwood, J.M. (1992b) Geographical variation. In: Elwood, J.M., Little, J. & Elwood, J.H., eds, *Epidemiology and Control of Neural Tube Defects*, Oxford, Oxford University Press, pp. 96–145

Little, J. & Nicoll, A. (1988) The epidemiology and service implications of congenital and constitutional anomalies in ethnic minorities in the United Kingdom. *Paediat. Perinatal Epidemiol.*, **2**, 161–184

Little, M.P., Wakeford, R. & Charles, M.W. (1994) A comparison of the risks of leukaemia in the offspring of the Sellafield workforce born in Seascale and those born elsewhere in West Cumbria with the risks in the offspring of the Ontario and Scottish workforces and the Japanese bomb survivors. *J. Radiol. Prot.*, **14**, 187–201

Little, J., Fishbein, L., Shuker, D.E.G. & Vainio, H. (1995) Teratogenicity of pharmaceutical agents established as having carcinogenic effects: review of effects and mechanisms. In: Ioannides, C., ed., *Drugs, Diet and Disease*, Volume 1. *Mechanistic Approaches to Cancer*, New York, Ellis Horwood, pp 98–149

Little, M.P., Wakeford, R., Charles, M.W. & Andersson, M. (1996) A comparison of the risks of leukaemia and non-Hodgkin's lymphoma in the first generation offspring ($F_1$) of the Danish Thorotrast patients with those observed in other studies of parental pre-conception irradiation. *J. Radiol. Prot.*, **16**, 25–36

Lock, S.P. & Merrington, M. (1967) Leukaemia in Lewisham (1957–63). *Br. Med. J.*, **3**, 759–760

London, S.J., Thomas, D.C., Bowman, J.D., Sobel, E., Cheng, T.C. & Peters, J.M. (1991) Exposure to residential electric and magnetic fields and risk of childhood leukemia. *Am. J. Epidemiol.*, **134**, 923–937

Love, R.R., Evans, A.M. & Josten, D.M. (1985) The accuracy of patient reports of a family history of cancer. *J. Chronic Diseases*, **38**, 289–293

Lowengart, R.A., Peters, J.M., Cicioni, C., Buckley, J., Bernstein, L., Preston-Martin, S. & Rappaport, E. (1987) Childhood leukemia and parents' occupational and home exposures. *J. Natl. Cancer Inst.*, **79**, 39–46

Lowenthal, R.M., Panton, J.B., Baikie, M.J. & Lickiss, J.N. (1991) Exposure to high tension power lines and childhood leukaemia: a pilot study. *Med. J. Aust.*, **155**, 347

Lucas, S.B. & Fischer, P.R. (1990) No neuroblastoma in Zaire. *Lancet*, **335**, 115

Lucie, N.P. (1991) Radon and acute lymphoblastic leukaemia. *Leuk. Lymph.*, **3**, 213–216

Lustbader, E.D., Williams, W.R., Bondy, M.L., Strom, S. & Strong, L.C. (1992) Segregation analysis of cancer in families of childhood soft-tissue-sarcoma patients. *Am. J. Hum. Genet.*, **51**, 344–356

Lyon, J.L., Klauber, M.R., Gardner, J.W. & Udall, K.S. (1979) Childhood leukemias associated with fallout from nuclear testing. *New Engl. J. Med.* **300**, 397–402

Lyons, R.A., Monaghan, S.P., Heaven, M., Littlepage, B.N.C., Vincent, T.J. & Draper, G.J. (1995) Incidence of leukaemia and lymphoma in young people in the vicinity of the petrochemical plant at Baglan Bay, South Wales, 1974 to 1991. *Occup. and Environ. Med.*, **52**, 225–228

MacDougall, L.G., Jankowitz, P., Cohn, R. & Bernstein, R. (1986) Acute childhood leukemia in Johannesburg. Ethnic differences in incidence, cell type and survival. *Am. J. Pediat. Hematol. Oncol.*, **8**, 43–51

Macfarlane, G.J., Evstifeeva, T., Boyle, P. & Grufferman, S. (1995) International patterns in the occurrence of Hodgkin's disease in children and young adult males. *Int. J. Cancer*, **61**, 165–169

Machado, S.G., Land, C.E. & McKay, F.W. (1987) Cancer mortality and radioactive fallout in Southwestern Utah. *Am. J. Epidemiol.*, **125**, 44–61

Macintyre, S. (1986) The patterning of health by social position in contemporary Britain: directions for sociological research. *Soc. Sci. Med.*, **23**, 393–415

MacMahon, B. (1962) Prenatal X-ray exposure and childhood cancer. *J. Natl. Cancer Inst.*, **28**, 1173–1191

MacMahon, B. (1972) Susceptibility to radiation-induced leukemia. *New Engl. J. Med.*, **287**, 144–145

MacMahon, B. (1981) More on Bendectin. *J. Am. Med. Assoc.*, **246**, 371–372

MacMahon, B. (1985) Prenatal X-ray exposure and twins. *New Engl. J. Med.*, **312**, 576–577

MacMahon, B. (1992a) Leukemia clusters around nuclear facilities in Britain. *Cancer Causes Control* **3**, 283–288

MacMahon, B. (1992b) Is acute lymphoblastic leukemia in children virus-related? *Am. J. Epidemiol.*, **136**, 916–924

MacMahon, B. & Levy, M.A. (1964) Prenatal origin of childhood leukemia. Evidence from twins. *New Engl. J. Med.*, **270**, 1082–1085

MacMahon, B. & Newill, V.A. (1962) Birth characteristics of children dying of malignant neoplasms. *J. Natl. Cancer Inst.*, **28**, 231–244

MacSween, J.M., Fernandez, L.A., Eastwood, S.L. & Pyesmany, A.F. (1980) Restricted genetic heterogeneity in families of patients with acute lymphocytic leukemia. *Tissue Antigens*, **16**, 70–72

Magee, P.N., Montesano, R. & Preussmann, R. (1976) N-nitroso compounds and related carcinogens. In: Searle, C.E., ed., *Chemical Carcinogens* (ACS Monograph No. 173), Washington DC, American Chemical Society, pp. 491–625

Magnani, C., Pastore, G., Luzzatto, L., Carli, M., Lubrano, P. & Terracini, B. (1989) Risk factors for soft tissue sarcomas in childhood: a case-control study. *Tumori*, **75**, 396–400

Magnani, C., Pastore, G., Luzzatto, L. & Terracini, B. (1990) Parental occupation and other environmental factors in the etiology of leukemias and non-Hodgkin's lymphomas in childhood: a case–control study. *Tumori*, **76**, 413–419

Magnani, C., Terracini, B., Cordero De Montezemolo, L., Gallone, G., Luzzatto, L., Mosso, M.L., Pastore, G. & Rosso, P. (1996) Incidence of second primary malignancies after a malignant tumor in childhood: A population-based survey in Piedmont (Italy). *Int. J. Cancer*, **67**, 6–10

Mainwaring, D. (1966) Epidemiology of acute leukaemia of childhood in the Liverpool area. *Br. J. Prev. Soc. Med.*, **20**, 189–194

Makata, A.M., Toriyama, K., Kamidigo, N.O., Eto, H. & Itakura, H. (1996) The pattern of pediatric solid malignant tumors in Western Kenya, East Africa, 1979–1994: an analysis based on histopathologic study. *Am. J. Trop. Med. Hyg.*, **54**, 343–347

Malamud, D. (1992) Saliva as a diagnostic fluid. Second now to blood? *Br. Med. J.*, **305**, 207–208

Malkin, D. (1994) p53 and Li–Fraumeni syndrome. *Biochim. Biophys. Acta*, **1198**, 197–213

Malkin, D. (1997) Cancers of childhood. In: DeVita, V.T., Jr, Hellman, S. & Rosenberg, S.A., eds, *Cancer: Principles and Practice of Oncology*, fifth edition, New York, Lippincott-Raven, pp. 2083–2091

Malkin, D., Li, F.P., Strong, L.C., Fraumeni, J.F., Jr, Nelson, C.E., Kim, D.H., Kassel, J., Gryka, M.A., Bischoff, F.Z., Tainsky, M.A. & Friend, S.H. (1990) Germ line p53 mutations in a familial syndrome of breast cancer, sarcomas, and other neoplasms. *Science*, **250**, 1233–1238

Malone, G.E., Roseman, J., Crist, W.M. & Acton, R.T. (1983) A review of evidence that the feline leukemia virus (FeLV) might be causative in childhood acute lymphocytic leukemia (ALL). In: Humphrey, G.B., Grindey, G.B. & Dehner, L.P., eds, *Adrenal and Endocrine Tumors in Children*, Boston, Martinus Nijhoff, pp. 45–65

Malvy, D.J.M., Burtschy, B., Arnaud, J., Sommelet, D., Leverger, G., Dostalova, L., Drucker, J. & Amedee-Manesme, O. (1993) Serum beta-carotene and antioxidant micronutrients in children with cancer. *Int. J. Epidemiol.*, **22**, 761–771

Mangano, J.J. (1997) Childhood leukaemia in US may have risen due to fallout from Chernobyl. *Br. Med. J.*, **314**, 1200

Mangino, M.M., Scanlan, R.A. & O'Brien, T.J. (1981) N-Nitrosamines in beer. In: Scanlan, R.A. & Tannenbaum, S.R., eds, *N-Nitroso Compounds*. Washington, DC, American Chemical Society, pp. 229–245

Mangoud, A., Hillier, V.F., Leck, I. & Thomas, R.W. (1985) Space-time interaction in Hodgkin's disease in Greater Manchester. *J. Epidemiol. Commun. Health*, **39**, 58–62

Mann, J.R. & Stiller, C.A. (1994) Changing pattern of incidence and survival in children with germ cell tumours (GCTs). *Adv. Biosci.*, **91**, 59–64

Mann, J.R., Dodd, H.E., Draper, G.J., Waterhouse, J.A.H., Birch, J.M., Cartwright, R.A., Hartley, A.L., McKinney, P.A. & Stiller, C.A. (1993) Congenital abnormalities in children with cancer and their relatives: results from a case–control study (IRESCC*). *Br. J. Cancer*, **68**, 357–363

Manning, M.D. & Carroll, B.E. (1957) Some epidemiological aspects of leukemia in children. *J. Natl. Cancer Inst.*, **19**, 1087–1094

Mantel, N. (1967) The detection of disease clustering and a generalized regression approach. *Cancer Res.*, **27**, 209–220

Marsden, H.B. (1988) The classification of childhood cancer. In: Parkin, D.M., Stiller, C.A., Draper, G.J., Bieber, C.A., Terracini, B. & Young, J.L., eds, *International Incidence of Childhood Cancer* (IARC Scientific Publications No. 87), Lyon, IARC, pp. 9–16

Marsden, H.B. & Steward, J.K. (1968) Tumours of the sympathetic system. In: *Tumours in Children (Recent Results in Cancer Research*, No. 13), Berlin, Springer, pp. 131–170

Martin, C.J. (1987) Monitoring maternity services by postal questionnaire: congruity between mothers' reports and their obstetric records. *Stat. Med.*, **6**, 613–627

Martos, M.C., Winther, J.F. & Olsen, J.H. (1993) Cancer among teenagers in Denmark, 1943–1987. *Int. J. Cancer*, **55**, 57–62

Maskarinec, G., Cooper, J. & Swygert, L. (1994) Investigation of increased incidence in childhood leukaemia near radio towers in Hawaii: preliminary observations. *J. Environ. Pathol. Toxicol. Oncol.*, **13**, 33–37

Massabi, M., Muaka, B.K. & Tamba, N. (1989) Epidemiology of childhood cancer in Zaire. *Lancet*, **ii**, 501

Mathieson, G. (1975) Pathologic aspects of epilepsy with special reference to the surgical pathology of focal cerebral seizures. *Adv. Neurol.*, **8**, 107–138

Mathur, G.P., Gupta, N., Mathur, S., Gupta, V., Pradhan, S., Dwivedi, J.N., Tripathi, B.N., Kushwaha, K.P., Sathy, N., Modi, U.J., Shendurnikar, N. & Mishra, P.K. (1993) Breastfeeding and childhood cancer. *Indian Pediat.*, **30**, 651–657

Matsui, I., Tanimura, M., Kobayashi, N., Sawada, T., Nagahara, N. & Akatsuka, J. (1993) Neurofibromatosis type 1 and childhood cancer. *Cancer*, **72**, 2746–2754

Matsunaga, E. (1981) Genetics of Wilms' tumor. *Human Genet.*, **57**, 231–246

Matsunaga, E., Minoda, K. & Sasaki, M.S. (1990) Parental age and seasonal variation in the births of children with sporadic retinoblastoma: a mutation-epidemiologic study. *Hum. Genet.*, **84**, 155–158

McCrea Curnen, M.G., Varma, A.A.O. & Christine, B.W. (1974) Childhood leukemia and maternal infectious diseases during pregnancy. *J. Natl. Cancer Inst.*, **53**, 943–947

McCredie, M., Høyer, A., Coates, M. & Tayor, R. (1992) *Trends in Cancer Incidence and Mortality in New South Wales 1972–1989*, New South Wales Central Cancer Registry, pp. 98–101

McCredie, M., Maisonneuve, P. & Boyle, P. (1994a) Antenatal risk factors for malignant brain tumours in New South Wales children. *Int. J. Cancer*, **56**, 6–10

McCredie, M., Maisonneuve, P. & Boyle, P. (1994b) Perinatal and early postnatal risk factors for malignant brain tumours in New South Wales children. *Int. J. Cancer*, **56**, 11–15

McDiarmid, M.A. & Weaver, V. (1993) Fouling one's own nest revisited. *Am. J. Ind. Med.*, **24**, 1–9

McDowall, M.E. (1985) Childhood kidney cancer and father's occupation. In: McDowall, M.E., *Occupational Reproductive Epidemiology. The Use of Routinely Collected Statistics in England and Wales 1980–82* (Studies on Medical and Population Subjects No. 50), London, HMSO, pp. 68–69

McIntyre, J.F., Smith-Sorensen, B., Friend, S.H., Kassell, J., Borresen, A.L., Yan, Y.X., Russo, C., Sato, J., Barbier, N., Miser, J., Malkin, D. & Gebhardt, M.C. (1994) Germline mutations of the p53 tumor suppressor gene in children with osteosarcoma. *J. Clin. Oncol.*, **12**, 925–930

McKinney, P.A. & Stiller, C.A. (1986) Maternal smoking during pregnancy and the risk of childhood cancer (letter). *Lancet*, **ii**, 519

McKinney, P.A., Cartwright, R.A., Stiller, C.A., Hopton, P.A., Mann, J.R., Birch, J.M., Hartley, A.L., Waterhouse, J.A. & Johnston, H.E. (1985) Inter-Regional Epidemiological Study of Childhood Cancer (IRESCC): Childhood cancer and the consumption of Debendox and related drugs in pregnancy. *Br. J. Cancer*, **52**, 923–929

McKinney, P.A., Cartwright, R.A., Saiu, J.M., Mann, J.R., Stiller, C.A., Draper, G.J., Hartley, A.L., Hopton, P.A., Birch, J.M., Waterhouse, J.A. & Johnston, H.E. (1987) The Inter-Regional Epidemiological Study of Childhood Cancer (IRESCC): a case-control study of aetiological factors in leukaemia and lymphoma. *Arch. Dis. Child.*, **62**, 279–287

McKinney, P.A., Alexander, F.E., Cartwright, R.A. & Parker, L. (1991) Parental occupations of children with leukaemia in west Cumbria, north Humberside, and Gateshead. *Br. Med. J.*, **302**, 681–687

McKinney, P.A., Ironside, J.W., Harkness, E.F., Arango, J.C., Doyle, D. & Black, R.J. (1994) Registration quality and descriptive epidemiology of childhood brain tumours in Scotland 1975–90. *Br. J. Cancer*, **70**, 973–979

McLaughlin, J.R., Anderson, T.W., Clarke, E.A. & King, W. (1992) *Occupational Exposure of Fathers to Ionizing Radiation and the Risk of Leukaemia in Offspring – a Case-Control Study* (AECB Project No. 7. 157. 1). A research report prepared for the Atomic Energy Control Board, Ottawa, Canada

McLaughlin, J.R., Clarke, E.A., Nishri, E.D. & Anderson, T.W. (1993a) Childhood leukemia in the vicinity of Canadian nuclear facilities. *Cancer Causes Control*, **4**, 51–58

McLaughlin, J.R., King, W.D., Anderson, T.W., Clarke, E.A. & Ashmore, J.P. (1993b) Paternal radiation exposure and leukaemia in offspring: the Ontario case–control study. *Br. Med. J.*, **307**, 959–966

McLaughlin, J.R., Kreiger, N., Sloan, M.P., Benson, L.N., Hilditch, S. & Clarke, E.A. (1993c) An historical cohort study of cardiac catheterization during childhood and the risk of cancer. *Int. J. Epidemiol.*, **22**, 584–591

McWhirter, W.R. (1982) The relationship of incidence of childhood lymphoblastic leukaemia to social class. *Br. J. Cancer*, **46**, 640–645

McWhirter, W.R. & Petroeschevsky, A.L. (1991) Incidence trends in childhood cancer in Queensland, 1973–1988. *Med. J. Aust.*, **154**, 453–455

McWhirter, W.R., McWhirter, K.M. & Taylor, D. (1983) Height and lymphoblastic leukaemia. *Arch. Dis. Child.*, **58**, 839

McWhirter, W.R., Dobson, C. & Ring, I. (1996) Childhood cancer incidence in Australia, 1982–1991. *Int. J. Cancer*, **65**, 34–38

Meadows, A.T., D'Angio, G.J., Miké, V., Banfi, A., Harris, C., Jenkin, R.D. & Schwartz, A. (1977) Patterns of second malignant neoplasms in children. *Cancer*, **40**, 1903–1911

Meadows, A.T., Baum, E., Fossati-Bellani, F., Green, D., Jenkin, R.D., Marsden, B., Nesbit, M., Newton, W., Oberlin, O., Sallan, S.G., Siegel, S., Strong, L.C. & Voute, P.A. (1985) Second malignant neoplasms in children: an update from the Late Effects Study Group. *J. Clin. Oncol.*, **3**, 532–538

Medical Research Council. (1972) BCG and vole bacillus vaccines in the prevention of tuberculosis in adolescence and early adult life. *Bull. WHO*, **46**, 371–385

Meighan, S.S. & Knox, G. (1965) Leukemia in childhood. Epidemiology in Oregon. *Cancer*, **18**, 811–814

Meinert, R., Kaatsch, P., Kaletsch, U., Krummenauer, F., Miesner, A. & Michaelis, J. (1996) Childhood leukaemia and exposure to pesticides: Results of a case–control study in northern Germany. *Eur. J. Cancer*, **32A**, 1943–1948

Memon, A. & Doll, R. (1994) A search for unknown blood-borne oncogenic viruses. *Int. J. Cancer*, **58**, 366–368

Mettler, F.A., Jr, Williamson, M.R., Royal, H.D., Hurley, J.R., Khafagi, F., Sheppard, M.C., Beral, V., Reeves, G., Saenger, E.L., Yokoyama, N., Parshin, V., Griaznova, E.A., Taranenko, M., Chesin, V. & Cheban, A. (1992) Thyroid nodules in the population living around Chernobyl. *J. Am. Med. Assoc.*, **268**, 616–619

Méhes, K., Signer, E., Plüss, H.J., Müller, H.J. & Stalder, G. (1985) Increased prevalence of minor anomalies in childhood malignancy. *Eur. J. Pediat.*, **144**, 243–249

Michaelis, J., Keller, B., Haaf, G. & Kaatch, P. (1992) Incidence of childhood malignancies in the vicinity of West German nuclear power plants. *Cancer Causes Control*, **3**, 255–263

Michaelis, J., Kaatsch, P. & Zöllner, I. (1994) Querschnittsuntersuchung zur Häufigkeit von Krebserkrankungen bei Kindern von beruflich strahlenex-ponierten Beschäftigten in westdeutschen kerntechnischen Anlagen. *Arbeitsmed. Sozialmed. Umweltmed.*, **29**, 324–330, 335

Michaelis, J., Haaf, H.G., Zollner, J., Kaatsch, P., Krummenauer, F. & Berthold, F. (1996) Case control study of neuroblastoma in west Germany after the Chernobyl accident. *Klinische Pädiatrie*, **208**, 172–178

Michaelis, J., Kaletsch, U., Burkart, W. & Grosche, B. (1997a) Infant leukaemia after the Chernobyl accident. *Nature*, **387**, 246

Michaelis, J., Schüz, J., Meinert, R., Menger, M., Grigat, J.P., Kaatsch, P., Kaletsch, U., Miesner, A., Stamm, A., Brinkmann, K. & Kärner, H. (1997b) Childhood leukemia and electromagnetic fields: results of a population-based case-control study in Germany. *Cancer Causes Control*, **8**, 167–174

Michalek, A.M., Buck, G.M., Nasca, P.C., Freedman, A.N., Baptise, M.S. & Mahoney, M.C. (1996) Gravid health status, medication use and risk of neuroblastoma. *Am. J. Epidemiol.*, **143**, 996–1001

Middleton, B., Byers, T., Marshall, J. & Graham, S. (1986) Dietary vitamin A and cancer – a multisite case–control study. *Nutr. Cancer*, **8**, 107–116

Mili, F., Khoury, M.J., Flanders, W.D. & Greenberg, R.S. (1993a) Risk of childhood cancer for infants with birth defects. I. A record-linkage study, Atlanta, Georgia, 1968–1988. *Am. J. Epidemiol.*, **137**, 629–638

Mili, F., Lynch, C.F., Khoury, M.J., Flanders, W.D. & Edmonds, L.D. (1993b) Risk of childhood cancer for infants with birth defects. II. A record-linkage study, Iowa, 1983–1989. *Am. J. Epidemiol.*, **137**, 639–644

Miller, R.W. (1963) Down's syndrome (mongolism), other congenital malformations and cancers among the sibs of leukemic children. *New Engl. J. Med.*, **268**, 393–401

Miller, R.W. (1966) Medical progress. Relation between cancer and congenital defects in man. *New Engl. J. Med.*, **275**, 87–93

Miller, R.W. (1968) Deaths from childhood cancer in sibs. *New Engl. J. Med.*, **279**, 122–126

Miller, R.W. (1971) Deaths from childhood leukemia and solid tumors among twins and other sibs in the United States, 1960–67. *J. Natl. Cancer Inst.*, **46**, 203–209

Miller, R.W. (1981) Contrasting epidemiology of childhood osteosarcoma, Ewing's tumor and rhabdomyosarcoma. *NCI Monogr.*, **56**, 9–14

Miller, R.W. (1989) No neuroblastoma in Zaire. *Lancet*, **ii**, 978–979

Miller, G. (1990) Epstein-Barr virus. Biology, pathogenesis and medical aspects. In: Fields, B.N. & Knipe, D.M., eds, *Virology*, 2nd edition, volume 2, New York, Raven Press, pp. 1921–1957

Miller, R.W. (1992) Childhood leukemia and neonatal exposure to lighting in nurseries. *Cancer Causes Control* 3, 581–582

Miller, R.W. & Rubinstein, J.H. (1995) Tumors in Rubinstein-Taybi syndrome. *Am. J. Med. Genet.*, **56**, 112–115

Miller, R.W., Fraumeni, J.F. & Manning, M.D. (1964) Association of Wilms' tumor with aniridia, hemihypertrophy and other congenital malformations. *New Engl. J. Med.*, **270**, 922–927

Miller, R.W., Fraumeni, J.F. & Hill, J.A. (1968) Neuroblastoma: epidemiologic approach to its origin. *Am. J. Dis. Child.*, **115**, 253–261

Miller, R.W., Young, J.L., Jr & Novakovic, B. (1995) Childhood cancer. *Cancer*, **75**, 395–405

Mills, A.E. (1979) Acute leukaemia in Bulawayo – experience with the FAB classification. *Cent. Afric. J. Med.*, **25**, 239

Mitchell, A.A., Cottler, L.B. & Shap[ ] questionnaire design on recall [ ] pregnancy. *Am. J. Epidemiol.*, **123**, 6[ ]

Mole, R.H. (1974) Antenatal irrad[ ] cancer: causation or coincidence? *B[ ]*

Mole, R.H. (1990a) Radon and leukae[ ]

Mole, R.H. (1990b) Childhood cancer [ ] to diagnostic X-ray examinations i[ ] 62, 152–168

Mole, R.H. (1991) Radiation from Ch[ ] leukemia. *Leukemia*, 5, 443–444

Moll, A.C., Imhof, S.M., Bouter, L.M.[ ] W., Bezemer, P.D., Koten, J.W. & [ ] Second primary tumors in pati[ ] retinoblastoma: A register-base[ ] 1945–1994. *Int. J. Cancer*, **67**, 515–519

Monaghan, H.P., Kratchik, B.R., MacGregor, D.L. & Fitz, C.R. (1981) Tuberous sclerosis complex in children. *Am. J. Dis. Child.*, **135**, 912–917

Monson, R.R. & MacMahon, B. (1984) Prenatal X-ray exposure and cancer in children. In: Boice, J.D., Jr & Fraumeni, J.F., Jr, eds, *Radiation Carcinogenesis: Epidemiology and Biological Significance*, New York, Raven Press, pp. 97–105

Morris, V. (1990) Space-time interactions in childhood cancers. *J. Epidemiol. Commun. Health*, **44**, 55–58

Morris, J.A., Butler, R., Flowerdew, R. & Gatrell, A.C. (1993a) Retinoblastoma in children of former residents of Seascale. *Br. Med. J.*, **306**, 650

Morris, J.A., Cowell, J.K. & Stiller, C.A. (1993b) Retinoblastoma: a possible link with low level radiation. *J. Med. Genet.*, **30**, 400–442

Morrow, R.H., Jr. (1985) Epidemiological evidence for the role of falciparum malaria in the pathogenesis of Burkitt's lymphoma. In: Lenoir, G., O'Conor, G. & Olweny, C.L.M., eds, *Burkitt's Lymphoma: a Human Cancer Model* (IARC Scientific Publications No. 60), Lyon, IARC, pp. 177–186

Morrow, R.H., Kisuule, A., Pike, M.C. & Smith, P.G. (1976) Burkitt's lymphoma in the Mengo districts of Uganda: epidemiologic features and their relationship to malaria. *J. Natl. Cancer Inst.*, **56**, 479–483

Morrow, R.H., Pike, M. & Smith, P.G. (1977) Further studies of space-time clustering of Burkitt's lymphoma in Uganda. *Br. J. Cancer*, **35**, 668–673

Moss, D.J., Burrows, S.R., Castelino, D.J., Kane, R.G., Pope, J.H., Rickinson, A.B., Alpers, M.P. & Heywood, P.F. (1983) A comparison of Epstein–Barr virus-specific T-cell immunity in malaria-endemic and -nonendemic regions of Papua New Guinea. *Int. J. Cancer*, **31**, 727–732

Mosso, M.L., Colombo, R., Giordano, L., Pastore, G., Terracini, B. & Magnani, C. (1992) Childhood Cancer Registry of the Province of Torino, Italy. *Cancer*, **69**, 1300–1306

Moutou, C., Hochez, J., Chompret, A., Tournade, M.F., Le Bihan, C., Zucker, J.M., Lemerle, J. & Bonaïti-Pellié, C. (1994) The French Wilms' tumour study: no clear evidence for cancer prone families. *J. Med. Genet.*, **31**, 429–434

MRC Vitamin Study Research Group (1991) Prevention of neural tube defects: results of the Medical Research Council Vitamin Study. *Lancet*, **338**, 131–137

Muir, C., Waterhouse, J., Mack, T., Powell, J., Whelan, S., Smans, M. & Casset, F. (1987) *Cancer Incidence in Five Continents*, Volume V (IARC Scientific Publications No. 88), Lyon, IARC

Muir, K.R., Huddart, S.N., Barrantes, J., Parkes, S.E. & Mann, J.R. (1990a) Relative occurrence of neuroblastoma and Wilms' tumour in ethnic subgroups in the West Midlands Health Authority Region. *Arch. Dis. Child.*, **65**, 1380

Muir, K.R., Parkes, S.E., Mann, J.R., Stevens, M.C.G., Cameron, A.H., Raafat, F., Darbyshire, P.J., Ingram, D.R., Davis, A. & Gascoigne, D. (1990b) 'Clustering' – real or apparent?: Probability maps of childhood cancer in the West Midlands Health Authority region. *Int. J. Epidemiol.*, **19**, 853–859

Muir, K.R., Parkes, S.E., Mann, J.R., Stevens, M.C.G. & Cameron, A.H. (1992) Childhood cancer in the West Midlands: Incidence and survival, 1980–1984, in a multi-ethnic population. *Clin. Oncol.*, **4**, 177–182

Muir, K.R., Parkes, S.E., Lawson, S., Thomas, A.K., Cameron, A.H. & Mann, J.R. (1995) Changing incidence and geographical distribution of malignant paediatric germ cell tumours in the West Midlands Health Authority Region, 1957–92. *Br. J. Cancer*, **72**, 219–223

Muirhead, C.R. (1995) Childhood leukemia in metropolitan regions in the United States: a possible relation to population density? *Cancer Causes Control*, **6**, 383–388

Muirhead, C.R., Butland, B.K., Green, B.M.R. & Draper, G.J. (1991) Childhood leukaemia and natural radiation. *Lancet*, **337**, 503–504

Muirhead, C.R., Butland, B.K., Green, B.M.R. & Draper, G.J. (1992) An analysis of childhood leukaemia and natural radiation in Britain. *Radiat. Protect. Dosim.*, **45**, 657–660

Mukiibi, J.M., Banda, L., Liomba, N.G., Sungani, F.C.M. & Parkin, D.M. (1995) Spectrum of childhood cancers in Malawi 1985–1993. *East Afric. Med. J.*, **72**, 25–29

Mulder, Y.M., Drijver, M. & Kreis, I.A. (1993) Patiënt-controle-onderzoek naar het verband tussen lokale milieufactoren en hematopoëtische maligniteiten bij jongeren in Aalsmeer. *Ned. Tijdschr. Geneeskd.*, **137**, 663–667

Mulder, Y.M., Drijver, M. & Kreis, I.A. (1994) Case-control study on the association between a cluster of childhood haematopoietic malignancies and local environmental factors in Aalsmeer, The Netherlands. *J. Epidemiol. Commun. Health*, **48**, 161–165

Mulvihill, M.J., Myers, M.H., Connelly, R.R., Byrne, J., Austin, D.F., Bragg, K., Cook, J.W., Hassinger, D.D., Holmes, F.F., Holmes, G.F., Krauss, M.R., Latourette, H.B., Meigs, J.W., Naughton, M.D., Steinhorn, S.C., Strong, L.C., Teta, M.J. & Weyer, P.J. (1987) Cancer in offspring of long-term survivors of childhood and adolescent cancer. *Lancet*, **ii**, 813–817

Munier, F., Spence, M.A., Pescia, G., Balmer, A., Gailloud, C., Thonney, F., van Melle, G. & Turz, H.P. (1992) Paternal selection favoring mutant alleles of the retinoblastoma susceptibility gene. *Hum. Genet.*, **89**, 508–512

Muñoz, N. & Bosch, F.X. (1987) Epidemiology of hepatocellular carcinoma. In: Okuda, K. & Purchase, I.F., eds, *Neoplasms of the Liver*, Tokyo, Springer, pp. 3–19

Murray, R., Heckel, P. & Hempelmann, L.H. (1959) Leukemia in children exposed to ionizing radiation. *New Engl. J. Med.*, **261**, 585–589

Myers, A., Cartwright, R.A., Bonnell, J.A., Male, J.C. & Cartwright, S.C. (1985) *Overhead Power Lines and Childhood Cancer. International Conference on Electric and Magnetic Fields in Medicine and Biology*, London, IEE Conference Publications, p. 257

Myers, A., Clayden, A.D., Cartwright, R.A. & Cartwright, S.C. (1990) Childhood cancer and overhead powerlines: a case–control study. *Br. J. Cancer*, **62**, 1008–1014

Myrianthopoulos, N.C. & Chung, C.S. (1974) Congenital malformations in singletons: epidemiologic survey. In: Bergsma, D., ed., *Birth Defects* (Orig. Art. Ser. X (11)), New York, Stratton, pp. 1–21

Nakissa, N., Constine, L.S., Rubin, P. & Strohl, R. (1985) Birth defects in three common pediatric malignancies; Wilms' tumor, neuroblastoma and Ewing's sarcoma. *Oncology, 42*, 358–363

Nambi, K.S.V., Mayya, Y.S., Rao, D.D. & Soman, S.D. (1992) A study on cancer mortality in Traput-based atomic energy community. *Arch. Environ. Health, 47*, 155–157

Nandakumar, A., Anantha, N., Appaji, L., Swamy, K., Mukherjee, G., Venugopal, T., Reddy, S. & Dhar, M. (1996) Descriptive epidemiology of childhood cancers in Bangalore, India. *Cancer Causes Control, 7*, 405–410

Narod, S.A. (1990) Radiation, genetics and childhood leukaemia. *Eur. J. Cancer, 26*, 661–664

Narod, S.A. & Lenoir, G.M. (1991) Are bilateral tumours hereditary? *Int. J. Epidemiol., 20*, 346–348

Narod, S.A., Stiller, C. & Lenoir, G.M. (1991) An estimate of the heritable fraction of childhood cancer. *Br. J. Cancer, 63*, 993–999

Narod, S.A., Hawkins, M.M., Robertson, C.M. & Stiller, C.A. (1997) Congenital anomalies and childhood cancer in Great Britain. *Am. J. Human Genet., 60*, 474–485

Nasca, P.C., Baptiste, M.S., MacCubbin, P.A., Metzger, B.B., Carlton, K., Greenwald, P., Armbrustmacher, V.W., Earle, K.M. & Waldman, J. (1988) An epidemiologic case–control study of central nervous system tumors in children and parental occupational exposures. *Am. J. Epidemiol., 128*, 1256–1265

Nass, C.C. (1989) *Parental Occupational Exposures and Astrocytoma in Children under Ten Years of Age in the Greater Delaware Valley.* PhD Thesis, Johns Hopkins University, Baltimore, MD

National Cancer Institute (1990) *Cancer Statistics Review, 1973–1987*, Bethesda, MD, National Institutes of Health

National Research Council Committee on Biological Effects of Ionizing Radiations (1990) *Health Effects of Exposures to Low Levels of Ionizing Radiation* (BEIR), Washington, DC, National Academy Press

Nebert, D.W. (1997) Polymorphisms in drug-metabolizing enzymes: what is their clinical relevance and why do they exist? *Am. J. Human Genet., 60*, 265–271

Neglia, J.P., Smithson, W.A., Gunderson, P., King, F.L., Singher, L.J. & Robison, L.L. (1988) Prenatal and perinatal risk factors for neuroblastoma. A case-control study. *Cancer, 61*, 2202–2206

Neglia, J.P., Meadows, A.T., Robison, L.L., Kim, T.H., Newton, W.A., Ruymann, F.B., Sather, H.N. & Hammond, G.D. (1991) Second neoplasms after acute lymphoblastic leukemia in childhood. *New Engl. J. Med., 325*, 1330–1336

Neumann, G. (1980) Zusammenhang zwischen Schutzimpfungen und bosartigen Neubildungen im Kindesalter? *Med. Klin., 75*, 72–75

Neutel, I.C. & Buck, C. (1971) Effect of smoking during pregnancy on the risk of cancer in children. *J. Natl. Cancer Inst., 47*, 59–63

NHMRC (National Health and Medical Research Council, Australian College of Paediatrics, Royal Australian College of Obstetricians & Gynaecologists. (1994) *Joint Statement and Recommendations. Vitamin K Prophylaxis for Haemorrhagic Disease in Infancy*, Canberra

Nikiforov, Y. & Gnepp, D.R. (1994) Pediatric thyroid cancer after the Chernobyl disaster. *Cancer, 74*, 748–766

Nimmagadda, R., Robb, D., Croucher, T., Thomson, D.H., Dryer, D.E. & Buehler, S.K. (1988) Atlantic Provinces, 1970–1979. In: Parkin, D.M., Stiller, C.A., Draper, G.J., Bieber, C.A., Terracini, B. & Young, J.L., eds, *International Incidence of Childhood Cancer* (IARC Scientific Publications No. 87), Lyon, IARC, pp. 73–76

Nishi, M. & Miyake, H. (1989) A case–control study of non-T cell acute lymphoblastic leukaemia of children in Hokkaido, Japan. *J. Epidemiol. Commun. Health, 43*, 352–355

Nishi, M., Miyake, H., Takeda, T. & Shimada, M. (1996) Epidemiology of childhood leukemia in Hokkaido, Japan. *Int. J. Cancer, 67*, 323–326

Noller, K.L., Decker, D.G., Lanier, A.P. & Kurland, L.T. (1972) Clear-cell adenocarcinoma of the cervix after maternal treatment with synthetic estrogens. *Mayo Clin. Proc., 47*, 629–630

Norman, M.A., Holly, E.A., Ahn, D.K., Preston-Martin, S., Mueller, B.A. & Bracci, P.M. (1996) Prenatal exposure to tobacco smoke and childhood brain tumours: results from the United States West Coast childhood brain tumor study. *Cancer Epidemiol. Biomarkers Prev., 5*, 127–133

Norris, F.D. & Jackson, E.W. (1970) Childhood cancer deaths in California-born twins. *Cancer, 25*, 212–218

Novakovic, B., Goldstein, A.M., Wexler, L.H. & Tucker, M.A. (1994) Increased risk of neuroectodermal tumors and stomach cancer in relatives of patients with Ewing's sarcoma family of tumors. *J. Natl. Cancer Inst., 86*, 1702–1706

NRPB (National Radiological Protection Board) (1984) *The Risks of Leukaemia and Other Cancers in Seascale from Radiation Exposure* (Chilton, NRPB-R171), London, HMSO

NRPB (National Radiological Protection Board) (1992) *Electromagnetic Fields and the Risk of Cancer. Report of an Advisory Group on Non-ionizing Radiation* (Documents of the NRPB, Vol 3, No. 1), Chilton, NRPB

O'Conor, G.T. (1970) Persistent immunologic stimulation as a factor in oncogenesis with special reference to Burkitt's tumor. *Am. J. Med., 48*, 279–285

O'Riordan, J., Finch, A., Lawlor, E. & McCann, S.R. (1992) Probability of finding a compatible sibling donor for bone marrow transplantation in Ireland. *Bone Marrow Transplant., 9*, 27–30

Oakley, A., Rajan, L. & Robertson, P. (1990) A comparison of different sources of information about pregnancy and childbirth. *J. Biosoc. Sci., 22*, 477–487

Obafunwa, J.O., Asagba, G.O. & Ezechukwu, C.C. (1992) Paediatric malignancies in Plateau State, Nigeria. *Cancer J., 5*, 211–215

Ogawa, O., Eccles, M.R., Szeto, J., McNoe, L.A., Yun, K., Maw, M.A., Smith, P.J. & Reeve, A.E. (1993) Relaxation of insulin-like growth factor II gene imprinting implicated in Wilms' tumour. *Nature, 362*, 749–751

Olney, J.W., Farber, N.B., Spitznagel, E. & Robins, L.N. (1996) Increasing brain tumor rates: is there a link to aspartame? *J. Neuropathol. Exper. Neurol., 55*, 1115–1123

Olsen, J.H., Winther, J. & de Nully Brown, P. (1990a) Risk of nonocular cancer in first-degree relatives of retinoblastoma patients. *Human Genet., 85*, 283–287

Olsen, J.H., Boice, J.D., Jr & Fraumeni, J.F., Jr (1990b) Cancer in children of epileptic mothers and the possible relation to maternal anticonvulsant therapy. *Br. J. Cancer, 62*, 996–999

Olsen, J.H., de Nully Brown, P., Schulgen, G. & Jensen, O.M. (1991) Parental employment at time of conception and risk of cancer in offspring. *Eur. J. Cancer, 27*, 958–965

Olsen, J.H., Garwicz, S., Hertz, H., Jonmundsson, G., Langmark, F., Lanning, M., Lie, S.O., Moe, P.J., Moller, T., Sankila, R. & Tulinius, H. (1993a) Second malignant neoplasms after cancer in childhood or adolescence. *Br. Med. J., 307*, 1030–1036

Olsen, J.H., Nielsen, A. & Schulgen, G. (1993b) Residence near high voltage facilities and risk of cancer in children. *Br. Med. J., 307*, 891–895

Olsen, J.H., Hertz, H., Blinkenberg, K. & Verder, H. (1994) Vitamin K regimens and incidence of childhood cancer in Denmark. *Br. Med. J., 308*, 895–896

Olsen, J.H., Boice, J.D., Jr, Seersholm, N., Bautz, A. & Fraumeni, J.F., Jr (1995) Cancer in the parents of children with cancer. *New Engl. J. Med., 333*, 1594–1599

Olsen, J.H., Hertz, H., Kjaer, S.K., Bautz, A., Mellemkjaer, L. & Boice, J.D., Jr (1996) Childhood leukemia following phototherapy for neonatal hyperbilirubinemia (Denmark). *Cancer Causes Control, 7*, 411–414

Olshan, A.F. (1986) Wilms' tumor, overgrowth, and fetal growth factors: a hypothesis. *Cancer Genet. Cytogenet., 21*, 303–307

Olshan, A.F., Breslow, N.E., Daling, J.R., Weiss, N.S. & Leviton, A. (1986) Childhood brain tumors and paternal occupation in the aerospace industry. *J. Natl. Cancer Inst., 77*, 17–19

Olshan, A.F., Breslow, N.E., Daling, J.R., Falletta, J.M., Grufferman, S., Robison, L.L., Waskerwitz, M. & Hammond, G.D. (1990) Wilms' tumor and paternal occupation. *Cancer Res., 50*, 3212–3217

.f., Breslow, N.E., Falletta, J.M., Grufferman, S., grass, T., Robison, L.L., Waskerwitz, M., Woods, , Vietti, T.J. & Hammond, G.D. (1993) Risk factors for .ns tumor. Report from the National Wilms Tumor udy. *Cancer, 72,* 938–944

son, J.M., Breslow, N.E. & Barce, N.E. (1993a) Cancer in twins of Wilms tumor patients. *Am. J. Med. Genet., 47,* 91–94

Olson, J.M., Breslow, N.E. & Beckwith, J.B. (1993b) Wilms' tumour and parental age: a report from the National Wilms' Tumour Study. *Br. J. Cancer, 67,* 813–818

Openshaw, S. & Craft, A. (1991) Using Geographical Analysis Machines to search for evidence of clusters and clustering in childhood leukaemia and non-Hodgkin lymphomas in Britain. In: Draper, G.J., ed., *The Geographical Epidemiology of Childhood Leukaemia and Non-Hodgkin Lymphomas in Great Britain, 1966–83* (Studies on Medical and Population Subjects No. 53), London, HMSO, pp. 109–122

Openshaw, S., Craft, A.W., Charlton, M. & Birch, J.M. (1988) Investigation of leukaemia clusters by use of a geographical analysis machine. *Lancet, i,* 272–273

Operskalski, E.A., Preston-Martin, S., Henderson, B.E. & Visscher, B.R. (1987) A case–control study of osteosarcoma in young persons. *Am. J. Epidemiol., 126,* 118–126

ORAU (Oak Ridge Associated Universities) (1992) *Health Effects of Low-Frequency Electric and Magnetic Fields. Report Prepared for the Committee on Interagency Radiation Research and Policy Coordination,* Washington, DC, US Government Printing Office

Orme, M.L.E. (1985) The Debendox saga. *Br. Med. J., 291,* 918–919

Osborne, R.H. & de George, F.V. (1964) Neoplastic diseases in twins: evidence for pre or perinatal factors conditioning cancer susceptibility. *Cancer, 17,* 1149–1154

Parker, L. & Craft, A.W. (1996) Radon and childhood cancers. *Eur. J. Cancer, 32A,* 201–204

Parker, L., Craft, A.W., Smith, J., Dickinson, H., Wakeford, R., Binks, K., McElvenny, D., Scott, L. & Slovak, A. (1993) Geographical distribution of preconceptional radiation doses to fathers employed at the Sellafield nuclear installation, West Cumbria. *Br. Med. J., 307,* 966–971

Parkes, S.E., Coad, N.A.G., Muir, K.R., Jones, T.J., Cameron, A.H. & Mann, J.R. (1994) Hodgkin's disease in children in the West Midlands, 1957–1986: A large population-based study. *Pediat. Hematol. Oncol., 11,* 471–486

Parkin, D.M., ed. (1986) *Cancer Occurrence in Developing Countries* (IARC Scientific Publications No. 75), Lyon, IARC

Parkin, D.M. (1990) The European Childhood Leukemia/Lymphoma Incidence Study. *Radiation Res., 124,* 370–371

Parkin, D.M. & Sanghvi, L.D. (1991) Cancer registration in developing countries. In: Jensen, O.M., Parkin, D.M., MacLennan, R., Muir, C.S. & Skeet, R.G., eds, *Cancer Registration: Principles and Methods* (IARC Scientific Publications No. 95), Lyon, IARC, pp. 185–198

Parkin, D.M., Sohier, R. & O'Conor, G.T. (1985) Geographic distribution of Burkitt's lymphoma. In: Lenoir, G., O'Conor, G. & Olweny, C.L.M., eds, *Burkitt's Lymphoma: a Human Cancer Model* (IARC Scientific Publications No. 60), Lyon, IARC, pp. 155–164

Parkin, D.M., Stiller, C.A., Draper, G.J., Bieber, C.A., Terracini, B. & Young, J.L., eds (1988a) *International Incidence of Childhood Cancer* (IARC Scientific Publications No. 87), Lyon, IARC

Parkin, D.M., Stiller, C.A., Draper, G.J. & Bieber, C.A. (1988b) The international incidence of childhood cancer. *Int. J. Cancer, 42,* 511–520

Parkin, M., Nectoux, J., Stiller, C. & Draper, G. (1989) L'incidence des cancers de l'enfant dans le monde. *Pédiatrie, 44,* 725–736

Parkin, D.M., Muir, C.S., Whelan, S.L., Gao, Y.T., Ferlay, J. & Powell, J. (1992) *Cancer Incidence in Five Continents,* Volume VI (IARC Scientific Publications No. 120), Lyon, IARC

Parkin, D.M., Cardis, E., Masuyer, E., Friedl, H.P., Hanslukwa, H., Bobev, D., Ivanov, E., Sinnaeve, J., Augustin, J., Plesko, I., Storm, H.H., Rahu, M., Karjalainen, S., Bernard, J.L., Carli, P.M., L'Huillier, M.C., Lutz, J.M., Schaffer, P., Schraub, S., Michaelis, J., Möhner, M., Staneczek, W., Vargha, M.,

Crosignani, P., Magnani, C., Terracini, B., Kriauciunas, R., Coebergh, J.W., Langmark, F., Zatonski, W., Merabishvili, V., Pompe-Kirn, V., Barlow, L., Raymond, L., Black, R., Stiller, C.A. & Bennett, B.G. (1993a) Childhood leukaemia following the Chernobyl accident: The European Childhood Leukaemia-Lymphoma Incidence Study (ECLIS). *Eur. J. Cancer, 29A,* 87–95

Parkin, D.M., Stiller, C.A. & Nectoux, J. (1993b) International variations in the incidence of childhood bone tumours. *Int. J. Cancer, 53,* 371–376

Parkin, D.M., Clayton, D., Black, R.J., Masuyer, E., Friedl, H.P., Ivanov, E., Sinnaeve, J., Tzvetansky, C.G., Geryk, E., Storm, H.H., Rahu, M., Pukkala, E., Bernard, J.L., Carli, P.M., L'Huillier, M.C., Ménégoz, F., Schaffer, P., Schraub, S., Kaatsch, P., Michaelis, J., Apjok, E., Schuler, D., Crosignani, P., Magnani, C., Terracini, B., Stengrevics, A., Kriauciunas, R., Coebergh, J.W., Langmark, F., Zatonski, W., Tulbure, R., Boukhny, A., Merabishvili, V., Plesko, I., Kramárová, E., Pompe-Kirn, V., Barlow, L., Enderlin, F., Levi, F., Raymond, L., Schüler, G., Torhorst, J., Stiller, C.A., Sharp, L. & Bennett, B.G. (1996) Childhood leukaemia in Europe after Chernobyl: 5 year follow-up. *Br. J. Cancer, 73,* 1006–1012

Passaro, K.T., Noss, J., Savitz, D.A., Little, R.E. & The ALSPAC Study Team. (1997) Agreement between self and partner reports of paternal drinking and smoking. *Int. J. Epidemiol., 26,* 315–320

Passmore, S.J., Draper, G.J. & Stiller, C.A. (1993) Vitamin K and childhood cancer. *Br. Med. J., 307,* 1140

Pastore, G., Mosso, M.L., Ghibaudo, P., Carli, M. & de Bernardi, B. (1985) Cancer mortality in relatives of children with soft tissue sarcomas and neuroblastoma: a national survey in Italy. In: Müller. H. & Weber, W., eds, *Familial Cancer* (1st Int. Res. Conf.), Basel, Karger, pp. 146–150

Pastore, G., Carli, M., Lemerle, J., Tournade, M.F., Voute, P.A., Rey, A., Burgers, J.M.V., Zucker, J.M., Burger, D., de Kraker, J. & Delemarre, J.F.M. (1988) Epidemiological features of Wilms' tumor: results of studies by the International Society of Paediatric Oncology (SIOP). *Med. Pediat. Oncol., 16,* 7–11

Pendergrass, T.W. & Hanson, J.W. (1976) Fetal hydantoin syndrome and neuroblastoma. *Lancet, ii,* 150

Pendergrass, T.W., Foulkes, M.A., Robison, L.L. & Nesbit, M.E. (1984) Stature and Ewing's sarcoma in childhood. *Am. J. Pediatr. Hematol. Oncol., 6,* 33–39

Pendergrass, T.W. (1985) Epidemiology of acute lymphoblastic leukaemia. *Semin. Oncol., 12,* 80–91

Penrose, M. (1970) Cat leukaemia. *Br. Med. J., i,* 755

Peris-Bonet, R., García, F.A., Alós, I.M., Ballester, E.G. & Medina, A.G. (1996) Childhood cancer incidence registration in the province of Valencia, Spain 1983–90. *J. Epidemiol. Biostat., 1,* 107–113

Perkkiö, M., Lie, S.O., Ekelund, H., Rajantie, J., Yssing, M., Läärä, E. & Siimes, M.A. (1990) Four pairs of siblings with acute leukemia during 1966–1985 in the Nordic countries: indication of an elevated familial risk? *Pediatr. Hematol. Oncol., 7,* 159–163

Pershagen, G. (1988) Health effects of Chernobyl. Important to measure among evacuees. *Br. Med. J., 297,* 1488

Pershagen, G., Ericson, A. & Otterblad-Olausson, P. (1992) Maternal smoking in pregnancy: does it increase the risk of childhood cancer? *Int. J. Epidemiol., 21,* 1–5

Peters, J.M., Preston-Martin, S. & Yu, M.C. (1981) Brain tumors in children and occupational exposure of parents. *Science, 213,* 235–237

Peters, J.M., Preston-Martin, S., London, S.J., Bowman, J.D., Buckley, J.D. & Thomas, D.C. (1994) Processed meats and risk of childhood leukemia (California, USA). *Cancer Causes Control, 5,* 195–202

Petridou, E., Hsieh, C.C., Kotsafakis, G., Skalkidis, Y. & Trichopoulos, D. (1991) Absence of leukaemia clustering on Greek Islands. *Lancet, 338,* 1204–1205

Petridou, E., Kassimos, D., Kalmanti, M., Kosmidis, H., Haidas, S., Flytzani, V., Tong, D. & Trichopoulos, D. (1993) Age of exposure to infections and risk of childhood leukaemia. *Br. Med. J., 307,* 774

Petridou, E., Proukakis, C., Tong, D., Kassimos, D., Athanassiadou-Piperopoulou, F., Haidas, S., Kalmanti, M., Koliouskas, D., Kosmidis, H., Louizi, A., Simopoulos, S. &

Trichopoulos, D. (1994) Trends and geographical distribution of childhood leukaemia in Greece in relation to the Chernobyl accident. *Scand. J. Soc. Med.*, **22**, 127–131

Petridou, E., Revinthi, K., Alexander, F.E., Haidas, S., Koliouskas, D., Kosmidis, H., Piperopoulou, F., Tzortzatou, F. & Trichopoulos, D. (1996a) Space–time clustering of childhood leukaemia in Greece: evidence supporting a viral aetiology. *Br. J. Cancer*, **73**, 1278–1283

Petridou, E., Trichopoulos, D., Dessypris, N., Flytzani, V., Haidas, S., Kalmanti, M., Koliouskas, D., Kosmidis, H., Piperopoulou, F. & Tzortzatou, F. (1996b) Infant leukaemia after *in utero* exposure to radiation from Chernobyl. *Nature*, **382**, 352–353

Petridou, E., Alexander, F.E., Trichopoulos, D., Revinthi, K., Dessypris, N., Wray, N., Haidas, S., Koliouskas, D., Kosmidis, H., Piperopoulou, F. & Tzortzatou, F. (1997) Aggregation of childhood leukemia in geographic areas of Greece. *Cancer Causes Control*, **8**, 239–245

Philips, A. (1994) Risk of cancer and exposure to power lines. Still no answers. *Br. Med. J.*, **308**, 1162–1163

Pike, M.C., Williams, E.H. & Wright, B. (1967) Burkitt's tumour in the West Nile District of Uganda. *Br. Med. J.*, **2**, 395–399

Pinkel, D. & Nefzger, D. (1959) Some epidemiological features of childhood leukemia in the Buffalo, N.Y. area. *Cancer*, **12**, 351–358

Pinkel, D., Dowd, J.E. & Bross, I.D.J. (1963) Some epidemiological features of malignant solid tumors of children in the Buffalo, N.Y. area. *Cancer*, **16**, 28–33

Pobel, D. & Viel, J.F. (1997) Case–control study of leukaemia among young people near La Hague nuclear reprocessing plant: the environmental hypothesis revisited. *Br. Med. J.*, **314**, 101–106

Polednak, A.P. (1986) Recent trends in incidence and mortality rates for leukemias and in survival rates for childhood acute lymphocytic leukemia, in upstate New York. *Cancer*, **57**, 1850–1858

Polhemus, D.W. & Koch, R. (1959) Leukemia and medical radiation. *Pediatrics*, **23**, 453–461

Pombo de Oliveira, M.S., Awad el Seed, F.E.R., Foroni, L., Matutes, E., Morilla, R., Luzzatto, L. & Catovsky, D. (1986) Lymphoblastic leukaemia in Siamese twins: evidence for identity. *Lancet*, **ii**, 969–970

Poole, C. (1996) Invited commentary: Evolution of epidemiologic evidence on magnetic fields and childhood cancers. *Am. J. Epidemiol.*, **143**, 129–132

Poole, C. & Trichopoulos, D. (1991) Extremely low-frequency electric and magnetic fields and cancer. *Cancer Causes Control*, **2**, 267–276

Potter, E.L. (1962) *Pathology of the Fetus and the Newborn*, Chicago, Year Book Publishers, pp. 155

Potthoff, R.F. & Whittinghill, M. (1966a) Testing for homogeneity. I. The binomial and multinomial distributions. *Biometrika*, **53**, 167–182

Potthoff, R.F. & Whittinghill, M. (1966b) Testing for homogeneity. II. The Poisson distribution. *Biometrika*, **53**, 183–190

Powell, J.E., Parkes, S.E., Cameron, A.H. & Mann, J.R. (1994) Is the risk of cancer increased in Asians living in the UK? *Arch. Dis. Child.*, **71**, 398–403

Powell, J.E., Kelly, A.M., Parkes, S.E., Cole, T.R.P. & Mann, J.R. (1995) Cancer and congenital abnormalities in Asian children: a population-based study from the West Midlands. *Br. J. Cancer*, **72**, 1563–1569

Pratt, J.A., Velez, R., Brender, J.D. & Manton, K.G. (1988) Racial differences in acute lymphocytic leukemia mortality and incidence trends. *J. Clin. Epidemiol.*, **41**, 367–371

Preston-Martin, S., Yu, M.C., Benton, B. & Henderson, B.E. (1982) N-Nitroso compounds and childhood brain tumors: a case–control study. *Cancer Res.*, **42**, 5240–5245

Preston-Martin, S., Navidi, W., Thomas, D., Lee, P.J., Bowman, J. & Pogoda, J. (1996a) Los Angeles study of residential magnetic fields and childhood brain tumors. *Am. J. Epidemiol.*, **143**, 105–119

Preston-Martin, S., Gurney, J.G., Pogoda, J.M., Holly, E.A. & Mueller, B.A. (1996b) Brain tumor risk in children in relation to use of electric blankets and water bed heaters. Results from the United States West Coast Childhood Brain Tumour Study. *Am. J. Epidemiol.*, **143**, 1116–1122

Preston-Martin, S., Navidi, W., Thomas, D., Lee, P.J., Bowman, J. & Pogoda, J. (1996c) Response to "Evolution of epidemiologic evidence on magnetic fields and childhood cancers". *Am. J. Epidemiol.*, **143**, 133–134

Preston-Martin, S., Pogoda, J.M., Mueller, B.A., Holly, E.A., Lijinsky, W. & Davis, R.L. (1996d) Maternal consumption of cured meats and vitamins in relation to pediatric brain tumors. *Cancer Epidemiol. Biomarkers Prev.*, **5**, 599–605

Preussman, R. (1984) Occurrence and exposure to N-nitroso compounds and nitrosatable precursors. In: O'Neill, I.K., Van Borstel, R.C., Miller, C.T., Long, J. & Bartsch, H., eds, *N-Nitroso Compounds: Occurrence, Biological Effects and Relevance to Human Cancer* (IARC Scientific Publications No. 57), Lyon, IARC, pp. 3–15

Price, C.H.G. (1958) Primary bone-forming tumors and their relationship to skeletal growth. *J. Bone Joint Surg.*, **40B**, 574–593

Prindull, G., Demuth, M. & Wehinger, H. (1993) Cancer morbidity rates of children from the vicinity of the nuclear power plant of Würgassen (FRG). *Acta Haematol.*, **90**, 90–93

Prisyazhiuk, A., Pjatak, O.A., Buzanov, V.A., Reeves, G.K. & Beral, V. (1991) Cancer in the Ukraine, post-Chernobyl. *Lancet*, **338**, 1334–1335

Pritchard-Jones, K. & Hastie, N.D. (1990) Wilms' tumour as a paradigm for the relationship of cancer to development. *Cancer Surv.*, **9**, 555–578

Pritchard-Jones, K. & Hawkins, M.M. (1997) Biology of Wilms' tumour. *Lancet*, **349**, 663–664

Pui, C.H., Dodge, R.K., George, S.L. & Green, A.A. (1987) Height at diagnosis of malignancies. *Arch. Dis. Child.*, **62**, 495–499

Rabkin, C.S., Hilgartner, M.W., Hedberg, K.W., Aledort, L.M., Hatzakis, A., Eichinger, S., Eyster, M.E., White, G.C., Kessler, C.M., Lederman, M.M., de Moerloose, P., Bray, G.L., Cohen, A.R., Andes, A., Manco-Jonson, M., Schramm, W., Kroner, B.L., Blattner, W.A. & Goedert, J.J. (1992) Incidence of lymphomas and other cancers in HIV-infected and HIV-uninfected patients with hemophilia. *J. Am. Med. Assoc.*, **267**, 1090–1094

Ragge, N.K. (1993) Clinical and genetic patterns of neurofibromatosis 1 and 2. *Br. J. Ophthalmol.*, **77**, 662–672

Rahman, N., Arbour, L., Tonin, P., Renshaw, J., Pelletier, J., Baruchel, S., Pritchard-Jones, K., Stratton, M.R. & Narod, S.A. (1996) Evidence for a familial Wilms' tumour gene (FWT1) on chromosome 17q12–q21. *Nature Genet.*, **13**, 461–463

Rainier, S. & Feinberg, A.P. (1994) Genomic imprinting, DNA methylation and cancer. *J. Natl. Cancer Inst.*, **86**, 753–759

Rainier, S., Johnson, L.A., Dobry, C.J., Ping, A.J., Grundy, P.E. & Feinberg, A.P. (1993) Relaxation of imprinted genes in human cancer. *Nature*, **362**, 747–749

Rallison, M.L., Dobyns, B.M., Keating, F.R., Jr., Rall, J.E. & Tyler, F.H. (1974) Thyroid disease in children. A survey of subjects potentially exposed to fallout radiation. *Am. J. Med.*, **56**, 457–463

Rallison, M.L., Dobyns, B.M., Keating, F.R., Rall, J.E. & Tyler, F.H. (1975) Thyroid nodularity in children. *J. Am. Med. Assoc.*, **233**, 1069–1072

Ramilo, J. & Harris, V.J. (1979) Neuroblastoma in a child with the hydantoin and fetal alcohol syndrome. The radiographic features. *Br. J. Radiol.*, **42**, 993–995

Ramot, B. & MacGrath, I. (1982) Hypothesis: the environment is a major determinant of the immunological sub-type of lymphoma and acute lymphoblastic leukaemia in children. *Br. J. Haematol.*, **52**, 183–189

Randolph, V.L. & Heath, C.W., Jr (1974) Influenza during pregnancy in relation to subsequent childhood leukemia and lymphoma. *Am. J. Epidemiol.*, **100**, 399–409

Raphael, K. (1987) Recall bias: A proposal for assessment and control. *Int. J. Epidemiol.*, **16**, 167–170

Reeves, J.D., Driggers, D.A. & Kiley, V.A. (1981) Household insecticide associated aplastic anaemia and acute leukaemia in children. *Lancet*, **ii**, 300–301

Rennie, J.M. & Kelsall, A.W.R. (1994) Vitamin K prophylaxis in the newborn – again. *Arch. Dis. Child.*, **70**, 248–251

Report to the Minister for Veterans' Affairs (1983) *Case-Control Study of Congenital Anomalies and Vietnam Service (Birth Defects Study)*, Canberra, Australian Government Publishing Service

Restrepo, M., Muñoz, N., Day, N., Parra, J.E., Hernandez, C., Blettner, M. & Giraldo, A. (1990) Birth defects among children born to a population occupationally exposed to pesticides in Colombia. *Scand. J. Work. Environ. Health*, **16**, 239–246

Richardson, S., Monfort, C., Green, M., Draper, G. & Muirhead, C. (1995) Spatial variation of natural radiation and childhood leukaemia incidence in Great Britain. *Stat. Med.*, **14**, 2487–2501

Robertson, C.M. & Hawkins, M.M. (1995) Childhood cancer and cystic fibrosis. *J. Natl. Cancer Inst.*, **87**, 1486–1487

Robison, L.L. (1993) Survivors of childhood cancer and risk of a second tumor. *J. Natl. Cancer Inst.*, **85**, 1102–1103

Robison, L.L., Swanson, T., Day, D.L., Ramsay, N.K.C., L'Heureux, P. & Nesbit, M.E., Jr (1982) Renal anomalies in childhood acute lymphoblastic leukemia. *New Engl. J. Med.*, **307**, 1086–1087

Robison, L.L. & Daigle, A. (1984) Control selection using random digit dialing for cases of childhood cancer. *Am. J. Epidemiol.*, **120**, 164–166

Robison, L.L., Nesbit, M.E., Sather, H.N., Level, C., Shahidi, N., Kennedy, A. & Hammond, D. (1984) Down syndrome and acute leukemia in children: a 10 year retrospective survey from Childrens' Cancer Study Group. *J. Pediat.*, **105**, 235–242

Robison, L.L., Nesbit, M.E., Jr, Sather, H.N., Meadows, A.T., Ortega, J.A. & Hammond, G.D. (1985) Height of children successfully treated for acute lymphoblastic leukemia: a report from the Late Effects Study Committee of Children's Cancer Study Group. *Med. Pediatr. Oncol.*, **13**, 14–21

Robison, L.L., Codd, M., Gunderson, P., Neglia, J.P., Smithson, W.A. & King, F.L. (1987) Birth weight as a risk factor for childhood acute lymphoblastic leukemia. *Pediat. Hematol. Oncol.*, **4**, 63–72

Robison, L.L., Buckley, J.D., Daigle, A.E., Wells, R., Benjamin, D., Arthur, D.C. & Hammond, G.D. (1989) Maternal drug use and risk of childhood nonlymphoblastic leukemia among offspring. *Cancer*, **63**, 1904–1911

Robison, L.L., Buckley, J.D. & Bunin, G. (1995) Assessment of environmental and genetic factors in the etiology of childhood cancers: the Childrens Cancer Group epidemiology program. *Environ. Health Perspect.*, **103**, 111–116

Rodrigues, L., Hills, M., McGale, P. & Elliott, P. (1991) Socio-economic factors in relation to childhood leukaemia and non-Hodgkin lymphomas: an analysis based on small area statistics for census tracts. In: Draper, G.J., ed., *The Geographical Epidemiology of Childhood Leukaemia and Non-Hodgkin Lymphomas in Great Britain, 1966–83* (Studies on Medical and Population Subjects No. 53), London, HMSO, pp. 47–56

Rodvall, Y., Pershagen, G., Hrubec, Z., Ahlbom, A., Pedersen, N.L. & Boice, J.D. (1990) Prenatal X-ray exposure and childhood cancer in Swedish twins. *Int. J. Cancer*, **46**, 362–365

Rodvall, Y., Hrubec, Z., Pershagen, G., Ahlbom, A., Bjurman, A. & Boice, J.D., Jr (1992) Childhood cancer among Swedish twins. *Cancer Causes Control*, **3**, 527–532

Rogan, W.J. (1986) An analysis of contaminated well water and health effects in Woburn, Massachusetts – comment. *J. Am. Stat. Assoc.*, **81**, 602–603

Roman, E., Beral, V., Carpenter, L., Watson, A., Barton, C., Tyder, H. & Aston, D.L. (1987) Childhood leukaemia in the West Berkshire and Basingstoke and North Hampshire District Health Authorities in relation to nuclear establishments in the vicinity. *Br. Med. J.*, **294**, 597–602

Roman, E., Watson, A., Beral, V., Buckle, S., Bull, D., Baker, K., Ryder, H. & Barton, C. (1993) Case–control study of leukaemia and non-Hodgkin's lymphoma among children aged 0–4 years living in West Berkshire and North Hampshire health districts. *Br. Med. J.*, **306**, 615–621

Roman, E., Watson, A., Bull, D. & Baker, K. (1994) Leukaemia risk and social contact in children aged 0–4 years in southern England. *J. Epidemiol. Commun. Health*, **48**, 601–605

Roman, E., Doyle, P., Ansell, P., Bull, D. & Beral, V. (1996) Health of children born to medical radiographers. *Occup. Environ. Med.*, **53**, 73–79

Roman, E., Ansell, P. & Bull, D. (1997) Leukaemia and non-Hodgkin's lymphoma in children and young adults: are prenatal and neonatal factors important determinants of disease? *Br. J. Cancer*, **76**, 406–415

Ron, E., Modan, B., Preston, D., Alfandary, E., Stovall, M. & Boice, J.D., Jr (1989) Thyroid neoplasia following low-dose radiation in childhood. *Radiation Res.*, **120**, 516–531

Ron, E., Lubin, J. & Schneider, A.B. (1992) Thyroid cancer incidence. *Nature*, **360**, 113

Ron, E., Lubin, J.H., Shore, R.E., Mabuchi, K., Modan, B., Pottern, L.M., Schneider, A.B., Tucker, M.A. & Boice, J.D., Jr (1995) Thyroid cancer after exposure to external radiation: a pooled analysis of seven studies. *Radiation Res.*, **141**, 259–277

Rosenthal, S.R., Crispen, R.G., Thorne, M.G., Piekarski, N., Raisys, N. & Rettig, P.G. (1972) BCG vaccination and leukemia mortality. *J. Am. Med. Assoc.*, **222**, 1543–1544

Ross, J.A., Davies, S.M., Potter, J.D. & Robison, L.L. (1994a) Epidemiology of childhood leukemia, with a focus on infants. *Epidemiol. Rev.*, **16**, 243–272

Ross, J.A., Potter, J.D. & Robison, L.L. (1994b) Infant leukemia, topoisomerase II inhibitors and the MLL gene. *J. Natl. Cancer Inst.*, **86**, 1678–1680

Ross, J.A., Perentesis, J.P., Robison, L.L. & Davies, S.M. (1996a) Big babies and infant leukemia: a role for insulin-like growth factor-1? *Cancer Causes Control*, **7**, 553–559

Ross, J.A., Potter, J.D., Reaman, G.H., Pendergrass, T.W. & Robison, L.L. (1996b) Maternal exposure to potential inhibitors of DNA topoisomerase II and infant leukemia (United States): A report from the Children's Cancer Group. *Cancer Causes Control*, **7**, 581–590

Ross, J.A., Potter, J.D., Shu, X.O., Reaman, G.H., Lampkin, B. & Robison, L.L. (1997) Evaluating the relationships among maternal reproductive history, birth characteristics, and infant leukemia: A report from the Children's Cancer Group. *Ann. Epidemiol.*, **7**, 172–179

Rosti, L., Lin, A.E. & Frigiola, A. (1996) Neuroblastoma and congenital cardiovascular malformations. *Pediatrics*, **97**, 258–261

Rothman, K.J. (1984) Significance of studies of low-dose radiation fallout in the western United States. In: Boice, J.D., Jr & Fraumeni, J.F., Jr, eds, *Radiation Carcinogenesis, Epidemiology and Biological Significance*, New York, Raven Press, pp. 73–82

Ruymann, F.B., Maddux, H.R., Ragab, A., Soule, E.H., Palmer, N., Beltangady, M., Gehan, E.A. & Newton, W.A., Jr (1988) Congenital anomalies associated with rhabdomyosarcoma: An autopsy study of 115 cases. A report from the Intergroup Rhabdomyosarcoma Study Committee (representing the Children's Cancer Study Group, the Pediatric Oncology Group, the United Kingdom Children's Cancer Study Group and the Pediatric Intergroup Statistical Centre). *Med. Pediat. Oncol.*, **16**, 33–39

Sahl, J.D. (1994) Viral contacts confound studies of childhood leukemia and high-voltage transmission lines. *Cancer Causes Control*, **5**, 279–283

Sala, E. & Oslen, J.H. (1993) Thyroid cancer in the age group 0–19: time trends and temporal changes in radioactive fallout. *Eur. J. Cancer*, **29A**, 1443–1445

Sali, D., Cardis, E., Sztanyik, L., Auvinen, A., Bairakova, A., Dontas, N., Grosche, B., Kerekes, A., Kusic, Z., Kusoglu, C., Lechpammer, S., Lyra, M., Michaelis, J., Petridou, E., Szybinski, Z., Tominaga, S., Tulbure, R., Turnbull, A. & Valerianova, Z. (1996) Cancer consequences of the Chernobyl accident in Europe outside the former USSR: A review. *Int. J. Cancer*, **67**, 343–352

Salonen, T. (1976) Prenatal and perinatal factors in childhood cancer. *Ann. Clin. Res.*, **7**, 27–42

Salonen, T. & Saxén, L. (1975) Risk indicators in childhood malignancies. *Int. J. Cancer*, **15**, 941–946

Sanders, B.M. & Draper, G.J. (1979) Childhood cancer and drugs in pregnancy. *Br. Med. J.*, **1**, 717–718

Sanders, B.M., White, G.C. & Draper, G.J. (1981) Occupations of fathers of children dying from neoplasms. *J. Epidemiol. Commun. Health*, **35**, 245–250

Sanders, B.M., Draper, G.J. & Kingston, J.E. (1988) Retinoblastoma in Great Britain 1969–80: incidence, treatment, and survival. *Br. J. Ophthalmol.*, **72**, 576–583

Sans, S., Elliott, P., Kleinschmidt, I., Shaddick, G., Pattenden, S., Walls, P., Grundy, C. & Dolk, H. (1995) Cancer incidence and mortality near the Baglan Bay petrochemical works, South Wales. *Occup. Environ. Medi.*, **52**, 217–224

Santibáñez-Koref, M.F., Birch, J.M., Hartley, A.L., Jones, P.H., Craft, A.W., Eden, T., Crowther, D., Kelsey, A.M. & Harris, M. (1991) p53 germline mutations in Li-Fraumeni syndrome. *Lancet*, **338**, 1490–1491

Sarasua, S. & Savitz, D.A. (1994) Cured and broiled meat consumption in relation to childhood cancer: Denver, Colorado (United States). *Cancer Causes Control*, **5**, 141–148

Satge, D., Sasco, A.J., Carlsen, N.L.T., Rubie, H. & Stiller, C.A. (1997) A negative association between Down's syndrome and neuroblastoma. *Arch. Dis. Child.*, **67**, 80

Savitz, D.A. (1988) *Case-Control Study of Childhood Cancer and Residential Exposure to Electric and Magnetic Fields. New York State Power Lines Project. Supplement to Contractor's Final Report* (cited in NRPB, 1992)

Savitz, D.A. & Ananth, C.V. (1994) Birth characteristics of childhood cancer cases, controls and their siblings. *Pediat. Hematol. Oncol.*, **11**, 587–599

Savitz, D.A. & Feingold, L. (1989) Association of childhood cancer with residential traffic density. *Scand. J. Work. Environ. Health*, **15**, 360–363

Savitz, D.A., Wachtel, H., Barnes, F.A., John, E.M. & Tvrdik, J.G. (1988) Case–control study of childhood cancer and exposure to 60-Hz magnetic fields. *Am. J. Epidemiol.*, **128**, 21–38

Savitz, D.A., Pearce, N.E. & Poole, C. (1989) Methodological issues in the epidemiology of electromagnetic fields and cancer. *Epidemiol. Rev.*, **11**, 59–78

Savitz, D.A., John, E.M. & Kleckner, R.C. (1990) Magnetic field exposure from electric appliances and childhood cancer. *Am. J. Epidemiol.*, **131**, 763–773

Savitz, D.A., Pearce, N. & Poole, C. (1993) Update on methodological issues in the epidemiology of electromagnetic fields and cancer. *Epidemiol. Rev.*, **15**, 558–566

Schinzel, A.A.G.L., Smith, D.W. & Miller, J.R. (1979) Monozygotic twinning and structural defects. *J. Pediat.*, **95**, 921–930

Schlehofer, B., Blettner, M., Geletneky, K., Haaf, H.G., Kaatsch, P., Michaelis, J., Mueller-Lantzsch, N., Niehoff, D., Winkelspecht, B., Wahrendorf, J. & Schlehofer, J.R. (1996) Sero-epidemiological analysis of the risk of virus infections for childhood leukaemia. *Int. J. Cancer*, **65**, 584–590

Schroeder, W.T., Chao, L.Y., Dao, D.D., Strong, L.C., Pathak, S., Riccardi, V., Lewis, W.H. & Saunders, G.F. (1987) Nonrandom loss of maternal chromosome 11 alleles in Wilms' tumors. *Am. J. Hum. Genet.*, **40**, 413–420

Schull, W.J. & Neel, J.V. (1965) *The Effects of Inbreeding on Japanese Children*, New York, Harper and Row

Schumacher, R., Mai, A. & Gutjahr, P. (1992) Association of rib anomalies and malignancy in childhood. *Eur. J. Pediat.*, **151**, 432–434

Schwartzbaum, J.A. (1992) Influence of the mother's prenatal drug consumption on risk of neuroblastoma in the child. *Am. J. Epidemiol.*, **135**, 1358–1367

Schymura, M.J., Zheng, D., Baptiste, M.S. & Nasca, P.C. (1996) A case–control study of childhood brain tumors and maternal lifestyle. *Am. J. Epidemiol.*, **143**, S8

Scranton, P.E., DeCicco, F.A., Totten, R.S. & Yunis, E.J. (1975) Prognostic factors in osteosarcoma. A review of 20 years' experience at the University of Pittsburgh Health Center Hospitals. *Cancer*, **36**, 2179–2191

Sculley, T.B., Apolloni, A., Hurren, L., Moss, D.J. & Cooper, D.A. (1990) Coinfection with A- and B-type Epstein–Barr virus in human immunodeficiency virus-positive subjects. *J. Infect. Dis.*, **162**, 643–648

Seeler, R.A., Israel, J.N., Royal, J.E., Kaye, C.I., Rao, S. & Abulaban, M. (1979) Ganglioneuroblastoma and fetal hydantoin-alcohol syndromes. *Pediatrics*, **63**, 524–527

Segi, M. (1960) *Cancer Mortality for Selected Sites in 24 Countries (1950–1957)*, Tohoku University School of Medicine, Japan

Seizinger, B.R. (1993) NF1: a prevalent cause of tumorigenesis in human cancers? *Nature Genet.*, **3**, 97–99

Selvin, S., Schulman, J. & Merrill, D.W. (1992) Distance and risk measures for the analysis of spatial data: a study of childhood cancers. *Soc. Sci. Med.*, **34**, 769–777

Sen, N.P., Seaman, S., Clarkson, S., Garrod, F. & Lalonde, P. (1984) Volatile N-nitrosamines in baby bottle rubber nipples and pacifiers. Analysis, occurrence and migration. In: O'Neill, I.K., Van Borstel, R.C., Miller, C.T., Long, J. & Bartsch, H., eds, *N-Nitroso Compounds: Occurrence, Biological Effects and Relevance to Human Cancer* (IARC Scientific Publications No. 57), Lyon, IARC, pp. 51–57

Severson, R.K., Buckley, J.D., Woods, W.G., Benjamin, D. & Robison, L.L. (1993) Cigarette smoking and alcohol consumption by parents of children with acute myeloid leukemia: an analysis within morphological subgroups – a report from the Childrens Cancer Group. *Cancer Epidemiol. Biomarkers Prev.*, **2**, 433–439

Shalat, S.L., Christiani, D.C. & Baker, E.L. (1987) Accuracy of work history obtained from a spouse. *Scand. J. Work. Environ. Health*, **13**, 67–69

Shapiro, S., Heinonen, O.P., Siskind, V., Kaufman, D.W., Monson, R.R. & Slone, D. (1977) Antenatal exposure to doxylamine succinate and dicyclomine hydrochloride (Bendectin) in relation to congenital malformations, perinatal mortality rate, birth weight, and intelligence quotient score. *Am. J. Obstet. Gynecol.*, **128**, 480–485

Sharp, L., Black, R.J., Harkness, E.F. & McKinney, P.A. (1996) Incidence of childhood leukaemia and non-Hodgkin's lymphoma in the vicinity of nuclear sites in Scotland, 1968–93. *Occup. Environ. Med.*, **53**, 823–831

Sharpe, C.R. & Franco, E.L. (1995) Etiology of Wilms' tumor. *Epidemio. Rev.*, **17**, 415–432

Sharpe, C.R., Franco, E.L., de Camargo, B., Lopes, L.F., Barreto, J.H., Johnsson, R.R. & Mauad, M.A. (1995) Parental exposures to pesticides and risk of Wilms' tumor in Brazil. *Am. J. Epidemiol.*, **141**, 210–217

Shaw, G., Lavey, R., Jackson, R. & Austin, D. (1984) Association of childhood leukemia with maternal age, birth order, and paternal occupation. *Am. J. Epidemiol.*, **119**, 788–795

Shaw, G.M., Malcoe, L.H., Croen, L.A. & Smith, D.F. (1990) An assessment of error in parental occupation from the birth certificate. *Am. J. Epidemiol.*, **131**, 1072–1079

Sherman, S. & Roizen, N. (1976) Fetal hydantoin syndrome and neuroblastoma. *Lancet*, **ii**, 517

Shigematsu, I. & Thiessen, J.W. (1992) Childhood thyroid cancer in Belarus. *Nature*, **359**, 681

Shimizu, Y., Kato, H. & Schull, W.J. (1990a) Studies of the mortality of A-bomb survivors. 9. Mortality, 1950–1985: Part 2. Cancer mortality based on the recently revised doses DS86. *Radiat. Res.*, **121**, 120–141

Shimizu, Y., Schull, W.J. & Kato, H. (1990b) Cancer risk among atomic bomb survivors. The RERF Life Span Study. *J. Am. Med. Assoc.*, **264**, 601–604

Shimizu, T., Chigira, M., Nagase, M., Watanabe, H. & Udagawa, E. (1990c) HLA phenotypes in patients who have osteosarcoma. *J. Bone Joint Surg.*, **72A**, 68–70

Shiono, P.H. & Klebanoff, M.A. (1989) Bendectin and human congenital malformations. *Teratology*, **40**, 151–155

Shiono, P.H., Chung, C.S. & Myrianthopoulos, N.C. (1980) Preconception radiation, intrauterine diagnostic radiation, and childhood neoplasia. *J. Natl. Cancer Inst.*, **65**, 681–686

Shiramizu, B., Barriga, F., Neequaye, J., Jafri, A., Dalla-Favera, R., Neri, A., Guttierez, M., Levine, P. & Magrath, I. (1991) Patterns of chromosomal breakpoint locations in Burkitt's lymphoma: relevance to geography and Epstein–Barr virus association. *Blood*, **77**, 1516–1526

Shore, R.E., Hildreth, N., Dvoretsky, P., Andresen, E., Moseson, M. & Pasternack, B. (1993) Thyroid cancer among persons given X-ray treatment in infancy for an enlarged thymus gland. *Am. J. Epidemiol.*, **137**, 1068–1080

Shu, X.O., Gao, Y.T., Linet, M.S., Brinton, L.A., Gao, R.N., Jin, F. & Fraumeni, J.F., Jr (1987) Chloramphenicol use and childhood leukaemia in Shanghai. *Lancet*, **ii**, 934–937

Shu, X.O., Gao, Y.T., Brinton, L.A., Linet, M.S., Tu, J.T., Zheng, W. & Fraumeni, J.F., Jr (1988) A population-based case–control study of childhood leukemia in Shanghai. *Cancer*, **62**, 635–644

Shu, X.O., Jin, F., Linet, M.S., Zheng, W., Clemens, J., Mills, J. & Gao, Y.T. (1994a) Diagnostic X-ray and ultrasound exposure and risk of childhood cancer. *Br. J. Cancer*, **70**, 531–536

Shu, X.O., Reaman, G.H., Lampkin, B., Sather, H.N., Pendergrass, T.W. & Robison, L.L. (1994b) Association of paternal diagnostic X-ray exposure with risk of infant leukemia. *Cancer Epidemiol. Biomarkers Prev.*, **3**, 645–653

Shu, X.O., Nesbit, M.E., Buckley, J.D., Krailo, M.D. & Robison, L.L. (1995a) An exploratory analysis of risk factors for childhood malignant germ-cell tumours: report from the Children's Cancer Group (Canada, United States). *Cancer Causes Control*, **6**, 187–198

Shu, X.O., Clemens, J., Zheng, W., Ying, D.M., Ji, B.T. & Jin, F. (1995b) Infant breastfeeding and the risk of childhood lymphoma and leukaemia. *Int. J. Epidemiol.*, **24**, 27–32

Shu, X.O., Ross, J.A., Pendergrass, T.W., Reaman, G.H., Lampkin, B. & Robison, L.L. (1996) Parental alcohol consumption, cigarette smoking and risk of infant leukemia: a Childrens Cancer Group Study. *J. Natl. Cancer Inst.*, **88**, 24–31

Sieber, W.K., Jr, Sundin, D.S., Frazier, T.M. & Robinson, C.F. (1991) Development, use and availability of a job exposure matrix based on national occupational hazard survey data. *Am. J. Ind. Med.*, **20**, 163–174

Siemiatycki, J. (1989) Friendly control bias. *J. Clin. Epidemiol.*, **42**, 687–688

Siemiatycki, J., Brubaker, G. & Geser, A. (1980) Space–time clustering of Burkitt's lymphoma in East Africa: analysis of recent data and a new look at old data. *Int. J. Cancer*, **25**, 197–203

Sigler, A., Lilienfeld, A., Cohen, B. & Westlake, J. (1965) Radiation exposure in parents of children with Down's syndrome. *Johns Hopkins Med. J.*, **117**, 374–399

Sinks, T.H., Jr (1985) *N*-Nitroso compounds, pesticides, and parental exposures in the workplace as risk factors for childhood brain cancer: a case–control study. *Dissertation Abst. Int.*, **46**, 1888–B

Skegg, D.C.G. (1978) BCG vaccination and the incidence of lymphomas and leukaemia. *Int. J. Cancer*, **21**, 18–21

Sklar, J.L. & Costa, J.C. (1997) Principles of cancer management: molecular pathology. In: DeVita, V.T., Jr, Hellman, S. & Rosenberg, S.A., eds, *Cancer: Principles and Practice of Oncology*, fifth edition, New York, Lippincott-Raven, pp. 259–284

Smith, P.G. (1982) Spatial and temporal clustering. In: Schottenfeld, D. & Fraumeni, J.F., eds, *Cancer Epidemiology and Prevention*, Philadelphia, Saunders, pp. 391–407

Smith, P.G. (1985) Rapporteur's report. In: Lenoir, G., O'Conor, G. & Olweny, C.L.M., eds, *Burkitt's Lymphoma: a Human Cancer Model* (IARC Scientific Publications No. 60), Lyon, IARC, pp. 225–228

Smith, P.G. (1991) Case–control studies of leukaemia clusters. *Br. Med. J.*, **302**, 672–673

Smith, P.J. (1992) Hereditary tumours of childhood. Messages for cancer in general. *Med. J. Aust.*, **156**, 232–233

Smith, P.G., Pike, M.C., Till, M.M. & Hardisty, R.M. (1976) Epidemiology of childhood leukaemia in Greater London: a search for evidence of transmission assuming a possibly long latent period. *Br. J. Cancer*, **33**, 1–8

Snider, D.E., Comstock, G.W., Martinez, I. & Caras, G.J. (1978) Efficacy of BCG vaccination in prevention of cancer: an update. *J. Natl. Cancer Inst.*, **60**, 785–788

Sofer, T., Goldsmith, J.R., Nusselder, I. & Katz, L. (1991) Geographical and temporal trends of childhood leukemia in relation to the nuclear plant in the Negev, Israel, 1960–1985. *Public Health Rev.*, **19**, 191–198

Sorahan, T. & Roberts, P.J. (1993) Childhood cancer and paternal exposure to ionizing radiation: preliminary findings from the Oxford survey of childhood cancers. *Am. J. Ind. Med.*, **23**, 343–354

Sorahan, T. & Stewart, A.M. (1993) Retinoblastoma and fetal irradiation. *Br. Med. J.*, **307**, 870

Sorahan, T., Lancashire, R., Prior, P., Peck, I. & Stewart, A. (1995a) Childhood cancer and parental use of alcohol and tobacco. *Ann. Epidemiol.*, **5**, 354–359

Sorahan, T., Lancashire, R., Stewart, A. & Peck, I. (1995b) Pregnancy ultrasound and childhood cancer: a second report from the Oxford Survey of Childhood Cancers. *Br. J. Obstet. Gynaecol.*, **102**, 831–832

Spiess, H. & Mays, C.W. (1970) Bone cancers induced by $^{224}$Ra(ThX) in children and adults. *Health Phys.*, **19**, 713–729

Spiess, H. & Mays, C.W. (1971) Erratum. *Health Phys.*, **20**, 543–545

Spiess, H. & Mays, C.W. (1973) Protraction effect on bone-sarcoma induction of $^{224}$Ra in children and adults. In: Sanders, C.L., Busch, R.H., Ballou, J.E. & Mahlum, D.D., eds, *Radionuclide Carcinogenesis. Proceedings of the Twelfth Annual Hanford Biology Symposium at Richland, Washington, May 10–12, 1972* (Atomic Energy Commission Symposium Series 29), Oak Ridge, TN, USAEC Technical Information Centre, CONF-720505, pp. 437–450

Spitz, M.R. & Johnson, C.C. (1985) Neuroblastoma and paternal occupation. A case–control analysis. *Am. J. Epidemiol.*, **121**, 924–929

Spitz, M.R., Sider, J.G., Cole Johnson, C., Butler, J.J., Pollack, E.S. & Newell, G.R. (1986) Ethnic patterns of Hodgkin's disease incidence among children and adolescents in the United States, 1973–82. *J. Natl. Cancer Inst.*, **76**, 235–239

Sriamporn, S., Vatanasapt, V., Martin, N., Sriplung, H., Chindavijak, K., Sontipong, S., Parkin, D.M. & Ferlay, J. (1996) Incidence of childhood cancer in Thailand 1988–1991. *Paediat. Perinatal Epidemiol.*, **10**, 73–85

Stark, C.R. & Mantel, N. (1966) Effects of maternal age and birth order on the risk of mongolism and leukaemia. *J. Natl. Cancer Inst.*, **37**, 687–698

Stark, C.R. & Mantel, N. (1967) Temporal-spatial distribution of birth dates for Michigan children with leukemia. *Cancer Res.*, **27**, 1749–1785

Stark, C.R. & Mantel, N. (1969) Maternal-age and birth-order effects in childhood leukemia: age of child and type of leukemia. *J. Natl. Cancer Inst.*, **42**, 857–866

Stein, A.D., Shea, S., Basch, C.E., Contento, I.R. & Zybert, P. (1992) Consistency of the Willett semiquantitative food frequency questionnaire and 24-hour dietary recalls in estimating nutrient intakes of preschool children. *Am. J. Epidemiol.*, **135**, 667–677

Steinberg, A.G. (1960) The genetics of acute leukemia in children. *Cancer*, **13**, 985–999

Sterling, T.D. & Arundel, A.V. (1986) Health effects of phenoxy herbicides. *Scand. J. Work. Environ. Health*, **12**, 161–173

Stevens, R.G., Jones, D.Y., Micozzi, M.S. & Taylor, P.R. (1988) Body iron stores and the risk of cancer. *New Engl. J. Med.*, **319**, 1047–1052

Stevens, W., Thomas, D.C., Lyon, J.L., Till, J.E., Kerber, R.A., Simon, S.L., Lloyd, R.D., Elghany, N.A. & Preston-Martin, S. (1990) Leukemia in Utah and radioactive fallout from the Nevada test site. *J. Am. Med. Assoc.*, **264**, 585–591

Stevens, M.C.G., Cameron, A.H., Muir, K.R., Parkes, S.E., Reid, H. & Whitwell, H. (1991) Descriptive epidemiology of primary central nervous system tumours in children: A population-based study. *Clin. Oncol.*, **3**, 323–329

Stewart, A.M. (1973) Cancer as a cause of abortions and stillbirths: the effect of these early deaths on the recognition of radiogenic leukaemias. *Br. J. Cancer*, **27**, 465–472

Stewart, A.M. (1980) Childhood cancers and the immune system. *Cancer Immunol. Immunother.*, **9**, 11

Stewart, A.M. & Hewitt, D. (1965) Aetiology of childhood leukaemia. *Lancet*, **ii**, 789–790

Stewart, A. & Kneale, G.W. (1971) Prenatal radiation exposure and childhood cancer. *Lancet*, **i**, 42–43

Stewart, A., Webb, J., Giles, D. & Hewitt, D. (1956) Malignant disease in childhood and diagnostic irradiation *in utero. Lancet*, **ii**, 447

Stewart, A., Webb, J. & Hewitt, D. (1958) A survey of childhood malignancies. *Br. Med. J.*, **1**, 1495–1508

Stiller, C.A. (1993a) Retinoblastoma and low level radiation. *Br. Med. J.*, **307**, 461–462

Stiller, C.A. (1993b) Trends in neuroblastoma in Great Britain: incidence and mortality, 1971–1990. *Eur. J. Cancer*, **29A**, 1008–1012

Stiller, C.A. (1994) International variations in the incidence of childhood carcinomas. *Cancer Epidemiol. Biomarkers Prev.*, **3**, 305–310

Stiller, C.A. & Boyle, P.J. (1996) Effect of population mixing and socioeconomic status in England and Wales, 1979–85, on lymphoblastic leukaemia in children. *Br. Med. J.*, **313**, 1297–1300

Stiller, C.A. & Bunch, K.J. (1990) Trends in survival for childhood cancer in Britain diagnosed 1971–85. *Br. J. Cancer*, **62**, 806–815

Stiller, C.A. & Draper, G.J. (1982) Trends in childhood leukaemia in Britain 1968–1978. *Br. J. Cancer*, **45**, 543–551

Stiller, C.A. & Nectoux, J. (1994) International incidence of childhood brain and spinal tumours. *Int. J. Epidemiol.*, **23**, 458–464

Stiller, C.A. & Parkin, D.M. (1990a) International variations in the incidence of childhood lymphomas. *Paediatr. Perinatal Epidemiol.*, **4**, 303–324

Stiller, C.A. & Parkin, D.M. (1990b) International variations in the incidence of childhood renal tumours. *Br. J. Cancer*, **62**, 1026–1030

Stiller, C.A. & Parkin, D.M. (1992) International variations in the incidence of neuroblastoma. *Int. J. Cancer*, **52**, 538–543

Stiller, C.A. & Parkin, D.M. (1994) International variations in the incidence of childhood soft-tissue sarcomas. *Paediat. Perinatal Epidemiol.*, **8**, 107–119

Stiller, C.A. & Parkin, D.M. (1996) Geographic and ethnic variations in the incidence of childhood cancer. *Br. Med. Bull.*, **52**, 682–703

Stiller, C.A., Lennox, E.L. & Kinnier-Wilson, L.M. (1987) Incidence of cardiac septal defects in children with Wilms' tumor and other malignant diseases. *Carcinogenesis*, **8**, 129–132

Stiller, C.A., McKinney, P.A., Bunch, K.J., Bailey, C.C. & Lewis, I.J. (1991a) Childhood cancer and ethnic group in Britain: a United Kingdom Children's Cancer Study Group (UKCCSG) study. *Br. J. Cancer*, **64**, 543–548

Stiller, C.A., O'Connor, C.M., Vincent, T.J. & Draper, G.J. (1991b) The national registry of childhood tumours and the leukaemia/lymphoma data for 1966–83. In: Draper, G.J., ed., *The Geographical Epidemiology of Childhood Leukaemia and Non-Hodgkin Lymphomas in Great Britain, 1966–83* (Studies on Medical and Population Subjects No. 55), London, HMSO, pp. 7–16

Stiller, C.A., Chessells, J.M. & Fitchett, M. (1994) Neurofibromatosis and childhood leukaemia/lymphoma: a population-based UKCCSG study. *Br. J. Cancer*, **70**, 969–972

Stiller, C.A., Allen, M.B. & Eatock, E.M. (1995) Childhood cancer in Britain: The National Registry of Childhood Tumours and Incidence Rates 1978–1987. *Eur. J. Cancer*, **31A**, 2028–2034

Stjernfeldt, M., Lindsten, J., Berglund, K. & Ludvigsson, J. (1986a) Maternal smoking during pregnancy and risk of childhood cancer. *Lancet*, **i**, 1350–1352

Stjernfeldt, M., Ludvigsson, J., Berglund, K. & Lindsten, J. (1986b) Maternal smoking during pregnancy and the risk of childhood cancer (letter). *Lancet*, **ii**, 687–688

Stjernfeldt, M., Samuelsson, L. & Ludvigsson, J. (1987) Radiation in dwellings and cancer in children. *Pediat. Hematol. Oncol.*, **4**, 55–61

Stowens, D., Cork, M.G. & Mallardi, A. (1961) La patologia della leucemia acuta infantile. *Minerva Pediat.*, **13**, 865–890

Strom, S.S. & Strong, L.C. (1991) Cancer among first-degree relatives of 383 childhood and adolescent osteosarcoma patients. *Am. J. Epidemiol.*, **134**, 766–767

Strong, L.C., Herson, J., Haas, C., Elder, K., Chakraborty, R., Weiss, K.M. & Majumder, P. (1984) Cancer mortality in relatives of retinoblastoma patients. *J. Natl. Cancer Inst.*, **73**, 303–311

Strong, L.C., Stine, M. & Norsted, T.L. (1987) Cancer in survivors of childhood soft tissue sarcoma and their relatives. *J. Natl. Cancer Inst.*, **79**, 1213–1220

Strong, L.C., Williams, W.R. & Tainsky, M.A. (1992) The Li–Fraumeni syndrome: From clinical epidemiology to molecular genetics. *Am. J. Epidemiol.*, **135**, 190–199

Stsjazhko, V.A., Tsyb, A.F., Tronko, N.D., Souchkevitch, G. & Baverstock, K.F. (1995) Childhood thyroid cancer since accident at Chernobyl. *Br. Med. J.*, **310**, 801

Suckling, R.D., Fitzgerald, P.H., Stewart, J. & Wells, E. (1982) The incidence and epidemiology of retinoblastoma in New Zealand: a 30-year survey. *Br. J. Cancer*, **46**, 729–735

Sussman, A., Leviton, A., Allred, E.N., Aschenbrener, C., Austin, D.F., Gilles, F.H., Hedley-Whyte, E.T., Kolonel, L.N., Lyon, J.L., Swanson, G.M. & West, D. (1990) Childhood brain tumor: presentation at younger age is associated with a family tumor history. *Cancer Causes Control*, **1**, 75–79

Sutton, R.N.P., Bishun, N.P. & Soothill, J.F. (1969) Immunological and chromosomal studies in first-degree relatives of children with acute lymphoblastic leukaemia. *Br. J. Haematol.*, **17**, 113–119

Swan, S.H., Shaw, G.M. & Schulman, J. (1992) Reporting and selection bias in case-control studies of congenital malformations. *Epidemiology*, **3**, 356–363

Swensen, A.R., Ross, J.A., Severson, R.K., Pollock, B.H. & Robison, L.L. (1997) The age peak in childhood acute lymphoblastic leukemia. *Cancer*, **79**, 2045–2051

Swerdlow, A.J., De Stavola, B., Maconochie, N. & Siskind, V. (1996) A population-based study of cancer risk in twins: Relationships to birth order and sexes of the twin pair. *Int. J. Cancer*, **67**, 472–478

Tabacchi, P., Chiricolo, M., Cenci, M., Barboni, F., Manfrini, M., Bacci, G., Picci, P., Campanacci, M., Licastro, F. & Franceschi, C. (1982) Frequency and prognostic value of HLA antigens in osteosarcoma patients. *Tissue Antigens*, **20**, 251–253

Taskinen, H.K. (1990) Effects of parental occupational exposures on spontaneous abortion and congenital malformation. *Scand. J. Work. Environ. Health*, **16**, 297–314

Taylor, A.M.R. (1992) Ataxia telangiectasia genes and predisposition to leukaemia, lymphoma and breast cancer. *Br. J. Cancer*, **66**, 5–9

Taylor, G.M., Robinson, M.D., Binchy, A., Birch, J.M., Stevens, R.F., Jones, P.M., Carr, T., Dearden, S. & Gokhale, D.A. (1995) Preliminary evidence of an association between HLA-DPB1*0201 and childhood common acute lymphoblastic leukaemia supports an infectious aetiology. *Leukemia*, **9**, 440–443

Teppo, L., Salonen, T. & Hakulinen, T. (1975) Incidence of childhood cancer in Finland. *J. Natl. Cancer Inst.*, **55**, 1065–1067

Thomas, T.L. & Waxweiler, R.J. (1986) Brain tumors and occupational risk factors – a review. *Scand. J. Work Environ. Health*, **12**, 1–15

Thompson, E.N., Dallimore, N.S. & Brook, D.L. (1988) Parental cancer in an unselected cohort of children with cancer referred to a single centre. *Br. J. Cancer*, **57**, 127–129

Thorne, R.N., Pearson, A.D.J., Nicoll, J.A.R., Coakham, H.B., Oakhill, A., Mott, M.G. & Foreman, N.K. (1994) Decline in incidence of medulloblastoma in children. *Cancer*, **74**, 3240–3244

Thorne, R., Foreman, N.K. & Mott, M.G. (1996) Radon in Devon and Cornwall and paediatric malignancies. *Eur. J. Cancer*, **32A**, 282–285

Tijani, S.O., Elesha, S.O. & Banjo, A.A. (1995) Morphological patterns of paediatric solid cancer in Lagos, Nigeria. *West Afric. J. Med.*, **14**, 174–180

Till, M.M., Hardisty, R.M., Pike, M.C. & Doll, R. (1967) Childhood leukaemia in Greater London: a search for evidence of clustering. *Br. Med. J.*, **3**, 755–758

Till, M., Rapson, N. & Smith, P.G. (1979) Family studies in acute leukaemia in childhood: a possible association with autoimmune disease. *Br. J. Cancer*, **40**, 62–71

Tjalma, R.A. (1966) Canine bone sarcoma: estimation of relative risk as a function of body size. *J. Natl. Cancer Inst.*, **36**, 1137–1150

Tomatis, L. (1989) Overview of perinatal and multigeneration carcinogenesis. In: Napalkov, N.P., Rice, J.M., Tomatis, L. & Yamasaki, H., eds, *Perinatal and Multigeneration Carcinogenesis* (IARC Scientific Publications No. 96), Lyon, IARC, pp. 1–15

Tomatis, L., Cabral, J.R.P., Likhachev, A.J. & Ponomarkov, V. (1981) Increased cancer incidence in the progeny of male rats exposed to ethylnitrosurea. *Int. J. Cancer*, **28**, 475–478

Tomenius, L. (1986) 50-Hz electromagnetic environment and the incidence of childhood tumors in Stockholm County. *Bioelectromagnetics*, **7**, 191–207

Tonini, G.P. (1993) Neuroblastoma: a multiple biological disease. *Eur. J. Cancer*, **29A**, 802–804

Totter, J.R. & MacPherson, H.G. (1981) Do childhood cancers result from prenatal X-rays? *Health Physics*, **40**, 511–524

Trotter, W.R. (1990) Is bracken a health hazard? *Lancet*, **336**, 1563–1565

Tucker, M.A., Meadows, A.T., Boice, J.D., Jr, Hoover, R.N. & Fraumeni, J.F., Jr (1984) Cancer risk following treatment of childhood cancer. In: Boice, J.D., Jr & Fraumeni, J.F., Jr, eds, *Radiation Carcinogenesis Epidemiology and Biological Significance*, New York, Raven Press, pp. 211–224

Tucker, M.A., Morris Jones, P.H., Boice, J.D., Jr, Robison, L.L., Stone, B.J., Stovall, M., Jenkin, R.D., Lubin, J.H., Baum, E.S., Siegel, S.E., Meadows, A.T., Hoover, R.N. & Fraumeni, J.F. (1991) Therapeutic radiation at a young age is linked to secondary thyroid cancer. *Cancer Res.*, 51, 2885–2888

Tulchinsky, T.H., Patton, M.M., Randolph, L.A., Meyer, M.R. & Linden, J.V. (1993) Mandating vitamin K prophylaxis for newborns in New York State. *Am. J. Pub. Health*, 83, 1166–1168

Turcot, J., Despres, J.P. & St Pierre, F. (1959) Malignant tumors of the central nervous system associated with familial polyposis of the colon: report of two cases. *Dis. Colon. Rectum*, 2, 465–468

Turnbull, B.W., Iwano, E.J., Burnett, W.S., Howe, H.L. & Clark, L.C. (1990) Monitoring for clusters of disease: application to leukemia incidence in upstate New York. *Am. J. Epidemiol.*, 132, S136–S143

Tynes, T. & Haldorsen, T. (1997) Electromagnetic fields and cancer in children residing near Norwegian high-voltage power lines. *Am. J. Epidemiol.*, 145, 219–226

Tyror, J.G. (1989) The medical implications of nuclear power plant accidents. In: Crosbie, W.A. & Gittus, J.H., eds, *Medical Response to Effects of Ionising Radiation*, London, Elsevier, pp. 1–36

UNSCEAR (United Nations Scientific Committee on the Effects of Atomic Radiation) (1982) *Ionizing Radiation: Sources and Biological Effects. 1982 Report to the General Assembly with annexes*, New York, United Nations, pp. 267–268

UNSCEAR (United Nations Scientific Committee on the Effects of Atomic Radiation). (1988) *Sources, Effects and Risks of Ionizing Radiation. 1988 Report to the General Assembly with Annexes*, New York, United Nations, pp. 29–293

Urquhart, J.D., Black, R.J., Muirhead, M.J., Sharp, L., Maxwell, M., Eden, O.B. & Jones, D.A. (1991) Case–control study of leukaemia and non-Hodgkin's lymphoma in children in Caithness near the Dounreay nuclear installation. *Br. Med. J.*, 302, 687–692

Ursin, G., Bjelke, E., Heuch, I. & Vollset, S.E. (1990) Milk consumption and cancer incidence: a Norwegian prospective study. *Br. J. Cancer*, 61, 454–459

US Congress Office of Technology Assessment. (1989) *Biological Effects of Power Frequency Electric and Magnetic Fields – Background Paper* (OTA-BP-E-53). Washington, DC, US Government Printing Office

Van den Bosch, C., Hills, M., Kazembe, P., Dziweni, C. & Kadzamira, L. (1993a) Time–space case clusters of Burkitt's lymphoma in Malawi. *Leukemia*, 7, 1875–1878

Van den Bosch, C., Griffin, B.E., Kazembe, P., Dziweni, C. & Kadzamira, L. (1993b) Are plant factors a missing link in the evolution of endemic Burkitt's lymphoma? *Br. J. Cancer*, 68, 1232–1235

van der Put, N.M.J., Steegers-Theunissen, R.P.M., Frosst, P., Trijbels, F.J.M., Eskes, T.K.A.B., van den Heuvel, L.P., Mariman, E.C.M., den Heyere, M., Rozen, R. & Blom, H.J. (1995) Mutated methylenetetrahydrofolate reductase as a risk factor for spina bifida. *Lancet*, 346, 1070–1071

Van der Wiel, H.J. (1960) *Inheritance of Glioma. The Genetic Aspects of Cerebral Glioma and its Relationship to Status Dysraphicus*, Amsterdam, Elsevier

van Duijn, C.M., van Steensel-Moll, H.A., Coebergh, J.W. & van Zanen, G.E. (1994) Risk factors for childhood acute non-lymphocytic leukemia: an association with maternal alcohol consumption during pregnancy? *Cancer Epidemiol. Biomarkers Prev.*, 3, 457–460

van Hoff, J., Schymura, M.J. & McCrea Curnen, M.G. (1988) Trends in the incidence of childhood and adolescent cancer in Connecticut, 1935–1979. *Med. Pediat. Oncol.*, 16, 78–87

van Steensel-Moll, H., Valkenburg, H.A., Vandenbroucke, J.P. & van Zanen, G.E. (1983) Time space distribution of childhood leukaemia in the Netherlands. *J. Epidemiol. Commun. Health*, 37, 145–148

van Steensel-Moll, H.A., Valkenburg, H.A., Vandenbroucke, J.P. & van Zanen, G.E. (1985a) Are maternal fertility problems related to childhood leukaemia? *Int. J. Epidemiol.*, 14, 555–560

van Steensel-Moll, H.A., Valkenburg, H.A. & van Zanen, G.E. (1985b) Childhood leukemia and parental occupation. A register-based case–control study. *Am. J. Epidemiol.*, 121, 216–224

van Steensel-Moll, H.A., Valkenburg, H.A. & van Zanen, G.E. (1986) Childhood leukemia and infectious diseases in the first year of life: a register-based case–control study. *Am. J. Epidemiol.*, 124, 590–594

van Steensel-Moll, H.A., van Duijn, C.M., Valkenburg, H.A. & van Zanen, G.E. (1992) Predominance of hospital deliveries among children with acute lymphocytic leukemia: speculations about neonatal exposure to fluorescent light. *Cancer Causes Control*, 3, 389–390

Vena, J.E., Bona, J.R., Byers, T.E., Middleton, E., Jr., Swanson, M.K. & Graham, S. (1985) Allergy related diseases and cancer: an inverse association. *Am. J. Epidemiol.*, 122, 66–74

Verkasalo, P.K., Pukkala, E., Hongisto, M.Y., Valjus, J.E., Jarvinen, P.J., Heikkila, K.V. & Koskenvuo, M. (1993) Risk of cancer in Finnish children living close to power lines. *Br. Med. J.*, 307, 895–899

Vessey, M.P. (1989) Epidemiological studies of the effects of diethylstilboestrol. In: Napalkov, N.P., Rice, J.M., Tomatis, L. & Yamasaki, H., eds, *Perinatal and Multigeneration Carcinogenesis* (IARC Scientific Publications No. 96), Lyon, IARC, pp. 335–348

Vianna, N.J. & Polan, A.K. (1976) Childhood lymphatic leukemia: prenatal seasonality and possible association with congenital varicella. *Am. J. Epidemiol.*, 103, 321–332

Vianna, N.J., Kovasznay, B., Polan, A. & Ju, C. (1984) Infant leukemia and paternal exposure to motor vehicle exhaust fumes. *J. Occup. Med.*, 26, 679–682

Viel, J.F. (1997) Leukaemia near La Hague nuclear plant. Authors reply. *Br. Med. J.*, 314, 1555

Viel, J.F. & Richardson, S.T. (1990) Childhood leukaemia around the La Hague nuclear waste reprocessing plant. *Br. Med. J.*, 300, 580–581

Viel, J.F., Richardson, S., Danel, P., Boutard, P., Malet, M., Barrelier, P., Reman, O. & Carre, A. (1993) Childhood leukaemia incidence in the vicinity of La Hague nuclear-waste reprocessing facility (France). *Cancer Causes Control*, 4, 341–343

Viel, J.F., Pobel, D. & Carré, A. (1995) Incidence of leukaemia in young people around the La Hague nuclear waste reprocessing plant: a sensitivity analysis. *Stat. Med.*, 14, 2459–2472

Villalobos-Salazar, J. (1989) Bracken derived carcinogens as affecting animal health and human health in Costa Rica. In: Taylor, J.A., ed., *Bracken Toxicity and Carcinogenicity as Related to Animal and Human Health* (International Bracken Group Special Publication No. 1), Aberystwyth, Institute of Earth Studies, University College of Wales, pp. 40–51

Vitamin K Ad Hoc Task Force (1993) Controversies concerning vitamin K and the newborn. *Pediatrics*, 91, 1001–1003

Vogel, F. (1979) Genetics of retinoblastoma. *Human. Genet.*, 52, 1–54

Volpe, J.J. (1992) Effect of cocaine use on the fetus. *New Engl. J. Med.*, 327, 399–407

Von Fliedner, V.E., Merica, H., Jeannet, M., Barras, C., Feldges, A., Imbach, P. & Wyss, M. (1983) Evidence for HLA-linked susceptibility factors in childhood leukemia. *Human Immunol.*, 8, 183–193

Von Kries, R. (1992) Vitamin K prophylaxis – a useful public health measure. *Paediat. Perinatal Epidemiol.*, 6, 7–13

Von Kries, R., Göbel, U., Hachmeister, A., Kaletsch, U. & Michaelis, J. (1996) Vitamin K and childhood cancer: a population based case–control study in Lower Saxony, Germany. *Br. Med. J.*, 313, 199–203

Waaler, H.T. (1970) BCG and leukaemia mortality. *Lancet*, ii, 1314

Wabinga, H.R., Parkin, D.M., Wabwire-Mangen, F. & Mugerwa, J.W. (1993) Cancer in Kampala, Uganda in 1989–91: changes in incidence in the era of AIDS. *Int. J. Cancer*, 54, 26–36

Wacholder, S., Silverman, D.T., McLaughlin, J.K. & Mandel, J.S. (1992a) Selection of controls in case–control studies. II. Types of controls. *Am. J. Epidemiol.*, 135, 1029–1041

Wacholder, S., Silverman, D.T., McLaughlin, J.K. & Mandel, J.S. (1992b) Selection of controls in case–control studies. III. Design options. *Am. J. Epidemiol.*, **135**, 1042–1050

Wakefield, M. & Kohler, J.A. (1991) Indoor radon and childhood cancer. *Lancet*, **338**, 1537–1538

Wakeford, R. (1997) Leukaemia near La Hague nuclear plant. Scientific context is needed. *Br. Med. J.*, **314**, 1553–1554

Wakeford, R. & Parker, L. (1996) Leukaemia and non-Hodgkin's lymphoma in young persons resident in small areas of West Cumbria in relation to paternal preconceptional irradiation. *Br. J. Cancer*, **73**, 672–679

Wakeford, R., Tawn, E.J., McElvenny, D.M., Binks, K., Scott, L.E. & Parker, L. (1994) The Seascale childhood leukaemia cases – the mutation rates implied by paternal preconceptional radiation doses. *J. Radiol. Protect.*, **14**, 17–24

Walker, A.H., Ross, R.K., Haile, R.W. & Henderson, B.E. (1988) Hormonal factors and risk of ovarian germ cell cancer in young women. *Br. J. Cancer*, **57**, 418–422

Waller, L.A., Turnbull, B.W., Gustafsson, G., Hjalmars, U. & Andersson, B. (1995) Detection and assessment of clusters of disease: an application to nuclear power plant facilities and childhood leukaemia in Sweden. *Stat. Med.*, **14**, 3–16

Wang, P.P. & Haines, C.S. (1995) Childhood and adolescent leukaemia in a North American population. *Int. J. Epidemiol.*, **24**, 1100–1109

Ward, E.M., Kramer, S. & Meadows, A.T. (1984) The efficacy of random digit dialing in selecting matched controls for a case–control study of pediatric cancer. *Am. J. Epidemiol.*, **120**, 582–591

Warren, R.P., Storb, R., Nguyen, D.D. & Thomas, E.D. (1977) Associations between leucocyte group-5a antigen and acute lymphoblastic leukaemia. *Lancet*, **i**, 509–510

Wartenberg, D. & Savitz, D.A. (1993) Evaluating exposure cutpoint bias in epidemiologic studies of electric and magnetic fields. *Bioelectromagnetics*, **14**, 237–245

Washburn, E.P., Orza, M.J., Berlin, J.A., Nicholson, W.J., Todd, A.C., Frumkin, H. & Chalmers, T.C. (1994) Residential proximity to electricity transmission and distribution equipment and risk of childhood leukemia, childhood lymphoma and childhood nervous system tumors: systematic review, evaluation and meta-analysis. *Cancer Causes Control*, **5**, 299–309

Wasserman, R., Galili, N., Ho, Y., Reichard, B.A., Shane, S. & Rovera, G. (1992) Predominance of fetal type DJH joining in young children with B precursor lymphoblastic leukemia as evidence for an *in utero* transforming event. *J. Exp. Med.*, **176**, 1577–1581

Watson, W.S. & Sumner, D.J. (1996) The measurement of radioactivity in people living near the Dounreay nuclear establishment, Caithness, Scotland. *Int. J. Radiation Biol.*, **70**, 117–130

Watson, M.S., Carroll, A.J., Shuster, J.J., Steuber, C.P., Borowitz, M.J., Behm, F.G., Pullen, D.J. & Land, V.J. (1993) Trisomy 21 in childhood acute lymphoblastic leukemia: A Pediatric Oncology Group study (8602). *Blood*, **82**, 3098–3102

Weinfeld, M.S. & Dudley, H.R. (1962) Osteogenic sarcoma. *J. Bone Joint Surg.*, **44a**, 269–276

Weinreb, M., Day, P.J.R., Niggli, F., Powell, J.E., Raafat, F., Hesseling, P.B., Schneider, J.W., Hartley, P.S., Tzortzatou-Stathopoulou, F., Khalek, E.R.A., Mangoud, A., El-Safy, U.R., Madanat, F., Al Sheyyab, M., Mpofu, C., Revesz, T., Rafii, R., Tiedemann, K., Waters, K.D., Barrantes, J.C., Nyongo, A., Riyat, M.S. & Mann, J.R. (1996) The role of Epstein–Barr virus in Hodgkin's disease from different geographical areas. *Arch. Dis. Child.*, **74**, 27–31

Weinstein, H.J. & Tarbell, N.J. (1997) Leukemias and lymphomas of childhood. In: DeVita, V.T., Jr, Hellman, S. & Rosenberg, S.A., eds, *Cancer: Principles and Practice of Oncology*, fifth edition, New York, Lippincott-Raven, pp. 2145–2165

Werler, M.M., Pober, B.R., Nelson, K. & Holmes, L.B. (1989) Reporting accuracy among mothers of malformed and nonmalformed infants. *Am. J. Epidemiol.*, **129**, 415–421

Werler, M.M., Lammer, E.J., Rosenberg, L. & Mitchell, A.A. (1990) Maternal vitamin A supplementation in relation to selected birth defects. *Teratology*, **42**, 497–503

Werner-Favre, C. & Jeannet, M. (1979) HLA compatibility in couples with children suffering from acute leukemia or aplastic anemia. *Tissue Antigens*, **13**, 307–309

Wertelecki, W. & Mantel, N. (1973) Increased birth weight in leukemia. *Pediat. Res.*, **7**, 132–138

Wertheimer, N. & Leeper, E. (1979) Electrical wiring configurations and childhood cancer. *Am. J. Epidemiol.*, **109**, 273–284

Wertheimer, N. & Leeper, E. (1980) Re: "Electrical wiring configurations and childhood leukemia in Rhode Island". *Am. J. Epidemiol.*, **111**, 461–462

Wertheimer, N. & Leeper, E. (1982) Adult cancer related to electrical wires near the home. *Int. J. Epidemiol.*, **11**, 345–355

Wertheimer, N. & Leeper, E. (1992) EMFs and cancer rates. *Microwave News*, **July/August**, 14

Wertheimer, N., Savitz, D.A. & Leeper, E. (1995) Childhood cancer in relation to indicators of magnetic fields from ground current sources. *Bioelectromagnetics*, **16**, 86–96

Wessels, G. & Hesseling, P.B. (1996) Unusual distribution of childhood cancer in Namibia. *Pediat. Hematol. Oncol.*, **13**, 9–20

West, R. (1984) Childhood cancer mortality: international comparisons 1955–1974. *World Health Stat. Quarterly*, **37**, 98–127

Westergaard, T., Andersen, P.K., Pedersen, J.B., Olsen, J.H., Frisch, M., Sørensen, H.T., Wohlfahrt, J. & Melbye, M. (1997) Birth characteristics, sibling patterns and acute leukemia risk in childhood: a population-based cohort study. *J. Natl. Cancer Inst.*, **89**, 939–947

Westphal, M., Morgan, S.K. & Grush, O.C. (1979) Nutrition and growth in children with acute lymphoblastic leukemia (ALL). *Clin. Res.*, **27**, 816A

White, L., Giri, N., Vowels, M.R. & Lancaster, P.A.L. (1990) Neuroectodermal tumours in children born after assisted conception. *Lancet*, **336**, 1577

Whitehead, A.S., Gallacher, P., Mills, J.L., Kirke, P.N., Burke, H., Molloy, A.M., Weir, D.G., Shields, D.C. & Scott, J.M. (1995) A genetic defect in 5,10 methylenetetrahydrofolate reductase in neural tube defects. *Q. J. Med.*, **88**, 763–766

Whittle, H.C., Brown, J., Marsh, K., Greenwood, B.M., Seidelin, P., Tighe, H. & Wedderburn, L. (1984) T-cell control of Epstein–Barr virus-infected B cells is lost during *P. falciparum* malaria. *Nature*, **312**, 449–450

WHO (World Health Organization). (1987) *Nuclear Accidents and Epidemiology* (Environmental Health Series No. 25), Copenhagen, WHO Regional Office for Europe

Whyte, P., Buchkovich, K.J., Horowitz, J.M., Friend, S.H., Raybuck, M., Weinberg, R.A. & Harlow, E. (1988) Association between an oncogene and an antioncogene: the adenovirus E1A proteins bind to the retinoblastoma gene product. *Nature*, **334**, 124–129

Wild, J., Schorah, C.J., Sheldon, T.A. & Smithells, R.W. (1993) Investigation of factors influencing folate status in women who have had a neural tube defect-affected infant. *Br. J. Obstet. Gynaecol.*, **100**, 546–549

Wilkey, I.S. (1973) Malignant lymphoma in Papua New Guinea: epidemiologic aspects. *J. Natl. Cancer Inst.*, **50**, 1703–1711

Wilkins, R.J. (1988) Genomic imprinting and carcinogenesis. *Lancet*, **i**, 329–331

Wilkins, J.R., 3rd & Hundley, V.D. (1990) Paternal occupational exposure to electromagnetic fields and neuroblastoma in offspring. *Am. J. Epidemiol.*, **131**, 995–1008

Wilkins, J.R., 3rd & Koutras, R.A. (1988) Paternal occupation and brain cancer in offspring: a mortality-based case–control study. *Am. J. Ind. Med.*, **14**, 299–318

Wilkins, J.R., 3rd & Sinks, T.H., Jr (1984a) Occupational exposures among fathers of children with Wilms' tumor. *J. Occup. Med.*, **26**, 427–435

Wilkins, J.R., 3rd & Sinks, T.H., Jr (1984b) Paternal occupation and Wilms' tumour in offspring. *J. Epidemiol. Commun. Health*, **38**, 7–11

Wilkins, J.R., 3rd & Sinks, T. (1990) Parental occupation and intracranial neoplasms of childhood: results of a case–control interview study. *Am. J. Epidemiol.*, **132**, 275–292

Wilkins, J.R., 3rd, McLaughlin, J.A., Sinks, T.H. & Kosnik, E.J. (1991) Parental occupation and intracranial neoplasms of childhood: anecdotal evidence from a unique occupational cancer cluster. *Am. J. Ind. Med.*, **19**, 643–653

Wilkins, J., Pickrel, C., Bunn, J. & Sinks, T. (1993) *N*-Nitroso compounds and risk of childhood brain tumour: mother's diet during pregnancy. *Am. J. Epidemiol.,* **138**, 615

Willett, W. (1990) *Nutritional Epidemiology*, Oxford, Oxford University Press

Williams, D. (1994) Chernobyl, eight years on. *Nature,* **371**, 556

Williams, E.H., Spit, P. & Pike, M.C. (1969) Further evidence of space–time clustering of Burkitt's lymphoma patients in the West Nile District of Uganda. *Br. J. Cancer,* **23**, 235–243

Williams, E.H., Day, N.E. & Geser, A.G. (1974) Seasonal variation in onset of Burkitt's lymphoma in the West Nile District of Uganda. *Lancet,* **ii**, 19–22

Williams, E.H., Smith, P.G., Day, N.E., Geser, A., Ellice, J. & Tukei, P. (1978) Space–time clustering of Burkitt's lymphoma in the West Nile District of Uganda: 1961–1975. *Br. J. Cancer,* **37**, 109–122

Williams, D., Pinchera, A., Karaoglou, A. & Chadwick, K.H. (1993) *Thyroid Cancer in Children Living near Chernobyl. Expert Panel Report on the Consequences of the Chernobyl Accident* (Report EUR 15248 EN), Luxembourg, Commission of the European Communities

Windham, G.C. & Bjerkedal, T. (1984) Malformations in twins and their siblings, Norway, 1967–79. *Acta Genet. Med. Gemellol.,* **33**, 87–95

Windham, G.C., Bjerkedal, T. & Langmark, F. (1985) A population-based study of cancer incidence in twins and in children with congenital malformations or low birth weight, Norway, 1967–1980. *Am. J. Epidemiol.,* **121**, 49–56

Winn, D.M., Li, F.P., Robison, L.L., Mulvihill, J.J., Daigle, A.E. & Fraumeni, J.F., Jr (1992) A case–control study of the etiology of Ewing's sarcoma. *Cancer Epidemiol. Biomarkers Prev.,* **1**, 525–532

Wolff, S.P. (1990) Child leukaemia – curies or cars? *Nature,* **346**, 517

Wolff, S.P. (1991a) Radon and socioeconomic indicators. *Lancet,* **337**, 1476

Wolff, S.P. (1991b) Leukaemia and wartime evacuation. *Nature,* **349**, 23

Wolff, S.P. (1992) Correlation between car ownership and leukaemia: is non-occupational exposure to benzene from petrol and motor vehicle exhaust a causative factor in leukaemia and lymphoma? *Experientia,* **48**, 301–304

Woods, W.G., Robison, L.L., Kim, Y., Schuman, L.M., Heisel, M., Smithson, A., Finley, J., Hutchinson, R. & Gibson, R.W. (1987) Association of maternal autoimmunity with childhood acute lymphocytic leukemia (ALL). *Proc. Am. Assoc. Cancer Res.,* **28**, 251

Woods, W.G., Tuchman, M., Robison, L.L., Bernstein, M., Leclerc, J.M., Brisson, L.C., Brossard, J., Hill, G., Shuster, J., Luepker, R., Byrne, T., Weitzman, S., Bunin, G. &

Lemieux, B. (1996) A population-based study of the usefulness of screening for neuroblastoma. *Lancet,* **348**, 1682–1687

Woodward, A. & McMichael, A.J. (1991) Passive smoking and cancer risk: the nature and uses of epidemiological evidence. *Eur. J. Cancer,* **27**, 1472–1479

Wulff, M., Högberg, U. & Sandström, A. (1996) Cancer incidence for children born in a smelting community. *Acta Oncol.,* **35**, 179–183

Yang, P., Grufferman, S., Khoury, M.J., Schwartz, A.G., Kowalski, J., Ruymann, F.B. & Maurer, H.M. (1995) Association of childhood rhabdomyosarcoma with neurofibromatosis type I and birth defects. *Genet. Epidemiol.,* **12**, 467–474

Yates, J.R.W., Fergusson-Smith, M.A., Shenkin, A., Guzman-Rodriguez, R., White, M. & Clark, B.J. (1987) Is disordered folate metabolism the basis for the genetic predisposition to neural tube defects? *Clin. Genet.,* **31**, 279–287

Yoshimoto, Y. (1990) Cancer risk among children of atomic bomb survivors: A review of RERF epidemiologic studies. *J. Am. Med. Assoc.,* **264**, 596–600

Yoshimoto, Y., Kato, H. & Schull, W.J. (1988) Risk of cancer among children exposed *in utero* to A-bomb radiations, 1950–84. *Lancet,* **ii**, 665–669

Yoshimoto, Y., Neel, J.V., Schull, W.J., Kato, H., Soda, M., Eto, R. & Mabuchi, K. (1990) Malignant tumors during the first 2 decades of life in the offspring of atomic bomb survivors. *Am. J. Hum. Genet.,* **46**, 1041–1052

Young, L.S., Yao, Q.Y., Rooney, C.M., Sculley, T.B., Moss, D.J., Rupani, H., Laux, G., Bornkamm, G.W. & Rickinson, A.B. (1987) New type B isolates of Epstein–Barr virus from Burkitt's lymphoma and from normal individuals in endemic areas. *J. Gen. Virol.,* **68**, 2853–2862

Zack, M., Cannon, S., Loyd, D., Heath, C.W., Jr, Falletta, J.M., Jones, B., Housworth, J. & Crowley, S. (1980) Cancer in children of parents exposed to hydrocarbon-related industries and occupations. *Am. J. Epidemiol.,* **111**, 329–336

Zack, M., Adami, H.O. & Ericson, A. (1991) Maternal and perinatal risk factors for childhood leukemia. *Cancer Res.,* **51**, 3696–3701

Zahalkova, M., Bilek, O., Kubikova, A. & Belusa, M. (1970) The incidence of leukaemias in children, and the clustering in space and time in South Moravian Province, Czechoslovakia. *Blut,* **21**, 180–185

Zaridze, D.G., Li, N., Men, T. & Duffy, S.W. (1994) Childhood cancer incidence in relation to distance from the former nuclear testing site in Semipalatinsk, Kazakhstan. *Int. J. Cancer,* **59**, 471–475

Zheng, W., Linet, M.S., Shu, X.O., Pan, R.P., Gao, Y.T. & Fraumeni, J.F., Jr (1993) Prior medical conditions and the risk of adult leukemia in Shanghai, People's Republic of China. *Cancer Causes Control,* **4**, 361–368

# Index

Achevé d'imprimer sur rotative par l'Imprimerie Darantiere à Dijon-Quetigny en février 1999
Dépôt légal : 1er trimestre 1999 - N° d'impression : 98-1057